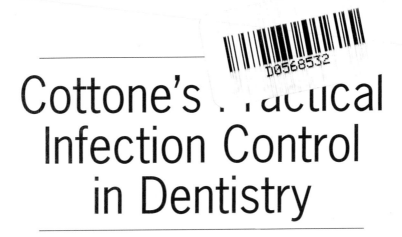

Cottone's Practical Infection Control in Dentistry

THIRD EDITION

Cottone's Practical Infection Control in Dentistry

THIRD EDITION

John A. Molinari, PhD

Professor and Chairman
Department of Biomedical Sciences
University of Detroit Mercy School of Dentistry
Detroit, Michigan

Jennifer A. Harte, DDS, MS

Director, Professional Services
USAF Dental Evaluation and Consultation Service
Great Lakes, Illinois

 Wolters Kluwer | Lippincott Williams & Wilkins
Health
Philadelphia • Baltimore • New York • London
Buenos Aires • Hong Kong • Sydney • Tokyo

Acquisitions Editor: Barrett Koger
Managing Editor: Matt Hauber / Laura Horowitz
Marketing Manager: Allison M. Noplock
Associate Production Manager: Kevin Johnson
Designer: Teresa Mallon
Compositor: Maryland Composition

Third Edition

351 West Camden Street   530 Walnut Street
Baltimore, MD 21201   Philadelphia, PA 19106

Printed in China

Library of Congress Cataloging-in-Publication Data

Molinari, John A.
  Cottone's practical infection control in dentistry / John A. Molinari, Jennifer A. Harte. —3rd ed.
    p. ; cm.
  Rev. ed. of: Practical infection control in dentistry / James A. Cottone. 2nd ed. 1996.
  Includes bibliographical references and index.
  ISBN 978-0-7817-6532-9
1. Dental offices—Sanitation. 2. Cross infection—Prevention. 3. Asepsis and antisepsis. I. Harte, Jennifer A. II. Cottone, James A. III. Cottone, James A. Practical infection control in dentistry. IV. Title. V. Title: Practical infection control in dentistry.
  [DNLM: 1. Dentistry. 2. Infection Control—methods. WU 29 M722c 2010]
  RK52.C685 2010
  617.6'01—dc22

                                                        2008021812

DISCLAIMER

To purchase additional copies of this book, call our customer service department at **(800) 638-3030** or fax orders to **(301) 223-2320**. International customers should call **(301) 223-2300**.

Visit Lippincott Williams & Wilkins on the Internet: http://www.lww.com. Lippincott Williams & Wilkins customer service representatives are available from 8:30 am to 6:00 pm, EST.

RRS0811

Acknowledgments

John dedicates this book to his wife, Gail, their children, and his parents, Ignazio and Clare Molinari. Their love, encouragement, and continued support were invaluable throughout preparation of this book. John also would like to thank Carol Grennan for her assistance in preparation of the manuscript.

Jennifer dedicates this text to the memory of her mother, Shirley Brukner Harte. Jennifer would like to thank the following individuals for their encouragement, support, and friendship over the years: John A. Molinari, William J. Davis, Stephen F. Robison, and William G. Kohn.

Last, but certainly not least, both authors want to acknowledge Dr. James A. Cottone, for whom this book has been re-named. As the amount of scientific and clinical knowledge about hepatitis B, HIV/AIDS, and healthcare occupational infectious disease risks expanded rapidly in the 1980s, Jim worked tirelessly to spearhead efforts in educating the dental profession in the principles and practices of infection control. His efforts in presenting leading edge information in seminars and numerous publications were major factors leading to the acceptance, utilization, and current success of standard infection control practices.

Preface to the Third Edition

Infection control education and practices have continued to evolve since the second edition of *Practical Infection Control in Dentistry*. In addition to numerous technological advances in equipment and other available products, dental professionals have demonstrated a willingness to respond to scientific and clinical evidence delineating occupational infectious disease risks. The routine application of former universal, and now standard, precautions has provided increased safety for all healthcare providers and their patients alike. As was mentioned in the Preface for the second edition, the routine use of effective infection control practices in dentistry actually led the way in addressing a number of infectious disease challenges confronting the health professions. This was illustrated by the profession's rapid acceptance of the hepatitis B vaccine in the early to mid-1980s before other healthcare workers adopted this preventive measure. Dental healthcare professionals should be rightly proud of their infection control progress.

Along with recognition of documented success in reducing the potential for many occupational infectious diseases must come the realization that emerging infectious diseases should also be considered when teaching and evaluating infection control precautions. The third edition of this book has been extensively modified from the previous editions to reflect many of these challenging issues for infection control. This should become initially apparent to the reader as one reviews the list of chapter titles. Included are expanded discussions on infectious diseases such as tuberculosis and influenza, which are transmitted by respiratory droplets and aerosols. The most current information and healthcare recommendations regarding the microbiology of airborne infectious diseases and their prevention are provided. In addition to updated chapters which present scientific and clinical knowledge about viral hepatitis, human immunodeficiency virus infection, and acquired immunodeficiency syndrome, readers will also find a separate chapter dealing with dental unit waterlines and infection control.

A substantial portion of this book addresses the most recent infection control recommendations for dentistry published by the Centers for Disease Control and Prevention in December 2003. The evidence-based approach used in the development of those guidelines has also been incorporated into the content for the third edition. Sections citing scientific and clinical evidence have been expanded to reinforce the rationale for specific infection control practices and protocols. Information found within chapters is presented in a manner which reflects a conscious effort by the authors to increase the profession's understanding of both the "why" and the "what" of infection control guidelines.

We hope you find this third edition of *Cottone's Practical Infection Control in Dentistry* to be a valuable textbook for infection control courses taught in schools and an important resource for dental care providers as you continue to refine your long-standing infection control commitment and efforts.

Additional Resources

The third edition of *Cottone's Practical Infection Control in Dentistry* includes additional resources for both instructors and students that are available on the book's companion website at http://thePoint.lww.com/Molinari3e.

Instructors

Approved adopting instructors will be given access to the following additional resources:

*PowerPoint presentations, with review questions
*Brownstone Test Generator
*Image bank
*WebCT and Blackboard Ready Cartridge

The PowerPoint presentations and Test Generator questions were created by David Cohen.

Students

Purchasers of the text can access the searchable full text online by going to the *Cottone's Practical Infection Control in Dentistry* website at http://thePoint.lww.com. See the inside front cover for more details, including the passcode you will need to gain access to the website.

Preface to the First Edition

Until recently the basic sources for infection control information for the dental practitioner were:

1. Advice from older practitioners whose knowledge was usually minimal or outdated.

2. Dental supply personnel who lack formal education in this area and could be biased towards their own products.

3. A trained assistant whose knowledge was variable depending on his or her experience.

4. A trained hygienist, who usually was the most knowledgeable but was discouraged once out in practice with statements such as "we don't do it that way here."

5. Miscellaneous articles and research reports in the literature, many of which perpetuate myths or sometimes are even misleading or wrong in their results and advice as they may have been authored by individuals who thought they knew the basics of something as "simple" as infection control.

In the past, few dental education institutions included sufficient classroom and clinical teaching of infection control. The basic information was usually discussed in microbiology or in a clinical introduction. Most schools prepared and sterilized the students' instruments for them, resulting in students graduating with little real experience in sterilization or other infection control procedures. The new graduate then embarked on a "do-it-yourself" project to develop some type of infection control system for their office. This system consisted of a blend of instrument disinfection, instrument sterilization, and household cleaning procedures adapted for the dental office, again depending on the quality of his or her staff.

Recent information regarding the transmission of hepatitis and herpes, and the emergence of Human Immunodeficiency Virus (HIV) infection and AIDS, along with the impact of standards from governmental agencies such as the Occupational Safety and Health Administration

(OSHA) and the Environmental Protection Agency (EPA), have led to an increased interest in infection control in general and as it relates to dentistry in particular. This interest is warranted because of the lack of traditional infection control procedures in dentistry over the years. In some instances, these events have led to the development of infection control protocols that are overly detailed and elaborate, incorporating every conceivable barrier, product, and procedure. Infection control procedures have gone too far in many facilities. There are some basic procedures that need to be followed.

The *GOAL* of good infection control in dentistry is to treat *every* patient as though he or she is infected with an incurable disease (universal precautions). The method to implement this goal is to develop *one* infection control protocol for use in the dental operatory that is simple and effective for use with *all* patients, including hepatitis B carriers, HIV antibody positive, and diagnosed AIDS patients. If appropriate measures are taken, infection control will then occur as a routine component of dental practice.

In order to assist in the development of one infection control protocol for all patients, this textbook has been divided into the following major areas:

1. Patient Assessment

2. Personal Protection

3. Sterilization and Chemical Disinfection

4. Environmental Surface and Equipment Disinfection

5. Aseptic Technique

Each of these areas is explored thoroughly in the chapters that follow, with a discussion of medical and legal considerations and today's minimum requirements in infection control at the end of the text.

This volume contains much information about infection control protocols and procedures. Although the authors, contributors and publisher have taken meticulous care to ensure the accuracy of the product formulations and manufacturer recommendations, the law requires the reader to consult information about changes in formulation and methods of product use printed in the package insert before using any product. The reader then can be certain that new data has not led to altered instructions.

Additionally, the area of infection control is changing daily with new products and techniques. The reader will need to become an evaluator of these advances. The use of this text as part of the reader's infection control education and training programs is encouraged because good infection control is a *philosophy*, not a series of "cookbook" steps. Practical infection control in dentistry is making a needed permanent change in the dental profession as we know it.

Contributors

NANCY ANDREWS, RDH, BS
Consultant
Costa Mesa, California

ROSS ANDREWS, AIA
Principal
Ross Andrews & Associates, Architects
Costa Mesa, California

HELENE BEDNARSH, RDH, MPH, BS
Director
HIV Dental Ombudsperson Program
Boston Public Health Commission
Boston, Massachusetts

EVELYN CUNY, MS, RDA
Assistant Professor
Department of Pathology & Medicine
University of the Pacific Arthur A. Dugoni School of Dentistry
San Francisco, California

LOUIS G. DePAOLA, DDS, MS
Professor
Department of Diagnostic Science & Pathology
Dental School
University of Maryland Baltimore
Baltimore, Maryland

KATHY J. EKLUND, RDH, MHP
Associate Professor and Director of Infection Control and
    Occupational Health
The Forsyth Institute
Boston, Massachusetts

VALLI I. MEEKS, DDS, MS
Assistant Professor
Department of Diagnostic Sciences & Pathology
Dental School
University of Maryland Baltimore
Baltimore, Maryland

VIRGINIA A. MERCHANT, DMD, MS
Professor
Department of Biomedical Sciences
University of Detroit Mercy School of Dentistry
Detroit, Michigan

SHANNON E. MILLS, DDS
Vice President
Professional Relations
Northeast Delta Dental
Concord, New Hampshire

GAIL E. MOLINARI, DDS, MS, MS
Associate Professor and Chairperson
Department of Pediatric Dentistry
University of Detroit Mercy School of Dentistry
Detroit, Michigan

KATHLEEN NEVEU, RDA, RDH, MS
Dental Hygiene Clinic Coordinator
Department of Periodontology & Dental Hygiene
University of Detroit Mercy School of Dentistry
Detroit, Michigan

GÉZA T. TERÉZHALMY, DDS, MA
Endowed Professor in Clinical Dentistry
The UTHSCSA Dental School
San Antonio, Texas

Contributors

Reviewers

BARBARA CROWLEY, MED, CDA
Department Chair (Retired)
Dental Studies Department
Pima Community College
Tucson, Arizona

CONNIE GROSSMAN, RDH, MED
Chairperson, Allied Health Profession
Columbus State Community College
Columbus, Ohio

KATHLEEN HARLAN, RDH, MS
Assistant Professor
Department of Dental Hygiene
Ferris State University
Big Rapids, Michigan

MARTHA MCCASLIN, CDA, BSBM
Program Director
Department of Dental Assisting
Dona Ana Community College
Las Cruces, New Mexico

R. HUNTER RACKLEY JR., RDH, BSDH, MHE
Assistant Professor
Department of Periodontics and Allied Dental Programs
Indiana University School of Dentistry
Indianapolis, Indiana

Contents

PART I
MICROBIOLOGICAL RATIONALE FOR PRACTICAL INFECTION CONTROL IN DENTISTRY 1

1. Historical Perspectives and Principles of Infection Control
   Helene Bednarsh and John A. Molinari   3

2. Viral Hepatitis and Hepatitis Vaccines
   John A. Molinari and Jennifer A. Harte   13

3. Human Immunodeficiency Virus, Acquired Immunodeficiency Syndrome, and Related Infections
   Louis G. DePaola and Valli I. Meeks   32

4. Tuberculosis and Other Respiratory Infections
   Géza T. Terézhalmy and John A. Molinari   45

5. Dental Unit Water and Air Quality Challenges
   Shannon Mills   63

PART II
PERSONAL PROTECTION 77

6. The Concept and Application of Standard Precautions
   Helene Bednarsh, Kathy Eklund, and John A. Molinari   79

7. Immunizations for Dental Healthcare Personnel
   John A. Molinari and Géza T. Terézhalmy   89

8. Personal Protective Equipment
   John A. Molinari and Jennifer A. Harte   101

PART III
ANTISEPSIS, STERILIZATION, AND DISINFECTION 121

9. Antisepsis and Hand Hygiene
   Nancy Andrews, Eve Cuny, John A. Molinari, and Jennifer A. Harte   123

10. Antimicrobial Preprocedural Mouth Rinses
    Gail Molinari   141

11. Sterilization Procedures and Monitoring
    Jennifer A. Harte and John A. Molinari   148

12. Environmental Surface Infection Control: Disposable Barriers and Chemical Disinfection
    John A. Molinari and Jennifer A. Harte   171

13. How to Choose and Use Environmental Surface Disinfectants
    John A. Molinari and Jennifer A. Harte   185

14. Asepsis Considerations of Office Design and Equipment Selection
    Nancy Andrews and Ross Andrews   194

PART IV
INFECTION CONTROL PROCEDURES AND PROTOCOLS 207

15. Management of Occupational Exposures to Blood and Other Body Fluids
    Jennifer A. Harte and John A. Molinari   209

16. Instrument Processing and Recirculation
    Jennifer A. Harte and John A. Molinari   221

17. Role for Single-Use Disposable Items
    Jennifer A. Harte and John A. Molinari   232

18. Infection Control in Dental Radiography
    Jennifer A. Harte and John A. Molinari   237

19. Infection Control in the Dental Laboratory
    Virginia A. Merchant   246

20. Medical Waste Management
    Kathy Neveu, Jennifer A. Harte, and John A. Molinari   261

PART V
ADDITIONAL RESOURCES 269

21. Evaluation of a Practical Dental Infection Control Program
    Jennifer A. Harte   271

22. Centers for Disease Control and Prevention
    Guidelines for Infection Control in Dental Health-Care Settings—2003   283

23. Occupational Safety and Health Administration (OSHA) Bloodborne Pathogens Standard   294

Appendix: Answers to the Review Questions   309

Glossary   311

Index   321

Color Insert follows page 206

Contents

Cottone's Practical Infection Control in Dentistry

THIRD EDITION

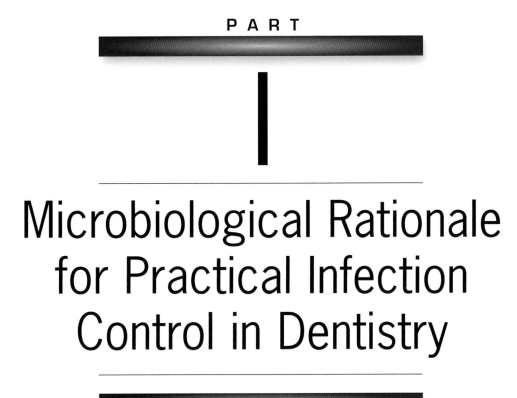

Microbiological Rationale for Practical Infection Control in Dentistry

1

Historical Perspectives and Principles of Infection Control

Helene Bednarsh
John A. Molinari

LEARNING OBJECTIVES

After completion of this chapter individuals should be able to:

1. List representative infectious diseases encountered in dental medicine.

2. Describe direct, indirect, and airborne modes of microbial transmission.

3. Describe representative historical milestones in the investigation of infectious diseases and their control in healthcare facilities.

4. Understand the rationale for effective and practical infection control precautions.

5. Describe the rationale for minimizing the potential for microbial cross-contamination and cross-infection in dental healthcare settings.

KEY TERMS

Airborne transmission: a means of spreading infection in which airborne droplet nuclei are inhaled by the susceptible host.

Asepsis: prevention from contamination with microorganisms. Includes sterile conditions on tissues, on materials, and in rooms, as obtained by excluding, removing, or killing organisms.

Aseptic technique: a procedure that breaks the cycle of cross-infection and ideally eliminates cross-contamination.

Cross-contamination: passage of microorganisms from one person or inanimate object to another.

Cross-infection: passage of microorganisms from one person to another.

Dental healthcare personnel (DHCP): refers to all paid and unpaid personnel in the dental healthcare setting who might be occupationally exposed to infectious materials, including body substances and contaminated supplies, equipment, environmental surfaces, water, or air. DHCP include dentists, dental hygienists, dental assistants, dental laboratory technicians (in-office and commercial), students and trainees, contractual personnel, and other persons not directly involved in patient care but potentially exposed to infectious agents (e.g., administrative, clerical, housekeeping, maintenance, or volunteer personnel).

Direct contact transmission: physical transfer of microorganisms between a susceptible host and an infected or colonized person.

Healthcare-associated infection: any infection associated with a medical or surgical intervention. The term "healthcare-associated" replaces "nosocomial," which is limited to adverse infectious outcomes occurring in hospitals.

Iatrogenic: induced inadvertently by healthcare personnel (HCP) or by medical treatment or diagnostic procedures. Used especially in reference to an infectious disease or other complication of medical treatment.

Indirect contact transmission: contact of a susceptible host with a contaminated, intermediate object, usually inanimate.

Infection control: policies and procedures used to prevent or reduce the potential for disease transmission.

Nosocomial infection: describes an infection acquired in a hospital as a result of medical care; now referred to as healthcare-associated infection (see definition for healthcare-associated infection).

Opportunistic infection: infection caused by normally nonpathogenic microorganisms in a host whose resistance has been decreased or compromised.

Spatter: visible drops of liquid or body fluid that are expelled forcibly into the air and settle out quickly, as distinguished from particles of an aerosol, which remain airborne indefinitely.

Standard precautions: universal precautions were based on the concept that all blood and body fluids that might be contaminated with blood should be treated as infectious because patients with bloodborne infections can be asymptomatic or unaware they are infected. The relevance of universal precautions to other aspects of disease transmission was recognized and, in 1996, the Centers for Disease Control and Prevention (CDC) expanded the concept and changed the term to standard precautions. Standard precautions integrate and expand the elements of universal precautions into a standard of care designed to protect healthcare personnel (HCP) and patients from pathogens that can be spread by blood or any other body fluid, excretion, or secretion. Standard precautions apply to contact with (a) blood; (b) all body fluids, secretions, and excretions (except sweat), regardless of whether they contain blood; (c) nonintact skin; and (d) mucous membranes. Saliva has always been considered a potentially infectious material in dental infection control; thus, no operational difference exists in clinical dental practice between universal precautions and standard precautions.

Universal precautions: set of practices and procedures based on the concept that all blood and all body fluids that might be contaminated with blood should be treated as infectious. (Also see standard precautions)

Dental healthcare personnel (DHCP) routinely are at an increased risk of **cross-infection** while providing treatment for their patients. This occupational potential for disease transmission becomes evident initially when one realizes that most human microbial pathogens have been isolated from oral secretions, and many of these can cause serious diseases in clinical

personnel via cross-infection from patients (Table 1-1). As a result of repeated exposure to the microorganisms present in blood and saliva, the incidence of certain infectious diseases was shown in the 1970s and early 1980s to be significantly higher among dental professionals than observed for the general population. Hepatitis B, hepatitis C, tuberculosis, herpes simplex virus infections, influenza,

Table 1-1 Representative Infectious Disease Risks in Dentistry

Disease	Etiologic Agent	Incubation Period
Bacterial		
Staphylococcal infections	*Staphylococcus aureus*	4–10 days
Tuberculosis	*Mycobacterium tuberculosis*	up to 6 months
Streptococcal infections	*Streptococcus pyogenes*	1–3 days
Pneumococcal infections	*Streptococcus pneumoniae*	1–3 days
Legionellosis	*Legionella pneumophila*	2–10 days
Viral		
Influenza	Influenza viruses	1–4 days
Common cold	Rhinoviruses (most common)	few days
Recurrent herpetic lesion	Herpes simplex, types 1 and 2	up to 2 weeks
Rubella	Rubella virus	9–11 days
Hepatitis B	Hepatitis B virus	6 weeks to 6 months
Hepatitis C	Hepatitis C virus	weeks to months
Delta hepatitis (hepatitis D)	Hepatitis D virus	weeks to months
Infectious mononucleosis	Epstein-Barr virus	4–7 weeks
Hand-foot-and-mouth disease	Primarily coxsackievirus A16	2 days to 3 weeks
Herpangina	Coxsackieviruses group A	5 days
Acquired immunodeficiency syndrome (AIDS)	Human immunodeficiency virus (HIV)	months to years
Fungal		
Dermatomycoses (superficial skin infections)	*Trichophyton, Microsporum, Epidermophyton,* and *Candida* genera	days to weeks
Candidiasis	*Candida albicans*	days to weeks
Miscellaneous		
Infections of fingers, hands, and eyes from dental plaque and calculus	Variety of microorganisms	1–8 days

and a variety of dermatological bacterial and mycotic diseases were well recognized. These and other occupational infections continue to serve as the rationale for increased understanding of modes of disease transmission and **infection control** procedures by dental care providers. As a result, DHCP are required to use appropriate infection control measures during patient care to reduce, as much as possible, potential risks of disease transmission to patients and themselves.

The general routes for transmission of microbial agents in dental medicine are as follows:

1. **Direct contact** with infectious lesions or infected saliva or blood

2. **Indirect contact** via transfer of microorganisms from a contaminated intermediate object

3. Spatter of blood, saliva, or nasopharyngeal secretions directly onto broken or intact skin or mucosa

4. Aerosolization, the **airborne transmission** of microorganisms

Part of the problem was that many practitioners and auxiliaries previously failed to comprehend or appreciate the infection potential presented by saliva and blood

during treatment. Neglecting to implement effective precautions and procedures also places others, including the practitioner's family and other patients, at an increased risk of disease. These dangers often were dismissed because much of the **spatter** coming from the patient's mouth is not readily noticed. Organic debris may be transparent or translucent and dries as a clear film on skin, clothing, and other surfaces.

A novel demonstration was first developed by Crawford in the 1970s using the premise "if saliva were red." He had practitioners dip their fingers into red poster paint before starting their normal clinical treatment. The paint subsequently was deposited on the various surfaces of the operatory as treatment progressed. This demonstrated the **cross-contamination** that occurred from the practitioner's "saliva-covered" fingers. This study was expanded by Glass, Cottone, and Leuke at the University of Texas Dental School at San Antonio by coating the surface of a dental (rubber) dam placed on a mannequin with the same type of poster paint as used by Crawford. A Class II operative preparation then was performed on a lower second molar by a dentist using a high-speed handpiece with air and water coolant. The practitioner and dental assistant were attired properly, using barrier precautions during the procedure. During treatment, dyed "saliva" was visible as spatter (Fig. I-1) that heavily contaminated the face, hair, protective eye wear, mask, chest, arms, and clothing of the dentist by the end of the procedure (Fig. I-2). In addition, the assistant and high-volume evacuator became laden with intraoral exudate (Fig. I-3). The use of a fluorescent light more graphically demonstrated the spatter (Fig. I-4). These figures dramatically show what occurs on a daily basis in the dental operatory and illustrate the challenge of infection control in dentistry.

Routine examinations and dental prophylaxis procedures also substantially expose the dental professional and patient to potentially infectious fluids. When Molinari, York, and others used red dye and water to simulate patient saliva at the University of Detroit Mercy, cross-contamination by the simulated saliva was evident as the gloved hands of the clinician became noticeably contaminated during the intraoral examination. As a result, secretions were transferred to the patient's chart when notations were written (Fig. I-5). Before the oral cavity was reentered, the gloved hands were washed. They were contaminated immediately, however, when the clinician continued the examination. When other procedures were started, such as periodontal probing and scaling and root planning, saliva also contaminated the instrument tray, instruments, and other equipment (Figs. I-6 to I-10). The unit light handle also was adjusted frequently throughout the session and showed obvious contamination from the clinician's hands (Fig. I-11). When the clinician repositioned her eye wear during the polishing procedure, oral fluids were transferred subsequently to her face, glasses, and mask (Fig. I-12). Finally, the "patient" showed dramatic evidence of the ease of oral fluid spread and the resultant accumulation of contamination at the conclusion of the appointment (Fig. I-13).

The documented exposure of practitioners, auxiliaries, and patients to a variety of bacterial, viral, and other microbial pathogens led to the development of a series of infection control protocols by the American Dental Association (ADA), Centers for Disease Control and Prevention (CDC), and, most recently, the Occupational Safety and Health Administration (OSHA). While the accomplishments from these recommendations are noteworthy, it is important to remember that the foundation principles and practices of **asepsis** were discovered and evolved long before the 20th century. It took many centuries of observation and investigation for scientists and clinicians to conclude that a vast array of microbial organisms were etiologies of most infectious diseases. Appreciation of major historical events and the chronology of infection control practices allow us to place current principles and recommendations into perspective. The timeline included in this chapter also reinforces a basic premise of infection control compliance, that is, *we need to understand how far we have come in order to ascertain where we are in the control of infectious diseases, so that we may investigate and develop effective approaches to address emerging issues* (Table 1-2). As a result of these and other numerous epidemiological, scientific, and clinical accomplishments, all patient care providers and their patients are far safer at the beginning of the 21st century than they were at the dawn of the previous century (Table 1-3).

When infection control recommendations are reviewed, a distinction must be made between sterilization and disinfection. Sterilization is defined as the destruction of *all* microbial forms. The limiting factor and the requirement for sterilization is the destruction of bacterial and mycotic spores. Disinfection properly refers only to inhibition or destruction of some but not all microbial pathogens. The term often is applied to the use of chemical agents and procedures that cannot destroy microbial endospores and certain pathogenic microorganisms, such as *Mycobacterium tuberculosis*. Cleaning simply refers to the removal of visible organic and inorganic contaminants from a surface. The use of chemical disinfectants in certain instances is warranted because it is neither possible nor necessary to sterilize all items and surfaces contaminated during dental treatment. The application of **aseptic technique** principles are at the heart of the healthcare professional's efforts to reduce cross-infection by ideally eliminating cross-contamination. With stringent application of fundamental principles, the wide range of occupational, **healthcare-associated** (i.e., **nosocomial**), **iatrogenic** and **opportunistic infections** can be dramatically reduced.

When the red-dye studies are viewed, one is tempted to institute every precaution available with no regard for the efficacy of various modes of transmission. Accumulated data has reinforced the CDC conclusion that hepatitis B virus is the most infectious occupational bloodborne pathogen. Thus hepatitis B is an excellent prototype when designing infection control procedures in dentistry. The principal transmission modes for this virus in order of efficiency are listed in Table 1-4.

When the efficiency of various modes of transmission is coupled with available products and techniques available today, the practitioner can make rational decisions as to which products and techniques are needed to formulate an appropriate, but not excessive, infection control program. Concern about asepsis in the dental office has increased in recent years because of the danger of disease transmission, although anxiety has been almost inversely proportional to the degree of transmissibility (Table 1-5). The need for accurate objective information on infection control procedures is greater than ever.

Demonstration of visible patient spatter on the hands, face, and clothes of the treatment provider, as well as on numerous surfaces in the treatment area, substantiates the need for an effective infection control program in the dental office. Routine examination and prophylaxis

(text continues on page 11)

Table 1-2 Infectious Disease and Infection Control Timeline

1546	Fracastoro—first reports of disease transmission by contagion.
1675	van Leeuwenhoek—first described bacteria and protozoa (animalcules) under microscope; built first simple microscope.
1750	Pringle—observed relationship of putrefaction to disease; performed studies with agents he called antiseptics.
1790s	Jenner—introduction of smallpox vaccine as effective method of preventing disease epidemics.
1827	Alcock—emphasized disinfectant properties of hypochlorite.
1840–70s	Nightingale—emphasized importance of sanitation; used statistics, surveillance, and data collection.
1843	Holmes—first to apply clinical epidemiologic methods to examine causal relationship between disease and practices of healthcare professionals. Demonstrated contagiousness of childbed fever (puerperal sepsis) from doctors and nurses.
1860s	Semmelweis—instituted hospital procedures to reduce mortality from puerperal septicemia; emphasized role of hand hygiene in prevention of cross-infection.
1860s	Lister—"Father of clean and decent surgery"; introduced aseptic technique for surgery and care of wounds; introduced phenols (carbolic acid).
1860–80s	Pasteur—established microbiology as a science; developed process of pasteurization.
1870–80s	Koch—isolated and demonstrated infectivity of anthrax bacillus; discovered *Mycobacterium tuberculosis*; formulated Koch's postulates for infectious disease investigation; examined effects of numerous disinfectants against bacteria.
1877	First isolation guidelines.
1890	Introduction of rubber gloves for use during surgery.
1929	Penicillin discovered by Sir Arthur Fleming.
1944	Public Health Service Act passed by Congress; included regulation of biologic products and control of communicable disease.
1949	First occupational case of serum hepatitis (later termed hepatitis B) reported in a healthcare worker. Infection developed following needlestick exposure to contaminated blood.
1952	First version of ADA infection control guidelines published in *Accepted Dental Remedies*; focus was on the use of chemical agents for disinfection and emphasized precleaning and heat sterilization.
1963	First published description of microbial contamination of dental unit waterlines; high levels of microbial contamination isolated in water samples taken from handpiece and syringe lines.
1970	OSHA created by Congress.
1970	EPA created; takes over pesticides program from FDA.
1973	General infection control recommendations released by the CDC.
1976	ADA Council on Dental Therapeutics publishes first consensus report delineating the role of the dentist and other dental personnel in preventing the transmission of type B hepatitis through dental practice.
1976	Congress passes amendments to the Medical Device Act; ensures safety and effectiveness of medical devices.
1976	Outbreak of pneumonia (later called Legionnaire's disease) occurs at Philadelphia hotel during an American Legion convention; 221 cases reported and 34 fatalities.
1978	First ADA report on infection control for dental offices published in the *Journal of the American Dental Association*: • suggested procedures for reducing contamination and cross-contamination • all instruments, burs, mirrors, bands, and other devices used in intraoral treatment should be routinely sterilized • initial consideration to waterline contamination and possible solutions suggested

(continued)

Table 1-2 Infectious Disease and Infection Control Timeline *(continued)*

1981	ADA Council on Dental Materials, Instruments, and Equipment publishes report to assist dentists in selecting and using devices and equipment for acceptable, effective, and controlled methods for the sterilization of instruments.
1981	First case reports of what is now known as AIDS but referred to as GRID reported by the CDC.
1982	CDC releases occupational infection control guidelines for HCW; guidelines included recommendations for dental HCW: (a) wear gloves, mask, and protective eyewear; and (b) sterilize instruments.
1982	Plasma-derived hepatitis B vaccine (Heptavax-B) becomes commercially available.
1983	HCW unions petition OSHA for emergency standard to make employers pay for HBV vaccine.
1983	Voluntary OSHA guidelines released for HCW receipt of hepatitis B vaccine.
1983–84	HIV identified.
1984	First case report of occupational HIV infection of a HCW; transmission occurred via accidental needlestick from an AIDS patient to a nurse in Africa.
1985	ADA Councils publish first comprehensive dental infection control guidelines; central recommendation was a shift from selective precautions to routine use of universal infection control precautions.
1986	CDC publishes first comprehensive dental infection control guidelines; central recommendation was a shift from selective precautions to routine use of universal infection control precautions.
1987	Last reported case of HBV transmission in a dental care setting, from an oral surgeon to 4 patients in New Hampshire; prior to this time, 20 clusters involving 300 patients reported; 9 of these clusters involved a dentist/oral surgeon.
1987	Recombinant HBV vaccine (Recombivax HB) becomes available in the United States; soon thereafter, Engerix B becomes available in many other countries for HBV vaccination.
1987	CDC reinforces universal precautions as basis for routine infection control. Agency emphasizes that blood, saliva, and gingival fluid in dentistry should be considered infectious; universal precaution recommendations also are published for HIV- and HBV-infected healthcare workers.
1987	OSHA publishes advance notice of rule-making for HCW infection control regulations.
1987	FDA approves AZT, first drug approved for treatment of AIDS.
1987	No further reports of HBV transmission from dentists to patients; outbreaks still reported from physicians to patients.
1988	OSHA releases draft of occupational exposure to bloodborne pathogens standard for review and comment.
1988	CDC releases Guidelines for Prevention of Transmission of HIV and HBV to Healthcare and Public-Safety workers.
1989	HCV identified; first form of NANBH identified; HCV believed to be major cause of hepatitis cases associated with blood transfusions.
1990	First case report of HIV transmission from a HCW to a patient (HIV-infected dentist).
1990	Americans with Disabilities Act passed, with implementation to occur in phases.
1990	First generation anti-HCV serologic blood test developed.
1990	OSHA revises enforcement procedures for draft of bloodborne pathogens standard.
1990	Reports of multiple drug-resistant *Mycobacterium tuberculosis* continue to increase.
1991	FDA sends Dear Colleague letter to dentists concerning sterilization of dental handpieces.
1991	FDA publishes initial recommendations for people with latex hypersensitivity.
1991	CDC releases infection control guidelines for HBV- and HIV-infected HCW; these include: (a) adherence to universal precautions; (b) acknowledgment that HIV is transmitted much less readily than HBV; and (c) recommendations for establishment of review panels in healthcare facilities.

Table 1-2 Infectious Disease and Infection Control Timeline *(continued)*

1991	OSHA Bloodborne Pathogens Standard becomes U.S. law.
1991	Reports of occupational dental injuries demonstrate downward trend from 12/year to 3–4/year.
1992	EPA regulations for tracking and management of medical waste standard become effective.
1992	CDC publishes report titled Management of Persons Exposed to Multidrug-Resistant Tuberculosis.
1992	OSHA petitioned by healthcare unions for workplace standard on TB control.
1992	HBV incidence continues to decline; down to 9% in general dentists and 20% in oral surgeons.
1993	CDC publishes updated dental infection control guidelines; included are TB precautions and recommendations for dental unit waterline infection control.
1993	CDC reports 55% decrease in rate of HBV infection.
1994	CDC finalizes guidelines on TB, guidelines for preventing transmission of *Mycobacterium tuberculosis* in healthcare facilities; occupational risk for dental healthcare workers generally considered to be low in most dental settings.
1995	ADA publishes statement on dental waterlines; suggestion of microbial target level for year 2000.
1995	CDC reports AZT reduces HIV infection risk by 79% in HCW when used as PEP.
1995–96	HIV protease inhibitors receive FDA approval; major successes of combination antiretroviral chemotherapeutic regimens in controlling HIV replication in infected patients.
1996	ADA Councils on Scientific Affairs and Dental Practice publish latest infection control recommendations for the dental office and the dental laboratory.
1996	CDC introduces standard precautions as the method of choice for infection control.
1996	CDC revises HIV PEP guidelines for occupational exposures to include use of reverse transcriptors and protease inhibitors in either mono or combination therapy.
1996	President signs Safe Drinking Water Act to improve U.S. water processing systems and water quality.
1997	FDA publishes latex policy statement requirement for manufacturers in product labeling; "hypoallergenic" label deemed inappropriate and misleading; regulations to go into effect in 1998.
1997	French Health Ministry issues findings of epidemiological investigation concerning HIV-infected orthopedic surgeon who transmitted HIV to patient during surgery.
1997	CDC releases Immunization of Healthcare Workers; Recommendations of the Advisory Committee on Immunization Practices (ACIP) and the Hospital Infection Control Practices Advisory Committee (HICPAC).
1998	CDC publishes recommendations for prevention and control of HCV infection and HCV-related chronic disease.
1998	FDA mandated latex regulations for manufacturers becomes effective.
1999	OSHA initiates drafting of legislation to reduce needlesticks among HCW.
2000	President signs Needlestick Safety and Prevention Act into law. This legislation calls for modifications to the federal OSHA Bloodborne Pathogens Standard: (a) to clarify the need for employers to evaluate and consider implementing safer sharps devices as they become available; and (b) to involve employees in identifying and choosing appropriate safety devices.
2000	CDC begins drafting updated dental infection control recommendations.
2001	OSHA releases new compliance directive for updated Bloodborne Pathogens Standard.
2001	CDC publishes updated guidelines and recommendcations for management of occupational exposures to HBV, HCV, and HIV and recommendations for PEP.

(continued)

Table 1-2 Infectious Disease and Infection Control Timeline *(continued)*

2002	CDC releases recommendations for hand hygiene in healthcare settings: Recommendations of the Healthcare Infection Control Practices Advisory Committee and the HICPAC/SHEA/APIC/IDSA Hand Hygiene Task Force.
2003	CDC releases Guidelines for Infection Control in Dental Health-Care Settings—2003; comprehensive update, includes other relevant guidelines and additional information; emphasis on standard precautions.
2005	CDC updates HIV PEP.
2007	CDC updates guidelines for isolation precautions regarding prevention of transmission of infectious agents in healthcare settings.

ADA, American Dental Association; AIDS, acquired immunodeficiency syndrome; AZT, azidothymidine; CDC, Centers for Disease Control and Prevention; EPA, Environmental Protection Agency; FDA, Food and Drug Administration; GRID, gay-related immune deficiency; HBV, hepatitis B virus; HCV, hepatitis C virus; HCW, healthcare workers; HIV, human immunodeficiency virus; NANBH, non-A, non-B hepatitis; OSHA, Occupational Safety and Health Administration; PEP, postexposure prophylaxis; TB, tuberculosis.

Table 1-3 Representative 20th Century Accomplishments in Infection Control

- Recognition of relationship between microbial pathogens and risk of occupational transmission of infectious disease: bloodborne, airborne, wound, acute, chronic infections

- Development and refinement of efficient aseptic techniques: hand-washing procedures, classes of antiseptics, infection-control cleaning procedures

- Conversion from chemical immersion to heat sterilization procedures for instrument reprocessing

- Adaptation to use of personal protective barriers during patient care: gloves, face masks, eyewear, clinic coats, and gowns

- Receipt of hepatitis B vaccine and other vaccines recommended for health professionals

- Application of universal precautions against bloodborne disease as infection control standard for patient treatment

- Adaptation of safer procedures to minimize accidental exposures to contaminated sharp items

- Development and use of newer technologies to prevent microbial cross-contamination and facilitate better infection control: sterilizers; personal and equipment barriers; automated instrument cleaning equipment; reusable, heat-stable dental instrumentation; single-use disposable needles; technical advancements in promoting dental unit water asepsis

- Provision of routine care to patients with increasing variety of immune system compromise

- Discovery and development of antimicrobial antibiotics to treat clinical infections

Adapted from Molinari JA. Dental infection control at the year 2000: Accomplishment recognized. J Am Dent Assoc 1999;130:1291–1298. Copyright © 1999 American Dental Association. All rights reserved. Reproduced by permission.

Table 1-4 Bloodborne Disease Transmission Efficiency

1. Direct or percutaneous inoculation by a contaminated needle or sharp object

2. Nonneedle percutaneous inoculation (scratches, burns, dermatitis; i.e., nonintact skin, especially on the hands)

3. Infectious blood or serum onto mucosal surfaces (intraoral, nasal, and ocular mucosa)

4. Other potentially infectious secretions (saliva) onto mucosal surfaces

5. Indirect transfer of potentially infectious blood via environmental surfaces (spatter)

6. Aerosol transfer of infectious blood (theoretical)

Adapted from Bond W. Modes of transmission of infectious diseases. From Proceedings of the National Symposium on Infection Control in Dentistry. Chicago, Illinois: May 13, 1986. U.S. Department of Health and Human Services.

Table 1-5 Infectious Agents of Concern to Healthcare Workers

	Transmissibility	Anxiety
Influenza	↑	↑
Herpes Simplex Virus		
Rubella virus		
Varicella-Zoster virus		
Hepatitis A virus		
Hepatitis B virus		
Hepatitis C virus		
Cytomegalovirus		
Human immunodeficiency virus		
Prions	↓	↓

expose the dental professional and patient to potentially infectious fluids. Recognition of the varying degrees of infection potential by microbial-laden secretions initially led to formulation of guidelines aimed at minimizing hepatitis B virus transmission. Similar protocols and procedures have been recommended regarding the routine treatment of patients with hepatitis C, human immunodeficiency virus, and acquired immune deficiency syndrome. Each of these guidelines mandates the use of the *same* appropriate infection control procedures in the care of *all* patients. In 1996, in an effort to prevent any potential infectious problems that might arise as a result of possible confusion between **universal precautions** (directed at bloodborne pathogens) and body substance isolation precautions (directed at other moist body substances), the CDC developed and published new guidelines for isolation procedures in hospitals. These guidelines incorporated the major features of universal and body substance isolation precautions into **standard precautions**. Since that time the use of standard precautions has replaced the use of both of its individual components. Just as with universal precautions, standard precautions should be used in the treatment of every patient regardless of their infection status. In the application of infection control principles, the images of "red saliva" should come to mind during any treatment procedure and serve as reinforcement for the routine use of effective, practical infection control procedures.

Critical Thinking

1. Explain the historical data which showed hand washing to be a fundamental infection control precaution.

SELECTED READINGS

ADA Councils on Dental Materials, Instruments, and Equipment; Dental Practice; and Dental Therapeutics. Infection control recommendations of the dental office and the dental laboratory. J Am Dent Assoc 1992;Suppl:1–8.

ADA Councils on Dental Therapeutics. Guidelines for infection control in the dental office and the commercial dental laboratory. J Am Dent Assoc 1985;110:969–972.

ADA Councils on Dental Therapeutics. Infection control in the dental office. J Am Dent Assoc 1978;97:673–677.

CDC. Guidelines for infection control in dental health-care settings. MMWR 2003;52:1–66.

CDC. Guidelines for prevention of transmission of HIV and HBV to health-care and public safety workers. MMWR 1989;38(S-6):1–37.

CDC. Provisional PHS interagency recommendations for screening donated blood and plasma for antibody to the virus causing AIDS. MMWR 1985;34:1.

CDC. Recommendations for preventing transmission of infection with human T lymphotropic virus type III/lymphadenopathy associated virus in the work place. MMWR 1985;34:682–686, 691–695.

CDC. Recommendations for prevention of HIV transmission in health-care settings. MMWR 1987;36:1S-18S.

CDC. Recommended infection control practices for dentistry. MMWR 1993;41(RR-8):1–12.

CDC. Update: Universal precautions of prevention of transmission of HIV, HBV, and other bloodborne pathogens in health-care settings. MMWR 1988;37:377.

Crawford JJ. Suggested guidelines for asepsis in the dental office environment, special supplement. N C Dent J 1980;63:4.

Department of Labor, Occupational Safety, and Health Administration. Enforcement procedures for the occupational exposure to bloodborne pathogens, CPL2-2.69. November 27, 2001.

Department of Labor, Occupational Safety, and Health Administration. Occupational exposure to bloodborne pathogens; final rule. Fed Reg 1991;56:64004–64182.

Environmental Protection Agency. Standards for the tracking and management of medical waste: interim final rule and request for comments. Fed Reg 1989;54:12371.

Garner JS. Guideline for isolation precautions in hospitals. The Hospital Infection Control Practices Advisory Committee. Infect Control Hosp Epidemiol 1996;17:53–80.

Glass BJ, Cottone JA, Leuke P. Contamination in dental radiology. Annual Meeting of the American Academy of Dental Radiology, Las Vegas, NV, 1987.

Molinari JA. Dental infection control in the year 2000. Accomplishment recognized. J Am Dent Assoc 1999;130:1291–1298.

Molinari JA. Infection control. Its evolution to the current standard precautions. J Am Dent Assoc 2003;134:569–574.

Molinari JA, Bednarsh H. Infectious disease and infection control timeline. Compend Contin Ed Dent 1998;19:640–650.

Molinari JA, Harte JA. Dental services. In: APIC Text of Infection Control and Epidemiology 2nd ed. Washington, DC: APIC; 2005:51-1–51-23.

Molinari JA, York J. Cross-contamination visualization. J Calif Dent Assoc 1987;15:12–16.

2

Viral Hepatitis and Hepatitis Vaccines

John A. Molinari
Jennifer A. Harte

LEARNING OBJECTIVES

After completion of this chapter individuals should be able to:

1 Define hepatitis and its symptomatology.

2 Distinguish between the various viruses associated with hepatitis.

3 Describe the general features of hepatitis A, hepatitis B, hepatitis C, hepatitis D, and hepatitis E, including the etiology, transmission, diagnosis, sequelae, and prophylaxis.

4 List and discuss the serologic markers used in the diagnosis of various forms of viral hepatitis.

5 Describe the implications of the carrier states for hepatitis B and hepatitis C.

6 List the risk factors associated with the different hepatitis viruses.

7 Comprehend the occupational considerations for viral hepatitis and transmission risks for healthcare workers.

8 Understand the chemotherapeutic approaches for management of persons infected with hepatitis viruses.

9 Describe the types and efficacy of available hepatitis A and hepatitis B vaccines.

INTRODUCTION

Two diseases have been primary occupational concerns over the past few decades for healthcare personnel (HCP): viral **hepatitis** and acquired immune deficiency syndrome (AIDS). Prior to the late 1970s, many dentists, hygienists, assistants, and dental lab technicians learned about viral hepatitis in school, but because there were only limited epidemiological studies and little infection control data available, people generally accepted the risk with little worry. Unfortunately, several dental professionals were infected, with some subsequently manifesting disease sequelae ranging from development of an infectious **carrier** state to **cirrhosis**, hepatocellular carcinoma, and even death. Viral hepatitis can have a short- or long-term incubation interval, depending on the etiologic agent involved. The possibility of prolonged symptomatic and asymptomatic sequelae to primary infection also exists. Fortunately, as much more is understood regarding modes of transmission, diagnosis, and prevention, approaches about viral etiologies, sensitive assays have been developed and effective vaccines have been produced against most of the major viral etiologies. This chapter examines the challenge that viral hepatitis continues to pose for the dental profession and places this challenge in proper perspective.

VIRAL HEPATITIS: THE MAJOR BLOODBORNE CHALLENGE

Hepatitis, or **inflammation** of the liver, can be caused by several viruses and a variety of other nonmicrobial etiologies. It can be caused by various disease states and drug reactions. It is therefore important for dental healthcare personnel (DHCP) to remember at the outset that a patient history of hepatitis does not automatically signify a case of viral hepatitis. While several different viruses can induce hepatic symptoms and abnormalities, currently at least seven distinct viruses have been identified as major causes of viral hepatitis, with manifestations ranging from acute to **chronic** disease. Table 2-1 lists these and other viruses that can cause hepatitis. Currently, at least six viruses are believed to account for the overwhelming majority of viral hepatitis infections (Table 2-2). While there are additional hepatitis viruses which could be added here, the following will discuss the five most extensively studied, the infections they cause, and the occupational implications for health professionals.

Hepatitis conditions in general are classically divided into prodromal, **icteric**, and convalescent phases. During the prodromal stage, nonspecific respiratory and/or gastrointestinal symptoms can develop. These can include malaise, loss of appetite, headaches, nausea, and flu-like

TABLE 2-1 Viruses That May Be Involved in Human Hepatitis

RNA Viruses
Picornaviruses (enteroviruses)
    Hepatitis A virus*
    Hepatitis D virus*
    Coxsackieviruses
    Echo viruses
Flaviviruses
    Hepatitis C virus*
Calciviruses
    Hepatitis E virus*
Togaviruses
    Yellow Fever Virus
    Rubella virus
Arenavirus
    Junin virus (Argentina)
    Machupo virus (Bolivia)
    Lassa virus (Lass fever–Africa)
    Rift Valley Fever virus (Africa)
Rhabdoviruses
    Marburg virus (Marburg disease—Africa)
    Ebola virus (Africa)
Paramyxovirus
    Measles virus

DNA Viruses
Hepadnavirus
    Hepatitis B virus*
Herpesviruses
    Cytomegalovirus
    Epstein-Barr virus
    Herpes Simplex viruses
Varicella-Zoster virus

Unclassified
Hepatitis F virus
Hepatitis G virus
Transfusion-Transmitted virus (TTV)

*Signifies major class of virus.

respiratory symptoms. When present, fever is usually low-grade. With specific regard to hepatitis B, arthritis and maculopapular skin rashes develop just prior to definitive positive diagnostic assays indicating viral infection. Since many cases of hepatitis are subclinical, all or none of these manifestations may occur. The subsequent icteric phase is characterized by onset of **jaundice** and dark, foamy urine. Stool color changes also may occur during this period, where it may be seen as lightening to a grayish-white appearance. Symptomatology of the icteric phase is also variable. While jaundice detected either on the skin, sclera, nail beds, or gingiva is generally considered to be the hallmark hepatitis manifestation, the majority of infections may only result in elevation of certain enzymes associated with liver cells (aminotrans-

ferase; transaminases). Elevation of these biochemical markers in a person's blood usually occurs a few days before or at the time of clinical symptoms. Other physical signs can include hepatitic tenderness, hepatomegaly, and splenomegaly. These manifestations disappear during the convalescent or recovery phase of infection. However, even in those individuals who recover normally without any long-term, chronic sequelae, malaise and fatigue may persist for weeks to months. Different types of viral hepatitis may present with variations from the above generalized description.

HEPATITIS A

Hepatitis A (Table 2-3) is caused by the hepatitis A virus (HAV), a small, single-stranded 27-nm ribonucleic acid (RNA) agent that shares properties with members of the picornavirus family. HAV has been shown to exhibit features similar to the enteroviruses. It is more stable to temperature and pH changes than the enteroviruses, however, and is also able to survive in feces and exudates, and for weeks on inanimate surfaces. The virus was first was described in 1973 and the disease was formerly known as "infectious hepatitis." This term is no longer considered an appropriate description. The illness caused by HAV characteristically has an abrupt onset with fever, malaise, anorexia, nausea, abdominal discomfort, icterus, inflammation of the liver, and jaundice. In approximately 20% of cases, relapse in liver inflammation may be seen, with some cases lasting approximately 6 months. Severity of illness is related to age. In children, most infections are asymptomatic and illness usually is not accompanied by jaundice. However, most infected adults become symptomatically ill, with jaundice. Death among patients with reported cases is infrequent (occurring in approximately 0.6% of patients) and is related to infection occurring during older age. HAV infection is self-limiting and recovery provides lifelong protection against recurrent disease.

HAV infection is common in many developing countries. In these areas most infections may occur during childhood, often manifesting little or no symptomatology. Although this disease typically has a low mortality rate, the morbidity of hepatitis A infection worldwide was approximately 1.4 million new cases per year. The incidence of hepatitis A has decreased in the United States over the past few decades. In 1980, 29,087 new cases were reported in the U.S. with an estimated 234,000 new infections occurring in the population. This is contrasted with recent Centers for Disease Control and Prevention (CDC) figures for 2005, showing 4,488 new reported cases with an estimated 42,000 new cases. Although the incidence of hepatitis A has decreased in the U.S., it still accounts for over 30% of the reported acute hepatitis cases.

TABLE 2-2 Comparison of Major Microbiological and Clinical Features of Viral Hepatitis

Feature	Hepatitis A Virus (HAV)	Hepatitis B Virus (HBV)	Hepatitis C Virus (HCV)	Hepatitis D Virus (HDV)	Hepatitis E Virus (HEV)	Hepatitis G Virus (HGV)
Family characteristics	Picornaviridae; nonenveloped single-stranded RNA	Hepadnaviridae; double-stranded DNA	Flaviviridae; enveloped single-stranded RNA	Satellite; nonenveloped single-stranded RNA	Caliciviridae; RNA	Flaviviridae; RNA
Incubation period	15–40 days	50–180 days	30–150 days	21–90 days	15–70 days	unknown
Onset	Usually acute	Usually insidious	Usually insidious	Usually acute	Usually acute	Acute disease spectrum unknown
Prodrome: Arthritis/rash	Not present	Sometimes	Sometimes	Unknown	Not present	unknown
Transmission	Fecal-oral; poor sanitation	Parenteral; sexual contact; perinatal; other secretions (i.e., saliva)	Usually parenteral; sexual contact less common; perinatal	Usually parenteral; sexual contact less common	Fecal-oral; waterborne (common in developing countries)	Parenteral; perinatal frequent coinfection with HCV
Carrier state	No	Yes (5% to 10%)	Yes (>85%)	Yes	No	Yes
Possible manifestations	None reported	Hepatocellular carcinoma; cirrhosis	Hepatocellular carcinoma; cirrhosis	Hepatocellular carcinoma; cirrhosis	None reported	None reported
Mortality	0.1% to 0.2%	1% to 2%; higher in adults >40 yrs	1% to 2%	2% to 20%	1% to 2% in general population; 20% in pregnant women	unknown
Homologous immunity	Anti-HAV	Anti-HBsAg	Not defined	Anti-HBsAg	Anti-HEV	Anti-HGV

Adapted from Krugman S. Viral hepatitis A, B, C, D, and E infection. Pediatr Rev 1992;13:203 and Molinari JA. Hepatitis C virus infection. Dent Clin North Am 1996;40:309.

TABLE 2-3 Hepatitis A Virus Characteristics

1. Picornavirus (RNA)

2. Humans are only natural host

3. Depending on conditions, can be stable in environment for months

4. Virus can remain stable and infectious at low ph and moderate temperatures

5. Inactivated by high temperatures, formalin, and chlorine

Transmission of HAV occurs primarily by person-to-person contact, generally through fecal-oral contamination. HAV is shed in the feces of persons with viral infection, with spread of the virus commonly occurring by a person putting something in their mouth which has been contaminated with feces from an HAV-infected individual. Transmission can thus occur by direct person-to-person contact, poor sanitation, and intimate (intrahousehold or sexual) contact. Among the risk factors are daycare center contact, international travel, intravenous drug use, men who have sex with men, and persons with chronic liver disease. Indirect transmission of HAV via contaminated water or food is common, most often from raw or inadequately cooked shellfish. Sharing utensils, sharing cigarettes, and kissing are *not* believed to transmit the infection. It must be noted that approximately 45% of the U.S. cases of hepatitis A for 2005 did not relate any known risk factors. While DHCP do not typically have occupational exposure to HAV, appropriate attention to hand hygiene procedures and personal hygiene are some of the factors DHCP should be aware of in their overall infection control practices.

The incubation period of hepatitis A is 15–40 days (average 28–30 days). Sudden onset of illness is characteristic of hepatitis A, with the clinical course of infection ranging from asymptomatic to severe. High concentrations of HAV are found in stools of infected people. Fecal virus excretion reaches its highest concentration late in the incubation period and early in the prodromal phase of illness; it diminishes rapidly once jaundice appears. Fever is often present during acute illness, but symptoms may only last 2–7 days. A person's greatest infectivity potential occurs during the 2-week period immediately before the onset of jaundice. Onset of symptoms is rapidly followed by a decrease in both **viremia** and infectiousness of the host. The virus has not been found in urine or other body fluids. Fortunately, a carrier state has not been demonstrated, nor has HAV been shown to induce chronic hepatitis. Instead, the virus is maintained in the population by serial propagation through human infection.

A reliable marker for immunity or even ongoing infection is the presence of anti-HAV in the serum. The diagnosis of acute hepatitis A is confirmed by finding anti-HAV of the immunoglobulin M (IgM) class in serum collected during the acute or early convalescent phase of disease. The antibodies persist for 4 to 6 weeks and are then replaced by high concentrations of IgG antibodies. These protective immunoglobulins appear in the convalescent phase of disease and remain detectable in serum thereafter, conferring lifelong protection against disease (Fig. 2-1). Commercial tests are available to detect IgM anti-HAV and total anti-HAV in serum.

Hepatitis A Vaccines

HAV has been grown successfully in culture and its genome has been cloned. A vaccine against hepatitis was developed and is being used in many countries. The rationale for development and use of a hepatitis A vaccine is the economic loss from prolonged convalescence associated with the infection. Development of HAV

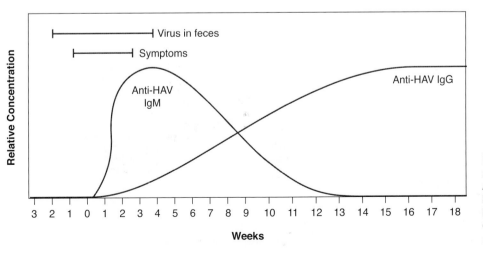

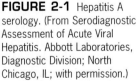

FIGURE 2-1 Hepatitis A serology. (From Serodiagnostic Assessment of Acute Viral Hepatitis. Abbott Laboratories, Diagnostic Division; North Chicago, IL; with permission.)

vaccines uses procedures designed to accomplish inactivation of the whole virus. Merck, Sharp & Dohme Research Laboratories was the first to release a hepatitis A vaccine, called VAQTA, which contains no detectable impurities and is free of residual formalin (which is used to inactivate the virus). This vaccine is very immunogenic and shows seroconversion in >95% of adults who receive one vaccine dose and approximately 100% of those who receive two doses. Children older than 12 months of age and adolescents demonstrate similar response rates (>97% after one dose and approximately 100% after two doses). Smith Kline Beecham also developed a formalin-inactivated vaccine, Havrix, which became available in 1995. Vaccination of groups of people known to be at high risk for HAV infection (i.e., travelers to HAV endemic countries, children in areas with high rates of hepatitis A, men who have sex with men, parenteral drug abusers, and recipients of clotting factors) has substantially reduced the disease burden. In addition, most cases of hepatitis A in the U.S. occur as community-wide outbreaks. Thus, prevention of disease also became a priority for widespread vaccination of children and adults. In 2001 a combination vaccine (Twinrix) became available to protect against both hepatitis A and hepatitis B.

In 1999 the CDC's Advisory Committee for Immunization Practices recommended that children living in states, counties, or communities with reported annual hepatitis A rates of 20 per 100,000 or higher between 1987 and 1997 be routinely vaccinated beginning at 2 years of age or older. Consideration of vaccination was also included for all children living in areas with reported hepatitis rates of between 10 and 20 cases per 100,000 population. The most recent public health recommendations for hepatitis A vaccination published in 2006 are summarized as follows:

1. All children should receive hepatitis A vaccine at 12–23 months of age.

2. Vaccination should be integrated into the routine childhood vaccination schedule.

3. Children who are not vaccinated by 2 years of age can be vaccinated at subsequent visits.

HEPATITIS B

Hepatitis B virus (HBV) infection is a major worldwide cause of acute and chronic hepatitis, cirrhosis, and primary hepatocellular carcinoma. The virus first was described in 1965. The frequency of HBV infection and patterns of transmission vary significantly in different parts of the world. In the United States, Canada, Western Europe, New Zealand, and Australia it is a disease of low endemicity, with only a 0.1% to 2.0% incidence, in contrast to areas which demonstrate a 10% to 20% seroprevalence (Southeast Asia, China, and subSaharan Africa). Hepatitis

B is most frequently acquired perinatally in the high prevalence regions, from infected mother to offspring, with a subsequent 90% risk of chronic HBV infection developing in those infants.

Globally, approximately 2 billion people have been infected, with estimates ranging from 350 to 400 million people being chronic carriers of the virus. Approximately 90% of the carriers live in less developed countries. HBV is the most frequent cause of chronic hepatitis in the world. This virus is also associated with as many as 80% of the cases of primary liver cancer with 1–1.5 million deaths each year attributable to hepatitis B sequelae. As a result this disease continues to be a leading cause of global infection and death. In the 1980s approximately 260,000 people were infected with HBV in the United States. Since the introduction of the hepatitis B vaccine and improved infection control precautions the estimated number declined to about 78,000 in 2001 and 51,000 for 2005. However, it is estimated that there are still approximately 1 million hepatitis B carriers in the United States of whom 20% to 40% will develop life threatening complications.

HBV Properties and Morphological Components

HBV infection is caused by HBV, a 42-nm, double-shelled DNA virus (Fig. 2-2, Table 2-4). The complete HBV virion is called the Dane particle. This particle is capable of replication and is the infectious agent. Several well-defined antigen–antibody systems have been associated with HBV infection. Hepatitis B surface **antigen** (HBsAg), formerly called "Australia antigen" or "hepatitis-associated antigen," is found on the surface of the virus and on accompanying 22-nm spherical and tubular forms. These particles represent excess HBsAg produced during viral replication. They also compose the major proportion of detectable HBsAg following HBV infection. HBsAg remains the major diagnostic antigen for viral infection. The various subtypes (adr, adw, ayw, ayr) of

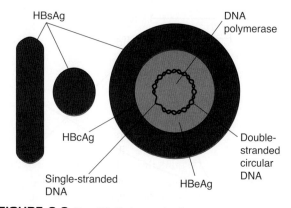

FIGURE 2-2 Hepatitis B virus and antigens.

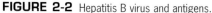

TABLE 2-4 Hepatitis Terminology

Abbreviation	Term	Comments
HAV	Hepatitis A virus	Etiologic agent of "infectious" hepatitis
Anti-HAV	Antibody to HAV virus	Detectable at onset of symptoms; lifetime persistence
IgM anti-HAV	IgM class antibody to HAV virus	Indicates recent infection with hepatitis A; tests positive up to 4–6 months after infection
HBV	Hepatitis B virus	Etiologic agent of "serum" or "long incubation" hepatitis; also known as Dane particle
HBsAg	Hepatitis B surface antigen	Surface antigen(s) of HBV detectable in large quantity in serum; several subtypes
HBeAg	Hepatitis Be antigen	Soluble antigen; antigen correlates with HBV replication, higher titer HBV in serum, and infectivity of serum
HBcAg	Hepatitis B core antigen	No commercial test available
Anti-HBs	Antibody to HBsAg	Indicates past infection with, and immunity to, HBV, passive antibody from HBIG, or immune response from hepatitis B vaccine
Anti-HBe	Antibody to HBeAg	Presence in serum of HBsAg carrier suggests lower titer of HBV
Anti-HBc	Antibody to HBcAg	Indicates past infection with HBV at some undefined time
IgM Anti-HBc	IgM class antibody to HBcAg	Indicates recent infection with HBV; tests positive for 4–6 months after infection
HCV	Hepatitis C virus	Name for one virus associated with PT-NANB
Anti-HCV	Antibody to Hepatitis C virus	Marker of previous HCV infection; does not specifically indicate immunity or viral carrier state
HEV	Hepatitis E virus	Proposed name for ET-NANB
HDV	Delta virus	Etiologic agent of delta hepatitis; only causes infection in presence of HBV
HDAg	Delta antigen	Detectable in early acute delta infection
Anti-HDV	Antibody to delta antigen	Indicates past or present infection with delta virus
Ig	Immune globulin (previously ISG, immune serum globulin, or **gamma globulin**)	Contains antibodies to HAV; lower titer antibodies to HBV
HBIG	Hepatitis B immune globulin	Contains high-titer antibodies to HBV

HBsAg provide useful epidemiologic markers. **Antibody** against HBsAg (anti-HBs) develops during recovery from infection and is responsible for long-term immunity. Antibody to the core antigen (anti-HBc) is produced against an internal component of the virus. This serologic marker is present in all HBV infections and persists indefinitely. IgM anti-HBc appears early in infection and persists for 6 or more months; it is a reliable marker of acute or recent HBV infection. The hepatitis Be antigen (HBeAg) is a third antigen, the presence of which correlates with HBV replication and high infectivity. Antibody to HBeAg (anti-HBe) develops in most HBV infections and correlates with lower infectiousness of the patient.

Figure 2-3 shows the typical serologic pattern of an acute HBV infection with subsequent recovery and immunity. This information is presented along interpretations of other HBV serologic profiles regarding immunity and carrier status in Table 2-5.

Onset of hepatitis B is generally insidious with clinical manifestations observed to vary for both acute and chronic infection. The incubation period of HBV is long: 50 to 180 days (average 60 to 120 days). This disease has a variety of ultimate outcomes including a carrier state, cirrhosis, acute hepatitis, and primary liver cancer (Fig. 2-4). Clinical symptoms and signs in acute cases include combinations of anorexia, malaise, nausea, vomiting,

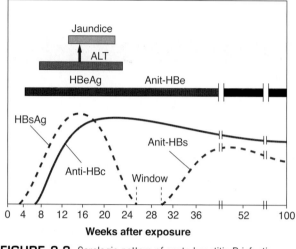

FIGURE 2-3 Serologic pattern of acute hepatitis B infection.

abdominal pain, and jaundice. Skin rashes, arthralgia, and arthritis also can occur. Several of these constitutional symptoms can precede the hallmark manifestation of jaundice by 1–2 weeks. Overall mortality rates for reported cases generally do not exceed 2%. In some instances these fatalities occur as a result of **fulminant** hepatitis which can progress rapidly.

Chronic hepatitis B is defined by the presence of HBsAg and persistence of HBV infection for at least 6 months. While viral chronic carriers can develop disease specific symptoms of cirrhosis or hepatotcellular carcinoma, many may present with severe fatigue, nausea, anorexia, and upper right quadrant tenderness. This chronic persistence of HBV infection develops in about 5% to 10% of adolescents and adults, which presents a significant occupational risk for nonimmune health professionals. The risks are even greater when an HBV chronically infected woman transfers the infection to newborn via the perinatal route. There can be as high as an 80% to 90% risk of infection for the newborn, of which 90% of those children will become chronic HBV carriers themselves. This condition greatly increases their risk for cirrhosis or hepatotcellular carcinoma as they age.

Modes of Transmission

HBV is capable of being transmitted parenterally, sexually, and vertically. The parenteral mode includes percutaneous and nonpercutaneous routes, both of which have significance in dentistry. Dental treatment involves the use of many small, sharp instruments which provide multiple opportunities for inadvertent percutaneous wounds to the operator. Performance of dental hygiene procedures, handling impressions, dental casts, and also while gathering contaminated instruments and cleaning them to remove debris before sterilization also provide potential occupa-

tional risks. Nonpercutaneous dental transmission includes the transfer of infectious body secretions such as blood, saliva, and a mixture of both.

The percutaneous route of virus transmission is more efficient in that the incubation period before HBsAg titer elevation can be as short as 7 days, whereas oral transmission involving intact mucosa usually involves a longer incubation period (approximately 54 days). In reality, this longer incubation period is advantageous for HBV transmission because it is then more difficult to associate the source of infection with any one patient or inanimate instrument. This can thus allow an infected care provider or patient a longer period of time to potentially transmit the virus to other practice personnel, patients, and family members.

HBV transmission in the dental operatory was shown to occur primarily via the horizontal mode—that is, among the staff, patients, and family members who associate with one another. Studies have shown that this transmission is predominantly from patient to healthcare provider and less often from healthcare provider to

TABLE 2-5 Interpretation of the Hepatitis B Serologic Profiles

Tests	Results	Interpretation
HBsAg	negative	
anti-HBc	negative	susceptible
anti-HBs	negative	
HBsAg	negative	
anti-HBc	positive	immune because of natural infection
anti-HBs	positive	
HBsAg	negative	
anti-HBc	negative	immune because of hepatitis B vaccination
anti-HBs	positive	
HBsAg	positive	
anti-HBc	positive	acutely infected
IgM anti-HBc	positive	
anti-HBs	negative	
HBsAg	positive	
anti-HBc	positive	chronically infected
IgM anti-HBc	negative	
anti-HBs	negative	
HBsAg	negative	
anti-HBc	positive	four interpretations possible*
anti-HBs	negative	

*(a) may be recovering from acute HBV infection; (b) may be distantly immune and test not sensitive enough to detect very low level of anti-HBs in serum; (c) may be susceptible with a false positive anti-HBc; or (d) may be undetectable level of HBsAg present in the serum and the person is actually a carrier.

From Centers for Disease Control and Prevention.

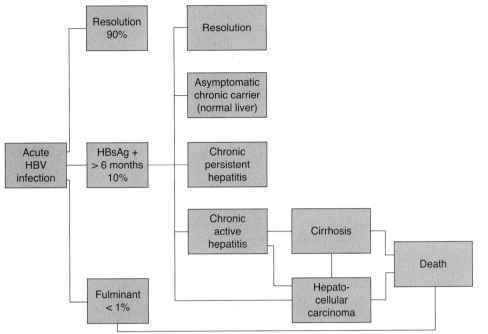

FIGURE 2-4 Outcomes of hepatitis B infection.

patient. While rare, transmission via this latter route does occur and has been documented. The most recent incident involved patient-to-patient HBV transmission in an oral surgery practice. This case was the only proven instance of patient-to-patient transmission in a dental setting and the first documented HBV transmission to dental patients since 1987.

Vertical transmission is also possible, with HBV passed perinatally from infected pregnant carriers or acutely infected mothers to their children via intimate, nonsexual contact. It can be transmitted during delivery, labor, or, less frequently, the gestational period. Perinatal HBV infections have a high infectivity rate of 70% to 90% compared with 10% to 40% during infancy. Perinatal transmission also has a high rate of progression into a carrier state. There is also the potential of transmission of HBV at birth from a woman who has progressed to the carrier state by infection from sexual contact, her own occupational exposure, or personal risk behavior. The development of the carrier state in the newborn infant is then possible, with a resultant increase in that child's ultimate risk for primary hepatocellular carcinoma later in life.

Frequency of Infection

Until the 1980s most dentists believed that there were few potential HBV carriers in their practice and, hence, that there was little chance of infection in their office or indeed in the profession as a whole. They were not alone because the majority of the medical profession, including staff members of most hospitals, believed the same myth. The number of patient population groups that have a significantly increased prevalence of HBV

infection, and hence an increased prevalence of the carrier state, is much larger than one would imagine. Many individuals remain unaware of their HBV infection. While the term "risk group" previously had the unfortunate consequence of causing some clinicians to use special "extra" infection control precautions for certain types of patients, delineation of certain populations with increased HBV risks was important in targeting groups of persons for receipt of hepatitis B vaccination soon after availability of the vaccine in 1982. These included providers of healthcare, patients in hemodialysis and hematology/oncology units, clients and staff of institutions for developmentally disabled persons, newborns of hepatitis B carrier mothers, and ethnic populations with a high incidence of disease (i.e., native born Alaskans and Pacific islanders). Please note that the dentist and the entire clinical dental staff are included in these high-risk populations. Why is this so?

HBV is an insidious disease, but fortunately with the widespread administration of the hepatitis B vaccine since its availability in 1982, the incidence has declined substantially in the U.S. and many other countries. Prior to 1982 there were approximately 300,000 new annual cases and the number of chronic HBV carriers was thought to be as high as 750,000. With the adoption of universal vaccination programs, the number of estimated new cases dropped to 78,000 in 2001. This decline has continued and for 2006 an estimated 46,000 persons, primarily young adults, were infected. One-quarter became ill with jaundice with approximately 5,000 people developing chronic liver disease. The U.S. still has approximately 1,000,000 HBV-infected carriers. Of major concern here is the progression of disease whereby chronic active hepatitis develops in approximately 25% of carriers, often leading to cirrhosis. HBV carriers also have a risk of primary liver cancer that is 12 to 300 times higher than that of other people. Most infections cause no symptoms or, at most, very nonspecific symptoms. This is because some of the symptoms of HBV are familiar to busy people: headache, mild gastrointestinal upset, general fatigue, and/or a few "stiff joints." It is easy to attribute these symptoms to too much coffee, late hours, overworking, or a mild case of the flu. Jaundice, the one presenting sign most believed to be pathognomonic of hepatitis, is unfortunately not routinely present as most HBV cases are **anicteric**. Depending on the route of transmission, virulence of the inoculum, and host resistance factors, only half or less of infected persons actually show jaundice. In addition, development of jaundice usually follows the appearance of HBsAg and HBeAg in the blood. Therefore even when jaundice develops the patient already has been potentially transmitting the disease. Thus, the major challenge in dental practice regarding HBV is to stop transmission from patient to dental staff, dental staff to practitioner, practitioner to patient, patient-to-patient, and dental staff to close intimate contacts (family) by using appropriate infection control measures.

As many as 80% of all HBV infections are undiagnosed. Unless patients have a history of immunity to HBV either from recovery of viral infection or a positive response to vaccination, a patient's medical history may therefore not be reliable. This realization serves as a basis for current standard infection control precautions—all patients must be regarded as potential HBV carriers and/or infected with other bloodborne pathogens. In this regard, the HBV carrier is central in the epidemiology of HBV transmission. A carrier is defined as a person who has HBsAg-positive serologic results on at least two occasions at least 6 months apart. In almost all instances anti-HBs is not detectable in viral carriers and, therefore, HBsAg titers in these patients remain positive. Figure 2-5 outlines the serologic profile of the carrier state in chronic hepatitis B. Although the degree of infectivity is best correlated with concentrations of HBeAg in blood, any person with positive results for HBsAg is potentially infectious. The likelihood of the carrier state developing varies inversely with the age at which infection occurs. During the perinatal period, HBV transmitted from HBeAg-positive mothers results in HBV carriage in as many as 90% of infected infants, whereas 6% to 10% of acutely infected adults become carriers. Unfortunately, the HBV carrier state develops more commonly with asymptomatic, **subclinical** HBV infection versus acute infection. Additionally, carriers with an asymptomatic, subclinical infection are more likely to be HBeAg positive, indicating that they are in a more infectious, contagious state and therefore are more liable to transmit the disease.

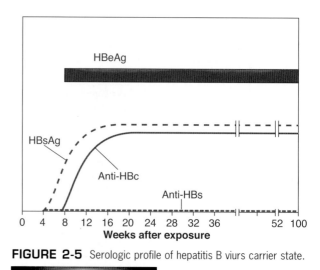

FIGURE 2-5 Serologic profile of hepatitis B viurs carrier state.

Prevalence of Infection in the Dental Profession

A historically important study that is often quoted as a resource for HBV occupational risks in the dental profession was performed in 1972 at the American Dental Association (ADA) annual session. At that time, 1,245 general practitioners were screened for HBsAg and anti-HBs. Of the dental students or dentists in private practice who were screened, 3.3% reported a positive hepatitis B history, whereas blood screening showed that 13.6% had positive serologic tests for previous HBV infection. More recent data from blood specimens collected at the 2005 ADA annual session indicated a decrease to 8.5% of dentists and 6.8% of dental hygienists demonstrating serum markers indicative of past or present hepatitis B infection. Six chronic hepatitis B carrier dentists (0.51%) and no hygienists or dental assistants were identified as HBV carriers during the 2005 ADA session. Although more dentists are becoming immunized against HBV via vaccine, this does not mean that the risk of infection for the *nonimmune* dental professional has decreased. Other studies in the mid-1980s focused on dental specialties and indicated that as many as 38.5% of oral surgeons had positive serologic results for HBV infection. When data from multiple reports were analyzed, results indicated that the general dentist had a three times greater risk of hepatitis exposure compared with the general U.S. population (Table 2-6). In addition, the risk of nonimmunized surgical specialists (i.e., oral surgeons) was approximately six times that of the general U.S. population.

Investigation assessing the presence of virus in oral fluids from known HBsAg carriers detected HBV in >70% of salivary samples collected from known carriers. The virus also has been transmitted by a human bite and can be detected in nasopharyngeal secretions and gingival

TABLE 2-6 Prevalence of Serologic Markers of Hepatitis B among Dental Personnel in Sera Collected from 1979 to 1981

Category	Number with Positive Results	Percentage with Positive Results (%)
Dental hygienists	10/59	16.9
Lab technicians	22/155	14.2
Dental assistants	45/350	12.9
Clerical	5/56	8.9
Other	0/9	0
Total	86/629	13.0

Adapted from Schiff ER, et al. Veterans Administration cooperative study on hepatitis and dentistry. J Am Dent Assoc 1986;113:390–396.

crevicular fluid. The greatest concentration of HBV detected intraorally is in the gingival sulcus. In many patients' mouths this area is inflamed routinely, easily allowing blood to mix with saliva and thus making the fluid potentially infectious for HBV. Despite these observations, however, the risk of HBV infection is more a factor of exposure to blood than general patient contact.

HBV Carrier State and Dentistry

Table 2-7 lists studies demonstrating that some dentists have transmitted HBV infection to their patients. Most often these cases were investigated by the CDC on finding clusters of HBV infections and determining a common factor of dental care by a single dentist within the previous 2 to 6 months before illness. The most outstanding case involved a 46-year-old male dentist from Pennsylvania who had no history of hepatitis or any disease with comparable symptoms but transmitted the same subtype of hepatitis that he was found to have to 55 of his patients. He rarely wore gloves while performing dental procedures before the incident occurred. He did wear gloves during the subsequent investigation and only two additional cases of hepatitis developed in more than 4,300 patients seen. Barrier techniques (mask, gloves, protective eyewear) have been shown time and again to be effective in preventing HBV transmission. Additionally, in 1984, 26 cases of HBV infection were reported in a dentist's practice in Indiana. The dentist had positive results for HBsAg with the same subgroup antigen as the infected patients but had no known history of HBV infection. Fulminant hepatitis developed in two patients, resulting in death. The dentist died of HBV infection sequelae in December 1988.

As can be noted from looking at Table 2-7, no documented cases of HBV transmission to dental patients were found from 1987–2001. Unfortunately a report in the May 1, 2007, issue of the *Journal of Infectious Diseases* quickly returned hepatitis B to the forefront of dental attention and concern. Although the CDC was able to document that a rare case of patient-to-patient transmission of HBV had occurred in an oral surgery practice in late 2001, public health investigators were unable to identify the specific mechanism of cross-infection. One possibility expressed was the thought that cross-contamination from an environmental source may have occurred. Even without the identification of the mode of HBV transfer, the rarity of such an event in dentistry attests to the overall success dentistry's infection control practices. The fact that it did occur, however, is a reminder that the stakes are high in preventing cross-infection and the necessity for performing everyday cleaning. This most recent case reinforces the principle that, even though appropriate standard precautions are

TABLE 2-7 HBV Transmission from Carrier Dentists to Patients

Author and Year	No. of Patients	Practice
Levin, Maddrey, Wands, and Mendeloff, 1974	13	General dentist
Williams, Panison, and Berquist, 1975	0	General dentist
Goodwin, Fannin, and McCracken, 1976	37	Oral surgeon
Watkins, 1976	15	Oral surgeon
Rimland, Parkin, Miller, and Schrank, 1977	55	Oral surgeon
Ahtone, et al, 1981	3	Oral surgeon
Hadler, et al, 1981	6	General dentist
Reingold, et al, 1982	12	Oral surgeon
Ahtone and Goodman, 1983	4	General dentist
Shaw, et al, 1986	26	General dentist
Centers for Disease Control, 1987	4	Oral surgeon
Redd, et al, 2007	1	Oral surgery (patient-to-patient viral transmission)

effective, they do not necessarily eliminate all risks. Despite what we would like to see as 100% protection, infection control precautions are not absolute. When all components are integrated into a total program, they function very well by *minimizing and reducing the potential for cross-infection*.

PREVENTION OF TRANSMISSION VIA IMMUNOPROPHYLAXIS

Active and Passive Immunity

Scientific and clinical evidence accumulated since the late 1970s strongly shows HBV transmission can be stopped in the dental office. Transmission can be prevented by neutralization of the host reservoir (eradication of all HBV sources), interruption of the modes of transmission (infection control practices), or immunization of susceptible hosts. Principles of immunization will be presented only briefly here, with further discussion included in Chapter 7. To understand immunoprophylaxis, one must understand active and passive immunization. *Passive immunity* occurs by transferring preformed antibodies from an actively immunized host to a person in need of immunity. The protection provided is transitory, onset is immediate, and examples are injection of immune serum globulin (ISG) or HBIG. In contrast, *active immunity* develops from stimulation of one's own immune response. Protection is provided only after a latent period, but benefits for the immunized person can be well worth it, as long-term immunity can develop and be maintained.

ISG primarily provides protection against HAV infection and is relatively inexpensive. Passive immunoprophylaxis via HBIG provides protection against HBV infection for approximately 2 months and is expensive. Active preincident immunity is preferable. Active immunity can be conferred through host recovery from acute infection or subclinical disease or through hepatitis B vaccination.

Hepatitis B Vaccines

Plasma-Derived Vaccine

The groundwork for the success of an immunizing preparation was set by Krugman, et al, in a classic series of studies that found that a 1:10 dilution of hepatitis B infective serum (strain MS-2) lost infectivity but retained its antigenicity when boiled for 1 minute. When used as a vaccine, this preparation prevented or modified the course of HBV in approximately 70% of subjects who were challenged later with HBV. MS-2 serum contained large quantities of HBsAg. Subsequent vaccine work focused on the extraction and purification of this noninfectious, viral coat protein for use as the antigen preparation in development of a component vaccine. This

effort was fostered by the observation that HBV replication in infected people was not as efficient as once thought because large amounts of excess HBsAg particles are synthesized and passed into the patient's circulation. As one recovers from infection, antibodies to this antigen (anti-HBs) are produced by the host's immune system and provide protection against a recurrent viral attack.

Accumulated evidence also indicated that these HBsAg forms are present in high concentrations in the circulation of carriers of HBV. Thus, carriers with high serum HBsAg titers were shown to provide a supply of viral antigen for vaccine production. This achievement was crucial to the overall effort because HBV could not be cultured in vitro. Clinical tests were started in 1975 for Heptavax-B, the original plasma-derived hepatitis B vaccine, and the vaccine was introduced in the U.S. in 1982. This vaccine was developed and manufactured by Merck Sharp & Dohme and represented a milestone in immunology as the first clinically available vaccine derived from human sources. Approximately 5.6 million people worldwide received the plasma-derived vaccine before it was discontinued in 1989. The vaccine is given in three separate intramuscular injections; the first two doses are administered 1 month apart and the third dose is given 6 months after the first dose. The immunogenicity potential of the vaccine is shown in Table 2-8. After the first dose, approximately 30% of normal, healthy, young adult vaccine recipients respond by the formation of antibodies. The response rate increases to 75% after the second dose, rising to a current response rate of 90% to 95% after the third dose. Most people assume erroneously that all vaccines have a 100% response rate; however, no vaccine produces absolute seroconversion in 100% of cases. Those who respond to the vaccine by the formation of protective levels of anti-HBs are completely protected against development of active HBV, asymptomatic HBV infection, and the carrier state.

TABLE 2-8 Antibody Responses* to Hepatitis B Three-Injection Vaccine Series by Age Group and Dose

Dose	Infants†	Teens and Adults‡
1	16% to 40%	20% to 30%
2	80% to 95%	75% to 80%
3	98% to 100%	90% to 95%

*Anti-HBs antibody titer of 10 mIU/mL or higher.
†Preterm infants less than 2 kg have been shown to respond to vaccination less often.
‡Factors that may lower vaccine response rates are age >40 years, male gender, smoking, obesity, and immune deficiency.

The vaccine production process was designed to thoroughly ensure a safe product. The collected serum, taken from human HBV carriers, was exposed to two biophysical purification steps and three chemical inactivation steps (pepsin at pH 2, 8 M urea, and 1:4,000 formalin), which virtually left an entirely safe suspension of HBsAg. Continued clinical monitoring of vaccine recipients by the CDC through 1984 and current monitoring by the Food and Drug Administration (FDA) indicate that there is no increased incidence of any severe side effects associated with the hepatitis B vaccine.

Recombinant DNA Vaccines

Advances in vaccine development continued to provide clinically useful preparations and in July 1986 the first vaccine made using recombinant DNA technology was licensed. Recombivax-HB, also from Merck Sharp & Dohme, became available for general use in the U.S. for the prevention of HBV infection in January 1987. This newer vaccine provided an alternative to the plasma-derived vaccine.

The recombinant vaccine is produced in cultures of *Saccharomyces cerevisiae* (common baker's yeast), into which a plasmid containing the gene for HBsAg has been inserted. HBsAg subsequently is harvested after lysis of cultured yeast cells. Purified HBsAg protein then undergoes sterile filtration and treatment with formalin before packaging. Administered vaccine is designed to contain 10 μg of HBsAg protein per milliliter, absorbed with 0.5 mg/mL of aluminum hydroxide (alum), with thimerosal as a preservative. Another recombinant DNA hepatitis B vaccine, Engerix-B, has been produced by SmithKline Biologicals in Belgium. The only stated contraindication for Recombivax-HB is for patients who are hypersensitive to yeast or any component of the vaccine.

At one time there was some concern about the possibility of the hepatitis B vaccine transmitting human immunodeficiency virus (HIV) infection. Several studies addressed this issue and supplied evidence confirming a lack of HIV transmission with this vaccine. The evidence concerns four significant areas:

1. Direct testing of the inactivation steps used in the vaccine-manufacturing process indicated that all three of the inactivation procedures (pepsin at pH 2, 8 M urea, and 0.1% formaldehyde) inactivated HIV. Thus, if HIV were in the vaccine plasma pool, it would be inactivated by the vaccine production process.

2. Studies were performed looking for HIV nucleic acid sequences in the vaccine itself, using an HIV probe. It was determined that the vaccine contained no AIDS virus–related amino acid sequences. All protein in the vaccine coded specifically for HBsAg.

3. The third approach attempted to detect seroconversion to anti-HIV in hepatitis B vaccine recipients. No seroconversion was detected in people who received vaccine manufactured from plasma pools that contained plasma of donors at high risk for HIV infection.

4. Monitoring of patients with AIDS reported to the CDC and FDA focused on epidemiologic evidence of an association between hepatitis B vaccine and AIDS. As of 1994, no relationship has been detected between receipt of hepatitis B vaccine and an increased incidence of HIV infection.

In addition, the incidence of AIDS for hepatitis B vaccine recipients in CDC vaccine trials among homosexually active men in Denver and San Francisco did not differ from that for men screened for possible participation in the trials but who received no hepatitis B vaccine because they were found to be immune. These and other reported observations clearly demonstrated that vaccination with the plasma-derived HBV vaccine posed no risk for HBV or HIV infection.

Pretesting

The issue of whether to pretest a person for anti-HBs immunity has been discussed at length since introduction of the vaccines. Pretesting can be cost-effective in large groups where the proportion expected to be antibody positive is substantial because those who are already anti-HBs positive are immune to HBV infection and therefore do not need the vaccine. Studies to date have shown that only 6.7% of vaccine recipients in dentistry were already immune. Thus, pretesting is not cost-effective in the average dental office, although it may be offered to potential vaccine recipients in an immunization program in accordance with the 1991 Occupational Safety and Health Administration (OSHA) standard. Unfortunately, there can be a significant number of false-positive reports for anti-HBs, particularly in a pretesting situation.

Post-testing

People electing to perform post-vaccination testing for anti-HBs should be aware of potential difficulties in interpreting the results. Serologic testing within 6 months of completing the primary series will differentiate people who respond to vaccine from those who fail to respond; however, the results of testing performed more than 6 months after completion of the primary series are more difficult to interpret. Therefore, post-testing should be scheduled soon after the last inoculation, preferably within 1–2 months.

A vaccine recipient who has negative results for anti-HBs several years after vaccination can be a primary nonresponder who remains susceptible to HBV or a vaccine responder whose antibody levels have decreased below detectability yet he or she is still protected against clinical disease. Should one not have responded, a second course of three additional doses of vaccine usually is prescribed by physicians. These extra doses will cause seroconversion in approximately 50% to 70% of the "first series" nonresponders.

Antibody Persistence and Booster Dose

Ongoing studies have shown that immunological memory in persons who have responded to vaccination with >10 U/mL of anti-HBs lasts for at least 23 years, and probably much longer. People who had demonstrable anti-HBs when initially tested, yet lost detectable anti-HBs on a subsequent blood test, have demonstrated a secondary anamnestic response that was protective against clinical infection when challenged with HBV. According to the CDC, it is not necessary to be tested routinely for anti-HBs each year after vaccination. The antibody response to properly administered vaccine is excellent for adults and children with a normal immune status and protection lasts as mentioned above because of the anamnestic response.

Site of Injection

There was some concern about a suboptimal response to the hepatitis B vaccine when it was administered into the buttocks. Post-testing of vaccine recipients early after vaccine introduction showed low seroconversion rates, with some response rates as low as 50%. A thorough follow-up of shipping techniques, vaccine storage techniques, retention of vaccine potency, and review of vaccine lots failed to identify any specific cause. A breakthrough occurred when the same vaccine lot was distributed to a general hospital and a health department in a large Canadian city. The health department had 100% seroconversion, whereas the general hospital had a much lower rate. The only difference was that the vaccine was administered into the deltoid muscle at the health department and the hospital administered the vaccine into the buttocks. Additional backtracking of the other sites reporting suboptimal responses indicated differences in site of injection to be the reason for the seroconversion discrepancies.

HEPATITIS C

In 1989, hepatitis C virus (HCV) was discovered using recombinant DNA technology. Until then and beginning in 1975, hepatitis C was previously termed parenterally transmitted non-A, non-B (NANB) hepatitis primarily because as many cases of bloodborne post-transfusion hepatitis could not be attributed to HAV, HBV, or any other known microorganism by serological assays. HCV has several characteristics similar to those of HBV: occurring after blood transfusions, parenteral drug use, and accidental sharps exposures. HCV is an RNA virus whose structure appears closely related to the general Flavivirus and Pestivirus. A major difference between

structural properties of HCV compared with those of other known hepatitis viruses is that different HCV strains can demonstrate extensive variations in genetic sequencing. This property, also called "genetic diversity," is related to HCV being able to mutate within a host during viral replication. As a result, several genotypes, or quasi-species, with significant differences in the RNA genome can be isolated within an infected individual. The ability of HCV to mutate and modify viral surface components is a major factor in the very high rate of chronic HCV infection.

Clinically, the features of HCV infection are variable as with other hepatitis viruses. Most (60% to 70%) individuals with acute HCV infection are asymptomatic or have nonspecific symptoms similar to hepatitis A and hepatitis B. Clinically, HCV infection often induces less hepatic inflammatory reactions and, thus, usually manifests milder symptoms. The incubation period ranges from 30–150 days. HCV RNA can be detected in the blood as soon as 1 week after initial exposure. Antibodies to HCV, or anti-HCV, can be detected within 3 months after onset of infection in approximately 90% of patients (Fig. 2-6). Unfortunately, more than 85% of hepatitis C cases progress to chronic HCV infection. Chronic HCV can take as long as 20 years to develop and progresses without signs or symptoms until patients have advanced liver disease. Almost 80% of chronic cases are stable with mild to moderate histologic disease. The other 20% eventually develop more serious sequelae such as cirrhosis and liver cancer. In the U.S., HCV is the leading cause of liver disease and may account for 8,000 to 13,000 deaths per year. In the U.S. approximately 3 to 4 million individuals are infected with HCV, with about 2.7 million being chronic carriers. This makes HCV the most common form of viral hepatitis today. The CDC estimates that the number of new cases of acute HCV infection in the U.S. has fallen from approximately 230,000 per year in the 1980s to its current level of about 20,000 cases per year.

The primary route of transmission of HCV is via the blood and although HCV traditionally had been considered a transfusion-associated disease, most reported cases have not been associated with a blood transfusion. In recent years less than 5% of the reported cases have been related to blood transfusions. Illegal intravenous drug use accounts for the majority (60%) of reported cases of acute HCV infections. In contrast to HBV transmission, sexual transmission of HCV appears less efficient. Perinatal and familial transmissions have also been documented. Studies have shown that HCV RNA is found in the saliva of approximately half the patients with chronic HCV, but the rate of transmission through saliva is low.

HCP are at risk for exposure to patient blood and possible subsequent infection from bloodborne diseases including HCV. However, HCV does not appear to be transmitted efficiently through occupational exposures

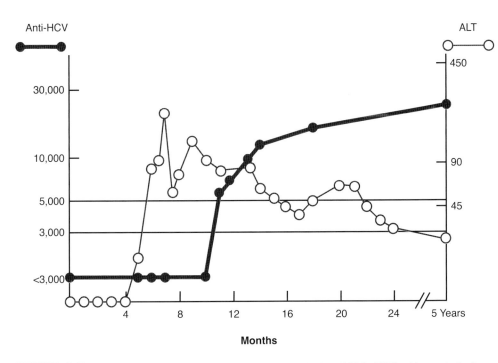

FIGURE 2-6 Acute hepatitis C virus infection. (From Stevens. Update, 3(2):2, 1989, with permission.)

to blood. The most recent follow-up studies of HCP exposed to HCV-infected blood through accidental percutaneous injury have determined an average low incidence of 1.8% (range, 0% to 7%) with one study determining that transmission occurred only from hollow-bore needles compared with other sharps. Although these studies have not documented seroconversion associated with mucous membrane or nonintact skin exposure, at least two cases of HCV transmission from a blood splash to the conjunctiva and one case of simultaneous transmission of HCV and HIV after nonintact skin exposure have been reported. Data are limited on survival of HCV in the environment. Compared with HBV, the epidemiologic data for HCV suggest that environmental contamination with blood containing HCV is not a significant risk for transmission in healthcare settings, with the possible exception of the hemodialysis setting where HCV transmission related to environmental contamination and poor infection-control practices has been documented.

The majority of studies indicate the prevalence of HCV infection among dentists, surgeons, and hospital-based HCP has declined and is currently similar to that among the general population, approximately 1% to 2%. In a study that evaluated risk factors for infection, a history of unintentional needlesticks was the only occupational risk factor independently associated with HCV infection. Unfortunately, multiple published reports have described transmission from HCV-infected

surgeons which apparently occurred during performance of invasive procedures with the overall risk for infection averaging 0.17%. There have not been any studies of the transmission from HCV-infected DHCP to patients reported and the risk for such transmission appears limited.

Presently, a vaccine is not available for HCV. This is primarily because there are six major genetic types, multiple subtypes, and HCV mutates frequently. Immunoglobulin and antiviral agents are not recommended for postexposure prophylaxis (PEP) after exposure to HCV-positive blood. In addition, no guidelines exist for administration of therapy during the acute phase of HCV infection. However, limited data indicate that antiviral therapy might be beneficial when started early in the course of HCV infection. When HCV infection is identified early, the person should be referred for medical management to a specialist knowledgeable in this area. Additional information about PEP after occupational exposure to HCV is presented in Chapter 15. Therefore, prevention of occupational transmission of HCV in healthcare settings continues to rely upon routine use of standard infection control precautions during patient care. This includes appropriate use of personal protective equipment (e.g., gloves, masks, protective eyewear), safe handling of sharp instruments to prevent occupational exposure to blood, and continued education of DHCP about the risk and prevention of blood-borne diseases.

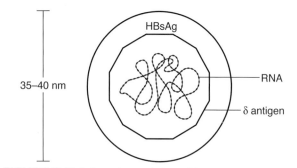

FIGURE 2-7 Schematic morphology of hepatitis D virus.

DELTA HEPATITIS

Hepatitis D virus (HDV) (Fig. 2-7), originally called the delta agent, was discovered in 1977 by Rizzetto and colleagues in Italy. Extensive investigations since that time have established the fact that delta hepatitis is unique and distinct from HBV, although HDV depends on HBV for clinical expression. HDV is defective in that it requires HBV as a helper virus for an outer protein coat (HBsAg), and thus for replication.

HDV infection is worldwide in distribution and occurs in two major epidemiologic patterns. Delta is endemic in Mediterranean countries such as southern Italy, the Middle East, and parts of Africa, as it is in parts of South America. Nonpercutaneous transmission of HBV and HDV is believed to occur primarily by intimate contact and transmucosal exchange of body fluids. In areas where HDV infection is nonendemic, including North America and Western Europe, HDV infection is confined to groups with frequent percutaneous exposures such as intravenous drug users and hemophiliacs. Current data indicates that HDV accounts for <5% of chronic hepatitis cases reported each year in the U.S. Earlier studies in the U.S. found HDV to be detectable in 24% of HBsAg-positive drug users and approximately 50% of HBsAg-positive hemophiliacs, although cases have been reported. Only limited information is available on the prevalence of HDV infection in DHCP.

Hepatitis relating to delta infection occurs in two primary modes. The first mode is simultaneous infection with HBV and HDV. When simultaneous infection occurs, the acute clinical course of hepatitis often is limited, with resolution of both HBV and delta infections, although fulminant hepatitis may develop. The second mode involves acute delta superinfection in HBsAg carriers. In this situation, the patient already has a high titer of circulating HBsAg. These patients are more likely to have a serious and possible acute fulminant form of hepatitis that more often leads to chronic HDV infection. Some of these patients will become carriers of HDV as well as HBsAg-positive. HDV has been associated with several hepatitis outbreaks in the U.S. The largest outbreak, in Worcester, Massachusetts, included a total of more than

700 cases, with more than 200 parenteral drug users, from 1983 to 1988. More than 65 of these people had positive results for prior infection with HDV. There were 14 deaths, with 11 of these people being delta positive. Four dentists and one physician were infected through this outbreak. One dentist died of fulminant hepatitis in 1986. Another dentist became an HBV carrier and infected at least four patients in his practice. Another outbreak of delta hepatitis occurred in Durham, North Carolina. Fortunately, this outbreak was limited in size; there were only 86 cases of hepatitis and at least 15% of these had markers for HDV infection.

Because all dental staff members are at an increased risk of HBV infection and of possibly becoming HBV carriers (unless immunized), members of the dental profession are at risk of simultaneous infection with HDV and HBV. Therefore, DHCP who are immune to HBV following hepatitis B vaccination or who have developed natural active immunity against HBV following viral infection are also protected against clinical exposure to HDV infection.

HEPATITIS E VIRUS

Hepatitis E is a viral infection caused by a single-stranded RNA calcivirus that is transmitted enterically via the fecal-oral route. This virus was first described in 1980 and is most frequently found in sporadic waterborne epidemics reported in developing countries. Most outbreaks have occurred in India, Asia, portions of Africa, and Mexico and none have been reported in Europe, the United States, and Australia. Current epidemiologic information indicates that the hepatitis E virus (HEV) is transmitted indirectly by ingestion of fecally contaminated water. The most prominent risks have been found for people who live or travel to an endemic area, those individuals having close personal contact with HEV-infected persons, and consumption of contaminated food or water representing the greatest risks. HEV is not considered a routine occupational infection for healthcare providers in particular because parenteral transmissons are, at most, very rare occurrences. In addition, at this time the U.S. is not considered to be endemic for HEV infection.

When viral infection is followed by symptomatic disease, onset is acute with an incubation period ranging from 15–70 days. Resultant signs and symptoms are similar to other viral hepatitis infections including loss of appetite, fatigue, nausea, abdominal pain, and fever. However, serologic tests are available to distinguish hepatitis E from other viral etiologies. Clinical manifestations are most frequently found in young to middle age adults. While most cases of HEV disease are self-limiting with no chronic state sequelae, pregnant women are at a much greater risk for developing fatal fulminant hepatitis. As many as 20% to 25% of pregnant women in the second or third trimester of pregnancy may develop this life-threatening condition and, unfortunately, the reasons for this remain unknown. This is in sharp contrast to the 1% to 2% mortality rate noted for the general population. Treatment for infection is supportive and an effective vaccine is not available.

SUMMARY

Several hepatitis viruses present a serious threat to members of the dental team. HBV and HDV infection represent the most life-threatening of these diseases; however, HCV has the highest carrier rate after infection. With the widespread application of hepatitis B vaccination in health professions since 1982, the overwhelming majority of dental and medical healthcare professionals are now immunologically protected against HBV and HDV. Presently, a vaccine is not available for HCV. Fortunately HCV does not appear to be transmitted efficiently through occupational exposures to blood. While the risk of HCV transmission appears very low in healthcare settings, standard infection control precautions must be used routinely to minimize occupational exposure and transmission.

Review Questions

1. Common hepatitis virus infections include hepatitis A, hepatitis B, and hepatitis C. Which is the least life-threatening and most mild of these diseases?
   A. Hepatitis A
   B. Hepatitis B
   C. Hepatitis C

2. The hepatitis A virus has which primary portal of entry?
   A. respiratory
   B. oral-fecal
   C. skin
   D. genital
   E. blood

3. This type of hepatitis may be traced to contaminated food or water, especially inadequately cooked shellfish.
   A. Hepatitis A
   B. Hepatitis B
   C. Hepatitis C
   D. All of the above
   E. Both A and B only

4. Which of the following characteristics applies to hepatitis A virus (HAV)?
   A. Antibodies against HAV have been shown to confer long-term protective immunity.
   B. Viral infection has a greater risk for development of a carrier state than hepatitis B virus infection.

   C. Cross-reactive immunity against HAV develops from receipt of the hepatitis B vaccine.
   D. HAV is a major occupational bloodborne infection risk for dental professionals.

5. The presence of _____ in a patient's serum is considered to represent recovery and immunologic protection from hepatitis B.
   A. Anti-HBc
   B. Anti-HBs
   C. HBeAg
   D. Anti-HAV
   E. None of the above

6. The presence of anti-HBc in a person's serum would indicate:
   A. the person is immune from reinfection with HBV.
   B. the person is a carrier of HBV.
   C. the person has been infected with HBV.
   D. the person has been vaccinated against HBV.
   E. the person is about to become jaundiced.

7. The greatest occupational healthcare worker risk for bloodborne infection is:
   A. hepatitis C virus.
   B. human immunodeficiency virus.
   C. hepatitis B virus.
   D. tuberculosis.

8. Which of the following have been involved in the transmission of hepatitis C?
   A. accidental needlesticks
   B. blood transfusions
   C. drug addicts sharing contaminated syringes
   D. all of the above

9. Which of the following statements is MOST appropriate for hepatitis D virus infection?
   A. common following ingestion of contaminated shellfish
   B. most common form of viral hepatitis from blood transfusion
   C. occurs as coinfection with HCV
   D. vaccine-preventable disease
   E. not involved in development of a carrier state

10. Artificial active immunization against HAV involves clinical use of a/an _____ vaccine, while the HBV vaccine is comprised of a/an _____.
    A. product/attenuated vaccine
    B. attenuated/product
    C. component/inactivated virus
    D. component/product
    E. inactivated virus/component

Critical Thinking

1. Using epidemiologic information, explain why hepatitis B virus is the bloodborne pathogen target for standard precautions.

2. You receive a copy of a patient's hepatitis B serological profile. It reads: HBsAg negative, anti-HBc positive, and anti-HBs positive. What is your opinion about the patient's possible history of hepatitis and immunity?

SELECTED READINGS

Ahtone JL. Hepatitis B association with an oral surgeon in Atlanta. Program and Abstracts: 109th Annual Meeting of the American Public Health Association. Washington, DC,1981.

Ahtone J, Goodman RA. Hepatitis B and dental personnel: Transmission to patients and prevention issues. J Am Dent Assoc 1983;106:219–222.

Alter MJ, Margolis HS, Krawczynski K, et al. The natural history of community-acquired hepatitis C in the United States. N Engl J Med 1992;327:1899–1905.

Andre F. Summary of safety and efficacy data on a yeast-derived hepatitis B vaccine. Am J Med 1889;87(Suppl 3A):3A–145A.

CDC. Guidelines for infection control in dental health-care settings—2003. MMWR 2003;52(No. RR-17):1–66.

CDC. Hepatitis B vaccine: evidence confirming lack of AIDS transmission. MMWR 1984;33:685–686.

CDC. Outbreak of hepatitis B associated with an oral surgeon—New Hampshire. MMWR 1987;36:132–133.

CDC. Protection against viral hepatitis. MMWR 1990;39(RR-2):1–26.

CDC. Update of hepatitis B prevention. MMWR 1987;36:353–366.

CDC. Updated U.S. Public Health Service guidelines for management of occupational exposures to HBV, HCV, and HIV and recommendations for post-exposure prophylaxis. MMWR 2001;50(RR-11):1–42.

Choo Q-L, Kuo G, Weiner AJ, et al. Isolation of a cDNA clone derived from a bloodborne non-A, non-B viral hepatitis genome. Science 1989;244:359–362.

Cleveland JL, Gooch BF, Shearer BG, et al. Risk and prevention of hepatitis C infection: implications for dentistry. J Am Dent Assoc 1999;130:641–647.

Cottone JA. Delta hepatitis: Another concern for dentistry. J Am Dent Assoc 1986;112:47–49.

Cottone JA. Hepatitis B virus infection in the dental profession. J Am Dent Assoc 1985;110:617–621.

Cottone JA. Recent developments in hepatitis: new virus, vaccine, and dosage recommendations. J Am Dent Assoc 1990;120:501–508.

Emerson SU, Purcell RH. Hepatitis E virus. Rev Med Virol 2003;13:145–154.

Feldman RE, Schiff ER. Hepatitis in dental professionals. J Am Med Assoc 1975;232:1228–1230.

Francis DP, Feorino PM, McDougal S, et al. The safety of the hepatitis B vaccine. Inactivation of the AIDS virus during routine vaccine manufacture. J Am Med Assoc 1986;256:869–872.

Goodwin D, Fannin SL, McCracken BB. An oral surgeon related hepatitis B outbreak. Calif Morbid 1976;14:1.

Hadler SC, Sorley DL, Acree KH, et al. An outbreak of hepatitis B in a dental practice. Ann Int Med 1981;95:133–138.

Hollinger FB, Grander JW, Nickel FR, et al. Hepatitis B prevalence within a dental student population. J Am Dent Assoc 1977;94:521–527.

Hoofnagle JH. Type D (delta) hepatitis. J Am Med Assoc 1989;261:1321–1325.

Hoofnagle JH, Di Bisceglie AM. Serologic diagnosis of acute and chronic viral hepatitis. Semin Liver Dis 1991;11:73–83.

Klein RS, Freeman K, Taylor PE, et al. Occupational risk for hepatitis C virus infection among New York City dentists. Lancet 1991;338:1539–1542.

Kuo G, Choo Q-L, Alter HJ, et al. An assay for circulating antibodies to a major etiologic virus of human non-A, non-B hepatitis. Science 1989;244:362–364.

Labrique AB, Thomas DL, Stoszek SK, et al. Hepatitis E: an emerging infectious disease. Epidemiol Rev 1999;21:162–179.

Lemon SM, Thomas DL. Vaccines to prevent viral hepatitis. New Engl J Med 1997;336:196–204.

Lettau LA, Smith JD, Williams D, et al. Transmission of hepatitis B with resultant restriction of surgical practice. J Am Med Assoc 1986;255:934–937.

Levin ML, Maddrey WC, Wands JR, et al. Hepatitis B transmission by dentists. J Am Med Assoc 1974;228:1139–1140.

Molinari JA. Hepatitis C: no longer a diagnosis by exclusion. Compend Cont Educ Dent 1994;15:682–684.

Molinari JA. Hepatitis C virus infection. Dent Clin N Am 1996;40:309–325.

Mosley JW, White E. Viral hepatitis as an occupational hazard of dentists. J Am Dent Assoc 1975;90:992–997.

Ohto H, Terazawa S, Sasaki N, et al. Transmission of hepatitis C virus from mothers to infants. New Engl J Med 1994;330:744–750.

Provost PJ, Hillman MR. An inactivated hepatitis A virus vaccine prepared from infected marmoset liver. Proc Exp Biol Med 1978;159:201–203.

Redd JT, Baumach J, Kohn W, et al. Patient-to-patient transmission of hepatitis B virus associated with oral surgery. J Infect Dis 2007;195:1311–1314.

Reingold AL. Transmission of hepatitis B by an oral surgeon. J Infect Dis 1982;145:262–263.

Rimland D, Parkin WE, Miller GB, et al. Hepatitis B outbreak traced to an oral surgeon. N Engl J Med 1977;296:953–958.

Rizzetto M. The delta agent. Hepatol 1983;3:729–737.

Schiff ER, de Medina MD, Kline SN, et al. Veterans Administration cooperative study on hepatitis and dentistry. J Am Dent Assoc 1986;113:390–396.

Shaw FE, Barrett CL, Hamm R, et al. Lethal outbreak of hepatitis B in a dental practice. J Am Med Assoc 1986;255:3260–3264.

Siew C, Gruninger SE, Miaw CL, et al. Percutaneous injuries in practicing dentists: a prospective study using a 20-day diary. J Am Dent Assoc 1995;126: 1227–1234.

Smith JL, Maynard JE, Berquist KR, et al. Comparative risk of hepatitis B among physicians and dentists. J Infect Dis 1976;133:705–706.

Sullivan DG, Bruden D, Deubner H, et al. Hepatitis C virus dynamics during natural infection are associated with long-term histological outcome of chronic hepatitis C disease. J Infect Dis 2007;196:239–248.

Szmuness W, Stevens C, Zang E, et al. A controlled clinic trial of the efficacy of the hepatitis B vaccine: a final report. Hepatol 1981;1:377–385.

Thomas DI, Gruninger SE, Siew C, et al. Occupational risk of hepatitis C infections among general dentists and oral surgeons in North America. Am J Med 1996;100:41–45.

Wasley A, Miller JT, Finelli L. Surveillance for acute viral hepatitis—United States, 2005. MMWR Surveill Summ 2007;56:1–45.

Werberger A, Mensch B, Kuter B, et al. A controlled trial of a formalin-inactivated hepatitis A vaccine in healthy children. N Engl J Med 1992;327:453–457.

West DJ. Clinical experience with hepatitis B vaccines. Am J Infect Control 1989;17:172–180.

Williams SV, Pattison CP, Berquist KR. Dental infections with hepatitis B. J Am Med Assoc 1975;232:1231–1233.

Winsom CJ, Kelly M. Medical/dental management of a chronic hepatitis C patient. Oral Surg Oral Med Oral Path 1993;75:786–790.

Winsom C, Siegel MA. Advances in the diagnosis and management of human viral hepatitis. Dent Clin N Am 2003;47:431–447.

Zajac BA, West D, Meibohm A. Improvements in the immunogenicity and purity of a genetically engineered hepatitis B vaccine. Hepatol 1988;8:1322–1329.

3

Human Immunodeficiency Virus, Acquired Immunodeficiency Syndrome, and Related Infections

Louis G. DePaola

Valli I. Meeks

LEARNING OBJECTIVES

After completion of this chapter individuals should be able to:

1 Discuss the emergence of the HIV/AIDS pandemic.

2 Clarify the differences between HIV infection and AIDS.

3 Discuss the epidemiology of HIV infection worldwide and in the United States.

4 Understand the virology of HIV.

5 List risk factors for transmission of HIV.

6 Understand the rationale and types of serologic assays used in diagnosis of HIV infection and AIDS.

7 Comprehend healthcare worker risks for acquiring HIV infection following accidental occupational exposure.

8 Describe opportunistic infections which can develop in HIV-infected persons.

9 Describe current strategies for medical management of HIV disease.

KEY TERMS

Acquired immunodeficiency syndrome (AIDS): a disease of the body's immune system caused by the human immunodeficiency virus (HIV). AIDS is characterized by the death of CD4 cells (an important part of the body's immune system), which leaves the body vulnerable to life-threatening conditions such as infections and cancers.

Acute retroviral syndrome (ARS): also known as primary HIV infection or acute HIV infection. The period of rapid HIV replication occurs 2 to 4 weeks after infection by HIV. Acute HIV infection is characterized by a drop in CD4 cell counts and an increase in HIV levels in the blood. Some, but not all, individuals experience flu-like symptoms during this period of infection. These symptoms can include fever, inflamed lymph nodes, sore throat, and rash. These symptoms may last from a few days to 4 weeks and then go away.

Antiretroviral therapy: treatment with drugs that inhibit the ability of retroviruses (such as HIV) to multiply in the body. The antiretroviral therapy recommended for HIV infection is referred to as highly active antiretroviral therapy (HAART), which uses a combination of medications to attack HIV at different points in its life cycle.

Highly active antiretroviral therapy (HAART): the name given to treatment regimens that aggressively suppress HIV replication and progression of HIV disease. The usual HAART regimen combines three or more anti-HIV drugs.

Human immunodeficiency virus (HIV): the virus that causes AIDS. HIV is in the retrovirus family and two types

have been identified: HIV-1 and HIV-2. HIV-1 is responsible for most HIV infections throughout the world, while HIV-2 is found primarily in West Africa.

Lymphocytes: a type of infection-fighting white blood cell found in the blood, lymph, and lymphoid tissue.

Opportunistic infection (OI): infection caused by normally nonpathogenic microorganisms in a host whose resistance has been decreased or compromised.

Retrovirus: a type of virus that stores its genetic information in a single-stranded RNA molecule, then constructs a double-stranded DNA version of its genes using a special enzyme called reverse transcriptase. The DNA copy is then integrated into the host cell's own genetic material. HIV is an example of a retrovirus.

Reverse transcriptase (RT): an enzyme found in HIV and other retroviruses. RT converts single-stranded HIV RNA into double-stranded HIV DNA. Some anti-HIV drugs interfere with this stage of HIV's life cycle.

Ribonucleic acid (RNA): chemical structure that carries genetic instructions for protein synthesis. Although DNA is the primary genetic material of cells, RNA is the genetic material for some viruses.

Seroconversion: the process by which a newly infected person develops antibodies to HIV. These antibodies are then detectable by an HIV test. Seroconversion may occur anywhere from days to weeks or months following HIV infection.

INTRODUCTION

Along with the evolution of modern-day society, infectious diseases are changing to become more resistant to standard treatment regimens and new diseases are constantly emerging. Some of these new diseases, such as severe acute respiratory syndrome (SARS), the first pandemic disease of the 21st century, have had relatively little impact. Emerging from November 2002 to July 2003, SARS caused a total of approximately 8,098 probable SARS cases and only 774 deaths. The worldwide spread of this disease, which was reported in 26 countries, however, was alarming. Other new diseases, such as the **acquired immunodeficiency syndrome (AIDS)** pandemic caused by infection with **human immunodeficiency virus (HIV)**, have been far more lethal and have had a significant, negative, global impact. HIV/AIDS have killed over 25 million people, dramatically illustrating the awesome capabilities of this disease even in the age of modern medical science. Since the first reports of this new infection in 1981, every country of the world has

reported cases of HIV/AIDS. By the end of 2007, the AIDS pandemic had infected an estimated 30–36 million people including almost 1 million Americans, of whom over 500,000 have died. Approximately 7,000 persons become newly infected with HIV each day and over 5,700 persons die from the immune suppression and/or **opportunistic infections (OI)** caused by AIDS.

The epicenter of the pandemic is subSaharan Africa where approximately 68% of those infected reside in that region. Although the prevalence of the HIV disease is very high, one in three infected Africans are unaware of their infection. In the early 1980s, the pandemic expanded rapidly and the number of new cases of HIV infection and AIDS deaths increased dramatically. AIDS hysteria began to gain momentum and very quickly raised the level of concern of acquiring this new and, in the 1980s, universally fatal disease. Healthcare providers were compelled to modify the delivery of medical and dental care to allay fears of both patients and health professionals and reduce the risk of HIV/AIDS transmission in hospitals, medical facilities, and dental offices throughout the world. As a result, the importance of infection control rose to unprecedented levels and the impact of HIV/AIDS on healthcare is monumental in scope. Clinical practice in the post-AIDS era changed dramatically, especially in the areas of infection control.

In addition, progression to HIV infection results in a dramatic decrease in the immune function and an increase in unusual and difficult to manage opportunistic infections. Many of these can present with oromaxillofacial lesions, thereby leading to the term *oral manifestations* of HIV disease. As the number of people infected with HIV continues to increase, so will the need for provision of oral healthcare for those with HIV disease. Consequently dental providers will need to have a thorough knowledge about HIV/AIDS and the medical/dental management of patients with HIV infection.

THE EMERGENCE OF HIV/AIDS

On June 5, 1981, the Centers for Disease Control and Prevention (CDC) reported an unusual cluster of *Pneumocystis carinii* pneumonia (PCP) infections and other unusual infections in five previously healthy, homosexual men. This cluster of five patients was very unique because each of them had PCP, abnormal ratios of **lymphocyte** subgroups, and was actively shedding cytomegalovirus. The presence of PCP, which previously had only been seen in patients with severe immune dysfunction, was accompanied by abnormal lymphocyte counts suggesting some sort of attack on the immune system resulting in a novel form of immune suppression. Shortly thereafter, other OI were documented including mycobacterial infections, toxoplasmosis, invasive fungal infections, non-Hodgkin's lymphoma, and an especially aggressive form of Kaposi's sarcoma (KS). The latter is a rare form of skin cancer that previously only had been seen in elderly Mediterranean men.

In a very short period of time additional cases were reported in gay men, injection drug users (IDU), Haitians, recipients of blood transfusions/products, infants, prisoners, and women who had sex with infected men. Because the initial cases of this new syndrome were reported in gay men this disease was first termed "gay-related immune deficiency" (GRID). However, it was soon recognized that anyone who came in contact with infected blood or body fluids could acquire the infection and in 1982 the term AIDS, acquired immune deficiency syndrome, was introduced. The cause of AIDS, however, remained elusive. Most felt that an undiscovered infectious agent, probably a virus, was responsible, especially since the disease was most common in gay men and hepatitis B virus infection was also very prevalent in this population. However, many other, and sometimes bizarre, theories abounded. It was not until 1983 that a new **retrovirus** was isolated and identified as the agent responsible for the development of AIDS. Some controversy surrounded the discovery of this new virus. It was initially called lymphadenopathy-associated virus (LAV) by the cofounder Luc Montagnier and human T-cell leukemia virus-III (HTLV-III) by Robert Gallo. It was eventually decided to name this new microorganism human immunodeficiency virus (HIV). Once HIV was isolated many people felt that continued rapid progress would soon lead to development of successful treatment regimens. Unfortunately, initial optimism was short lived and, at this time, neither a cure nor a preventive vaccine is available. However, substantial progress has been made, as accomplishments in **antiretroviral therapy** have contributed to improved medical management of HIV disease, thereby significantly extending the life expectancy of those infected with HIV.

It is now widely recognized that oral health is essential to general health and well-being of the general population. Since HIV-infected persons tend to have much higher levels of oral, dental, and periodontal diseases, maintenance of good oral health is a major health goal for this group. Therefore, dental healthcare personnel (DHCP) need to recognize the importance of establishing and maintaining oral health in this ever increasing segment of the population. These treatment strategies also have to be employed in conjunction with an infection control program that ensure practice safety for DHCP and minimize the risk of disease transmission in the dental office by complying with appropriate government regulations and recommendations.

PATHOGENESIS AND NATURAL HISTORY OF HIV DISEASE

HIV is an **ribonucleic acid (RNA)** virus and is classified as a retrovirus. Retroviruses are unique because they contain the enzyme **reverse transcriptase**. This enzyme is essential in performing in a retrograde step, converting viral RNA into an intermediary DNA to reproduce new, infectious virions. Infection occurs when gp120, a viral glycoprotein, contacts and attaches onto a cell that has a specific surface CD4 molecule, which functions as a high affinity surface virus receptor. This receptor is primarily found on the surfaces of CD4+ T-lymphocytes. Monocytes and macrophages can also be infected and provide reservoirs for large quantities of viable HIV, especially in the lymph nodes. These infected cells can remain latent for years or, alternatively, can enter active virus production, leading to the release of infectious virions. Whether HIV in the cell becomes latent or productive depends on complex interactions between the virus and host regulatory systems and this phenomenon significantly contributes to an infected host's inability to effectively eliminate HIV from the human body post-infection.

Following binding of gp120 with a receptor cell CD4 molecule, a complex interaction with other viral co-

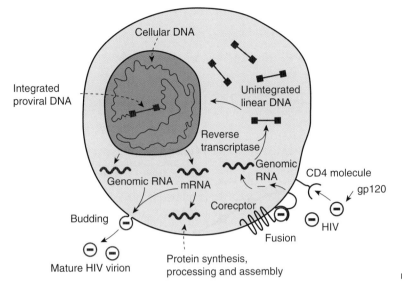

CD4 molecule

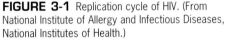

gp120

FIGURE 3-1 Replication cycle of HIV. (From National Institute of Allergy and Infectious Diseases, National Institutes of Health.)

receptor proteins occurs, which subsequently allows HIV to fuse with the outer lipid layer of the lymphoid cell. This early component of the replication cycle is called fusion (Fig. 3-1). Once the virus binds to the CD4 molecule and co-receptor it passes through the cell membrane. Upon entry into the host CD4+ cell, HIV RNA is converted by the enzyme reverse transcriptase to HIV-DNA. This proviral copy of DNA can then be integrated into the host cell's genetic material making that cell capable of producing progeny HIV particles. As viral replication proceeds, long chains of viral protein are produced which are cleaved by a protease enzyme to produce necessary viral proteins, enzymes, and genomic RNA. In a complex, not completely understood process, proteins and other molecules in the host cell direct the accumulation of HIV components in special intracellular sacks that normally function to carry proteins out of the cell. Budding and release of viable HIV is thought to occur by this process, once again demonstrating the ability of HIV to manipulate cellular mechanisms. The host cell is killed during the process of replication. Production of new virions rapidly leads to infection of additional lymphoid cells, which in turn yields more virus. Thus, once initiated, there is a relentless production of HIV causing the death of an increasing number of immune competent cells. This directly translates to a gradual decline in immune function to the point where opportunistic infections overwhelm the ability of the immune system to control them. Eventually, the patient succumbs to the infection. Blocking or inhibition of any of the critical binding sites or enzymes would result in incomplete, noninfectious HIV particles and, therefore, they have become targets for antiretroviral therapy.

The natural history of untreated HIV proceeds in six stages and the average time from infection to death is 10 years. These are: viral transmission; primary HIV infection/acute retroviral syndrome; recovery and **seroconversion**; asymptomatic chronic HIV infection; symptomatic HIV infection/AIDS; and death (Fig. 3-2). Once HIV infection is established, the virus reproduces in very large numbers (high plasma viremia/viral load) and disseminates throughout the body, seeding the lymph nodes. This is accompanied by a dramatic drop in CD4+ cells (Fig. 3-2). Within 2–3 weeks, primary HIV infection, also known as **acute retroviral syndrome** develops. The symptoms, which are very variable from mild to profound, primarily consist of fever (96%); adenopathy (74%); pharyngitis (70%); an erythematous maculopapular rash on the face, trunk, and sometimes extremities (70%); myalgia (54%); and headache (32%). Because of the benign presentation in many cases, the diagnosis of HIV at this time is frequently overlooked. Within 2–3 more weeks, the infected person's cytotoxic T cell response results in reduction of plasma viremia and clinical recovery. Symptoms resolve, in most cases spontaneously, and 95% of individuals will seroconvert and develop detectable HIV antibody (anti-HIV). This serum marker was very important in the early years of the pandemic because, with the serologic sensitivity available in the 1980s, HIV was not detectable until seroconversion took place. Equilibrium between the immune system and HIV follows seroconversion, resulting in decline in the viral load from the peak level of HIV viremia, to the point where levels remain for months to years (Fig. 3-2). This is known as the viral set point and it has been shown to be an important marker of HIV infection, since the higher the viral load is at this point in the disease, the poorer the prognosis and the more rapid the progression to the development of AIDS. Chronic HIV infection follows and is characterized by a gradual degradation of immune function that continues for an average of 8 years (Fig. 3-2).

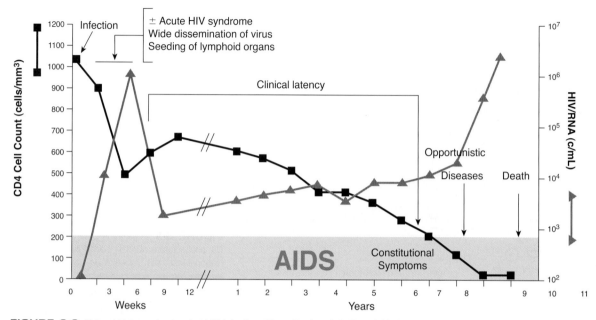

FIGURE 3-2 Natural history of untreated HIV infection. (From Bartlett J, Gallant J. Medical Management of HIV Infection. Baltimore: Johns Hopkins University, 2007. Reproduced with permission from Dr. Bartlett.)

Infected individuals are asymptomatic and appear immunologically healthy at this time. As immune function continues to decline (CD4 <500), OIs begin to occur and this marks the beginning of symptomatic HIV infection. Within 1–2 years the CD4 cell count falls below 200 and/or appearance of one or more AIDS defining illnesses (Table 3-1) marks the disease progression to a diagnosis of AIDS. The progression to death in untreated disease is 1–3 years.

EPIDEMIOLOGY OF HIV DISEASE

By most estimates, approximately 45 million people are living with HIV infection worldwide. In 2007 there were about 2.5 million deaths that were directly attributable to AIDS. HIV/AIDS has severely impacted many countries and those who cannot access and/or afford quality healthcare are particularly vulnerable. More than 96% of the cases are in low and middle income countries. Women account for almost 50% of cases and 40% are among young people. Most deaths are attributable to inadequate access to HIV prevention and treatment services. Sixty-eight percent of all people living with HIV live in subSaharan Africa. This region alone suffered 76% of all AIDS deaths in 2007. Asia also bears a very large burden of HIV/AIDS with an estimated 4.9 million people living with HIV infection in 2007. Since the first reports of AIDS in 1981 more than 25 million people have died of the disease. Africa alone has 12 million AIDS orphans. In underdeveloped countries, that have >90% of the cases, 7.1 million people are in immediate need of life-saving AIDS drugs, but only 28% are receiving these life-saving medications.

A cumulative total of 956,018 AIDS cases have been reported in the U.S. from the beginning of the epidemic in June 1981 to the end of 2005. Of this number, 769,635 were men and 186,383 were women. The number of people living with AIDS (PLWA) has steadily increased since 1985, with 433,760 PLWA reported in 2005. Approximately 1 million people in the U.S. are currently living with HIV/AIDS of which >400,000 have AIDS. In addition, 20,000 people die each year in the U.S. from AIDS. Unfortunately, despite advances in antiretroviral treatment, new technologies, and rapid testing, 24% to 27% of the people infected with HIV do not know they are infected. Furthermore, an estimated 42% to 59% of those infected with HIV/AIDS are not receiving medical care.

There are 40,000 new infections of HIV/AIDS per year, down from an annual incidence of 150,000 reported in the 1980s. After peaking at 69,242, the number of new U.S. AIDS cases declined from 42,832 in 1995–1998 to 41,993 in 2005. The decline in AIDS cases observed in the late 1990s may correspond to the introduction of **highly active antiretroviral therapy (HAART)** and protease inhibitors (PI) to the ART regimens, with saquinavir being the first PI approved by the Food and Drug Administration (FDA) in 1995.

In terms of the demographics in the U.S., HIV/AIDS disproportionately affects certain subsets of the population. Current trends regarding the infection show that despite an apparent leveling off in the number of new AIDS cases over the past 10 years, African Americans and Latinos account for a disproportionate rise in the number of new AIDS cases when compared to the racial and ethnic demographics of the total U.S. population. In

TABLE 3-1 AIDS Defining Illnesses

Candidiasis of esophagus, trachea, bronchi, or lungs	Herpes simplex with mucocutaneous ulcer for >1 month or bronchitis, pneumonitis, esophagitis
Cervical cancer, invasive	Histoplasmosis, extrapulmonary
Coccidioidomycosis, extrapulmonary	HIV-associated dementia: disabling cognitive and/or motor dysfunction interfering with occupation or activities of daily living
Cryptococcosis, extrapulmonary	HIV-associated wasting: involuntary weight loss of >10% of baseline plus chronic diarrhea (>2 loose stools/day for >30 days) or chronic weakness and documented enigmatic fever for >30 days
Cryptosporidiosis with diarrhea for >1 month	Isoporosis with diarrhea for >1 month
Cytomegalovirus of any organ other than liver, spleen, or lymph nodes	Kaposi's sarcoma in patient younger than 60 (or older than 60 with positive HIV serology)
Lymphoma of brain in patient younger than 60 (or older than 60 with positive HIV serology)	*Pneumocystis carinii* pneumonia
Lymphoma, non-Hodgkin's	Pneumonia, recurrent bacterial with positive HIV serology
Mycobacterium avium or *M. kansasii*, disseminated	Progressive multifocal leukoencephalopathy
Mycobacterium tuberculosis, disseminated	*Salmonella septicemia* (nontyphoid), recurrent with positive HIV serology
Mycobacterium tuberculosis, pulmonary	Toxoplasmosis of internal organ

(Modified from Bartlett J, Gallant J. Medical Management of HIV Infection. Baltimore: Johns Hopkins University, 2007.)

1985 Caucasians accounted for 60% of the persons with AIDS, followed by African Americans (25%), and Latinos (15%). These numbers can be compared to AIDS figures for 2005 which indicated a 29% incidence in Caucasians, 48% in African Americans, and 20% in Latinos. Thus while African Americans represent only 12.2% of the U.S. population; they account for almost 50% of the cases.

The CDC has developed one of the most comprehensive surveillance systems for collected AIDS case data and routinely updates the impact of HIV/AIDS in the U.S. Monitoring continues to improve with newly developed technologies, which can distinguish recent infections from infections older than 160 days. Use of these assays is expected to track the epidemic more precisely in the U.S. Such scrutiny of the disease has allowed documentation of trends in the mortality and morbidity of the AIDS epidemic.

TRANSMISSION OF HIV

HIV is spread by contact with blood and body fluids (semen, vaginal secretions, and breast milk) that have been infected with the virus. The routes of transmission of HIV are well described. These are:

- Sexual contact
- Injection drug use (IDU)
- Mother to child
  - Perinatal
  - Breast feeding
- Exposure to blood/blood products
  - Blood/blood product transfusion or infusion
  - Organ transplantation
  - Occupational exposure

Sexual contact accounts for the majority of cases in adults. Mucosal linings of the vagina, vulva, penis, rectum, or the oral cavity are lined with immune system cells (dendritic cells) and present receptors on which HIV can bind. These cells then migrate to the regional lymph nodes, initiating HIV infection. The virus can enter the body through mucosal surfaces during sexual contact. HIV transmission is enhanced in any circumstance that causes damage (breaks or tears) to mucosal surfaces such as genital herpes or other sexually transmitted diseases that cause ulceration and/or inflammation. It is well documented that blood transmits HIV and any behavior, medical/dental treatment, or occupational activity where there is contact with blood, blood products, or body fluids puts an unprotected individual at risk for acquiring HIV infection. In the early part of the pandemic, before adequate tests for detection of HIV were developed, transfusion of blood/blood products was problematic.

With more sensitive and sophisticated tests available today, however, transfusion-related transmission of HIV is very rare in the U.S. and other developed countries. Unfortunately, blood transfusion still accounts for HIV transmission in underdeveloped regions where testing is not available. IDU accounts for almost one third of the cases of HIV in the U.S., primarily because of sharing syringes and other equipment for drug injection contaminated with minute quantities of blood infected with HIV. Children born to mothers who contracted HIV through sharing needles or having sex with an IDU may become infected as well. Women who are infected can pass the disease onto their unborn children and this mother-to-child transmission of HIV is the most significant source of HIV infection in young children. In 1994 accumulated evidence suggested that zidovudine (ZDV) given to pregnant women infected with HIV and their newborns significantly reduced the risk of perinatal transmission. This strategy, accompanied with improved counseling and testing, has dramatically reduced perinatal HIV transmission incidence in the U.S. to about 100–200 infants/year. Many of these infections involve women who were not tested early enough in pregnancy or who did not receive prevention services. In contrast, other areas of the world that have the most number of cases, fewer resources, and the inability to access ZDV and other antiretroviral drugs have about a 30% the incidence of perinatal transmission.

It is important to note here that current knowledge about the stability and viability of HIV continues to show that this retrovirus does not survive well in the environment, is unable to replicate outside of the body, and is rapidly inactivated. Thus, the possibility of environmental transmission is considered remote. Also, there is no scientific evidence to suggest or support possible HIV transmission by casual contact, air, water, insects, or other animal bites. While colds and flu may be transmitted by shaking hands or talking, sharing food, eating utensils, plates, drinking glasses, household items, or by hugging and kissing on the cheek or lips, HIV is not.

RISK FOR OCCUPATIONAL TRANSMISSION OF HIV

Clinical and scientific evidence supports the belief that the risk of HIV transmission after percutaneous exposure of healthcare personnel (HCP) to HIV-infected blood is quite low. Although the data are encouraging, the risk of acquiring HIV infection from an occupational exposure remains real for both medical and dental professionals. The transmission rate has been estimated to be approximately 0.3% after a percutaneous injury and approximately 0.09% after a mucous membrane exposure. Viral infection after a non-intact skin exposure is estimated to be less than the risk for mucous membrane exposures. As of December 2002, CDC had confirmed 57 American HCP with documented HIV seroconversion resulting from accidental occupation-

al exposures. These affected HCP included 19 laboratory workers (16 of whom were clinical laboratory workers), 24 nurses, 6 physicians, 2 surgical technicians, 1 dialysis technician, 1 respiratory therapist, 1 health aide, 1 embalmer/morgue technician, and 2 housekeeper/maintenance workers. Routes of exposure in these cases included: percutaneous (puncture/cut injury) exposure (48), mucocutaneous (mucous membrane and/or skin) exposure (5), both percutaneous and mucocutaneous exposure (2), and unknown (2). Body fluids involved in these accidents consisted of: HIV-infected blood (49), concentrated virus in a laboratory (3), visibly bloody fluid (1), and unspecified fluid (4). To date, no DHCP have been documented to have been occupationally infected with HIV during provision of dental care. With regard to the 57 known cases, several factors have been found to play a role in occupational HIV transmission in healthcare settings. Increased risk was associated with exposure to larger quantities of blood from the source person, deeper injuries, and the higher titer of HIV in donor blood.

DIAGNOSTIC TESTING

Although the virus was discovered and isolated in 1983, it was not until 1985 that reliable serologic tests were available to detect HIV antibody. While crude by today's standard, these were invaluable at the time and formed the basis for a nationwide HIV screening program. Standard HIV testing consists of an initial enzyme linked immunoassay (EIA) followed by a confirmatory Western blot (WB). The EIA spectrophotometrically detects the presence of antibody binding to HIV antigens. Current assays are extremely accurate with a sensitivity of 99.5% and a specificity of 99.994% 3 months after HIV transmission. Despite this level of accuracy, no test is 100% sensitive and specific and tests can yield an occasional false negative or false positive result. While the EIA is recommended for screening for HIV, the WB test is the confirmatory test. WB detects antibodies to HIV including those produced against the viral core, polymerase, and envelope antigens. Positive tests require confirmation with repeat testing. Most people (95%) develop detectable HIV antibodies within 6 months of infection, but a small percentage may take much longer to develop detectable immunoglobulins. Since serologic tests cannot rule out infection that occurs before antibody appearance (i.e., a window period), a negative EIA result does not rule out the possibility of HIV infection. More recent technological improvements in testing have resulted to the ability to quantify the viral load in the blood. As a result use of the polymerase chain reaction (PCR) and quantitative plasma HIV RNA or viral load testing have improved the possibility of diagnosing early HIV infection, predicting the probability of transmission, predicting the progression in the chronically infected, and assessing the need for and monitoring ART. More recently, rapid HIV tests have been approved by the FDA. Four of these use blood/plasma/serum as a test medium. The test result is available within 10–40 minutes depending on the manufacturer. The fast turn around time is very valuable especially after possible exposure to HIV from an occupational exposure or sexual episode/assault. One rapid test uses saliva instead of blood, with the obvious advantages of ease of collection and no need for venipuncture or fingerstick. Most states have specific laws that require counseling before tests for HIV are performed and anyone who would require HIV testing should be referred to an approved test site.

MEDICAL MANAGEMENT OF HIV DISEASE

Antiretroviral Therapy

Although a cure for HIV/AIDS remains elusive, enormous progress has been made in the medical management of HIV. Perhaps the most significant accomplishment has been the ability to control HIV replication through the use of HAART. Controlled clinical trials have been shown to suppress the viral load, sustain this suppression, significantly improve immune function, and markedly reduce morbidity and mortality of HIV/AIDS. HAART also has been shown to reduce new AIDS defining illnesses, hospitalizations, and deaths by 60% to 80%. These very favorable clinical improvements are a direct result of inhibition of HIV replication and sustained reduction of viral load. Upon HIV infection, the virus reproduces at a very high rate infecting and killing T-4 helper lymphocytes. When the normal CD4 count of 1,000 falls to 500, then 200 and below, OIs begin to appear and can be very difficult to treat, especially with progressively declining immune function. The key to the control of OI is controlling HIV replication and preventing continued decrease in immune function. In the 1980s, ART was in its infancy and no effective, long-term therapy existed that could suppress HIV reproduction and progression to AIDS. The diagnosis of AIDS had a mortality rate approaching 100%. In early clinical trials a reverse transcriptase inhibitor, zidovudine (ZDV), was shown to be efficacious and was licensed by the FDA in 1987. Initially, ZDV seemed effective, but this drug and subsequent drugs used in monotherapy regimens failed to sustain viral suppression as resistant strains of HIV rapidly emerged, and did not significantly improve the prognosis of AIDS. Subsequent FDA approval in 1995 of saquinavir (Inverase), the first of a new class of antiretroviral drugs called protease inhibitors (PIs), dramatically improved the ability to suppress HIV reproduction, sustain the suppression, and reduce immune suppression. Since then, over 30 ART drugs have been approved by the FDA (Table 3-2) and many more agents are in various phases of clinical trials. Some have been withdrawn because of adverse side effects or toxicity.

The principle of HAART is to use combinations of drugs which attack HIV at different points of its reproductive cycle. The goals of HAART are to: (a) prolong and improve the quality of life; (b) reduce HIV viral load as much as possible for as long as possible; (c) improve immune function; (d) minimize drug interaction/toxicity; and (e) reduce vertical transmission of HIV. HAART has evolved into the standard of care for the treatment of HIV infection and recently two new classes of ART (entry and integrase inhibitors) have been introduced into the HAART regimens that will give clinicians additional agents to manage HIV disease.

OPPORTUNISTIC INFECTIONS

It is understood that in disease progression to AIDS, HIV infects CD41 lymphocytes and eventually destroys the body's cellular immune system and its ability to fight diseases. Early in the HIV/AIDS epidemic, systemic complications and OI predictably occurred as immune function decreased. These continue to be frequent causes of death in people infected with HIV (Table 3-2).

While treating OI is critical in the short term to maintain the patient's life, prevention of OI is paramount for long-term survival. Prevention of OI with primary and secondary chemoprophylaxis (Table 3-2) evolved to become the current standard of care. Although OI are still the cause of mortality and morbidity in areas of the world where access to ART is limited, HAART has reduced the incidence of OI for patients with access to the medications. OI notably occur as the CD4 cell count falls below 200, with the absolute CD4 cell count used as a predictor of susceptibility to OI. Maintaining a CD4 cell count above 200 is considered a primary strategy in prevention of OIs. HAART instituted when a patient experiences HIV-related symptoms or when the CD4 cell count nears 200 is therefore strongly recommended. The success of HAART in reducing the incidence of AIDS-related OI ultimately prompted the reevaluation of prophylaxis against OI in patients where ART has created a stable, reconstituted immune system. Because HIV replicates more when the body's immune system is fighting an infection, it is imperative to treat OI promptly to prevent destruction of the body's defenses.

SUMMARY

More than 25 years have passed since the first report of AIDS was published in 1981. Although tremendous progress has been made in reducing the morbidity and mortality of HIV/AIDS, the pandemic, short of a major scientific breakthrough, is expected to persist well into the future. Providers of oral healthcare should expect to see more patients infected with HIV and should be familiar with the pathogenesis, management, and infection control procedures necessary to provide oral/dental care to this population.

TABLE 3-2 HIV/AIDS Associated Opportunistic Infections Seen in Adults

Opportunistic Infection	Symptoms	Primary Prophylaxis	Treatment	Alternative
Pneumocystic carinii Pneumonia (also called *P. jiroveci* pneumonia)	Parasitic infection of lung; fever, cough, difficulty breathing, night sweats, fatigue, weight loss	• Trimethoprim/Sulfamethoxazole (TMP/SMX) po qd • TMP/SMX double strength po 3×/week • Dapsone 50 mg po bid • Dapsone 100 mg po qd • Aerosolized Pentamidine 300 mg once a month	• TMP/SMX double strength, 2 tablets tid × 21 days • IV TMP/SMX	• Aerosolized pentamidine • Dapsone 100 mg po qd + TMP 15 mg/kg po tid
Candida Oral, Oropharyngeal	Fungal infection; often presents as white or yellow plaques on oral mucosa; can also present as red maculae or patches	Not recommended because of risk of developing azole-resistant candida	• Clotrimazole troches 10 mg, 5×/day; 10–14 days • Nystatin pastilles 200,000 units, 4–5× daily × 14 days • Fluconazole 100 mg po qd; 7–14 days • Itraconazole 200 mg oral suspension; po qd swish and swallow, empty stomach	• Amphotericin B 0.3–0.7 mg/kg IV: bid • Voriconazole 200 mg po qd; 7–14 days
Cryptococcal Meningitis	Fungal infection of brain and spinal column; nausea, headache, fever, fatigue	Not recommended	IV Amphotericin B 0.7 mg/kg + Flucytosine 25 mg/kg po qid × 14 days; then Fluconazole 400 mg po qd × 8 weeks or until CSF cultures are sterile	• IV Amphotericin B 0.7 mg/kg qd × 14 days then Fluconazole 400–800 mg qd • Fluconazole + flucytosine 25 mg/kg qid × 4–6 weeks
Histoplasmosis	Fungal infection with fever, fatigue, weight loss, difficulty breathing, swollen lymph nodes	Itraconazole 200 mg qd; recommended with CD4 cell count <100 and risk of infection	• Amphotericin B • Itraconazole 200 mg po bid	• Itraconazole 400 mg IV qd • Fluconazole 800 mg po qd
Aspergillosis	Fungal infection with wheezing, fever, cough, shortness of breath; also can be disseminated infection	Not recommended	Voriconazole 6 mg/kg IV q12h × 2 then 4 mg/kg IV q12h for ≥1 week then 200 mg bid	IV Amphotericin B
Toxoplasmosis	Parasite primarily infecting the brain causing altered mental state; severe headaches, fever, seizures	• TMP/SMX (ds) qd • TMP/SMX qd	Pyrimethamine 200 mg po, then 50–75 mg po qd and sulfadiazine 1 g po qid plus leucovorin 10–20 mg po qd × 6 weeks	• IV TMZ/SMX • Pyrimethamine + Leucovorin + Clindamycin 600 mg IV or po qid
Cryptosporidosis	Parasitic infection causing diarrhea	Avoid exposure to organism found in feces, feces-contaminated drinking water	Manage undetectable viral load and CD4 cell count ≥100 with HAART	• Nitazoxanide 500 mg po bid • Paromomycin 25–35 mg/kg po • Supportive care for hydration

(continued)

TABLE 3-2 HIV/AIDS Associated Opportunistic Infections Seen in Adults (continued)

Opportunistic Infection	Symptoms	Primary Prophylaxis	Treatment	Alternative
Mycobacterium Avium Complex	Bacterial infection causing night sweats, fever, fatigue, weight loss, diarrhea, weakness, anemia	• Clarithromycin 500 mg bid • Azithromycin 1,200 mg once a week	• Clarithromycin 500 mg po bid + Ethambutol 15 mg/kg po qd	Azithromycin 500–600 mg po qd + Ethambutol
Herpes Simplex Virus Disease	Viral infection; vesicular lesions which rupture becoming painful, irregular ulcerations	Suppressive regime or treat each episode; early treatment of episodic occurrence recommended to shorten duration of lesions/ulceration	• Acyclovir 400 mg po tid • Famciclovir 250 mg po tid • Valacyclovir 1 g po bid All for 7–10 days	• Foscarnet 120–200 mg/kd/day IV • Cidofovir mg/kd IV weekly
Herpes Zoster Dermatomal (Shingles)	Viral infection; activation of Varicella zoster virus, which has been dormant in sensory nerve; unilateral, often vesicular lesions	Varicella zoster immunoglobulin within 48–96 hrs of exposure to chicken pox or V. zoster virus	• Famciclovir 500 mg po tid • Valacyclovir 1 g po tid Both 7–10 days or until lesions crust • Acyclovir 10 mg/kg IV q8h followed by Valacyclovir	Foscarnet IV 120–200 mg/kg/d
Cytomegalovirus (CMV)	Viral infection transmitted through close contact; can infect all body tissues/organs	Ganciclovir 1 g tid	• Ganciclovir intraocular implant and Valganciclovir 900 mg po qd for CMV retinitis • IV Ganciclovir or IV Foscarnet × 21–28 days • Valganciclovir 900 mg po bid × 14–21 days, then 900 mg qd	• IV Ganciclovir 5 mg/kd q12h × 14–21 days, then 5 mg/kg qd • Cidofovir 5 mg/kg IV once a week for 2 weeks + Probenecid 2 g po 3 hr before then 1 g po 2 hr after Cidofovir, then 1 g po 8 hr later

bid, two times a day; IV, intravenous; po, by mouth; qd, once a day; qid, four times a day; tid, three times a day.
(Modified from Treating Opportunistic Infections Among HIV-Infected Adults and Adolescents. MMWR Morb Mortal Weekly Rep 2004;53(RR-15):1–112.

TABLE 3-3 Antiretroviral Drugs 2007

Nucleoside Reverse Transcriptase Inhibitor (NRTI)	Nonnucleoside Reverse Transcriptase Inhibitor (NNRTI)	Protease Inhibitors (PI)	Entry Inhibitor
zidovudine, AZT, ZDV (Retrovir)	nevirapine, NVP (Viramune)	saquinavir, SQV (Invirase)	enfuvirtide, T-20 (Fuzeon)
didanosine, ddi (Videx)	delavirdine, DLV (Rescriptor)	ritonavir, RTV (Norvir)	mavaviroc, MVC (Selzentry)
stavudine, d4T (Zerit)	efavirenz, EFV (Sustiva)	indinivir, IDV (Crixivan)	**Integrase Inhibitor**
lamivudine, 3TC (Epivir)		nelfinavir, NFV (Viracept)	raltegravir, MK-0518 (Isentress)
abacavir, ABC (Ziagen)		atazanavir (ATV) (Reyataz)	**ART Combination Formulations**
emtricitabine (FTC) (Emtriva)		fosamprenavir (FPV) (Lexiva)	zidovudine + lamivudine, 3TC/AZT (Combivir)
Nucleotide Reverse Transcriptase Inhibitor (NRTI)		tipranavir (TPV) (Aptivus)	abacavir + lamivudine + zidovudine ABC/3TC/AZT (Trizivir)
tenofovir DF, (TDF) (Viread)		durunavir (DRV) (Prezista)	lopinavir/ritonavir, LPV/RTV (Kaletra)
		lopinavir (LPV) Only available in combination lopinavir/ritonavir, LPV/RTV (Kaletra)	efavirenz/ tenofovir/ emtricitabine EFV/TDV/FTC (Atripla)

Other ART drugs that were withdrawn from the market: zalcitabine, ddc (Hivid); saquinavir (Fortovase); amprenavir, APV (Agenerase)
(Modified from Bartlett J, Gallant J. Medical Management of HIV Infection. Baltimore: Johns Hopkins Unversity, 2007; and Panel on Antiretroviral Guidelines for Adult and Adolescents. Guidelines for the use of antiretroviral agents in HIV-1-infected adults and adolescents. Washington, DC: Department of Health and Human Services, 2007.)

Review Questions

1. HIV is a(n) _____ virus and is classified as a retrovirus.

A. DNA

B. RNA

C. reverse transcriptase

D. retrograde

2. The natural history of untreated HIV proceeds in six stages. Which is not a stage in this progression?

A. viral transmission

B. acute retroviral syndrome

C. recovery and seroconversion

D. adenopathy

3. Which of the following are routes of transmission of HIV?

A. sexual contact

B. injection drug use

C. occupational exposure

D. sharing household items

E. A, B, C

F. all of the above

4. Blood transfusion still accounts for HIV transmission in underdeveloped countries where testing is not available. Injection drug use accounts for almost one third of the cases of HIV in the United States.

A. The first statement is true. The second statement is false.

B. The first statement is false. The second statement is true.

C. Both statements are true.

D. Both statements are false.

5. The risk of HIV transmission after percutaneous exposure in the dental setting to HIV-infected blood is _____.

A. high

B. moderate

C. low

6. The most significant accomplishment regarding the medical management of HIV/AIDS is

A. the discovery of a cure.

B. the ability to control HIV replication through the use of highly active antiretroviral therapy.

C. the discovery of opportunistic infections.

D. the use of enzyme linked immunoassays to control HIV replication.

Critical Thinking

1. Describe the most common oral manifestations observed in patients diagnosed with AIDS.

2. Describe how HIV infection leads to suppression of host cellular immunity.

SELECTED READINGS

AETC National Resource Center, Guidelines for the use of antiretroviral agents in adults and adolescents: comprehensive summary. Available online at http://www.aidsetc.org/aidsetc?page=etres display&resource=etres-6. Accessed May 6, 2008.

Barre-Sinoussi F, Cherman J, Rey F, et al. Isolation of a T-lymphotropic retrovirus from a patient at risk for acquired immune deficiency syndrome (AIDS). Science 1983;220:868–871.

Bartlett JG. HIV: Twenty years in review. The Hopkins HIV Rep 2001;13:8–9.

Bartlett J, Gallant J. Medical Management of HIV Infection. Baltimore: Johns Hopkins University, 2003.

Bartlett J, Gallant J. Medical Management of HIV Infection. Baltimore: Johns Hopkins University, 2007.

Brown J. Impact of intensified dental care on outcomes in human immunodeficiency virus Infection. AIDS Patient Care and STDs 2002;16:479–486.

Cardo DM, Culver DH, Ciesielski CA, et al. A case-control study of HIV seroconversion in healthcare workers after percutaneous exposure. N Engl J Med 1997;337:1485–1490.

CDC. Acquired immune deficiency syndrome (AIDS) in prison inmates—New York, New Jersey. MMWR 1983;31:700–701.

CDC. Drug-associated HIV transmission continues in the United States. Available online at http://www.cdc.gov/ hiv/resources/factsheets/idu.htm. Accessed May 6, 2008.

CDC. Epidemiological notes and reports. *Pneunocystis* pneumonia—Los Angeles. MMWR 1981;30:1–3.

CDC. Guidelines for national human immunodeficiency virus case surveillance, including monitoring for human immunodeficiency virus infection and acquired immune deficiency syndrome. MMWR 1999;48(RR-13):1–28.

CDC. HIV and its transmission. Available online at http://www.cdc.gov/hiv/resources/factsheets/ transmission.htm. Accessed May 6, 2008.

CDC. HIV/AIDS surveillance report, Volume 17, Revised Edition, June 2007. Available online at http://www.cdc.gov/hiv/topics/surveillance/resources/ reports/2005report/default.htm. Accessed May 6, 2008.

CDC. Immunodeficiency among female sexual partners of males with acquired immune deficiency syndrome (AIDS)—New York. MMWR 1983;31:697–698.

CDC. Mother-to-child (perinatal) HIV transmission and prevention. Available online at http://www.cdc.gov/hiv/ topics/perinatal/resources/factsheets/perinatal.htm. Accessed May 6, 2008.

CDC. Opportunistic infections and Kaposi's sarcoma among Haitians in the United States. MMWR 1982;31: 353–354,360–361.

CDC. *Pneumocystis carinii* pneumonia among persons with hemophilia A. MMWR 1982;31:365–367.

CDC. Possible transfusion-associated acquired immune deficiency syndrome (AIDS)—California. MMWR 1982;31:652–654.

CDC.Treating Opportunistic Infections Among HIV-Infected Adults and Adolescents. MMWR 2004;53(RR-15): 1–112. Available online at http://www.cdc.gov/mmwr/ preview/mmwrhtml/rr5315a1.htm. Accessed May 6, 2008.

CDC. Unexplained immunodeficiency and opportunistic infections in infants—New York, New Jersey, California. MMWR 1982;31:665–667.

CDC. Guidelines for infection control in dental health-care settings—2003. MMWR 2003;52(RR-17):1–66.

CDC. Updated U.S. public health service guidelines for the management of occupational exposures to HBV, HCV, and HIV and recommendations for postexposure prophylaxis. MMWR 2001;50(RR-11):1–52.

CDC. Updated U.S. public health service guidelines for the management of occupational exposures to HIV and recommendations for postexposure prophylaxis. MMWR 2005;54(RR-9):1–17.

Connor EM, Sperling RS, Gelber R, et al. Reduction of maternal-infant transmission of human immunodeficiency virus type with zidovudine treatment. N Eng J Med 1994;331:1173–1180.

Clumeck N, Mascart-Lemone F, deMaubeuge J, et al. Acquired immune deficiency syndrome (AIDS) in black Africans. Lancet 1983;1:642.

Department of Child and Adolescent Health and Development (CAH), World Health Organization. HIV and infant feeding data analysis. Available online at http://www.who.int/child_adolescent_health/ documents/fch_cah_04_9/en/. Accessed May 6, 2008.

Fauci A, Pantaleo G, Stanley S, et al. Immunopathogenic mechanisms of HIV infection. Ann Intern Med 1996;124: 654–663.

Fischl M, Richman D, Grieco M, et al. The efficacy of azidothymidine (AZT) in the treatment of patients with AIDS and AIDS-related complex: a double-blind, placebo-controlled trial. N Eng J Med 1987;317:185–191.

Joint United Nations Programme on HIV/AIDS (UNAIDS) and World Health Organization (WHO). UNAIDS, WHO. AIDS epidemic update. Available online at http://data.unaids.org/pub/EPISlides/2007/2007_epiup date_en.pdf. Accessed May 6, 2008.

Joint United Nations Programme on HIV/AIDS (UNAIDS) and World Health Organization (WHO). UNAIDS, WHO. Overview of the global AIDS epidemic: 2006. Available online at http://data.unaids.org/pub/GlobalReport/2006/ 2006_GR_CH02_en.pdf. Accessed May 6, 2008.

Masur H, Michelis M, Wormser G, et al. Opportunistic infection in previously healthy women: initial manifestations of a community-acquired cellular immunodeficiency. Ann Intern Med 1982;97:533–539.

Mocroft A, Vella S, Benfiels T, et al. Changing patterns of mortality across Europe in patients with HIV-1. Euro SIDA Study Group. Lancet 1998;352(9142): 1725–1730.

National Institute of Allergy and Infectious Diseases, National Institutes of Health. How HIV causes AIDS. Available online at http://www.niaid.nih.gov/factsheets/ howhiv.htm. Accessed May 6, 2008.

Niu M, Stein D, Schnittman S. Primary human immunodeficiency virus type 1 infection: review of pathogenesis and early treatment intervention in humans and animal retrovirus infections. J Infect Dis 1993;168: 1490–1501.

Palella F, Delany K, Moorman A, et al. Declining morbidity and mortality among with advanced human immunodeficiency virus infection. New Engl J Med 1998;338: 853–860.

Panel on Antiretroviral Guidelines for Adult and Adolescents. Guidelines for the use of antiretroviral agents in HIV-1-infected adults and adolescents. Department of Health and Human Services. Available online at http://aidsinfo.nih.gov/contentfiles/ AdultandAdolescentGL.pdf. Accessed May 6, 2008.

Sepkowitz K. AIDS—The first 20 years. N Engl J Med 2001;344:1764–1772.

Teshale E. Estimated Number of HIV-infected Persons Eligible for and Receiving HIV Antiretroviral Therapy, 2003—United States. Abstract #167, 12th Conference on Retroviruses and Opportunistic Infections. Boston, MA: February 2005. Note, among those ages 15–49.

The Henry J. Kaiser Family Foundation. The HIV/AIDS Epidemic in the United States. Available online at http://www.kff.org/hivaids/upload/3029-06.pdf. Accessed May 6, 2008.

U.S. Department of Health and Human Services. Oral health in America: A report of the surgeon general. Rockville, MD: U.S. Department of Health and Human Services, National Institute of Dental and Craniofacial Research, National Institutes of Health. Available online at http://www.nidcr.nih.gov/DataStatistics/ SurgeonGeneral/sgr/. Accessed May 6, 2008.

United States Public Health Service and the Infectious Diseases Society of America. Guidelines for the prevention of opportunistic infections in persons infected with human immunodeficiency virus. Available online at http://aidsinfo.nih.gov/contentfiles/OIpreventionGL.pdf. Accessed May 6, 2008.

World Health Organization (WHO). Severe acute respiratory syndrome. Available online at http://www.wpro. who.int/sars/. Accessed May 6, 2008.

CHAPTER

4

Tuberculosis and Other Respiratory Infections

Géza T. Terézhalmy

John A. Molinari

LEARNING OBJECTIVES

After completion of this chapter individuals should be able to:

1 Comprehend the generation of microbial aerosols and airborne droplets from patients' mouths during provision of dental treatment.

2 Describe representative bacterial, viral, and other disease conditions which can develop via aerosolized microorganisms.

3 Discuss the continuing mutation and adaptation of influenza viruses as they relate to viral infection and the occurrence of epidemic and pandemic outbreaks.

4 Discuss the reemergence of tuberculosis in the United States and other countries, including epidemiological factors, infection versus active disease, and infection control recommendations to healthcare professionals

5 Describe the rationale and application of respiratory infection control measures to protect exposed dental healthcare personnel.

KEY TERMS

Antigenic drift: a minor change in surface antigens that results from point mutations in a gene segment; may result in an epidemic since the protection that remains from past exposure to similar viruses is incomplete.

Antigenic shift: a major change in one or both surface antigens (hemagglutinin or neuraminidase) that occurs at varying intervals; may result in a worldwide pandemic if the virus is efficiently transmitted from person to person.

Caseation necrosis: necrosis that transforms tissue into a dry, cheese-like mass.

Droplet nuclei: particles 5 μm diameter or less that are formed by dehydration of airborne droplets containing microorganisms that can remain suspended in the air for long periods of time.

Tubercle: a small rounded nodule produced by infection with *Mycobacterium tuberculosis*, consisting of a mass of inflammatory cells and bacteria surrounded by connective tissue.

INTRODUCTION

Respiratory infections are the most common microbial diseases found in humans. In addition, disease resulting from acute respiratory illness, such as influenza, tuberculosis, and pneumonia, are responsible for over 10% of the global deaths following microbial infection. Etiologies are quite varied, as numerous viruses, bacteria, fungi, and parasitic microbes are involved. While each airborne or droplet infection exhibits its own distinctive manifestations, a few generalizations can be made (Table 4-1). The breadth of these syndromes can be readily appreciated by reviewing a representative list-

ing of airborne and droplet-mediated microbial diseases (Table 4-2).

Many of the microorganisms responsible for upper respiratory tract infections have been isolated in dental aerosols. The release of these airborne fluids is routinely visible to dental healthcare personnel (DHCP) and patients alike during most treatments. While their infectious potential for was historically overlooked, accumulated evidence has led to a dramatic increase in health professional and public concern over the past 20 years. In a specific application for dentistry, dental students have been shown to experience a consistently higher incidence of upper respiratory tract infections than their counterparts in medical and pharmacy schools. A positive correlation also has been demonstrated between the incidence of common cold epidemics in patients and in DHCP who treated them. A survey of the incidence of upper respiratory tract infections in dental hygienists and dietitians during a 1-year period showed that hygienists experienced significantly more colds than did dietitians. Dental hygienists, however, did not miss significantly more workdays, suggesting the potential for transmission of their infection to others.

While there is a paucity of data linking dental instrumentation to the generation of **droplet nuclei** containing *Mycobacterium tuberculosis*, it can be anticipated that DHCP and patients with infectious tuberculosis (TB) will generate droplet nuclei by coughing, sneezing, laughing, and talking. In one recent study conducted after the introduction of standard body fluid precautions, the tuberculin skin test conversion rates over 12 months in dentists, dental hygienists, and dental assistants were reported to be 1.7%. The population baseline positive tuberculin skin test prevalence was 4.6%. The probable transmission of multiple drug-resistant tuberculosis (MDRTB) disease from patients to 2 DHCP has been documented and there is evidence of TB disease transmission from an oral surgeon to 15 patients following extractions.

TABLE 4-1   General Features of Microbial Respiratory Infections

Bacterial Infection
- Inflammation of site of local infection for noninvasive disease
- More severe invasive disease associated with fever and white cell infiltration
- Syndromes range from localized infections to aggressive pneumonias
- Examples include tuberculosis, pneumococcal pneumonia, legionellosis, tularemia, plague, anthrax
- Most can be effectively treated with appropriately administered antibiotics

Viral Infection
- Leading cause of human disease, hospitalization, mortality
- Syndromes range in severity from mild colds to acute and chronic pneumonias
- Single most frequent cause of acute illness in U.S.
- Most can not be treated with antimicrobial chemotherapy
- Leading cause of inappropriate antibiotic use

Mycotic and Parasitic Infections
- Many are associated with chronic infection and pneumonias
- Increased susceptibility found with immune compromised persons

TABLE 4-2 Representative Airborne or Droplet Microbial Infections

Disease	Transmission
Pneumonic plague (*Yersinia pestis*)	Patient-to-patient without insect vector; inhalation
Tuberculosis (*Mycobacterium tuberculosis*)	Droplet nuclei from coughing
Influenza (influenza viruses)	Coughing, but can also occur from direct contact
Legionellosis (*Legionella pneumophila*)	Aerosolization; inhalation
Common cold (multiple viruses)	Aerosols; virus-contaminated hands and fomites
Severe acute respiratory syndrome (SARS-coronavirus)	Aerosolized droplets; direct contact
Anthrax (*Bacillus anthracis*)	Inhalation of spores; inoculation; ingestion (rare)
Chickenpox (Varicella-Zoster virus)	Predominately via respiratory route
Measles (Measles virus)	Airborne respiratory droplets
Mumps (Mumps virus)	Direct person-to-person contact; respiratory droplets
German measles (Rubella virus)	Airborne respiratory secretions

UPPER RESPIRATORY TRACT INFECTIONS

It is conventional to divide the respiratory tract into two parts: upper and lower. The upper respiratory tract is comprised of the nasal cavity, nasopharynx, and larynx. The trachea, bronchi, and lungs constitute the lower respiratory tract. Infections of the upper respiratory tract are more common than any other microbial disease. This is probably due in part to the large number of different, potentially pathogenic microbial forms involved. Many infections are self-limiting but can lead to more serious secondary sequelae in certain susceptible individuals. Because they may also be difficult to diagnose the potential for ineffective mistreatment of conditions occurs in many instances.

Common Cold

Etiology and Epidemiology

Approximately 1 billion cases of the common cold occur in the United States each year. Several viruses can cause the common cold, but rhinoviruses are by far the most common. These organisms are spread by aerosols and direct person-to-person contact via contaminated hands. Viruses from infected people are airborne in droplet nuclei that are emitted during respiration, talking, sneezing, and coughing. Predisposing factors for susceptibility include physical and emotional stress and allergic nasopharyngeal disorders. These RNA viruses are also able to remain viable on skin and environmental surfaces for hours. Rhinovirus infection has an incubation period of 1 to 4 days leading to onset of acute symptoms. They are transmitted by aerosols from infected persons, direct person-to-person contact via contaminated hands, and environmental surfaces. Actual shedding of the virus usually precedes the onset of clinical symptoms by 1 to 2 days, but peak viral secretion occurs during the symptomatic phase.

Clinical Manifestations

Rhinoviruses cause localized infections where nasal ciliated epithelial cells are target sites for attachment, penetration, and viral replication. Because the virus replicates best at 33°C, it does not spread to deeper respiratory tissues. The main anatomic location of infection is the muscular, membranous area behind the nasal cavity and above the nasopharynx. Because the nasopharynx is continuous with the oral cavity and larynx, the site of infection can involve any or all of these areas and give rise to the terms rhinitis, nasopharyngitis, pharyngitis, and laryngitis. Signs and symptoms include profuse nasal discharge, sneezing, headache, fever, malaise, dryness, soreness, hoarseness, and tickling of the throat. Nasal secretions during the symptomatic period are clear or mucoid in appearance. As the illness progresses, a cough may appear as an increasingly prominent symptom lasting up to 2 weeks. Smell and taste are frequently impaired. In the absence of complications, signs and symptoms resolve in 4 to 10 days. Secondary bacterial infections are frequent and consist of suppuration in the nasopharynx with involvement by direct extension from the nose to the accessory sinuses, ears, mastoids, pharynx, larynx, trachea, bronchi, and lungs.

Diagnosis

Diagnosis is primarily presumptive. Infection with picornaviruses (rhinoviruses, coxsackievirus, and echoviruses) in the fall and winter months is rare, when myxovirus (influenza, parainfluenza, and respiratory syncytial viruses) infections predominate. When a specific diagnosis is needed, biochemical and molecular biologic procedures with good sensitivity and specificity are available. In a differential diagnosis one must also consider bacterial infections and allergic rhinorrhea as possible causes of symptoms.

Treatment and Prevention

Treatment of the common cold includes rest, sufficient fluids to prevent dehydration, and a light, palatable, well-balanced diet. Nasal decongestants may provide temporary relief. An analgesic/antipyretic agent may be given for the relief of headache, fever, and associated muscular aches and pains. Cough may be reduced by steam inhalation, with antitussive syrups containing codeine or dextromethorphan, or with an expectorant, an agent that promotes the ejection of mucus or exudates from the trachea, bronchi, and lungs. Covering coughs and sneezes, hand washing, and the use of environmental surface disinfectants reduce the spread of infection.

Influenza

Etiology and Epidemiology

Historical and current epidemiologic characteristics of influenza outbreaks graphically illustrate the ongoing challenge influenza viruses present to public health. Influenza is an acute respiratory infection caused by influenza viruses. They are single-stranded, helical-shaped RNA viruses classified in the family Orthomyxoviridae; commonly referred to as "the flu," in most cases infection results in self-limited disease. However, some viral strains have the capacity to cause more severe disease, thereby leading to potentially life-threatening pneumonia in susceptible people. There are three influenza virus types, termed A, B, and C, which are distinguished by specific antigenic differences in viral components (Table 4-3).

In the United States, epidemics of influenza typically occur during the late fall and winter months. Influenza type A subtypes, categorized on the basis of hemagglutinin (HA) or neuraminidase (NA) surface proteins, and influenza type B viruses, separated into two genetic lineages but not categorized into subtypes, cause human

---

TABLE 4-3 Comparison of Influenza Types

Type A
Natural hosts are wild birds
- Can infect birds, people, pigs, and other animals
- Subtypes based on antigenic differences of hemagglutinin (HA) and neuraminidase (NA) surface proteins
- Can cause moderate to severe disease
- Can undergo antigenic shift and antigenic drift
- Can cause large pandemics with high mortality

Type B
- Human infection only
- Primarily infects children
- Generally cause milder disease than type A viruses
- Severe cases of flu generally found in elderly or high-risk persons
- Do not cause pandemics, only seasonal epidemics

Type C
- Rarely reported as cause of human influenza
- Most infections are asymptomatic
- No epidemics seen

Adapted from Molinari JA. Fighting the flu. Dimen Dent Hyg 2005;3:22–26.

---

disease. Epidemics typically occur in the late fall and winter months. It is estimated that approximately 10% to 20% of the population get the flu each year with up to 40 million individuals requiring outpatient medical visits. These result in approximately 226,000 hospitalizations and 36,000 deaths annually, with the highest rates of influenza complications and hospitalizations seen in young children and persons >65 years of age.

A unique feature of influenza viruses is their ability to undergo antigenic drift and/or antigenic shift. **Antigenic drift** is a minor change in surface HA and NA antigens resulting from point mutations that occur during viral replication. Influenza A virus undergoes antigenic drift more rapidly than influenza B. The frequent emergence of new antigenic variants is the virologic basis for seasonal influenza epidemics. **Antigenic shift**, however, involves a different genetic mechanism and can have worldwide and life-threatening consequences. This involves recombination between segments of viral nucleic acid from different strains of influenza type A viruses. Major antigenic changes occur in both HA and NA at varying intervals as a result of the integration/recombination of RNA strands between human strains of influenza A viruses and those strains that infect birds. If the progeny influenza viruses establish themselves in humans, infected persons have little or no protective immunity, primarily because these new strain has never been seen before. If the worst-case scenario occurs and these strains are passed efficiently via the airborne person-to-person route, there is a distinct potential for onset of a widespread influenza pandemic.

Influenza viruses are spread from person to person primarily through large-particle (≥5 μm) respiratory droplet transmission when an infected person coughs and sneezes near a susceptible person. Transmission via large-particle droplets requires close contact between source and recipient persons, because droplets do not remain suspended in the air and generally travel only a short distance (≤1 meter) through the air. Infectious viral concentrations can survive evaporation of aerosolized respiratory particles and remain suspended in the air for extended intervals. Thus, viral transmission may occur to susceptible persons who are within the same room, but not in close proximity to infected, symptomatic individuals. Contact with respiratory-droplet contaminated surfaces is another potential source of transmission. The typical incubation period for influenza is 1–4 days. Adults can be infectious from the day before symptoms begin through approximately 5 days after onset of illness. Children can be infectious for ≥10 days after onset of symptoms.

Clinical Manifestations

Uncomplicated influenza illness is characterized by the abrupt onset of fever, myalgia, headache, nonproductive cough, sore throat, and rhinitis. In children otitis media, nausea, and vomiting are also common. Uncomplicated influenza typically resolves after 3–7 days, although cough and malaise can persist for more than 2 weeks. Influenza virus infections can cause primary influenza viral pneumonia, exacerbate underlying pulmonary or cardiac disease, lead to secondary bacterial sinusitis, otitis, and pneumonia, or predispose to coinfections with other viral and bacterial pathogens. Rarely, encephalopathy, myositis, myocarditis, pericarditis, and Reye syndrome have been reported.

Diagnosis

In the absence of laboratory confirmation, respiratory illnesses caused by influenza viruses are difficult to distinguish from illnesses caused by other respiratory pathogens on the basis of signs and symptoms alone. Consequently, the diagnosis of influenza should be considered in any patient with respiratory symptoms or fever during the influenza season.

Prevention and Treatment

Annual immunization against current influenza A and B subtypes is the most effective method of preventing infection and has been shown to reduce associated complications. Influenza vaccines contain strains of influenza viruses that are antigenically equivalent to one influenza A (H3N2) virus, one influenza A (H1N1) virus, and one influenza B virus. Since antibody against one influenza virus type or subtype confers limited or no protection against another type or subtype of influenza virus and antibody to one antigenic type or subtype of influenza virus might not protect against infection with a new anti-

genic variant of the same type or subtype, each year one or more virus strains in the vaccine might be changed on the basis of global surveillance of influenza viruses and the emergence and spread of new strains.

Antiviral agents with activity against influenza viruses can be effective for the chemoprophylaxis and treatment of influenza. Four licensed influenza antiviral agents are available in the United States: amantadine, rimantadine, zanamivir, and oseltamivir. Because of influenza A virus resistance to amantadine and rimantadine, these agents should not be used unless evidence of susceptibility to these antiviral medications has been established among circulating influenza A viruses. While chemoprophylaxis is no substitute for vaccination both zanamivir and oseltamivir appear to be effective in the treatment of influenza A and B infection when treatment is instituted within 2 days of the onset of illness.

Rhinosinusitis

Etiology and Epidemiology

Rhinosinusitis affects more than 10% of the U.S. population. It is characterized by inflammation of the paranasal sinuses because of viral (upper respiratory tract infection), bacterial, or fungal infections or allergic conditions. The initial viral infection of the common cold may be followed by a secondary bacterial infection. *Streptococcus pneumoniae*, *Haemophilus influenzae*, and *Moraxella catarrhalis* are the predominant organisms recovered in acute bacterial rhinosinusitis. Anaerobic bacteria may play a role in chronic rhinosinusitis. *S. pneumoniae*, *H. influenzae*, and anaerobes have been identified in dental aerosols and contaminated water lines.

Clinical Manifestations

Acute and chronic rhinosinusitis produce similar clinical signs and symptoms. Maxillary sinusitis produces pain over the affected sinus, toothache, and a frontal headache. Frontal sinusitis produces pain over the frontal sinus and a frontal headache. Ethmoid sinusitis produces pain behind the eyes and a frontal headache. Sphenoid sinusitis is characterized by malaise and pain referred to the frontal and/or occipital areas. These sinus infections rarely occur without rhinitis, hence the term rhinosinusitis. Fever and chills suggest an extension of the infection beyond the infected sinus.

Diagnosis

In both acute and chronic rhinosinusitis, the edematous mucous membrane and retained exudates cause the affected sinus to appear radiographically radiopaque. Periapical dental radiographs may be useful to rule out odontopathic and/or periodontopathic infection as a cause of chronic rhinosinusitis.

Treatment

Ttreatment of acute rhinosinusitis may include steam inhalation, which promotes vasoconstriction and drainage, and topical use of vasoconstrictors, such as phenylephrine. The empirical administration of penicillin or erythromycin is indicated for both acute and chronic rhinosinusitis. The susceptibility of the pathogens isolated from sinus exudates and the patient's response guide subsequent therapy. Rhinosinusitis not responding to antibiotic therapy may require surgical intervention.

Pharyngitis

Etiology and Epidemiology

Acute pharyngitis is usually of viral origin (i.e., rhinovirus, coronavirus, influenza A and B viruses, parainfluenza virus, enterovirus, adenivirus, Epstein Barr virus [EBV], herpes simplex virus [HSV], cytomegalovirus, and human immunodeficiency virus [HIV]) but it may also be caused by group A beta-hemolytic streptococci, *Mycoplasma pneumoniae*, *Chlamydia pneumoniae*, or other bacteria. Infection with *Streptococcus pyogenes*, isolated from dental aerosols, can produce classical bacterial pharyngitis.

Clinical Manifestations

The hallmark of pharyngitis is a sore throat and pain when swallowing. The pharyngeal mucosa is erythematous and edematous and may be covered by pseudomembraneous purulent exudates. Fever and cervical lymphadenopathy are present. *Herpesvirus hominis* may cause ulcerative pharyngitis and subsequent recurrent herpetic infections. Coxsackievirus may cause herpangina, especially in children, and infectious mononucleosis (EBV) in adolescents may cause similar clinical manifestations. Gonococcal pharyngitis is commonly asymptomatic, but may resemble viral or streptococcal disease.

Diagnosis

Differentiating viral and bacterial pharyngitis on the basis of clinical examination alone is difficult. Definitive diagnosis and successful management require culture and susceptibility testing.

Treatment

Treatment includes rest and the administration of acetaminophen to relieve pain. A regimen of penicillin or erythromycin is initiated to prevent rheumatic fever for those patients with clinical evidence of bacterial pharyngitis, while awaiting the results of culture and susceptibility testing.

Laryngitis

Etiology and Epidemiology

Laryngitis is defined as inflammation of the larynx. Acute laryngitis may occur during the course of a common cold or as a complication of measles, pertussis, bronchitis, or pneumonia. Chronic laryngitis is likely to occur in people who constantly use their voices. Chronic rhinosinusitis also may make the patient susceptible to chronic laryngitis.

Clinical Manifestations

In acute laryngitis, the throat is sore and the voice is hoarse. Later, the patient may lose his or her voice altogether. A cough is usually present but is nonproductive unless there is associated tracheitis and bronchitis. Small children may have a brassy cough with associated swelling of the mucous membrane, which can cause obstruction of the airway. Malaise, fever, and/or dysphasia may be present in more severe infections. Hoarseness is the chief symptom of chronic laryngitis. Pain is absent or minimal.

Diagnosis

Direct laryngoscopy may reveal mild to moderate erythema and edema of the mucous membranes. In chronic laryngitis, the vocal cords may be thickened and red. It is essential to refer patients with persistent hoarseness that has been present for more than 3 weeks to an otorhinolaryngologist to exclude papilloma, cord paralysis, carcinoma, or, more rarely, tuberculosis or syphilis as a diagnosis.

Treatment

Resting the voice and use of steam inhalations promote relief of symptoms associated with acute viral laryngitis.

LOWER RESPIRATORY TRACT INFECTIONS

Acute Tracheobronchitis

Etiology and Epidemiology

Acute tracheobronchitis affects approximately 5% of the U.S. population annually. It is an inflammatory response of the tracheobronchial tree to infections. Environmental pollutants and the inhalation of various allergens are predisposing or contributory factors. Viruses are by far the most common etiologies and specific causative agents may vary according to time of year. Between fall and spring, influenza and respiratory syncytial viruses are common, whereas coxsackieviruses and echoviruses are common in the summer, and rhinovirus infections occur throughout the year. In young adults acute bronchitis may be associated with *Mycoplasma pneumoniae*, *Bordetella pertussis*, and *Chlamydia pneumoniae* infections.

Clinical Manifestations

Acute tracheobronchitis causes soreness behind the sternum and a dry, painful, nonproductive cough. The patient wheezes and has difficulty breathing. As secondary bacterial infection occurs, thick, purulent sputum is produced. Malaise and fever for up to 5 days is common. Persistent fever suggests complicating pneumonia.

Diagnosis

Diagnosis is usually based on clinical signs and symptoms. Gram stain and culture should be performed to identify the causative organism. A chest x-ray is also indicated to rule out other diseases for patients presenting with severe disease symptoms.

Treatment

Rest, oral fluids, and an antipyretic are indicated during the febrile stage. Antibiotics are indicated when purulent sputum is present, when high fever persists, and in patients with chronic obstructive pulmonary disease.

Pneumonia

Etiology and Epidemiology

Bacteria are the most common causes of pneumonia. Defective leukocyte activity predisposes patients to infections with pneumococci, streptococci, *Haemophilus influenzae*, and *Pneumocystis carinii*. *Streptococcus pneumoniae* (pneumococci) strains are responsible for 98% of the infections, with staphylococci accounting for 1%, *Klebsiella pneumoniae* for 0.6%, and *H. influenzae* for 0.3% of the bacterial pneumonias. Friedlander's pneumonia (*K. pneumoniae*) is most common among alcoholic men between the ages of 40 to 60 years, with high mortality rates of 40% to 60% compared with 5% for pneumococcal infections. *H. influenzae* pneumonia is also very common in alcoholic men.

Staphylococcal pneumonia occurs primarily in children, patients with altered pulmonary function, and hospitalized patients. This life-threatening secondary infection is frequently noted during influenza epidemics, and is associated with an overall mortality rate ranging from 25% to 60%. Other pathogens include anaerobic bacteria, *Chlamydia*, *Legionella pneumophila*, *Klebsiella pneumoniae*, and other Gram-negative bacilli. The organisms are spread by droplet nuclei (inhalation) and by aspiration from the upper respiratory tract.

Clinical Manifestations

Signs and symptoms include a rapidly rising fever, a painful cough, and the production of purulent sputum sometimes mixed with blood (hemoptysis). The patient experiences pain on respiration and, as a result, breathing becomes rapid and shallow.

Diagnosis

Diagnosis is based on clinical signs and symptoms in conjunction with the radiographic distribution of the infiltrate. Culturing expectorated sputum is the most practical method of identifying bacterial pathogens. However, special culture techniques, special stains, and a lung biopsy may be required to determine a specific etiological agent.

Treatment

Treatment consists of respiratory support and the administration of appropriate antimicrobial agents.

Tuberculosis

Etiology and Epidemiology

Tuberculosis (TB) is primarily a chronic disease of humans. *Mycobacterium tuberculosis*, the causative organism, is carried in airborne particles called droplet nuclei that are generated when persons with infectious TB disease cough, sneeze, shout, sing, or talk. These droplet nuclei are 1–5 microns in size, can remain suspended in air for hours, and can be carried in normal air currents throughout a room or building. The probability that a person who is exposed to *M. tuberculosis* will become infected depends on the concentration of infectious droplet nuclei in the air and the duration of the exposure to a person with infectious, active disease. Environmental factors such as exposure in confined spaces, inadequate ventilation, and recirculation of air containing infectious droplet nuclei further increase the likelihood of transmission. Persons at highest risk for exposure to and infection with *M. tuberculosis* are close contacts of persons who share air space in a household or other enclosed environment with a person with pulmonary tuberculosis (Table 4-4).

An estimated 2 billion persons are infected globally with *M. tuberculosis*. While most infections do not lead to symptomatic TB, each year, approximately 9 million persons become ill and nearly 2 million die of the disease. This chronic infection is therefore the single most frequent cause of death in the world from one infectious agent. Other sobering statistics reinforce the devastating impact of *M. tuberculosis* infection and TB: (a) active, symptomatic disease is curable, yet TB kills 5,000 people every day; (b) TB is the leading cause of death in HIV-infected persons (250,000 deaths/year); and (c) 1 symptomatic person infects 10–15 others each year.

In the United States, a total of 13,767 cases (4.6 cases per 100,000) of symptomatic TB were reported in 2006. These findings indicate that although the TB rate in 2006

TABLE 4-4 Persons at Highest Risk for Exposure to and Infection with *M. tuberculosis*

Foreign-born persons from countries with a high incidence of TB disease who arrived in the U.S. within the past 5 years	Africa, Asia, Eastern Europe, Latin America, and Russia
Persons who frequently travel to countries with a high incidence of TB disease	
Residents and employees of settings that are high risk	Correctional facilities, long-term care facilities, and homeless shelters
Populations at high risk who are defined locally as having an increased incidence of TB disease	Foreign-born persons Hispanics Blacks Asians Patients untreated for LTBI HIV-infected patients Patients receiving immunosuppressive therapy
Populations at high risk who are defined locally as medically underserved and who have low income	
Infants, children, and adolescents exposed to adults in high-risk categories	
Healthcare personnel who serve patients who are at high risk	
Healthcare personnel with unprotected exposure to a patient with TB disease	

was the lowest recorded since national reporting began in 1953, the decline has slowed from an average annual rate of 7.3% (1993–2000) to an average rate of 3.8% per year (2000–2006). The rate of TB in foreign-born persons was 9.5 times that of those born in the United States. In addition, Hispanics, African Americans, and Asians had TB rates 7.6, 8.4, and 21.2 times higher than Caucasians, respectively. The number of multidrug-resistant TB cases (MDR-TB) remained constant at 1.2% from 2004 to 2005, the most recent year for which complete drug-susceptibility data are available. The slower deceleration of TB rate nationally, the disparity of TB rates between Caucasians and racial/ethnic minorities, and the increased incidence of MDR-TB cases all threaten progress toward the goal of eliminating TB in the United States.

Transmission and Infection

TB is not a highly contagious disease in that *M. tuberculosis* requires prolonged or frequent close contact with an infectious source for transmission to a susceptible host. Casual or sporadic contact with an infectious TB patient usually will not result in microbial transmission. This statement has direct application to the observed low TB risk associated with most dental procedures. The overwhelming majority lead to acute sporadic exposure and the intervals are too brief to allow sufficient aerosolized concentrations of mycobacteria to infect those DHCP providing care.

When droplet nuclei are inhaled, the bacilli travel to the alveoli where a local infection is established. The immune response to such infections is predominantly cell-mediated, involving both CD4+ and CD8+ T-cells. Pulmonary macrophages process the antigens and pres-

ent them to both major-histocompatibility-complex (MHC) class II molecules, which activate CD4+ cells; and to MHC class I molecules, which activate CD8+ T cells. Within 2–10 weeks following exposure the immune response will limit further multiplication of *M. tuberculosis*; however, not all bacilli are eliminated from the body.

Latent TB Infection

M. tuberculosis bacilli that are not eliminated by the immune system are incarcerated in tuberculous granulomas at foci of infection where they can remain viable for many years. At this stage the person infected is said to have latent tuberculosis infection (LTBI). This condition is also termed asymptomatic primary TB. Although immunological test results for *M. tuberculosis* infection are positive, these patients have no symptoms, no radiographic abnormalities compatible with tuberculosis, and no positive bacteriologic culture tests. Patients with LTBI are asymptomatic and are not contagious. In these people the protective cell-mediated immune response prevents continued multiplication and dissemination of the bacteria, but does not destroy all the microorganisms present. The remaining mycobacteria can become sequestered in affected tissues and can be the source reactivation TB which can develop decades later.

Tuberculosis (TB disease)

Approximately 5% to 10% of the people who become infected with *M. tuberculosis* and who are not treated for LTBI will develop TB disease during their lifetime (Table 4-5). *M. tuberculosis* is spread via the lymphatics to cause granulomatous inflammation in both the lung periphery and hilar nodes, accompanied by respiratory symptoms. Classic symptoms include chronic ill health, coughing

TABLE 4-5 Diseases and Conditions That Increase the Risk of Progression from LTBI to TB Disease

HIV infection

History of infection with *M. tuberculosis* within the past 2 years

History of untreated or inadequately treated TB disease

Infants and children aged <4 years

Diabetes mellitus

Chronic renal failure

Immunosuppressive therapy

Silicosis

Malignancies (carcinoma of the head, neck, lung; leukemia; lymphoma)

Intestinal bypass or gastrectomy

Body weight =10% below ideal weight

with hemoptysis (i.e., bloody sputum), low-grade fever, weight loss, and night sweats. While the lungs are the most common sites for TB disease, about 15% of patients present with an extrapulmonary site of infection. This occurrence is especially common in patients who have both TB disease and HIV infection. In a few instances, **tubercle** bacilli may spread via the bloodstream to many organs giving rise to miliary tuberculosis.

Lesions may appear anywhere in the lung parenchyma but usually are present in the periphery. Microscopically, mycobacteria can be seen within alveolar macrophages where they are resistant to phagocytic destruction. They can even multiply within the phagocytic cells, thereby fostering dissemination in tissues. Host macrophages and lymphocytes are attracted by chemotactic factors to the infection site, which contains acid-fact bacilli and cell debris. The histological appearance of the lesion is one of multinucleated giants consisting of fused macrophages (i.e., Langhans cells). These eventually work to wall off the infection site, but bacteria can continue to replicate inside host phago-

cytic cells. Microscopically, the bacteria are present as intracellular bacteria within the center of the developing chronic CD4+ and CD8+ lymphochyte response. Tissue necrosis occurs during the immunopathological process with a loss of individual cellular outline. Because necrosis was historically seen as transforming affected tissue into a dry, cheese-like mass, the term **caseation necrosis** has been applied to this response in TB. The distinctive lesion seen on radiographs is called a tubercle.

Infected sputum may cause tuberculous tracheitis, laryngitis (hoarseness, coughing, and pain), and tuberculous ulcers on the tonsils (dysphagia) and nasal cavity (obstruction, perforation, nasal discharge). Oral tuberculous lesions are not commonly observed (prevalence 0.05% to 5%), but they present as nonspecific ulcerative or papillomatous lesions. Less frequently they may be observed as erythematous patches or indurations. Pain and cervical lymphadenopathy are common but not universal findings. When the cervical lymph nodes are involved, they may caseate (form tuberculous abscesses) or undergo fibrosis and calcification. The usual result for most patients with active, TB disease is one of healing and development of cellular immunity.

Diagnosis

Latent TB Infection

Preseumptive diagnosis of *M. tuberculosis* infection clinically relies on conversion of the infected person to a positive Type IV (delayed) hypersensitivity state, as shown by the tuberculin skin test (TST). The antigenic preparation used for skin testing is derived from in vitro *M. tuberculosis* cultures. The routinely used antigen in intradermal testing for tuberculin hypersensitivity is called purified protein derivative (PPD). This intradermal (Mantoux) test is the traditional method of diagnosing LTBI. The antigen is injected intracutaneously into either the volar or dorsal surface of the forearm. In patients with LTBI, the TST evokes a Type IV hypersensitivity reaction to the tuberculin mediated by CD4+ T-lymphocytes producing an area of redness and swelling. The test is read at 48 hours. The presence of any erythema is disregarded with the diameter of induration measured instead (Table 4-6). While the relative specificity of the TST skin test is high, both false positive and false negative reactions have been reported.

TABLE 4-6 Interpreting the Tuberculin Skin Test Reaction

Induration of ≥5 mm	Induration of ≥10 mm	Induration of ≥15 mm
People with HIV infection	Foreign-born persons	People with no risk factors for TB
Close contacts of people with TB	HIV-negative persons who use illicit drugs	
People who have had TB disease before	People in residential facilities	
Illicit drug users	Children ≤4 years of age	

The Centers for Disease Control and Prevention (CDC) recommends that persons with a positive TST undergo further evaluation, including a chest radiograph to determine whether the person has TB disease. In recent years several in vitro diagnostic tests, blood assays for *Mycobacterium tuberculosis* (BAMT), have been developed. One of these tests approved by the Food and Drug Administration (FDA) for the detection of latent TB infection is the QuantiFERON®-TB Gold (QFT-G) test. The sensitivity of QFT-G is statistically similar to that of TST. However, the QFT-G has greater selectivity as it measures the cell-mediated response to peptides from two *M. tuberculosis* proteins, which are not present in any Bacille Calmette-Guerin (BCG) vaccine strains and are absent from the majority of other mycobacteria.

TB Disease

Definitive diagnosis of active TB disease requires the demonstration of bacteria in the patient's tissues or secretions. Bacteriologic examination includes obtaining a specimen of sputum. Detection of acid-fast bacilli (AFB) in stained (Ziehl-Neelsen method) smears examined microscopically can provide the first bacteriologic clue to clinical disease. However, not all AFB are tubercle bacilli and a positive bacteriologic culture for *M. tuberculosis* is essential to confirm the diagnosis. DNA probes specific for the genus *Mycobacterium* now are used routinely to identify specific bacteria.

Treatment

Latent TB infection

The risk for progression from LTBI to TB disease is highest during the first 2 years after infection, and is often predicated on concomitant medical conditions that alter the ability of the immune system to maintain the isolation of *M. tuberculosis* (see Table 4-5). HIV infection is the most important risk factor. It has been estimated that persons co-infected with *M. tuberculosis* and HIV have a 6% to 10% risk per year of developing TB disease. This compares with a 10% lifetime risk for an immunocompetent person infected only with *M. tuberculosis*.

Isoniazid (Table 4-7) given for 6–9 months in a single daily dose, is the anti-tuberculin drug of choice for the treatment of LTBI. Patients who become TST positive following exposure to patients with tubercle bacilli who are resistant to isoniazid, and those patients with intolerance to isoniazid, may be treated with rifampin for 4 months. For patients with known exposure to MDR TB disease, a regimen with two drugs to which *M. tuberculosis* is susceptible is recommended for 9 to 12 months.

TB Disease

All isolates of *M. tuberculosis* are tested for anti-mycobacterial drug susceptibility, but results generally do not become available for at least 2 weeks. Until susceptibility results are available, the empirical initial phase of treatment consists of isoniazid, rifampin, pyrazinamide, and ethambutol. When the infection proves to be caused by fully susceptible *M. tuberculosis* strains, the initial phase of treatment continues for 2 months with isoniazid, rifampin, and pyrazinamide.

The continuation phase of treatment, predicated on the results of sputum cultures at 2 months, may last for an additional 4 to 7 months. Disseminated TB disease, tuberculous meningitis, and infections in children are usually treated for 9 to 12 months. Osteomyelitis is usually treated for 6 to 9 months.

Drug-Resistant TB Disease

Resistance to isoniazid is the most common pattern to mycobacterial drug resistance. These infections are treated with rifampin, pyrazinamide, and ethambutol for 6 to 9 months. Streptomycin is an alternative to ethambutol and a fluoroquinolone is often added to the regimen if there is extensive disease. MDR TB disease is treated with ≥4 drugs to which the organisms are susceptible. Three drugs are usually given by mouth and the fourth by injection. AFB smears and cultures are performed monthly and treatment is continued for 18 to 24 months, or 12 to 18 months after the microbiological studies become negative. The parenteral drug is continued for 6 months after culture conversion.

TB Disease in Patients with HIV Infection

The treatment of TB disease is complicated by co-infection with HIV. CD4+ cell counts <100 cells/mL have been associated with rifamycin resistance. Furthermore, rifamycins induce hepatic CYP3A4 enzymes and can accelerate the metabolism of protease inhibitors and some non-nucleoside reverse transcriptase inhibitors, decreasing their bioavailability to sub-therapeutic levels.

RESPIRATORY TRACT INFECTIONS: INFECTION CONTROL STRATEGIES IN THE DENTAL HEALTHCARE SETTING

Standard precautions provide a hierarchy of preventive strategies to prevent or reduce the risk of occupational exposure to bloodborne pathogens and other potentially infectious material. While standard precautions reduce the risk of occupational exposure to most organisms responsible for upper respiratory tract infections, they are inadequate to prevent the spread of *M. tuberculosis*. To prevent the cross-infection in these instances, transmission-based precautions are necessary based on a three-level hierarchy of administrative, environmental, and respiratory-protection controls.

TABLE 4-7 Antimycobacterial Agents

First-Line Drugs		
Drug	**Mechanism of Action**	**Adverse Drug Effects**
Ethambutol	Inhibits arabinosyl tranferase	Optic neuritis Loss of visual acuity
Pyrazinamide	Inhibits fatty acid synthetase 1	Morbilliform rash Arthralgias Hyperuricemia
Isoniazid	Inhibits fatty acid synthetase 2	Hepatitis Peripheral neuropathy Inhibits CYP450 enzymes

Rifamycins
  Rifampin
  Rifabutin
  Rifapentin
	Bind to RNA polymerase and inhibit transcription	Hepatitis
		Flu-like symptoms
		Morbilliform rash
		GI disturbances
		Induce CYP450 enzymes

Second-Line Drugs		
Drug	**Mechanism of Action**	**Adverse Drug Effects**
Cycloserine	Inhibits monomer synthesis	Psychosis Seizures Peripheral neuropathy
Ethionamine	Inhibits fatty acid synthetase 2	Hepatitis Hypothyroidism

Aminoglycosides
  Streptomycin
  Capreomycin
  Kanamycin
  Amikacin
	Bind to the 30S ribosomal subunit and inhibit translation	Ototoxicity
		Nephrotoxicity
		Neuromuscular blockade

Fluoroquinolones
  Ciprofloxacin
  Ofloxacin
  Gatifloxacin
  Levofloxacin
  Moxifloxacin
	Inhibit topoisomerase II (DNA gyrase), thereby releasing DNA with staggered double-stranded breaks	Nausea
		Abdominal pain
		Restlessness
		Confusion

Aminosalicylic acid	Competitive para-aminobenzoic acid antagonist	GI disturbances
Combination Drugs		
Rifamate	isoniazid + rifampin	
Rifater	isoniazid + rifampin + pyrazinamide	

Administrative Controls

The first and most important level is the implementation of administrative controls (Table 4-8). Administrative controls can reduce the risk of exposure to persons who might have infectious TB disease and are essential prerequisites for effective environmental and respiratory-protection controls in all settings where patients with suspected or confirmed TB disease are expected to be encountered.

TABLE 4-8 Administrative Controls

- Implement an initial and ongoing (annual) TB education and training program for DHCP

- Conduct an annual TB risk assessment for the dental healthcare setting

- Develop, implement, and enforce a written TB infection control plan to ensure prompt detection, airborne infection isolation, and treatment of persons with suspected or confirmed TB disease

- Implement an initial and ongoing TB infection control surveillance program for DHCP

TB Education and Training Program for DHCP

Education and training of DHCP is an essential part of administrative controls in a TB infection-control program. DHCP include all paid and unpaid persons working in the dental healthcare setting who have the potential for exposure to *M. tuberculosis* through air space shared with persons with suspected or confirmed infectious TB disease. Table 4-9 presents suggested elements of a TB education and training program for DHCP. The level of training will vary according to the risk classification of the setting. Training may be combined with other required infection control-related education and training programs and should be documented.

TB Risk Assessment for the Dental Healthcare Setting

The overall risk of DHCP for exposure to a patient with infectious TB disease is probably low. Nevertheless, every dental healthcare setting should conduct initial

---

TABLE 4-9 Suggested Components of a TB Education and Training Program for DHCP

- Epidemiology of TB in the local community, the U.S., and worldwide

- Basic concepts of *M. tuberculosis* transmission, pathogenesis, clinical signs and symptoms, diagnosis of LTBI and TB disease, and treatment of LTBI and TB disease
  - TB and impaired immunity

- The hierarchy of TB infection control measures in the dental healthcare setting
  - Administrative controls
  - Environmental controls
  - Respiratory-protection controls

- Potential for occupational exposure to infectious TB disease in the dental healthcare setting
  - TB infection control surveillance

---

and ongoing (annual) evaluations of TB risk for the setting; i.e., determine the demographics of the patient population served in the setting (see Tables 4-4 and 4-5). Consult with the local or state health department.

TB Infection Control Program in the Dental Healthcare Setting

The primary risk of exposure to *M. tuberculosis* in the dental healthcare setting is contact with patients with undiagnosed or unsuspected infectious disease. A high index of suspicion and rapid implementation of precautions are essential to prevent and interrupt cross-infection. Specific precautions will vary depending on the setting, i.e., patient population served (see Table 4-4), and the type of services provided in a particular setting.

Minimum requirements in a community-based dental healthcare setting is implementation and enforcement of a TB infection-control protocol that provides for prompt: (a) identification of patients with suspected or confirmed infectious TB disease, (b) isolation of patients with suspected and confirmed TB disease from other patients and DHCP, and (c) referral of patients with suspected or confirmed symptomatic disease for a medical evaluation who require dental healthcare procedures, to a facility with appropriate environmental controls and respiratory protection controls.

Identification of Patients with Suspected or Confirmed TB Disease

When reviewing medical histories (initial and periodic updates), including a review of organ systems, all patients should be routinely asked about (a) a history of (i) exposure to TB, (ii) LTBI, and (iii) symptomatic TB; (b) medical conditions that increase the risk of TB disease (see Table 4-5); and (c) signs and symptoms of active disease (see Clinical Manifestations). Patients with a history of LTBI and confirmed TB disease should be questioned about the status of their anti-mycobacterial treatment. A provisional diagnosis of respiratory TB disease should be considered for any patient with signs and symptoms of infection in the lungs or airways, coughing for >3 weeks, loss of appetite, unexplained weight loss, night sweats, bloody sputum or hemoptysis, hoarseness, fever, fatigue, and chest pain.

Isolation of Patients with Suspected or Confirmed TB Disease from Other Patients and DHCP

Patients suspected of having TB disease and patients with documented infectious TB who have not completed antimycobacterial treatment should not be kept in the community-based dental healthcare setting any longer than required. While in such a setting, these patients should be promptly isolated from other patients and DHCP, and they should be instructed to observe strict respiratory hygiene and cough etiquette procedures. If possible, they should wear a surgical mask. When coughing or sneezing, they should turn their heads away from other persons and cover their mouth and nose with their hands or preferably a cloth of tissue.

Referral of Patients with Suspected or Confirmed TB Disease for a Medical Evaluation and/or Required Urgent Dental Care

Routine dental care should be postponed until a physician confirms that the patient does not have infectious TB disease or until it is confirmed that the patient is no longer infectious. Dental healthcare settings in which patients with suspected or confirmed TB disease are rarely seen. Consequently, patients with suspected or confirmed TB disease requiring urgent dental care must be promptly referred to a dental healthcare facility that meets the requirements for appropriate environmental respiratory-protection controls.

Environmental Controls

Environmental controls are physical or mechanical measures (as opposed to administrative measures) intended to prevent the spread and reduce the concentration of infectious droplet nuclei 1–5 μm in diameter in ambient air. Patients with suspected or confirmed TB disease requiring urgent dental care must be treated in a room that meets requirements for airborne infection isolation (AII) room. AII rooms provide negative pressure in the room (air flows under the door gap into the room), an air exchange rate of 6–12 ACH (air exchange rate as the number of air exchange units per hour), and direct exhaust of air from the room to the outside of the building or recirculation of air through a high efficiency particulate air (HEPA) filter.

Respiratory-Protection Controls

Administrative and environmental controls minimize the number of areas in which exposure to *M. tuberculosis* might occur and, therefore, the number of persons exposed. However, they do not eliminate the risk of exposure in limited areas. Surgical masks do not prevent inhalation of *M. tuberculosis* droplet nuclei and, therefore, standard precautions are not sufficient to prevent transmission of this organism. DHCP performing urgent dental care on a patient with suspected or confirmed TB disease must wear at least N95 disposable respirators. N95 disposable respirators are nonpowered, air-purifying, particulate-filter respirators. The N (not resistant to oil)-series respirators are available with filtration efficiencies of 95% (N95), 99% (N99), and 99.7% (N100) when challenged with 0.3 μm particles. When respirators are used they should be used in the context of a complete respiratory protection program. This program should include

training and fit testing to ensure an adequate seal between the edges of the respirator and the wearer's face. Additional information can be found in Chapter 8 (Personal Protective Equipment) and from the National Institute for Occupational Safety and Health (NIOSH).

TB Infection Control Surveillance Program for DHCP

Baseline and Follow-up Screening for LTBI and TB Disease

The CDC guidelines explicitly identify dental healthcare facilities as settings in which patients with suspected or confirmed TB disease are expected to be encountered. Consequently, all DHCP who have the potential for exposure to *M. tuberculosis* through air space shared with persons with suspected or confirmed infectious TB disease or to clinical specimens that might contain tubercle bacilli, shall receive baseline TB screening at the time of hire, using the two-step TST or a single BAMT such as the QFT-G. The administration, reading, and interpretation of TST or other tests are to be performed by trained personnel. The facility's level of TB risk will determine the need for routine follow-up TST.

All DHCP with positive test results should be evaluated promptly for active disease. A thorough history of exposure to *M. tuberculosis* should be obtained to determine whether the infection is occupational or community acquired. Baseline-positive and newly positive DHCP and those with documented treatment for LTBI or TB disease should receive one chest radiographic as part of the evaluation to rule out TB disease. If the result of the initial radiographic examination is negative, no further radiographs are necessary unless symptoms suggestive of TB disease develop. Periodically, DHCP with positive test results should be reminded about the signs and symptoms of TB disease and the need for prompt evaluation of any pulmonary symptoms. Routine chest radiographs are not required on TST- or BAMT-negative personnel.

Preventive Therapy

Preventive therapy (see Treatment of LTBI) should be offered to all personnel with positive TST or BAMT results if they are younger that 35 years. It should further be offered to the all personnel, regardless of age, who have conversion of their TST or BAMT results. Preventive therapy may be provided through the local or state health department or by other healthcare providers, as appropriate.

Post-Exposure Management of DHCP

As soon as possible after an exposure to *M. tuberculosis* (i.e., exposure to a person with pulmonary or laryngeal

TABLE 4-10 Work Restrictions: Respiratory Tract Infections

Infectious State		Restrictions
Influenza and respiratory syncytial viruses	Acute infection with fever	Exclude from contact with patients at high-risk until acute symptoms resolve (approximately 5 days after onset of illness)
Group A streptococci	Acute infection	Restrict from duty until 24 hours after antibacterial chemotherapy is initiated
Mycobacterium tuberculosis	LTBI (TST or QFT-G positive)	No restrictions
	TB disease (pulmonary or laryngeal)	Exclude from duty until documentation is provided that they are noninfectious

TB for whom proper isolation precautions have not been implemented), TST or BAMT testing should be done on DHCP known to have had negative results from previous testing. If the initial post-exposure test is negative, repeat the test 12 weeks after exposure. Do not perform TST or BAMT testing or chest radiographs on personnel with previous positive test results, unless they have symptoms suggestive of active disease.

WORKPLACE RESTRICTIONS FOR DHCP WITH RESPIRATORY TRACT INFECTIONS

Since standard precautions are inadequate to prevent the spread of *M. tuberculosis* and some DHCP and patients are at higher risk for the consequences of infection caused by influenza, respiratory syncytial viruses, and group A streptococci, additional administrative controls (i.e., work restrictions) are necessary (Table 4-10).

All DHCP with active TB disease (pulmonary or laryngeal) should be excluded from the workplace until documentation is provided from their healthcare provider that they are (a) receiving adequate therapy, (b) their cough has resolved, and (c) that they have had three consecutive sputum smears collected with negative results for AFB. The sputum specimens should be collected in an 8- to 24-hour interval, with at least one being an early morning specimen. After returning to work, they should obtain periodic documentation from their healthcare provider that effective drug therapy has been maintained for the recommended period of time and that sputum smears remain negative for AFB.

Promptly evaluation of DHCP for infectiousness is necessary for those with TB disease who discontinue treatment before being cured. Exclude from duty those who are found to remain infectious until: (a) treatment is resumed, (b) an adequate response to therapy is documented, and (c) sputum smear results are negative for AFB. In addition, consideration should be given to imple-

ment direct observed therapy for DHCP with TB diseases that have not been compliant with drug regiments.

Do not exclude those DHCP from the workplace who have TB only at sites other than the lung or larynx or who are receiving preventive chemotherapy because of positive TST results, even if they are unable or unwilling to accept or complete a full course of preventive therapy. All such DHCP should be instructed to seek prompt evaluation if symptoms suggestive of TB disease develop.

Immune Compromised DHCP

DHCP who are known to be immune compromised should be referred to their personal health professionals who can individually counsel them regarding their risk of respiratory tract infections. At the request of immune compromised DHCP, accommodations for work settings in which they would have the lowest possible risk for occupational exposure should be offered. Consider the provisions of the Americans with Disabilities Act of 1990 and other federal, state, and local regulations in evaluating these situations.

SUMMARY

A wide variety of microorganisms can be detected in aerosols and droplet spatter produced by numerous dental procedures. There is potential for cross-contamination and cross-infection to dental personnel and their patients. Many of the common respiratory infections, such as colds and influenza, are often overlooked because of their frequency of occurrence within the population and the fact that "everyone gets them." Unfortunately, these and other droplet-mediated infections can occasionally predispose an infected person to more serious systemic conditions. The institution of standard precautions, has helped to protect those who are at the greatest risk of occupational exposure and cross-infection, the DHCP.

Review Questions

1. Which of the following statements about *Mycobacterium* is false?

   A. Mycobacteria are intracellular organisms.

   B. The most common mode of transmission of *M. tuberculosis* is inhalation of infectious aerosols.

   C. Humans are the only natural reservoir for *M. tuberculosis.*

   D. The bacteria are spore-formers.

   E. *M. tuberculosis* can remain dormant in hosts for years and reactivate.

2. Antimicrobial drugs used in the treatment of active, symptomatic tuberculosis include all of the following, EXCEPT:

   A. ethambutol

   B. isoniazid

   C. pyrazinamide

   D. penicillin

   E. both B and C only

3. A dental patient in your practice is found to have a positive PPD skin test result, and a negative follow-up chest x-ray. The most plausible diagnosis would be:

   A. *M. tuberculosis* infection without active disease

   B. a false-positive skin test for TB

   C. reactivation TB in its early stages

   D. primary symptomatic TB

4. Caseous lesions containing inflammatory cells and found as a result of *Mycobacteria* infection, are called:

   A. pseudomembranes

   B. tubercules

   C. abscesses

   D. terminal necrosis

5. The classical manifestation of latent tuberculosis infection is:

   A. abscess

   B. tubercle

   C. positive PPD skin test only

   D. miliary tuberculosis

6. Hemagglutinin and neuraminidase are structural components on the surfaces of:

   A. rhinoviruses

   B. *M. truberculosis*

   C. influenza viruses

   D. respiratory synctial virus

7. Which of the following statements is associated with acute rhinosinusitis?

   A. Secondary infection with *Streptococcus pneumoniae* can develop.

   B. Most often caused by anaerobic bacteria.

   C. Symptoms include night sweats, bloody sputum, and high fever.

   D. Etiologic viruses continue to mutate via antigenic drift.

8. Antigenic drift, a minor change in HA and NA antigens resulting from point mutations which occur during viral replication, is found with:

   A. all *M. tuberculosis* strains

   B. influenza viruses

   C. rhinoviruses

   D. only multiple drug resistant *M. tuberculosis* strains

9. The primary site of influenza virus infection is:

   A. respiratory ciliated epithelial cells

   B. alveolus

   C. phagocytic monocyte

   D. none of the above

10. Which of the following occurs as a result of antigenic shift in influenza A virus?

    A. recombination of RNA segments between human and bird viral strains

    B. single point mutations in hemagglutinin

    C. single point mutations in neuraminidase

    D. morphologic shift from influenza A to influenza B virus

---

Critical Thinking

1. An apparently healthy patient comes into the practice for a routine dental appointment. During the update of his medical history, the patient informs you that he recently had a positive skin test for tuberculosis (TB). The assistant who is working with you suddenly becomes visibly nervous and asks to see you away from the patient. She informs you that she is very concerned about catching TB from this patient.

   a. What would be the potential risk occupational infection with *Mycobacterium tuberculosis* during a routine 45–60 minute dental appointment?

   b. What can you tell her about infection versus active disease concerning tuberculosis?

c. Describe the most common symptoms found in patients who have primary active TB.

d. What types of respiratory precautions would be needed if you ever were faced with treating a patient who was symptomatic for active TB.

2. Influenza viruses have a high rate of genetic mutation during replication and an ability to exchange genetic material between viral strains. How does this apply to the influenza characteristics of antigenic drift and antigenic shift leading to seasonal influenza and pandemic influenza?

SELECTED READINGS

Abramowicz M. Drugs for tuberculosis. Treatment guidelines. Med Letter 2004;2:83–88.

Al-Serhani AM. Mycobacterial infection of the head and neck: presentation and diagnosis. Laryngoscope 2001;111:2012–2016.

American Thoracic Society. Targeted tuberculin testing and treatment of latent tuberculosis infection. Am J Respir Crit Care Med 2000;161:S221–S247.

American Thoracic Society, CDC, Infectious Disease Society of America. Diagnostic standards and classification of tuberculosis in adults and children. An J Respir Crit Care Med 2000;161:1376–1395.

American Thoracic Society, CDC, Infectious Disease Society of America. Treatment of tuberculosis. MMWR 2003;52(RR-11):1–78.

Barnes PF, Bloch AB, Davidson PT, et al. Tuberculosis in patients with human immunodeficiency virus infection. N Engl J Med 1991;234:1644–1650.

Belting C, Haberfelde GC, Juhl LK. Spread of organisms from dental air rotor. J Am Dent Assoc 1964;68:648–651.

Bhatt AP, Jayakrishnan A. Tuberculous osteomyelitis of the mandible: a case report. Int J Paediatr Dent 2001;11:304–308.

Block AB, Cauthen GM, Hayden CH, et al. The epidemiology of tuberculosis in the United States. Semin Respir Infect 1989;4:157–170.

Brennan PJ. The envelope of mycobacteria. Ann Rev Biochem 1995;64:29–63.

Bull TR. Tuberculosis of the larynx. Brit Med J 1966;2:991–992.

Cantwell MF, Shehab ZM, Costello AM, et al. Brief report: congenital tuberculosis. N Engl J Med 1994;330:1051–1054.

CDC. Congenital pulmonary tuberculosis associated with maternal cerebral tuberculosis. MMWR 2005:54:249–250.

CDC. Guidelines for infection control in dental healthcare settings-2003. MMWR 2003:52(RR-17):1–66.

CDC. Guidelines for preventing the transmission of *Mycobacterium tuberculosis* in health-care facilities, 1994. MMWR 1994;43(RR-13):1–132.

CDC. Guidelines for preventing the transmission of *Mycobacterium tuberculosis* in health-care facilities, 2005. MMWR 2005;54(RR-17):1–141.

CDC. Guidelines for using QuantiFERON®-TB Gold test for detecting *Mycobacterium tuberculosis* infection in the United States. MMWR 2005;54(RR-15):49–55.

CDC. Outbreak of multidrug-resistant tuberculosis at a hospital—New York City, 1991. MMWR 1993;42:427,433–434.

CDC. Preventing and control of tuberculosis in U.S. communities with at-risk minority populations: recommendations of the Advisory Council for the Elimination of Tuberculosis. MMWR 1992;41(RR-5):1011.

CDC. Self-reported tuberculin testing among Indian Health Service and Bureau of Prisons dentists, 1993. MMWR 1994;43:209–211.

CDC. Trends in tuberculosis—United States, 2005. MMWR 2006;55:305–308.

CDC. Tuberculosis and acquired immunodeficiency syndrome—Florida. MMWR 1986;35:587–590.

CDC. Tuberculosis and human immunodeficiency virus infection: recommendations of the Advisory Committee for the Elimination of Tuberculosis (ACET). MMWR 1989;38:236–238;243–250.

CDC. Tuberculosis morbidity—United States, 1997. MMWR 1998;47:253–272.

CDC. World TB day—March 24, 2004. MMWR 2004;53:209–214.

Chaparas SD. Tuberculin test. Variability with the Mantoux procedure. Ann Rev Respir Dis 1985;132:175–177.

Cleveland JL, Gooch BF, Boylard EA, et al. TB infection control recommendations from the CDC, 1994. J Am Dent Assoc 1995;126:593–597.

Cleveland JL, Kent J, Gooch BF, et al. Multidrug-resistant *Mycobacterium tuberculosis* in an HIV dental clinic. Infect Cont Hosp Epidemiol 1995;16:7–11.

Colditz GA, Brewer TF, Berkey CS, et al. Efficacy of BCG vaccine in the prevention of tuberculosis: meta-analysis of the published literature. J Am Med Assoc 1994;271:698–702.

Comstock GW, Lovesay VT, Woolpert SF. The prognosis of a positive tuberculin reaction in childhood and adolescence. Am J Epidemiol 1974;99:131–138.

Dimitrakopoulos I, Zoulounis L, Lazaridis N, et al. Primary tuberculosis of the oral cavity. Oral Surg Oral Med Oral Pathol 1991;72:712–715.

Duell RC, Madden RM. Droplet nuclei produced during dental treatment of tubercular patients. A preliminary study. Oral Surg Oral Med Oral Pathol 1970;30:711–715.

Eng HL, Lu S-Y, Yang C-H, et al. Oral tuberculosis. Oral Surg Oral Med Oral Pathol 1996;81:415–420.

Ferebee SH. Controlled chemoprophylaxis trials in tuberculosis. A general overview. Adv Tuberc Res 1970;17:28–106.

Frieden TR, Sherman LF, Maw KL, et al. A multi-institutional outbreak of highly drug-resistant tuberculosis: epidemiology and clinical outcomes. JAMA 1996;276:1259–1260.

Friedman TR, Sterling T, Pablos-Mendez A, et al. The emergence of drug-resistant tuberculosis in New York City. N Engl J Med 1993;328:521–526.

Glassroth J, Robins AG, Snider DE. Tuberculosis in the 1980s. N Engl J Med 1980;302:1441–1450.

Glickman MS, Jacobs WR. Microbial pathogenesis of Mycobacterium tuberculosis: dawn of a discipline. Cell 2001;104:477–485.

Goble M, Iseman MD, Madsen LA, et al. Treatment of 171 patients with pulmonary tuberculosis resistant to isoniazid and rifampin. N Engl J Med 1993;328: 527–532.

Grode L, Seiler P, Baumann S, et al. Increased vaccine efficacy against tuberculosis of recombinant Mycobacterium bovis bacilli Calmette-Guerin mutants that secrete listeriolysin. J Clin Invest 2005;115:2472–2479.

Haddad NM, Zaytoun GM, Hadi U. Tuberculosis of the soft palate: an unusual presentation of tuberculosis. Otolaryngol Head Neck Surg 1987;97:91–92.

Harrel SK, Molinari JA. Aerosols and spatter in dentistry. A brief review of the literature in infection control implications. J Am Dent Assoc 2004;135:429–437.

Hashomoto Y, Tanioka H. Primary tuberculosis of the tongue: report of a case. J Oral Maxillofac Surg 1989;47:744–746.

Havlir DV, Barnes PF. Tuberculosis in patients with human imminuodeficiency virus infection. New Engl J Med 1999;340:367–373.

Hock-Liew E, Shin-Yu L, Chuang-Hwa Y, et al. Oral tuberculosis. Oral Surg Oral Med Oral Pathol Oral Radiol Endod 1996;81:415–420.

Holmes S, Gleeson MJ, Cawson RA. Mycobacterial disease of the patotid gland. Oral Surg Oral Med Oral Pathol Oral Radiol Endod 2000;90:292–298.

Iseman MD. Treatment of multidrug-resistant tuberculosis. N Engl J Med 1993;329:784–791.

Jasmer RM, Nahid P, Hopewell PC. Latent tuberculosis infection. New Engl J Med 2002;347:1860–1866.

Johanson WG, Pierce AK, Sanford JP, et al. Nosocomial infections with gram-negative bacilli: the significance of colonization of the respiratory tract. Ann Intern Med 1972;77:701–706.

Kenyon TA, Valway SE, Ihle WW, et al. Transmission of multidrug-resistant mycobacterium tuberculosis during a long airplane flight. N Eng J Med 1996;334(15):933–938.

Lazarevic V, Flyn J. CD8+ T cells in tuberculosis. Am J Respir Crit Care Med 2002;166:1116–1121.

Li CK, Chan YF, Har CY. Congenital tuberculosis. Aust Paediartr J 1989;25:366–367.

Mignogna MD, Muzio LLO, Favia G, et al. Oral tuberculosis: a clinical evaluation of 42 cases. Oral Dis 2000;6:25–30.

Mikitka D, Mills SE, Dazey SE, et al. Tuberculosis infection in U.S. Air Force dentists. Am J Dent 1995;8:33–36.

Milburn HJ. Primary tuberculosis. Curr Opin Pulm Med 2001;7:133–141.

Miziara ID. Tuberculosis tuberculosis affecting the oral cavity in Brazilian HIV-infected patients. Oral Surg Oral Med Oral Pathol Oral Radiol Endod 2005;100:179–182.

Molinari JA. Fighting the flu. Dimen Dent Hyg 2005;3(1):22–26.

Molinari JA. The implications of influenza. Dimen Dent Hyg 2005;3(2):22–24.

Molinari JA, Cottone JA, Chandrasekar, PH. Tuberculosis in the 1990s: current implications for dentistry. Compend Contin Educ Dent 1993;14:276–290.

Nardell EA. Environmental control of tuberculosis. Med Clin N Amer 1993;77:1315–1334.

Nichol KL, Margolis KL, Wuorenma J, et al. The efficacy and cost effectiveness of vaccination against influenza among elderly persons living in the community. N Eng J Med 1994;331:778–784,807–808.

Onorato IM, McCray E. Prevalence of human immunodeficiency virus among patients attending tuberculosis clinics in the United States. J Infect Dis 1992;165:87–92.

Pablos-Mendez A, Sterling, TR, Frieden TR, et al. The relationship between delayed or incomplete treatment and all-cause mortality in patients with tuberculosis. J Am Med Assoc 1996;276:1223–1228.

Pierce J, Sims SL, Holman GH. Transmission of tuberculosis to hospital workers by a patient with AIDS. Chest 1992;101:581–582.

Porteous NB, Brown JP.Tuberculin skin test conversion rate in dental healthcare workers—results of a prospective study. Am J Infect Cont 1999;27:385–387.

Rattan A, Kalia A, Ahmad N. Multidrug-resistance *Mycobacterium tuberculosis*: molecular perspectives. Emerg Infect Dis 1998;4:195–209.

Saunders BM, Cooper AM. Restraining mycobacteria: role of granulomas in mycobacterial infections. Immunol Cell Biol 2000;78:334–341.

Sbarbaro JA. Skin testing in the diagnosis of tuberculosis. Res Inf 1986;1(4):234–238.

Selwyn PA, Hartel D, Lewis VA, et al. A prospective study of the risk of tuberculosis amond intravenous drug users with human immunodeficiency virus infection. N Engl J Med 1989;320:545–550.

Sepkowitz KA. Tuberculosis and the healthcare worker: a historical perspective. Annals of Internal Medicine 1994;120(1):71–77.

Small PM, Fujiwara PI. Management of tuberculosis in the United States. New Engl J Med 2001;345:189–200.

Small PM, Scheter GF, Goodman PC, et al. Treatment of tuberculosis in patients with advanced human immunodeficiency virus infection. N Engl J Med 1991;324:289–294.

Smith I. *Mycobacterium tuberculosis* pathogenesis and molecular determinants of virulence. Clin Microbiol Rev 2003;16:463–496.

Smith WHR, Mason KD, Davis D, et al. Intaoral and pulmonary tuberculosis following dental treatment. Lancet 1982;1:842–844.

Suleiman AM. Tuberculous parotitis: report of 3 cases. Brit J Oral Maxillofac Surg 2001;39:320–323.

Sunderman G, McDonald RJ, Maniatis T, et al. Tuberculosis as a manifestation of the acquired immunodeficiency syndrome (AIDS). J Am Med Assoc 1986;256:362–366.

Theuer CP, Hopevell PC, Elias D, et al. Human immunodeficiency virus infection in tuberculosis patients. J Infect Dis 1990;162:8–12.

Valway SE, Sanchez MPC, Shinnick TF, et al. An outbreak involving extensive transmission of a virulent strain of *Mycobacterium tuberculosis*. N Eng J Med 1998;338:633–644.

Wagner W. Changing diagnostic and treatment strategies for chronic sinusitis. Cleveland Clinic J Med 1996;63:396–405.

Wald ER. Sinusitis in children. N Eng J Med 1992; 326:319–23.

Weinberger SE. Recent advances in pulmonary medicine (Part I). N Eng J Med 1993;328:1389–1397.

Weinberger SE. Recent advances in pulmonary medicine (Part II). N Engl J Med 1993;328:1462–1470.

Yonemaya T, Yoshida M, Matsui T, et al. Oral care and pneumonia. Lancet 1999;354:515.

Zuber PLF, McKenna MT, Binkin NJ, et al. Long-term risk of tuberculosis among foreign-born persons in the United States. J Am Med Assoc 1997;278:304–307.

5

Dental Unit Water and Air Quality Challenges

Shannon Mills

LEARNING OBJECTIVES

After completion of this chapter individuals should be able to:

1 Understand biofilm bacteria colonize dental units and other dental devices that use water for cooling and irrigating dental operative sites.

2 Become familiar with potential routes of exposure to contaminated water, aerosols, and other airborne hazards in the dental environment.

3 Describe the potential health consequences of acute and chronic exposure to microbial contaminated dental water, aerosols, and other airborne hazards in the dental environment.

4 Apply basic infection control principles to the problem of biofilm colonization in dental equipment and devices.

5 Implement effective engineering and work practice controls in the dental setting to prevent exposure to waterborne and airborne hazards.

6 Make evidence-based choices in the selection of dental equipment and products designed to remediate water-borne and airborne hazards to reduce exposure risks to patients and dental healthcare professionals.

KEY TERMS

Aerosol: particles of respirable size generated by both humans and environmental sources that can remain viable and airborne for extended periods in the indoor environment; commonly generated in dentistry during use of handpieces, ultrasonic scalers, and air/water syringes.

Bacteria: tiny one-celled organisms present throughout the environment that require a microscope to be seen. While not all bacteria are harmful, some cause disease. Examples of bacterial disease include diphtheria, pertussis, tetanus, *Haemophilus influenza*, and pneumococcus (pneumonia).

Bacterial count: a method of estimating the number of bacteria per unit sample. The term also refers to the estimated number of bacteria per unit sample, usually expressed as colony forming units (CFUs) per square centimeter (cm^2) per milliliter (mL).

Biofilm: a microbially derived sessile community characterized by cells that are irreversibly attached to a substratum or interface to each other, are embedded in a matrix of extracellular polymeric substances that they have produced, and exhibit an altered phenotype with respect to growth rate and gene transcription.

Boil water advisory: a public health announcement that the public should boil tap water before drinking it; when issued, the public should assume the water is unsafe to drink.

Colony forming unit (CFU): the minimum number of separable cells on the surface of or in semi-solid agar medium which gives rise to a visible colony of progeny is on the order of tens of millions. CFUs may consist of pairs, chains, and clusters as well as single cells and are often expressed as colony forming units per milliliter (CFU/mL).

Dental treatment water: nonsterile water used for dental therapeutic purposes, including irrigation of nonsurgical operative sites and cooling of high speed rotary and ultrasonic instruments.

Endotoxin: the lipopolysccharide of Gram-negative bacteria, the toxic character of which reside in the lipid protein. Endotoxins can produce pyrogenic reactions in persons exposed to their bacterial component.

Glycocalyx: a gelatinous polysaccharide and/or polypeptide outer covering. The glycocalyx can be identified by negative staining techniques. The glycocalyx is referred to as a capsule if it is firmly attached to the cell wall, or as a slime layer if loosely attached. This material produced by bacteria forms the structural matrix of biofilm.

Heterotrophic bacteria: those bacteria that require an organic carbon source for growth (i.e., they derive energy and carbon from organic compounds). The modifier "mesophilic" describes bacteria that grow best within the middle ranges of environmental temperature.

Independent water reservoir: a container used to hold water or other solutions and supply it to handpieces and air/water syringes attached to a dental unit. The independent reservoir, which isolates the unit from the public water system, may be provided as original equipment or as a retrofit device on all modern dental units.

Oral surgical procedure: involves the incision, excision, or reflection of tissue that exposes normally sterile areas of the oral cavity. Examples include biopsy, periodontal surgery, apical surgery, implant surgery, and surgical extractions of teeth (e.g., removal of erupted or nonerupted tooth requiring elevation of mucoperiosteal flap, removal of bone or sectioning of tooth, and suturing if needed).

Planktonic: collective name free-floating microbiological organisms dispersed in solution, as in the case of free-swimming plankton.

Potable (drinking) water: water suitable for drinking per applicable public health standards.

Retraction: the entry of oral fluids and microorganisms into waterlines through negative water pressure.

Spatter: visible drops of liquid or body fluid that are expelled forcibly into the air and settle out quickly, as distinguished from particles of an aerosol, which remain airborne indefinitely.

Sterile water: water that is sterilized and contains no antimicrobial agents.

While we may often take for granted that the air we breathe and the water we drink are safe, we are constantly reminded that chemical and biological contaminants in water, and particulates and toxic gases in air, can pose potential health risks. The dental office is no exception and can present unique challenges to ensuring a safe and healthy practice environment. In this chapter we will explore the potential hazards that water and air can present and learn how these risks can be avoided.

DENTAL WATERLINE CONTAMINATION

Modern dental units equipped with air turbine–powered handpieces and ultrasonic scalers are sophisticated engineering marvels that enable the delivery of high quality restorative and surgical treatment with exceptional comfort for both the patient and the dental treatment team. Major changes in dental unit design in the 1960s were driven by the need to provide coolant water for the new generation of high-speed air-powered and ultrasonic dental instruments. As a result, dental units contain lengths of narrow bore plastic tubing that deliver compressed air to power handpieces and water to cool and irrigate the operative site. Although usually unseen by both clinician and patient, this maze of small bore plastic tubing offers an optimal environment for the proliferation of complex microbial communities known as **biofilm** (Fig. 5-1).

Since the phenomenon of bacterial colonization of dental water delivery systems was first described in 1963, numerous reports have confirmed that water produced by dental units and other dental equipment (i.e., **dental treatment water**) can contain very high levels of **bacteria**. While most dental unit water samples exhibit colony counts ranging from 1,000 to 10,000 **colony forming units** per milliliter (CFU/mL), counts greater than 1,000,000 CFU/mL have been documented. In contrast, the standard established by the Environmental Protection Agency (EPA), American Public Health Association (APHA), and the American Waterworks Association (AWWA) for **potable** and recreational water is only 500 CFU/mL of noncoliform bacteria. To understand this phenomenon and its implications for dentistry, we must first gain some insights into the nature of biofilm.

What is Biofilm?

Biofilm exists on this planet in virtually all environments where there is water and a suitable solid substrate for

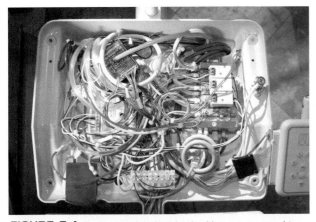

FIGURE 5-1 Representative dental unit with cover removed to show multiple narrow bore plastic tubings that deliver water and compressed air to handpieces and air/water syringes. (Courtesy of Michael F Neubauer, DDS, MS.)

attachment. In fact, the vast majority of microorganisms in nature probably exist as biofilm. While at first glance, biofilm appears to be nothing more than random, amorphous collections of bacteria and other microorganisms, closer investigation reveals highly complex microbial architecture and ecology.

Natural biofilms are heterogeneous in both species and morphology and may have surprisingly complex structure. Fungi, algae, protozoa, and even larger organisms such as microscopic worms also reside in or adjacent to biofilms in aquatic and marine environments as well as in municipal water systems. Biofilms begin when free-floating (**planktonic**) bacteria attach themselves to solid surfaces and adapt to a sessile existence. As they replicate, the bacteria release signaling compounds that stimulate other bacteria in the environment to undergo phenotypic changes in a process known as quorum sensing. An important function of quorum sensing is to initiate the production of long chain oligopolysaccharides that form a protective matrix known as a **glycocalyx** or slime layer. The glycocalyx provides a structural framework that protects the organisms within the biofilm from desiccation, chemical insult, and predation. Protected by the slime coating, bacteria continue to replicate—initially forming microcolonies that later coalesce to produce continuous sheets of biofilm. Microstructural architecture forms within biofilm as a result of signaling compound mediated interactions between and among various species of microorganisms. These architectural features appear to facilitate transport of nutrients and waste products using processes that in many respects mimic the complexity of multicellular organisms (Fig. 5-2A,B). If the previous description of a biofilm sounds familiar to dentists, it may be because dentistry's traditional adversary—dental plaque—is a classic biofilm.

Once formed, a biofilm provides a protected microenvironment that may dramatically amplify the numbers of microorganisms and microbial by-products present in water used for dental treatment. Dental waterlines provide an excellent environment for microbial growth. The plastics typically used in dental unit construction readily support the formation of biofilm. Furthermore, the small diameter of the tubing creates a high surface to volume ratio that increases the surface area available for biofilm formation in relation to the volume of water coursing through the lines. Because of a property of fluid dynamics known as laminar flow, the rate of water flow is greatest in the center of the tubing and decreases to near zero at the tubing surface. Virtually stagnant conditions therefore exist at the tubing wall interface even when water is flowing. For this reason, it is nearly impossible to create flow rates with shear forces great enough to remove biofilms by flushing. Because of this unfortunate convergence of biology, physics, and geometry, the water exiting dental

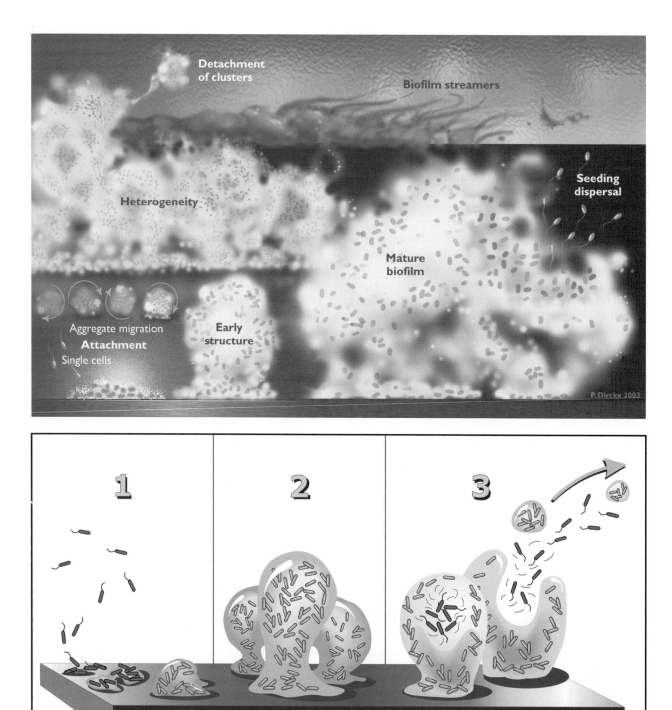

FIGURE 5-2 (A) Conceptual illustration of the heterogeneity of biofilm structure and function. *Foreground*: biofilm life cycle. *Midground*: heterogeneity in bacterial activity and communities make-up. *Background*: Streamer formation and detachment. (Illustration used with permission of the Center for Biofilm Engineering, Montana State University, Bozeman, Montana, and P. Dirckx.) **(B)** The biofilm life cycle in three steps: attachment, growth of colonies, swarming phenomenon and detachment in clumps or "seeding dispersal." (Illustration used with permission of the Center for Biofilm Engineering, Montana State University, Bozeman, Montana, and P. Dirckx.)

units is often hundreds or thousands of times more contaminated than the incoming tap water.

Most of the organisms isolated from dental water systems are aquatic noncoliform water bacteria. These predominantly Gram-negative water microorganisms usually enter the dental unit from the public water supply. Although oral flora may be isolated from dental water systems, they are less well adapted to flourish in the low temperature, low nutrient environment found in waterlines. Oral flora may however, enter waterlines during treatment if **retraction** of oral fluids into handpieces or air-water syringes occurs. Subsequent patients may thereby be exposed to these retracted microbes. Incorporation of engineering features to prevent water retraction reduces the likelihood of this occurrence.

Potential Effects on Health

A large body of scientific evidence exists to document waterborne infections and disease in hospital settings. While numerous microorganisms have been associated with hospital-related waterborne infections, *Pseudomonas*, nontuberculous *Mycobacterium* species, and *Legionella* species are the most commonly cited pathogens. Medical devices associated with waterborne infections include nebulizers, endoscopes, otologic equipment, and hemodialysis units.

Most organisms isolated from dental water systems originate from the public water supply and do not usually pose a high risk of disease for healthy persons. The increasing numbers of patients with weakened immune systems who seek dental treatment, however, provide reasons for concern about dental water quality. Potential human pathogens including *Pseudomonas*, *Klebsiella*, *Legionella*, and nontuberculous *Mycobacterium* species have been isolated from dental water supplies. For immune compromised individuals, these organisms could potentially cause infection and illness.

Despite the presence of potentially pathogenic bacteria in numbers greatly exceeding levels established for drinking and recreational waters, few cases of illness among patients or dental healthcare workers have been documented. Because most dental offices are located in outpatient settings, however, epidemiologic links between an infection and recent exposure to contaminated dental water are difficult to establish. Nevertheless, there are published reports documenting exposure or adverse health effects from contaminated dental unit water.

Two independent investigations detected higher titers of antibodies to *Legionella*, the genus of bacteria responsible for outbreaks of Legionnaires' disease, in the blood of dental personnel compared to demographically similar control populations. Chronic exposure to *Legionella* contaminated aerosols generated from dental units was cited as the most likely cause. Nevertheless, no cases of *Legionella* pneumonia among the exposed workers were documented.

Contaminated dental unit water was implicated as the source for localized *Pseudomonas* infections in two immune-compromised patients and carriage of the same strain of bacteria in 78 additional individuals. A retrospective analysis of case records, however, failed to show infections in healthy patients attributable to contaminated dental unit water.

A possible reason for the infrequent occurrence of infections may be the small quantity of coolant water used in most dental procedures combined with the use of high-speed evacuation. Nevertheless, contaminated water can still enter the patient via ingestion or inhalation of contaminated aerosols. Contaminated water may also contact open wounds and provide a portal for microorganisms to enter into the bloodstream.

Bacterial **endotoxin** (a lipopolysaccharide found in the cell walls of Gram-negative bacteria) may also be present in water from colonized dental units. Endotoxin can produce potent physiologic effects on susceptible individuals including fever, tachycardia, exacerbation of asthma, and septic shock. Persons undergoing hemodialysis with contaminated dialysis fluid may experience potentially serious reactions to endotoxin. To prevent these so-called "pyrogenic reactions" only very low levels of endotoxin are permitted in **sterile water** used in surgery or hemodialysis. The United States Pharmacopeia (USP) sets a limit of only 0.25 endotoxin units per milliliter (EU/mL). In contrast, researchers have found levels as high as 2,560 EU/mL in water from dental units. A tentative link has been reported between bacterial contamination of dental units and new onset of asthma in dentists that may be related to exposure to endotoxin.

Despite the high numbers of potentially pathogenic organisms reported in water used for dental treatment, and evidence of waterborne infections and other complications associated with medical treatment, there is little data on dental post-treatment or occupationally acquired infections. Nevertheless, the use of water of poor microbiologic quality for dental procedures is inconsistent with generally accepted infection control principles. This is particularly true when methods to assure better water quality are readily available.

Guidelines and Policy

In response to concerns about the quality of water used in dental treatment, the American Dental Association (ADA) convened an expert panel in 1995 to address the issue. Based on the panel's findings, the ADA Council of Scientific Affairs published a white paper that acknowledged the

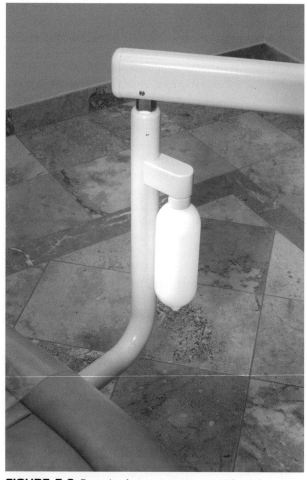

FIGURE 5-3 Example of separate water reservoir used as an approach to improve water quality. (Courtesy of Michael F Neubauer, DDS, MS.)

poor microbiologic quality of dental unit water and established goals for improving dental unit water quality. Suggested prevention strategies to improve water quality included separate water reservoirs independent of the public water supply (Fig. 5-3), chemical disinfection of the waterline tubing, daily draining and air purging regimens, and waterline filters.

In December of 2003, the Centers for Disease Control and Prevention (CDC) published *Guidelines for Infection Control in Dental Healthcare Settings—2003*. The new guidelines updated 1993 CDC recommendations that recommended flushing of dental waterlines at the beginning of the day and between patients, and the use of sterile water or saline for irrigation of surgical sites where bone is exposed. The 2003 CDC guidelines provide more comprehensive guidance regarding water used in dentistry by addressing three specific areas: (a) general recommendations, (b) boil water advisories, and (c) oral

surgical procedures. Some state dental boards have adopted the following recommendations as the standard of care or have incorporated the recommendations into state dental practice regulations. These are excerpted below:

VIII. Dental Unit Waterlines, Biofilm, and Water Quality

  A. General Recommendations

    1. *Use water that meets EPA regulatory standards for drinking water (i.e., ≤500 CFU/mL of **heterotrophic water bacteria**) for routine dental treatment output water (IB, IC).*

    2. *Consult with the dental unit manufacturer for appropriate methods and equipment to maintain the recommended quality of dental water (II).*

    3. *Follow recommendations for monitoring water quality provided by the manufacturer of the unit or waterline treatment product (II).*

    4. *Discharge water and air for a minimum of 20–30 seconds after each patient, from any device connected to the dental water system that enters the patient's mouth (e.g., handpieces, ultrasonic scalers, and air/water syringes) (II).*

    5. *Consult with the dental unit manufacturer on the need for periodic maintenance of antiretraction mechanisms (IB).*

  B. Boil Water Advisories

    1. *The following apply while a boil water advisory is in effect:*

      a. *Do not deliver water from the public water system to the patient through the dental operative unit, ultrasonic scaler, or other dental equipment that uses the public water system (IB, IC).*

      b. *Do not use water from the public water system for dental treatment, patient rinsing, or hand washing (IB, IC).*

      c. *For hand washing, use antimicrobial-containing products that do not require water for use (e.g., alcohol-based hand rubs). If hands are visibly contaminated, use bottled water, if available, and soap for hand washing or an antiseptic towelette (IB, IC).*

    2. *The following apply when the boil water advisory is canceled:*

      a. *Follow guidance given by the local water utility regarding adequate flushing of waterlines. If no guidance is provided, flush dental waterlines and faucets for 1–5 minutes before using for patient care (IC).*

      b. *Disinfect dental waterlines as recommended by the dental unit manufacturer (II).*

IX. Special Considerations

   F. Oral Surgical Procedures

      1.c. Use sterile saline or sterile water as a coolant/irrigant when performing oral surgical procedures. Use devices specifically designed for delivering sterile irrigating fluids (e.g., bulb syringe, single-use disposable products, and sterilizable tubing) (IB).

CDC/HICPAC Ranking Scale

Each recommendation is categorized on the basis of existing scientific data, theoretical rationale, and applicability. Rankings are based on the system used by CDC and the Healthcare Infection Control Practices Advisory Committee (HICPAC) to categorize recommendations.

Indications for Use of Sterile Irrigating Solutions

Dental unit water that meets drinking water standards is presumably safe for most routine dental procedures. This includes routine oral prophylaxis, restorative procedures, and initial access into the dental pulp. The use of sterile irrigating solutions for surgery, however, is a well-accepted principle of medical practice. The fact that the oral cavity is colonized with endogenous bacteria does not relieve dentists from their obligation to incorporate this principle into their clinical practice when performing invasive procedures.

The 1993 CDC infection control recommendations required the use of sterile irrigating solutions only for procedures that involve the cutting of bone. The 2003 guideline, however, provides a more comprehensive definition of **oral surgical procedures** to include "the incision, excision, or reflection of tissue that exposes the normally sterile areas of the oral cavity." The guidelines permit the use of water with fewer than 500 CFU/mL for deep scaling and tooth extractions that do not involve reflection of mucoperiosteal flaps or manipulation of bone. Sterile irrigating solutions are required for biopsies, periodontal surgery, apical surgery, implant surgery, removal of erupted or nonerupted teeth requiring elevation of a mucoperiosteal flap, removal of bone or sectioning of tooth, and suturing.

Improving Dental Treatment Water

Although flushing water through dental waterlines can clear planktonic organisms suspended in the bulk fluid, research has shown that the effects are transient. **Bacterial counts** may quickly rise to levels equal to or exceeding preflush levels as pieces of biofilm are dislodged as water flows through the lines. Flow rates high enough to create the shear forces needed to dislodge biofilm are not attainable in clinical settings. The CDC recommends flushing waterlines between patients to eliminate any patient material that may have been retracted into handpieces and air water syringes during dental procedures, but does not consider flushing to be an effective means to reliably improve dental water quality.

A range of engineering and work practice controls have been evaluated to improve dental water quality and a wide range of commercial products are currently available to the profession to control or eliminate biofilm in dental waterlines. Currently available products include:

- chemical germicides or cleaners that inactivate or remove biofilms (sometimes described as intermittent or "shock" treatment).

- chemical germicides or cleaners that prevent attachment of biofilm in new or cleaned systems (sometimes described as continuous treatment). These products may be added to or used as the irrigating solution for clinical treatment.

- slow-release resin cartridges or metering devices that release low concentrations of agents designed to prevent attachment of biofilm including antimicrobial reservoirs and tubing.

- antimicrobial materials that inhibit biofilm formation that are incorporated into the plastics used to make tubing and reservoirs.

- sterile water delivery systems for use in surgical procedures that bypass the dental unit and employ sterile disposable or sterilizable tubing.

An ideal antibiofilm agent would be nontoxic, nonpyrogenic, and nonsensitizing to humans; noncorrosive to metals; have no deleterious effect on rubber or synthetics; and not interfere with the performance of any dental restorative or therapeutic agents. It would also have to have rapid, broad-spectrum antimicrobial activity against bacteria, fungi, and protozoa. Its mode of action should be bactericidal and it should also be capable of breaking up biofilm. A degree of substantivity would confer resistance to biofilm reformation on water system surfaces. It should also be inexpensive. Although no such ideal product exists at this time, products claiming many of the attributes of the hypothetical ideal are now being marketed. Before introducing any chemical agent into a dental water system, the user must seek assurance from the manufacturer that the product is nontoxic, will not damage the dental unit, and—if continuously present in treatment water—that it will not harm the patient or dental healthcare professional or interfere with restorative bonding agents.

All products commercially available in the United States should have appropriate regulatory approvals. The U.S. Food and Drug Administration (FDA) clears or grants exemptions to devices intended to improve the quality of water used in dental treatment. The U.S. EPA registers antimicrobial agents (see Chapter 12 for more information on EPA procedures). State regulatory agencies may also require additional regulatory clearance for germicidal chemicals.

Clinical monitoring of water quality can ensure that procedures are properly performed and that devices are working in accordance with the manufacturer's previously validated protocol. Monitoring dental unit water quality can assist in identifying problems in performance or compliance, and also provides documentation. There is no need to identify specific organisms unless investigating a waterborne illness or a unit that is refractory to treatment. Testing should accurately detect a wide concentration range and type of aerobic, mesophilic, heterotrophic, waterborne bacteria within a reasonable incubation time at room temperature. Generally, there are two options to monitor dental unit water quality: commercial self-contained test kits or commercial water testing laboratories. Dentists should consult with the manufacturer of their dental unit or water delivery system to determine the best method for maintaining acceptable water quality (i.e., ≤500 CFU/mL) and the recommended frequency of monitoring.

Source Water Concerns

The quality of water delivered by dental units depends on the quality of water entering the system. Since dental devices cannot produce unfiltered output that is cleaner than the water that enters it, the process must begin with clean source water of acceptable quality. If source water is generated on site, water distillers and storage containers must be properly maintained to avoid bacterial contamination. Both large storage vessels and water reservoirs need to be periodically cleaned and disinfected. Water conditioning systems that treat water by filtration, sedimentation, and/or ultraviolet germicidal irradiation (UVGI) can improve input water quality, but have no residual effect on planktonic bacteria or biofilm within the dental unit.

Retraction

Although most modern dental units are designed to be nonretracting, researchers have recovered oral flora from dental water lines. Older units may be equipped with antiretraction devices that require periodic inspection and replacement. Because retracted oral fluids may contain human pathogens, including viruses that can be transmitted to subsequent patients, taking measures to avoid this cross-infection risk are warranted. The CDC guidelines recommend flushing dental waterlines for 20 to 30 seconds between patients to expel any retracted material. Users should contact the dental unit manufacturer for guidance on the need for periodic maintenance of dental antiretraction devices.

Boil Water Advisories

In recent years there has been an increase in the numbers of **"boil water advisories"** resulting from microbial contamination of public drinking water systems. One notable event was the sickening of nearly 400,000 residents of Milwaukee, Wisconsin, in 1993 when the municipal water system was contaminated with the parasitic protozoan *Cryptosporidium parvum*.

In response, the CDC has issued guidance on actions to take during such events. Water from the public water system should not be used for dental treatment or hand washing until the boil water advisory is cancelled. Waterless hand wash agents, such as alcohol hand rubs, may be used. Patients should not rinse with water from the public water system. Dental units equipped with **independent water reservoir** systems may be used during boil water advisories as long as reservoirs are filled with uncontaminated water. After the advisory has been canceled, all water lines and faucets should be flushed according to guidance given by the local water utility. If no guidance is provided, the CDC recommends flushing dental waterlines and faucets for 1 to 5 minutes before patient care. The dental waterlines should be disinfected as recommended by the dental unit manufacturer.

DENTAL AIR QUALITY

Dental rotary and ultrasonic instruments can generate liquid airborne particles that may contain infectious microorganisms. Larger particles, described as **spatter**, consist of droplets greater than 50 microns in diameter that behave ballistically and fall to the floor with a 2-foot range of the point of origin. Although protective garments, eyewear, and surgical masks can protect skin, eyes, and mucous membranes from direct exposure, particles that fall to the floor mix with dust to create particles that can become airborne and settle on skin, clothing, and surfaces. Ranging in size from 5 to 50 microns in diameter, mists settle gradually and can remain suspended in air for longer periods of time. While suspended, evaporation can transform them and their microbial cargo into smaller particles known as residual droplet nuclei.

Aerosols consist of particles usually smaller than 10 μm diameter. Droplet nuclei and aerosols can remain suspended in air for long periods of time and can be inhaled and reach the terminal pulmonary alveoli. While alpha streptococci form the bulk of organisms present in dental aerosols, staphylococci, diphtheroids, pneumococci, *Mycobacterium tuberculosis*, influenza virus, hepatitis virus, *Herpesvirus hominis*, and *Neisseria* species have also been recovered. Examples of diseases that are spread by aerosols or droplets include tuberculosis, influenza, pneumonic plague, measles, severe acute respiratory syndrome (SARS), and Legionnaires' disease. There is no evidence, however, that bloodborne pathogens including hepatitis B, hepatitis C, or HIV can be spread by these routes.

The number of bacterial particles permissible in the air in hospital operating rooms is 1 viable particle per cubic foot (VP/cuft) of air. In contrast, counts ranging from 109 to 300 VP/cuft of air have been measured during dental procedures using a high speed handpiece. Airborne bacterial counts have been shown to increase by up to 250% following 1.5 to 50 minute operative procedures. Measurements of operatory air taken 30 minutes after use of an ultrasonic scaler contained 5,000 VP/cuft—an increase of approximately 3,000% over preprocedural levels.

Measures that can reduce the amount of potentially infectious spatter, mists, and aerosols present in operatory air include the liberal use of high-volume evacuation and use of dental dam or other effective means of isolation. Preprocedural rinsing with an antimicrobial mouth rinse has been shown to reduce oral bacterial counts by up to 90% and may also help control the microbial content of aerosols generated during dental procedures. Regular surgical masks protect nasal and oral mucosa from exposure to spatter containing blood or saliva, but may not provide adequate protection from aerosols or respiratory droplet nuclei. CDC recommendations for preventing exposure to *Mycobacterium tuberculosis* require the use of fit-tested "Surgical N-95 Respirators" that meet requirements established by the National Institute for Occupational Safety and Health (NIOSH) and have been cleared to market by the FDA for use in healthcare.

Microbial Quality of Dental Compressed Air

Although the process of air compression is lethal to microorganisms, moisture condensing in air lines can create conditions hospitable to the growth of bacteria and fungi. Keeping air lines dry appears to be the best means to prevent growth of microorganisms from occurring. Dental offices should install oil-free compressors with either desiccant or refrigerant dryers designed specifically for medical or dental applications. Periodic maintenance must be performed as directed by the manufacturer to assure optimum performance.

Controlling Nitrous Oxide Exposure

Nitrous oxide is a clear, odorless, noncombustible gas that has been used for over 150 years as a safe and effective means to control pain and anxiety for dental patients. Chronic occupational exposure to nitrous oxide, however, has been linked to a range of potentially serious medical conditions including reduced fertility, spontaneous abortions, and neurological, renal, and liver disease by epidemiologic data and animal studies. Exposure to nitrous oxide may occur as a result of leaks from the anesthetic administration system and improper scavenging of waste anesthetic gas. Warnings about potential neurological and reproductive risks associated with chronic exposure to nitrous oxide were first issued in a 1977 report from NIOSH—a branch of the CDC. The report found levels of nitrous oxide in dental offices greater than 1,000 ppm and proposed methods to lower the amount of waste gas present to 50 ppm. Properly operating scavenging systems were shown to be able to reduce nitrous oxide concentrations in operatory air by more than 70%.

In 1994, the agency issued a *NIOSH Alert* that provided updated information on health risks and proposed a series of measures to reduce occupational exposure to healthcare professionals. The recommended exposure limit (REL) was set at 25 ppm as a time weighted average (TWA) during periods of anesthetic administration to prevent decreases in mental performance and manual dexterity. A REL to prevent adverse reproductive effects could not be established because of insufficient dose-effect data from epidemiological investigations. The Occupational Safety and Health Administration (OSHA) has not set an exposure limit for nitrous oxide, but does require that exposed workers be informed about potential hazards associated with the use of nitrous oxide under the OSHA "Hazard Communications Standard."

NIOSH research indicated that concentrations of nitrous oxide in dental operatories could be reduced to approximately 25 ppm by implementing methods of control including system maintenance, ventilation, and work practices. In 1997, the ADA convened an expert panel to review the NIOSH recommendations and the existing scientific data regarding the safe use of nitrous oxide in the dental office. The ADA published an "Association Report" that agreed with the NIOSH recommendations for inspection, maintenance, scavenging systems, ventilation, and work practices, but did not endorse the NIOSH REL of 25 ppm citing lack of scientific consensus. The 1997 Association Report recommended:

- properly installing nitrous oxide delivery systems including scavenging equipment with a readily visible and accurate flow meter, a vacuum pump with a capacity for up to 45 liters of air per minute (L/min) at each workstation, and a variety of well-fitting masks.

- venting of exhaust to the outside, not in proximity to air intake vents.

- ventilating to provide good room air mixing.

- checking the pressure connections for leaks each time the machine is turned on or when the gas cylinder is changed. Checking high-pressure line connections on a quarterly basis. Either a soap solution or infrared spectrophotometer can be used to diagnose leaks.

- inspecting reservoir bags, masks, and connectors for worn parts, holes, or tears prior to the first daily use.

- using masks and scavenging equipment with appropriate flow rates (up to 45 L/min or according to manufacturer's recommendations).

- selecting well-fitting masks and proper inflation of the reservoir bag.
- minimizing talking and mouth breathing during procedures.
- checking for changes in tidal volume and vacuum flow rates during procedures
- delivering 100% oxygen to the patient at the end of the procedure to purge the patient's lungs and the system of residual nitrous oxide. (Do not use an oxygen flush.)
- conducting periodic (semiannual) personal sampling of chair side personnel exposed to nitrous oxide.

Other Respiratory Hazards

In addition to biological contaminants and waste anesthetic gases, other chemicals and materials found in dental offices and dental laboratories may pose respiratory hazards to the dental team. These include volatile chemicals such as methyl methacrylate and glutaraldehyde, toxic or sensitizing metals including nickel and beryllium, and particulates such as silica dust. Dental healthcare professionals must become knowledgeable about these hazards and take appropriate measures to prevent exposure.

DIRECTIONS FOR FUTURE RESEARCH AND DEVELOPMENT

Although considerable progress has been made in our understanding of aquatic biofilm in dental unit water systems and indoor air quality, much remains to be learned. A wide variety of technical approaches for the control or eradication of biofilm and improvement of dental treatment water have shown promise and many are already commercially available. Unfortunately, the data necessary to develop a truly evidence-based approach to improving dental water quality is in short supply. There is a lack of consensus on standard test methods to validate the safety and efficacy of methods to improve air and water quality. In addition, there are few epidemiological studies of possible health effects. Additional research is essential to assure that water and air used in dental treatment is consistently of the highest quality.

Much remains unknown about the risks associated with airborne biological and chemical contaminants in the dental environment. While studies continue to suggest that chronic exposure to nitrous oxide may have detrimental health effects on dental healthcare professionals, there are still insufficient data to characterize what constitutes a safe level of exposure.

SUMMARY

Ensuring a safe clinical environment by taking measures to provide clean water and air during dental procedures is consistent with well-established infection control principles. Device manufacturers must meet their obligation to design and market safe, effective, and economical products. Prudent dentists, mindful of their obligation to protect the health and safety of their patients and staff, will take measures improve the quality of water and air in clinical practice.

✓ Practical Dental Infection Control Checklist

General Considerations

❑ Is water that meets EPA regulatory standards for drinking water (i.e., ≤500 CFU/mL of heterotrophic water bacteria) used for routine dental treatment output water?

❑ Do DCHP use sterile saline or sterile water as a coolant/irrigant when performing oral surgical procedures?

❑ Does the dental office/clinic consult with the dental unit manufacturer for appropriate methods and equipment to maintain the recommended quality of dental water?

❑ Are recommendations for monitoring water quality provided by the manufacturer of the unit or waterline treatment product followed?

❑ Is water and air discharged for a minimum of 20–30 seconds after each patient, from any device connected to the dental water system that enters the patient's mouth (e.g., handpieces, ultrasonic scalers, and air/water syringes)?

❑ Does the dental office/clinic consult with the dental unit manufacturer on the need for periodic maintenance of antiretraction mechanisms?

Boil Water Advisories

❑ If a boil water advisory is in effect, does the dental office/clinic have a written protocol to follow? If yes, does it include:

  ❑ not delivering water from the public water system to the patient through the dental operative unit, ultrasonic scaler, or other dental equipment that uses the public water system?

  ❑ not using water from the public water system for dental treatment, patient rinsing, or hand washing?

  ❑ using antimicrobial products that do not require water for use (e.g., alcohol-based hand rubs) for hand washing? Note: If hands are visibly contaminated, use bottled water, if available, and soap for hand washing or an antiseptic towelette.

❑ When the boil water advisory is canceled does the dental clinic/office have a written protocol to follow? If yes, does it include:

  ❑ following guidance given by the local water utility regarding adequate flushing of waterlines? Note: If no guidance is provided, are dental waterlines and faucets flushed for 1–5 minutes before using for patient care?

❏ disinfecting/cleaning dental waterlines as recommended by the dental unit manufacturer?

Review Questions

1. Most organisms isolated from dental water systems originate from the public water supply and do not usually pose a high risk of disease for healthy individuals. However, there are published reports documenting exposure or adverse health effects from contaminated dental water.

   A. The first statement is true. The second statement is false.

   B. The first statement is false. The second statement is true.

   C. Both statements are true.

   D. Both statements are false.

2. For nonsurgical dental procedures, use water with less than _____ CFU/mL.

   A. 200

   B. 300

   C. 400

   D. 500

3. Which of the following statements regarding improving dental unit water quality is true?

   A. Flushing water through dental unit waterlines clears planktonic organisms and is an acceptable means of permanently improving dental unit water quality.

   B. Using chemical germicides or cleaners, periodically or continuously, can prevent the attachment of biofilm in new or cleaned systems.

   C. Antimicrobial materials incorporated into the waterline tubing or bottles can inhibit biofilm formation.

   D. Slow-release resin cartridges that release low concentrations of agents are designed to prevent attachment of biofilm.

   E. B, C, and D are correct

4. An ideal antibiofilm agent would be

   A. nontoxic

   B. nonpyrogenic

   C. nonsensitizing to humans

   D. noncorrosive to metals

   E. all of the above

5. Which of the following statements is true regarding dental unit waterlines?

   A. If municipal water is the source that enters the dental unit waterline, output will always meet drinking water quality.

   B. Flushing the waterlines for >2 minutes at the beginning of the day reduces the biofilm in the waterlines.

   C. Dentists should consult with the manufacturer of the dental unit or water delivery system to determine the best method for maintaining optimal water quality.

   D. Dental unit waterlines can reliably deliver optimal water quality when used for irrigation during a surgical procedure.

   E. All of the above.

   F. A, B, and D are correct.

6. The CDC recommends the use of sterile irrigation solutions for

   A. scaling and root planning.

   B. biopsy procedures.

   C. periodontal surgery.

   D. surgical extractions of teeth.

   E. A, C, and D

   F. B, C, and D

   G. all of the above

7. Which of the following infectious agents is not known to be transmitted by the respiratory route?

   A. Hepatitis C virus

   B. *Mycobacterium tuberculosis*

   C. *Legionella pneumophila*

   D. Severe acute respiratory syndrome

8. Which of the following may be effective in reducing exposure to contaminated aerosols in the dental setting?

   A. Use of a dental dam and high volume evacuation

   B. Antibiotic prophylaxis

   C. Use of OSHA-approved face shields and protective eyewear

   D. Good aseptic surgical technique

Critical Thinking

1. Earlier in the week, a news show had a story about contaminated water from a dental office. A patient calls your office and asks you what you're doing to keep the water used during his dental treatment clean. How do you respond?

2. You heard on the morning news that the city in which your dental office is located is under a boil water advisory. What will you do when you arrive at the dental office? What will you do when the boil water advisory is canceled?

3. What type of procedures are performed in your dental office requiring the use of sterile irrigating solutions? How do you deliver sterile irrigating solutions during patient treatment in your dental office/clinic?

4. Do you monitor the quality of the dental treatment water in your office/clinic? How do you accomplish this? Do you keep written records documenting the water monitoring? Why or why not?

5. What measures do you take to reduce the amount of potentially infectious spatter, mists, and aerosols in the dental operatory?

SELECTED READINGS

Dental Unit Water Lines

Barbeau J, Tanguay R, Faucher E, et al. Multiparametric analysis of waterline contamination in dental units. Appl Environ Microbiol 1996;62:3954–3959.

Bartoloni JA, Porteous NB, Zarzabal LA. Measuring the validity of two in-office water test kits. J Am Dent Assoc 2006;137:363–371.

Cohen ME, Harte JA, Stone ME, et al. Statistical modeling of dental unit–water bacterial test kit performance. J Clin Dent 2007;18:39–44.

Depaola LG, Mangan D, Mills SE, et al. A review of the science regarding dental unit waterlines. J Am Dent Assoc 2002;133:1199–1206.

Donlan RM. Biofilms: microbial life on surfaces. Emerg Infect Dis 2002;8:881–890.

Fotos PG, Westfall, HN, Snyder IS, et al. Prevalence of *Legionella*-specific IgG and IgM antibody in a dental clinic population. J Dent Res 1985;64:1382–1385.

Karpay RI, Plamondon TJ, Mills SE. Comparison of methods to enumerate bacteria in dental unit water lines. Curr Microbiol 1999;38:132–134.

Karpay RI, Plamondon TJ, Mills SE, et al. Validation of an in-office dental unit water monitoring technique. J Am Dent Assoc 1998;129:207–211.

Martin M. The significance of the bacterial contamination of dental water systems. Br Dent J 1987;163:152–153.

Mills S. The dental unit waterline controversy-defusing the myths, defining the solutions. J Am Dent Assoc 2000;131:1427–1441.

Mills SE. Waterborne pathogens and dental waterlines. Dent Clin North Am 2003;47:545–557.

Putnins EE, Di Giovanni D, Bhullar AS. Dental unit–waterline contamination and its possible implications during periodontal surgery. J Periodontol 2001;72:393–400.

Santiago JI, Huntington MK, Johnston AM, et al. Microbial contamination of dental unit waterlines: short- and long-term effects of flushing. Gen Dent 1994;42:528–544.

Shearer BG. Biofilm and the dental office [published erratum appears in J Am Dent Assoc 1996;127(4):436]. J Am Dent Assoc 1996;127(2):181–189.

Smith RS, Pineiro SA, Singh R, et al. Discrepancies in bacterial recovery from dental unit water samples on R2A medium and a commercial sampling device. Curr Microbiol 2004;48:243–246.

Williams HN, Kelley J, Folineo D, et al. Assessing microbial contamination in clean water dental units and compliance with disinfection protocol. J Am Dent Assoc 1994;125:1205–1211.

Williams JF, Johnston AM, Johnson B, et al. Microbial contamination of dental unit waterlines: prevalence, intensity, and microbiological characteristics. J Am Dent Assoc 1993;124:59–65.

Kohn WG, Collins AS, Cleveland JL, et al. Guidelines for infection control in dental healthcare settings—2003. MMWR Recomm Rep 2003;52:1–66.

Indoor Air Quality

ADA Council on Scientific Affairs; ADA Council on Dental Practice. Nitrous oxide in the dental office. J Am Dent Assoc 1997;128:364–365.

American Academy of Pediatric Dentistry Clinical Affairs Committee; American Academy of Pediatric Dentistry Council on Clinical Affairs. Policy on minimizing occupational health hazards associated with nitrous oxide. Pediatr Dent 2005;27:49–50.

Barnes JB, Harrel SK, Rivera-Hidalgo F. Blood contamination of the aerosols produced by in vivo use of ultrasonic scalers. J Periodontol 1998;69:434–438.

Bentley CD, Burkhart NW, Crawford JJ. Evaluating spatter and aerosol contamination during dental procedures. J Am Dent Assoc 1994;125:579–584.

Control of nitrous oxide in dental operatories. National Institute for Occupational Safety and Health. Appl Occup Environ Hyg 1999;14:218–220.

Drisko CL, Cochran DL, Blieden T, et al. Position paper: sonic and ultrasonic scalers in periodontics. Research, Science, and Therapy Committee of the American Academy of Periodontology. J Periodontol 2000;71:1792–1801.

Fine DH, Yip J, Furgang D, Barnett ML, et al. Reducing bacteria in dental aerosols: preprocedural use of an antiseptic mouthrinse. J Am Dent Assoc 1993;124:56–58.

Harrel SK, Barnes JB, Rivera-Hidalgo F. Aerosol and splatter contamination from the operative site during ultrasonic scaling. J Am Dent Assoc 1998;129:1241–1249.

Harrel SK, Molinari J. Aerosols and splatter in dentistry: a brief review of the literature and infection control implications. J Am Dent Assoc 2004;135:429–437.

Logothetis DD, Martinez-Welles JM. Reducing bacterial aerosol contamination with a chlorhexidine gluconate prerinse. J Am Dent Assoc 1995;126:1634–1639.

NIOSH. Control of nitrous oxide in dental operatories. Centers for Disease Control and Prevention, 1994.

NIOSH. Hazard Controls, Control of Nitrous Oxide in Dental Operatories. Centers for Disease Control and Prevention, 1998.

PART

II

Personal Protection

6

The Concept and Application of Standard Precautions

Helene Bednarsh

Kathy Eklund

John A. Molinari

LEARNING OBJECTIVES

After completion of this chapter individuals should be able to:

1 Distinguish between isolation (transmission-based), universal, and standard precautions.

2 Describe the evolution of infection-control practices in healthcare settings up to the current standard precautions.

3 Differentiate the roles of the Centers for Disease Control and Prevention (CDC) and the Occupational Safety and Health Administration (OSHA).

4 Discuss the modifications in CDC guideline recommendations.

Bloodborne pathogens: disease-producing microorganisms spread by contact with blood or other body fluids contaminated with blood from an infected person. Examples include hepatitis B virus (HBV), hepatitis C virus (HCV), and human immunodeficiency virus (HIV).

Bloodborne pathogens standard: a standard developed, promulgated, and enforced by OSHA directing employers to protect employees from occupational exposure to blood and other potentially infectious material.

Centers for Disease Control and Prevention (CDC): one of the 13 major operating components of the Department of Health and Human Services (HHS), which is the principal agency in the United States government for protecting the health and safety of all Americans and providing essential human services, especially for those people who are least able to help themselves.

Occupational Safety and Health Administration (OSHA): established in 1971, OSHA aims to ensure worker safety and health in the United States by working with employers and employees to create better working environments; setting and enforcing standards; providing training, outreach, and education; establishing partnerships; and encouraging continual improvements in workplace safety and health.

Standard precautions: universal precautions (UP) were based on the concept that all blood and all body fluids that

might be contaminated with blood should be treated as infectious because patients with bloodborne infections can be asymptomatic or unaware they are infected. The relevance of UP to other aspects of disease transmission was recognized, and in 1996 the CDC expanded the concept and changed the term to "standard precautions." Standard precautions integrate and expand the elements of UP into a standard of care designed to protect healthcare personnel (HCP) and patients from pathogens that can be spread by blood or any other body fluid, excretion, or secretion. Standard precautions apply to contact with (a) blood; (b) all body fluids, secretions, and excretions (except sweat), regardless of whether they contain blood; (c) nonintact skin; and (d) mucous membranes. Saliva has always been considered a potentially infectious material in dental infection control; thus, no operational difference exists in clinical dental practice between UP and standard precautions.

Transmission-based precautions: a set of practices that apply to patients with documented or suspected infection or colonization with highly transmissible or epidemiologically important pathogens for which precautions beyond the standard precautions are needed to interrupt transmission in healthcare settings.

Universal precautions (UP): set of practices and procedures based on the concept that all blood and all body fluids that might be contaminated with blood should be treated as infectious. (Also see Standard Precautions.)

Infection control is a critical component of quality dental care. The fundamental principle of infection control—to prevent disease transmission—provides the foundation for any infection-control guideline. Today infection-control guidelines are developed using an evidence-based approach that integrates scientific information; governmental and professional recommendations; federal, state, and local regulations; and practice-specific considerations. Infection-control guidelines can be used by individual healthcare practices and healthcare institutions to develop site/practice-specific policies and standard operating procedures (SOPs).

Prevention of infection and disease transmission has been a subject of medical research since the 1800s. As medical research became more formalized and the body of scientific literature concerning infectious disease increased, theories regarding infection control evolved. Early research identified methods to prevent transmission of infection and focused on the "behavior of healthcare professionals, expansion of infection control practice . . . and the increasing application of epidemiologic methods." The first strategy to prevent infections in

hospitals involved the quarantine of infectious patients. This strategy was followed by isolation precautions, **universal precautions (UP)**, blood and body fluid precautions, and, most recently, standard precautions. This chapter discusses the evolution of these precautions and the manner in which evidence of the efficacy of these interventions was used to develop current guidelines and recommendations. A comparison of the more recent precaution approaches since 1970 is presented in Table 6-1.

Infection-control precautions can be broken down into three main areas: (a) assumption-based, (b) isolation and/or transmission-based, and (c) universal/standard. These precautions evolved over time and are based in epidemiologic and applied sciences.

EVOLUTION OF ASSUMPTION-BASED INFECTION-CONTROL GUIDELINES

There is evidence that infection-control practices began as early as the 19th century, when a pharmacist published a paper stating that physicians and other persons

TABLE 6-1 Historical Summary of Isolation Precautions Used in Hospitals to Prevent Cross-Transmission of Infections, Particularly Bloodborne Infections, 1970 to Present

Characteristics	Blood Precautions	Blood and Body Substance Isolation	Universal Precautions	Body Substance Isolation	Standard Precautions (Current Recommendations)
Year published	1970	1983	1985, 1987, 1988	1987	1996, 2007
Purpose	To prevent cross-infection of patients and personnel from infection transmissible by contact with blood or items contaminated with blood.	To prevent infections transmitted by direct or indirect contact with infective blood or body fluids.	To prevent transmission of all bloodborne infectious diseases to people exposed in the course of their duties to blood from persons who may be infected with HIV.	To reduce cross-transmission of organisms among patients and to reduce caregiver exposure to moist body substances of patients.	To reduce the risk of transmission of blood-borne pathogens and the risk of transmission of pathogens from moist body substances.
Applicable population	Patients in the hospital with certain etiologic agents in their blood.	Patients in the hospital with infectious diseases that result in the production of infective blood or body fluids.	All patients, especially those in emergency-care settings. Also applicable in the workplace and other healthcare settings where invasive procedures are performed (such as dentistry, autopsies or morticians' services, dialysis), and laboratories.	All patients, whether or not infections have been identified.	All patients receiving care in hospitals, ambulatory care, long-term care, home care, and infusion services regardless of their diagnosis or presumed infection status.
Infective material	Blood.	Infective blood or body fluids.	Blood and other body fluids.	Any moist body substance.	Blood; all body fluids, secretions, and excretions, except sweat, regardless of whether or not they contain visible blood; nonintact skin; and mucous membranes.
Distinguishing features	Needle and syringe precautions to prevent accidental injury after their use on patients with certain bloodborne infections. Cap or bend needles and put into impervious bag.	Gloves indicated if touching blood or body fluids. Private room and gown necessary under certain conditions. Avoid needlestick injuries by disposing used needles in labeled puncture-resistant containers. Do not recap or bend needles before disposing.	Use appropriate barrier precautions to prevent skin and mucous membrane exposure when contact with blood or other body fluids of any patient is anticipated.	Wear gloves for anticipated contact with blood, secretions, mucous membranes, nonintact skin, and moist body substances for all patients. Use additional barriers to keep moist body substances off the skin, clothing, and particularly the mucous membranes.	Synthesizes the major features of UP and BSI, and is the recommended strategy for preventing nosocomial infections (referred to as healthcare-associated infections in 2007) because of cross-transmission. To be used in conjunction with transmission-based precautions for patients documented or suspected to be infected with highly transmissible or epidemiologically important pathogens.

(Adapted from Emori, TG. Isolation Systems. *APIC TEXT of Infection Control and Epidemiology*, 2000. Association for Professionals in Infection Control and Epidemiology, Inc., Washington, DC, 2000.)

attending patients with contagious disease should moisten their hands with a liquid chloride solution. This was based on the assumption that contamination led to infection, and infection to disease and potentially death. Early attempts at infection control during the delivery of healthcare relied on strategies to prevent transmission of infections. These strategies were based less on methodological research and more on observations or coincidental circumstances.

Oliver Wendell Holmes was the first to apply "clinical epidemiologic methods to examine a causal association [between diseases] and the practices of healthcare professionals." As a result of his observations and investigation, he surmised that birth attendants spread puerperal fever. Even though the exact mechanism was not known, once hand contamination was removed there was less detectable infection. This intervention subsequently led to less illness and lower mortality. Holmes's theory also predated both Pasteur's germ theory and Semmelweis's theories on hand hygiene.

As mentioned above, the practice of cleaning hands with an antiseptic agent probably began in the early 19th century. In 1822, a French pharmacist reported that solutions containing chlorides of lime or soda could eradicate the foul odors associated with human corpses, and that such solutions could be used as disinfectants and antiseptics. In a paper published in 1825, this pharmacist stated that physicians and other persons attending patients with contagious diseases would benefit from moistening their hands with a liquid chloride solution. Later, in 1846, Ignaz Semmelweis was the first to observe and report health outcomes associated with antiseptic hand cleansing. An intervention trial using historical controls demonstrated in 1847 that the mortality rate among mothers who delivered in the First Obstetrics Clinic at the General Hospital of Vienna was substantially lower when hospital staff cleaned their hands with an antiseptic agent than when they washed their hands with plain soap and water. He observed that women whose babies were delivered by students and physicians in the First Clinic at the General Hospital of Vienna consistently had a higher mortality rate than those whose babies were delivered by midwives in the Second Clinic. Semmelweis observed that physicians who went directly from the autopsy suite to the obstetrics ward had a disagreeable odor on their hands despite washing their hands with soap and water upon entering the obstetrics clinic. He postulated that the puerperal fever that affected so many parturient women was caused by "cadaverous particles" transmitted from the autopsy suite to the obstetrics ward via the hands of students and physicians. Perhaps because of the known deodorizing effect of chlorine compounds, in May of 1847 he insisted that students and physicians clean their hands with a chlorine solution between each patient contact in the clinic. The maternal mortality rate in the First Clinic subsequently dropped

dramatically and remained low for years. This intervention by Semmelweis represents the first evidence indicating that cleansing heavily contaminated hands with an antiseptic agent between patient contacts may reduce healthcare-associated transmission of contagious diseases more effectively than hand washing with plain soap and water.

In 1843, Oliver Wendell Holmes concluded, independently of Semmelweis, that puerperal fever was spread by the hands of healthcare personnel. Although Semmelweis and Holmes described procedures that could be taken to limit the spread of infection, their recommendations had little impact on obstetrics practices at the time. Gradually, however, these seminal studies by Semmelweis and Holmes began a movement in healthcare infection-control guidance. Hand washing became accepted as one of the most important measures for preventing transmission of pathogens in healthcare facilities.

EVOLUTION OF ISOLATION OR TRANSMISSION-BASED GUIDELINES

Quarantine was another measure of infection control in the mid to late 1800s. In 1877, placing patients with infectious disease in separate facilities, commonly referred to as quarantine, had become a common recommendation and practice. It was assumed that isolating sick people who shared certain symptoms from those without the symptoms would somehow manage the spread of disease. However, this practice of separating patients with contagious diseases from noncontagious patients failed to stop the transmission of microbial infections. Transmission continued to occur because patients were not separated or segregated according to specific diseases, and few if any aseptic practices were followed. By the late 1960s, most infectious-disease hospitals had closed, and patients were placed in either individual rooms or disease-specific wards.

In 1970, the **Centers for Disease Control and Prevention (CDC)** published "Isolation Techniques for Use in Hospitals," which was later revised in 1975. These guidelines recommended that hospitals use one of several categories of isolation (e.g., Respiratory Isolation, Protective Isolation, Enteric Precautions, and Blood Precautions), none of which were rigorously evaluated for their effectiveness in preventing transmission of infections or their cost-effectiveness. In addition, isolation precautions relied heavily on being able to identify patients with an infectious disease and were not always a safeguard against the spread of infection.

With regard to **bloodborne pathogens** such as HBV, HIV, and HCV, infection-control precautions are not based solely on recent risks for HBV as described in the 1970s and HIV since the early 1980s. Transmission of bloodborne infections was documented even before some other occupational pathogens were isolated and identified. Examples include instances of major breaches in infection control linked to transmission of HBV and what is now known as HCV. One such example occurred during World War II. A campaign of mass inoculation within the military was linked to transmission of HBV because of the failure to routinely change needles during vaccination of recruits. Another example occurred in Egypt, where the high prevalence of HCV, and possibly HBV, has been linked to the use of parenteral antischistomal therapy (PAT), which was practiced from the 1960s through the early 1980s. PAT involved a form of mass inoculation, and there is a high probability that contaminated injection devices spread the disease.

During subsequent decades, more attention was given to disease-specific epidemiology and how this affected decisions for isolation precautions as an approach to interrupt the spread of infection. During this time, hospitals were also reporting new nosocomial infection issues. The CDC described these as being caused by newly recognized pathogens, or drug-resistant organisms. It also was suggested that commonly used isolation precautions might not have been appropriate and that modifications were indicated. For example, Blood Precautions became Blood and Body Fluid Precautions, and were expanded to include other potentially infectious fluids besides blood. Persons with AIDS were a group of target patients for this series of precautions. The concept of Protective Isolation was replaced with categories of isolation. Other recommendations and guidelines were also updated as new epidemiologic data became available.

CDC Guidelines and Universal Precautions

In 1985, epidemiologic evidence involving bloodborne pathogens supported the development and implementation of new infection-control precautions. In part because of the availability of the hepatitis B vaccine and health professionals' concerns regarding the HIV/AIDS epidemic, healthcare emphasis changed from isolation to UP. Evidence of subclinical or asymptomatic infection with HBV and HIV made it clear that medical history and examination were not reliable tools for identifying all patients with potentially infectious bloodborne pathogens. The concept of UP applied Blood and Body Fluid Precautions to *all* patients, regardless of their infection status. Reports of hospital personnel acquiring HIV through needlestick and other accidents with contaminated sharps spurred a renewed emphasis on preventing percutaneous injuries, along with the routine use of gloves, masks, protective eyewear, and other personal protective equipment to prevent mucous membrane exposures. Later CDC recommendations emphasized that blood was the most important source of HIV and HBV transmission. Hepatitis B immunization and UP, such as engineering, work practice, and administrative

controls, were able to prevent blood contact, and thus were determined to be the best protective strategies.

Specific infection-control precautions for dentistry were first published by the CDC in 1986 in "Recommended Infection Control Practices for Dentistry," and later updated in 1993. Before dental-specific guidelines were established, protection from bloodborne disease transmission in dental facilities was addressed within guidelines for other healthcare groups (i.e., medical) and consisted of a few sentences to a few paragraphs. Early recommendations were not very specific. The 1986 guidelines represented a major step in the evolution of dental-specific recommendations to prevent the transmission of disease in dental facilities. These recommendations were based on the concept of UP, were specific to bloodborne routes of disease transmission, and were procedurally based. As early as 1983 it was expected that dental healthcare personnel (DHCP) would no longer place their bare hands into a body cavity, but after 1983 and indeed by 1986, there was epidemiological and clinical evidence to support this and other appropriate preventive practices. The use of effective healthcare work practices, the safety of the instruments and devices used to deliver care, and the use of personal protective equipment and other barriers became minimum standards for infection control in dental facilities.

In 1987, Body Substance Isolation (BSI) was introduced to allow an increased focus on moist and potentially infectious body fluids from all patients regardless of their known or suspected infection status. The primary focus of BSI was on the use of gloves. Unlike UP, however, hand washing was not emphasized. In addition, there were no protective provisions for diseases transmitted by routes other than bloodborne (i.e., contact, droplet, and airborne transmission).

Occupational Safety and Health Administration (OSHA) Regulations

It is sometimes assumed that the **OSHA Bloodborne Pathogens Standard** was a result of the discovery of the HIV/AIDS epidemic and its potential risks to healthcare personnel. The actual impetus was HBV infection risks for healthcare personnel and the availability of a hepatitis B vaccine since 1982. Unions representing healthcare workers petitioned OSHA requesting an emergency temporary standard under the General Duty Clause. This clause requires employers to have a workplace free from recognized harm and, in this particular instance, to protect employees from HBV transmission. The unions requested that OSHA require employers to provide the HBV vaccination free of charge. Instead of issuing an emergency temporary standard for the vaccine only, OSHA began what was to be a 5-year process to develop a standard to protect healthcare workers from risks associated with bloodborne disease transmission.

In 1991, following a series of public hearings, OSHA published the Bloodborne Pathogens Standard based on the UP concept introduced in 1986. The final standard was published on December 6, 1991, and went into effect in early 1992. It has since been amended, as discussed further below. The 1991 standard imposed obligations on employers to provide safe and healthful work environments for all healthcare employees. Requirements to protect employees included work practice controls, engineering controls, personal protective equipment, and administrative controls. Such controls in the dental setting can be described as:

1. Work practice controls relating to the manner in which a task is performed and advising the use of safer work practices designed to minimize the risk of disease transmission.

2. Engineering controls that are technology-based and refer to items or instruments that isolate a hazard, such as a sharps disposal container.

3. Personal protective equipment, including gloves, masks, protective eyewear, and protective clothing (e.g., long-sleeved gowns), to prevent contamination of the individual during the delivery of oral healthcare services.

4. Administrative controls that represent the policies, procedures, and practices within a dental facility to reduce risks associated with bloodborne disease transmission.

In 2001, revisions to OSHA's Bloodborne Pathogens Standard became effective as mandated by the Needlestick Safety and Prevention Act of 2000. The revisions clarified the need for employers to consider safer needle devices as they become available, and to involve employees who are directly responsible for patient care (e.g., dentists, hygienists, and dental assistants) in identifying and choosing such devices.

It is important to realize that OSHA and the CDC are two completely different governmental agencies with different mandates. In differentiating OSHA from CDC publications that relate to healthcare, the CDC develops guidelines designed to protect both the patient and the healthcare personnel, while OSHA regulations apply only to the latter. Also, guidelines published by the CDC or other advisory agencies do not carry the weight of law that a regulatory agency such as OSHA has. OSHA also relies on appropriate authorities, including the CDC, as they formulate standards. Thus, it is important to be aware of updates or changes to recommended infection-control practices to remain in compliance with OSHA regulations. Therefore, as either a standard of practice or a matter of law, it is incumbent upon DHCP to become familiar with the new guidelines and seek to incorporate the recommendations as indicated. In summary, OSHA has the authority to require and enforce compliance with recommended infection-control practices and procedures.

CURRENT CDC GUIDELINES AND STANDARD PRECAUTIONS

In the past several years, the structure of published guidelines has continued to evolve to include, whenever possible, evidence-based recommendations, linkages to other "like" guidelines, and consistency with other published guidelines, regulations, and recommendations. Most recommendations are ranked according to categories of existing scientific data, theoretical rationale, and opinions of experts. Guidelines, as defined for clinical practice by the Institute of Medicine (IOM), should be "systematically developed statements to assist practitioner and patient decisions about appropriate healthcare for specific clinical circumstances." Mindful of the fact that not all guidelines are clinical in nature, the IOM expanded the definition to include public health circumstances to assist policy makers, health agencies, and others as well.

Before 1996, guidelines were developed by panels of experts, were narrative in design, and contained random errors and other bias. The current approach used by the CDC is to use systematic reviews to attempt to reduce bias. The CDC has guidelines prepared by a supervised, recognized group or committee that writes or at least approves a guideline. Recommendations should be based on evidence from available literature. Furthermore, in determining when to update a guideline, it is important to consider new evidence and to establish a research agenda. Finally, in 1996 the development of new guidelines attempted to minimize bias by undergoing a transition to use evidence-based information and policy.

The most current CDC recommendations for dental infection control were released on December 19, 2003, and were entitled "Guidelines for Infection Control in Dental Health-care Settings–2003." Since the previous update for dental infection control in 1993, the landscape had changed in knowledge, practice, devices, epidemiology, and the format of guidelines development. Therefore, dental professionals should note these differences. The rationale for published recommendations is more detailed than in past guidelines and is reflected in the range of recommendations. The 2003 CDC guidelines use five categories to rank specific recommendations:

Category IA: Strongly recommended for implementation and strongly supported by well-designed experimental, clinical, or epidemiologic studies.

Category IB: Strongly recommended for implementation and supported by experimental, clinical, or epidemiologic studies and a strong theoretical rationale.

Category IC: Required for implementation, as mandated by federal or state regulation or standard. When IC is used, a second rating can be included to provide the basis of existing scientific data, theoretical rationale, and applicability. Because of state differences, the reader should not assume that the absence of a IC designation implies the absence of state regulations.

Category II: Suggested for implementation and supported by suggestive clinical or epidemiologic studies or a theoretical rationale.

Unresolved issue: No recommendation. Insufficient evidence or no consensus regarding efficacy exists.

Commensurate with the design of the new generation of guidelines, recommendations from other appropriate CDC infection-control guidelines, such as those for environmental infection control and hand hygiene, are currently incorporated into one comprehensive document. Other significant issues are also addressed in this update that were not included in earlier guidelines, including the use of lasers and considerations for protection against prions.

A change in terminology is evident when one compares the 2003 CDC guidelines with those published earlier. The 1986 and 1993 CDC dental infection-control guidelines focused on the risk of transmission of bloodborne pathogens among dental health professionals and patients, and recommended the use of UP to reduce that risk. UP were based on the concept that all blood and all body fluids that might be contaminated with blood should be treated as infectious, because patients with bloodborne infections can be asymptomatic or unaware they are infected. Preventive practices used to reduce blood exposures, particularly percutaneous exposures, include (i) careful handling of sharp instruments, (ii) use of rubber dams to minimize blood spattering, (iii) hand washing, and (iv) use of protective barriers (e.g., gloves, masks, protective eyewear, and gowns).

The CDC recognized the relevance of UP to other aspects of non-bloodborne disease transmission, and in 1996 the CDC expanded the concept and changed the term to **standard precautions**. Standard precautions integrate and expand the elements of UP into a standard of care designed to protect healthcare personnel and patients from pathogens that can be spread by blood or any other body fluid, excretion, or secretion. Standard precautions apply to contact with (i) blood; (ii) all body fluids, secretions, and excretions (except sweat), regardless of whether they contain blood; (iii) nonintact skin; and (iv) mucous membranes. Because saliva has always been considered a potentially infectious material in dental infection control by the CDC and OSHA, no operational difference exists in clinical dental practice between UP and standard precautions.

Standard precautions apply to all patients. As mentioned above, they are designed to integrate and expand UP to include:

- organisms spread by blood and also body fluids, secretions, and excretions, whether or not they contain blood
- nonintact or broken skin
- mucous membranes

The major elements of standard precautions include:

- hand washing
- use of gloves, eye and face protection (mask, eyewear, and face shields), and gowns
- aseptic management of patient-care equipment
- environmental infection control
- injury prevention and management
- respiratory hygiene/cough etiquette
- safe injection practices

Although the 2003 CDC guidelines use the term "standard precautions" to replace UP, to date OSHA still continues to use the term "universal precautions." This is because the Bloodborne Pathogens Standard specifically applies to the prevention and management of exposure to blood and serum body fluids and related substances that may be contaminated with bloodborne pathogens, such as HIV, HBV, and HCV.

The CDC also provides guidance for **transmission-based precautions** in addition to standard precautions. Transmission-based precautions might be necessary to prevent the potential spread of certain diseases (e.g., tuberculosis, influenza, and varicella) that are transmitted through airborne transmission, droplets, or contact transmission (e.g., sneezing, coughing, and contact with skin). When acutely ill with these diseases, patients do not usually seek routine dental outpatient care. Nonetheless, a general understanding of precautions for diseases transmitted by all routes is critical because (a) some dental care providers are hospital-based or work part-time in hospital settings, (b) patients infected with these diseases might seek urgent treatment at outpatient dental offices, and (c) DHCP might become infected with these diseases. Necessary transmission-based precautions might include patient placement (e.g., isolation), adequate room ventilation, respiratory protection (e.g., N-95 masks) for dental personnel, or postponement of non-emergency dental procedures.

SUMMARY

An important lesson to be learned from the previous discussion is that it is imperative for dental professionals to review individual state laws and consult with their Board of Registration in Dentistry to determine their legal obligations concerning infection-control guidelines and regulations. Although it has been noted that the CDC is not a regulatory agency, many state boards have adopted CDC infection-control recommendations into their practice acts and/or states have legislated compliance with current United States Public Health Service guidelines. This was illustrated in the autumn of 1993 when Massachusetts adopted the obligation to comply with the 1993 CDC dental infection-control recommendations and all future updates as published by the CDC.

At a minimum, a dental facility should review and revise its infection-control policies and procedures, and update its exposure control plan (ECP). An ECP must be updated annually and any time there is a significant change in knowledge, practices, or policy. These new guidelines present a unique opportunity for all staff members to review the manner in which they deliver dental services and to implement recommended measures that can minimize further the already low risk of disease transmission in dental settings.

✓ Practical Dental Infection-Control Checklist

Program Administration

❑ Does the dental office/clinic have a written infection-control program for DHCP to prevent or reduce the risk of disease transmission that includes

   ❑ establishment and implementation of policies, procedures, and practices (in conjunction with the selection and use of technologies and products) to prevent work-related injuries and illnesses among DHCP, and

   ❑ healthcare-associated infections among patients?

❑ Does the infection-control program:

   ❑ embody the principles of infection control and occupational health,

   ❑ reflect current science, and

   ❑ adhere to relevant federal, state, and local regulations and statutes?

❑ Does the dental office/clinic have access to the most current copies of the

   ❑ CDC dental infection-control guidelines (available by visiting http://www.cdc.gov/oralhealth)?

   ❑ OSHA regulations (both federal OSHA [available by visiting http://www.osha.gov] and if applicable, state OSHA)?

   ❑ Appropriate state and local requirements (e.g., state dental board requirements)?

❑ Are standard precautions used for all patient encounters?

   ❑ Are transmission-based precautions applied when patients requiring additional precautions receive treatment in the dental office/clinic?

❑ Does the dental office/clinic have a written exposure control plan (ECP)?

❑ Does the dental office/clinic have an assigned infection-control coordinator (e.g., dentist or other DHCP) who is knowledgeable, or willing to be trained, managing the program?

Personnel Health Elements of an Infection-Control Program

❑ Does the dental office/clinic have a written health program for DHCP including policies, procedures, and guidelines for

   ❑ education and training;

   ❑ immunizations;

   ❑ exposure prevention;

   ❑ postexposure management;

   ❑ medical conditions, work-related illness, and associated work restrictions;

   ❑ contact dermatitis and latex hypersensitivity; and

   ❑ maintenance of records, data management, and confidentiality?

Review Questions

1. OSHA develops regulations to protect the employee. The CDC develops guidelines to protect both the patient and the healthcare worker.

   A. The first statement is true. The second statement is false.

   B. The first statement is false. The second statement is true.

   C. Both statements are true.

   D. Both statements are false.

2. OSHA's Bloodborne Pathogen Standard requires employers to protect employees by implementing

   A. Work practice controls.

   B. Engineering controls.

   C. Personal protective equipment.

   D. Administrative controls.

   E. A, B, and C.

   F. All of the above.

3. Which of the following is true regarding standard infection-control precautions?

   A. Standard precautions are strategies used to reduce the risk of transmission of pathogens in the healthcare setting.

   B. Standard precautions should be used in caring for all patients, regardless of their infectious status.

   C. Transmission-based precautions are used beyond standard precautions to interrupt the spread of certain pathogens.

   D. Standard precautions apply to exposure to blood, all body fluids and secretions (except sweat), nonintact skin, and mucous membranes.

   E. All of the above.

   F. None of the above.

4. The major elements of standard precautions include

A. Hand washing.

B. Using personal protective equipment.

C. Environmental infection control.

D. Injury prevention and injury management.

E. A and B.

F. All of the above.

Critical Thinking

1. Does your dental office/clinic have a copy of the most current:

   a. OSHA Bloodborne Pathogens Standard?

   b. CDC Guidelines for Infection Control in Dental Healthcare Settings?

2. Are these documents readily accessible to all employees?

3. Do you use standard precautions for all patient encounters? What are the major elements of standard precautions?

4. Does your office have a written infection-control policy in your office/clinic? Do you know where it is located? When was the last time it was updated?

5. Do you have a written ECP in your office/clinic? When was the last time it was updated? Is it updated at least once a year?

SELECTED READINGS

CDC. CDC guidelines: improving the quality. Atlanta, GA: CDC; 1996.

CDC. Guidelines for infection control in dental health-care settings–2003. MMWR 2003;52(RR-17):1–66.

CDC. Guidelines for prevention of transmission of human immunodeficiency virus and hepatitis B virus to health-care and public-safety workers: a response to P.L. 100-607 The Health Omnibus Programs Extension Act of 1988. MMWR 1989;38(suppl 6S).

CDC. Hospital infection control practices advisory committee. Part 1. Evolution of isolation practices. Atlanta, GA: CDC; 1997.

CDC. Isolation techniques for use in hospitals. 2nd ed. HHS publication no. (CDC) 80-8314. Washington, DC: U.S. Government Printing Office; 1975.

CDC. Perspectives in disease prevention and health promotion update: universal precautions for prevention of transmission of human immunodeficiency virus, hepatitis B virus, and other bloodborne pathogens in health-care settings. MMWR 1988;38:377–382, 387–388.

CDC. Recommendations for preventing transmission of infection with human T-lymphotropic virus type III/ lymphadenopathy-associated virus during invasive procedures. MMWR 1985;34:681–695.

CDC. Recommendations for prevention of HIV transmission in health-care settings. MMWR 1987;36(suppl 2S)1S–19S.

CDC. Recommended infection control practices for dentistry, 1993. MMWR 1993;41(RR-8):1–12.

CDC. Recommended infection control practices for dentistry. MMWR 1986;35:237–242.

CDC. Update: universal precautions for prevention of transmission of human immunodeficiency virus, hepatitis B virus, and other bloodborne pathogens in health-care settings. MMWR 1988;37:377–382, 387–388.

Frank C, Mohamed K, Lavanchy D, et al. The role of parental antischistomal therapy in the spread of hepatitis C virus in Egypt. Lancet 2000;355:887–891.

Garner JS. Hospital infection control practices advisory committee. Guideline for isolation precautions in hospitals. Infect Control Hosp Epidemiol 1996;17: 53–80.

Garner JS, Favero MS. CDC guideline for handwashing and hospital environmental control, 1985. Infect Control 1986;7:231–243.

IOM (Institute of Medicine). Clinical Practice Guidelines: Directions for a New Program. Washington, DC: National Academy Press; 1992.

Labarraque AG. Instructions and Observations Regarding the Chlorides of Soda and Lime [in French]. New Haven, CT: Baldwin and Treaway; 1829.

Larson E. A retrospective on infection control. Part 1: Nineteenth century—consumed by fire. Am J Infect Control 1997;25:236–241.

Larson E. A retrospective on infection control. Part 2: Twentieth century—the flame burns. Am J Infect Control 1997;25:340–349.

Lynch T. Communicable Disease Nursing. St. Louis, MO: Mosby; 1949.

National Communicable Disease Center. Isolation Techniques for Use in Hospitals. PHS publication 2054. Washington, DC: U.S. Government Printing Office; 1970.

Rotter M. Hand washing and hand disinfection. In: Mayhall CG, ed. Hospital Epidemiology and Infection Control. 2nd ed. Philadelphia, PA: Lippincott Williams & Wilkins, 1999.

Semmelweis I. Etiology, Concept, and Prophylaxis of Childbed Fever. Madison, WI: University of Wisconsin Press; 1983.

Siegel JD, Rhinehart E, Jackson M, et al; and the Healthcare Infection Control Practices Advisory Committee. Guideline for isolation precautions: preventing transmission of infectious agents in healthcare settings. CDC 2007:1–219.

United States Dept. of Labor, Occupational Safety and Health Administration, 29 CFR Part 1910.1030 occupational exposure to bloodborne pathogens, final rule. Fed Regist 1991;56:64174–64182.

United States Dept. of Labor, Occupational Safety, and Health Administration 29, CFR part 1910.1030 occupational exposure to bloodborne pathogens; needlestick and other sharps injuries, final rule. Fed Regist 2001;66;5317–5325. [As amended from and includes Fed Regist 1991, 29 CFR Part 1910.1030.]

7

Immunizations for Dental Healthcare Personnel

John A. Molinari

Géza T. Terézhalmy

LEARNING OBJECTIVES

After completion of this chapter individuals should be able to:

1 Comprehend the historical role vaccines have played in the prevention of infectious diseases.

2 Understand the principles of immunization as applied to currently available vaccines.

3 Describe the major categories of vaccine preparations.

4 Discuss updated scientific and clinical knowledge concerning current vaccine recommendation for healthcare professionals.

5 Be aware of the most current vaccination recommendations for dental healthcare personnel (DHCP).

Active immunization: see vaccination.

Attenuated (live) vaccines: preparations derived from live, wild-type, disease-causing microorganisms. They are modified in vitro by repeated culturing with resultant weakening of their virulence before their use in immunization. After vaccination into immune-competent hosts they are able to replicate in the body for a period of time, but do not cause disease.

Cellular immunity (cell-mediated immunity): immune responses and effects caused sensitized lymphocytes or activated macrophages.

Humoral immunity: immunity because of specific immunoglobulins (i.e., antibodies) in blood or other tissues.

Immunization: the act of artificially inducing immunity or providing protection against a disease.

Inactivated (killed) vaccines: produced by growing bacteria or viruses in vitro and then inactivating the whole organisms with chemicals or heat. They cannot replicate in the body after administration as an immunizing agent.

Product vaccine: detoxified antigenic products produced by bacteria that are used in certain vaccine regimens. Detoxification of microbial exotoxins with formalin yields a toxoid that is used for immunization.

Subunit (component) vaccines: preparations used for immunization that use a portion of the bacteria or virus that is able to stimulate host protective immunity.

Vaccination (or immunization): the act of artificially inducing immunity against a disease.

Vaccine: an administered immunologic preparation that stimulates the body's immune system to produce protective humoral immunity (antibodies) or cell-mediated immunity (sensitized T lymphocytes), or both against a disease.

INTRODUCTION

One of the earliest infection-control milestones occurred near the end of the 18th century, more than a half century before Lister's revolutionary investigations of asepsis and hand washing were conducted. This achievement in 1796 involved the successful introduction of vaccination as an effective way to prevent disease. Dr. Edward Jenner was an English physician who had observed that milk maids who contracted cowpox from milking infected dairy cows did not develop smallpox during outbreaks of the deadly disease that periodically ravaged the English countryside. Subsequently, Jenner was able to induce similar protective immunity by transferring vesicular fluid from cowpox lesions on milk maids' hands into the skin of unprotected recipients. These subjects did not develop smallpox when the disease reappeared in the surrounding area. By 1800, approximately 6,000 people had been administered purulent material from similar cowpox lesions, with resultant protection against smallpox. This induced protection against one of the most feared infectious scourges and introduced the "era of immunization." After publication of his work in 1798, Jenner was forever credited as being the first to control an infectious disease by using procedures that did not transmit the disease (i.e., vaccination).

Widespread use of **vaccines** as a major public health innovation has proven to be extremely successful in protecting the population from many childhood and adult infectious diseases. By the end of the 20th century, the benefits were so dramatic in reducing the incidence of many previously common infections that the Centers for Disease Control and Prevention (CDC) cited **vaccination** as the number one public health achievement of the century. This impact against vaccine-preventable diseases is summarized in Table 7-1. Of these, the greatest achievement to date has been the global eradication of smallpox as a human infectious disease.

Routine **immunization** has become an integral part of pediatric preventive medicine, and although the incidence of many vaccine-preventable diseases has been reduced significantly by childhood immunization, they have not been eliminated. Today, a substantial percentage of the remaining morbidity and mortality from several of these diseases occurs in adults or older adolescents. Adults who escaped natural infection or immunization as children are at increased risk for measles, rubella, mumps, and poliomyelitis. Protection against tetanus and diphtheria after childhood vaccination needs to be boosted every 10 years, whereas other immunizations, such as influenza vaccines, are indicated primarily for adults.

Despite the availability of safe and effective vaccines, many adults still acquire vaccine-preventable diseases. For example, each year an estimated 50,000 adults die of complications from *Streptococcus pneumoniae* infection, influenza virus infection, and hepatitis B virus (HBV) disease. Various reports have identified multiple barriers to achievement of high vaccination levels among adults, including (a) missed opportunities to vaccinate during contacts with healthcare providers for unrelated office visits; (b) lack of perceived risk to vaccine-preventable diseases; (c) mistaken perception that vaccine-preventa-

TABLE 7-1 Decrease in Cases of Vaccine-Preventable Diseases in the United States Through 1998 as Reported by the CDC*

Disease	No. of Cases		Reduction (%)
	Baseline[†]	1998	
Smallpox	48,164	0	100
Diphtheria	175,885	0	100
Pertussis	147,271	7,405	95
Tetanus	1,314	41	97.9
Paralytic polio	16,316	0	100
Measles	503,282	100	100
Mumps	152,209	666	99.6
Rubella	47,745	364	99.3
Haemophilus influenzae type b	20,000	63	99.7

*Reported in CDC. Impact of vaccines universally recommended for children—United States, 1990–1998. MMWR 1999;48:243–248.
[†]Baseline = 20th century annual prevaccine infection rate.

ble diseases have been virtually eliminated from many developed countries, especially the United States; and (d) patient and provider fears concerning adverse events after vaccination. In contrast, vaccination regimens against hepatitis B and influenza have been associated positively with a history of vaccinations, evidence-based recommendations by the CDC and other health professional agencies for hepatitis B and influenza vaccinations, and an expressed response by healthcare professionals and others at risk to comply with published recommendations.

Healthcare workers are at particular risk for several vaccine-preventable diseases. Responsible professional organizations have been obligated to educate, continuously inform, and provide balanced assessments of benefits, costs, and risks on the antigens that are recommended routinely for the immunization of healthcare personnel. Expansion of earlier recommendations was accomplished in 1997 when the CDC published comprehensive immunization recommendations for all healthcare workers. Updated recommendations for DHCP were provided in the CDC *Guidelines for Infection Control in Dental Health-care Settings*–2003.

PRINCIPLES OF IMMUNIZATION

Immunization is the act of artificially inducing immunity or providing protection against disease. A person can become immune to a microbial disease by one of three mechanisms. They can (a) develop a symptomatic or asymptomatic infection and recover with their immune system actively producing a protective immune response (i.e., natural active immunity); (b) receive injection(s) of antibodies from an immune person to prevent onset of infection (i.e., artificial passive immunity); and (c) be administered a specific antigen and have their immune system stimulated to produce an immune response without manifesting disease (i.e., artificial active immunity).

Artificial passive immunization does not stimulate the person's own immune system. The classic form of this immune procedure is the use of whole human serum or hyperimmune human globulin to treat or prevent certain infectious diseases. The basic premise involves injection of antibodies from an immune person into a nonimmune host. The antibody preparation is obtained from donors who have either recovered from a clinical or subclinical microbial disease, or been immunized by vaccination. The rationale is that the transferred immunoglobulins will help inactivate or clear the infectious agent or toxin from the recipient's body before symptomatic or asymptomatic infection results. Passive immunization is almost always performed after a nonimmune individual has been exposed to a specific disease (e.g., after possible exposure to tetanus). The exogenously administered antibodies are thus immediately available to protect the recipient, thereby filling the gap between the exposure to antigen and the appearance of a protective response. However, because the injected antibodies can be rapidly cleared from the system, the recipient's own immune apparatus may not have time to respond. Passive immunity provides protection against some diseases; however, it is only temporary in that the antibody concentrations typically decline rapidly within 14 to 28 days. The previous description is different from the most common form of passive immunization, termed "natural passive immunity." In this instance a fetus or an infant receives immunoglobulins from the mother. The immunoglobulins cross the placenta during the last trimester of pregnancy and can provide protection from certain diseases for at least 3 to 4 months postpartum.

With regard to **active immunization**, the immune system is able to develop antigen-specific **humoral immunity** (antibodies or immunoglobulins) or **cell-mediated immunity** sensitized CD4+ T lymphocytes after administration of a specific antigen. A critical factor in applying active immunization principles is to use antigens that do not cause illness, yet are immunologically identical or similar to the disease-causing agent in nature. Once artificial active immunization has been mounted against the relatively innocuous vaccine antigen, the expectation is that little or no clinical infection will develop when virulent microorganisms are encountered by the vaccinated individual. The use of vaccines is also the preferred approach for disease prevention because in addition to stimulating protective antibodies or sensitized T cells, vaccination produces immunologic memory that can last for many years post-vaccination. This concept has been shown to be valid in controlling many serious infectious diseases. It should also be stressed that active immunization is most effective when instituted before an individual is exposed to the natural disease or its etiologic agent. The primary emphasis of this chapter will focus on this form of immunization for healthcare professionals.

PROPERTIES OF AN IDEAL VACCINE

The development and preparation of vaccines strive to meet basic requirements for an ideal preparation (Table 7-2). First and foremost, a vaccine must be proven safe for human use. The basic rule of "do no harm" applies to immunizations as it does to health professionals. Ongoing monitoring and assessment of possible vaccine-related adverse effects continue long after any vaccine has been tested in trials and received governmental clearance for administration to the population. Vaccine safety is therefore a primary evaluation factor. All healthcare professionals should be aware of ongoing vaccine evaluations by the CDC and other public health agencies. This is an important aspect of being a health professional, so appropriate scientific and clinical information can be provided to those who inquire about vaccine safety.

Although vaccinations are among the most widely used preventive measures against many infectious diseases, no vaccine is perfect and adverse effects do occur. Although vaccines today are remarkably safe, effective, and free of major adverse effects, frequent minor local irritations and extremely rare severe systemic illnesses have been reported. The National Childhood Vaccine

TABLE 7-2 Properties and Requirements of an Ideal Vaccine

- Safe
- Immunogenic: stimulating the proper type of host immune response
- Provide lifelong immunity
- Require only a single administration
- Should not induce side effects
- Should be nonallergenic
- Nonimmunosuppressive: should not make recipient more susceptible to other diseases
- Inexpensive

Injury Act of 1986 requires that healthcare providers report to the United States Department of Health and Human Services postimmunization events serious enough to require medical attention.

The overwhelming majority are relatively minor, including injection site soreness, temporary myalgia, fatigue, and fever. Information is continuously collected on suspected vaccine-related side effects in an effort to weigh risks versus benefits. In a few instances, vaccines have been removed from the marketplace and reformulated in an effort to significantly reduce real or perceived adverse reactions. One such example involved an earlier form of the pertussis (i.e., whooping cough) vaccine for children. Immunization originally used a vaccine composed of killed *Bordetella pertussis*. This preparation was highly effective in dramatically reducing the incidence of disease; however, rare toxicity reactions caused several parents to refuse vaccination for their children. The current acellular pertussis vaccine made up of purified microbial components and detoxified pertussis toxin has greatly reduced the incidence of adverse effects and is well accepted. The efficacy of immune protection with the acellular vaccine is comparable to the whole cell vaccine and the incidence of adverse effects after receipt of the acellular preparation is significantly lower than after administration of the whole cell vaccine. A second example involved the live, **attenuated** rotavirus vaccine. As will be discussed in the following section, attenuated strains of viruses have been treated to greatly reduce their pathogenicity and yet still be able to replicate in the vaccinated host for a period of time for enhanced immune stimulation. In the case of the rotavirus vaccine, rare instances of an intestinal obstruction were noted after the preparation passed the trial period and the vaccine was withdrawn within 2 years after being licensed.

The immunogenicity of a vaccine is fundamentally important if protection against a specific disease is going to develop in an immunized host. The preparation must not only use the microbial antigen(s) that will protect against infection and disease but also be administered via a route that will stimulate the host to produce artificial active immunity post-immunization. The number of times a vaccine must be administered to immunize a recipient is important along with the duration of protection. Vaccination protocols that require numerous injections for the primary regimen and frequent booster doses, such as that noted for vaccination against anthrax, can have lower compliance than immunization with fewer doses.

Scientists and vaccine manufacturers are very cognizant of reducing as much as possible the hypersensitivity potential of vaccines. Despite multiple efforts to develop nonallergenic preparations, many adverse reactions to vaccines are caused by hypersensitivity to one or more vaccine components, such as residual animal proteins, antibiotics, preservatives, or stabilizers. The most common allergenic component is egg protein found in vaccines prepared in embryonated chicken eggs or chicken embryonal cultures (i.e., measles, mumps, influenza). People who can eat eggs or egg-containing products can receive these vaccines, but vaccination is contraindicated for people with a history of anaphylactic reaction to eggs or egg proteins. On rare occasions, patients will have an anaphylactic reaction to neomycin found in trace amounts in the measles, mumps, and rubella vaccine and streptomycin found in the oral polio vaccine (OPV). Allergic reactions against the preservative thimerosal have also been noted. Until recently, thimerosal was used as the preservative in most nonviable vaccines, but it has been removed because of the increasing frequency of reported hypersensitivity reactions.

In general, immunizations with live virus vaccines should be avoided in immune-compromised patients. This has become a major consideration for routine public health immunization recommendations, because the percentage of people who are immune compromised and living longer has increased rapidly in recent decades (Table 7-3). With regard to vaccination of healthcare personnel, the substantial number of working immune-compromised clinicians places increased importance on the above recommendation. Two obvious concerns to consider here are (a) the immune system of an immune-compromised person may not be able to control attenuated vaccine organisms, and the person can actually develop the disease; and (b) immunization of immune-compromised persons may not stimulate protective immunity. In addition, although there is no direct evidence of increased risk to a fetus from vaccination, most live, attenuated vaccines are not generally administered to a pregnant woman.

TYPES OF VACCINES

Two broad types of vaccines have been successfully used in immunizing people. These are live, attenuated microbial vaccines and inactivated microorganisms or components of microbes. The following brief discussion will consider these as classified into four major classes: (a) inactivated, (b) attenuated, (c) product, and (d) component vaccines. A representative list of vaccines in each class is provided in Table 7-4. In addition to these broad groups, some vaccines are routinely administered as combined preparations, especially for children. Examples include the measles, mumps, rubella and diphtheria, acellular pertussis, and tetanus vaccine regimens.

TABLE 7-3 Representative Immune-Compromising Diseases and Conditions

1. Neoplasia or antineoplastic therapy
2. Congenital immune suppression
3. Alcoholic cirrhosis or chronic hepatitis carrier
4. Anatomic or functional asplenia
5. Autoimmune diseases (i.e., systemic lupus erythematosus, rheumatoid arthritis)
6. Arthritis
7. Conditions resulting in renal failure
8. Persons infected with human immunodeficiency virus or who have acquired immune deficiency syndrome
9. Diabetes
10. Effects of aging

TABLE 7-4 Representative Examples of Human Vaccines

Inactivated Whole Pathogen
- hepatitis A
- influenza
- poliomyelitis (IPV)
- Japanese encephalitis
- cholera (*Vibrio cholerae*)
- typhoid fever (*Salmonella typhi*)

Live, Attenuated Microorganisms
- vaccinia virus for immunization against smallpox
- poliomyelitis (OPV)
- influenza—live attenuated influenza virus
- measles
- mumps
- rubella
- varicella
- zoster

Microbial Product Vaccines
- tetanus
- diphtheria
- anthrax

Component Vaccines
- hepatitis B (hepatitis B surface antigen)
- pneumococcal pneumonia (capsular polysaccharides from *Streptococcus pneumoniae*)
- *Haemophilus influenzae* type b (capsular polysaccharide and polysaccharide/protein conjugate vaccines available)
- acellular pertussis (purified bacterial components and inactivated pertussis toxin)
- meningococcal meningitis (capsular polysaccharides from *Neisseria meningitides*)

TABLE 7-5 Characteristics of Inactivated Vaccines

Advantages
- inexpensive to manufacture; only requires propagation of pathogen
- highly immunogenic
- do not cause infection
- well tolerated by most recipients
- cannot multiply or revert to virulent form
- no danger to immune-compromised people
- provide known available antigen concentration
- primarily induce humoral immunity—primarily immunoglobulin-G in blood

Disadvantages
- requires propagation of the pathogen
- chemical treatment required for inactivation may reduce immunogenicity
- must be certain of microbial inactivation
- may require high antigen concentrations to immunize host
- usually do not produce immunity with single dose
- antibody titer may diminish with time
- often must use recommended booster injections
- inclusion of all antigenic types may not occur

Inactivated Vaccines

Inactivated vaccines contain whole bacteria or viruses that have been killed by exposure to heat, formalin, or other cidal chemicals (Table 7-5). Many early vaccines used to immunize the population were in this class, including the original *Bordetella pertussis* vaccine for whooping cough, influenza, inactivated polio vaccine (IPV), rabies, and hepatitis A vaccine. A major advantage for this class of vaccine is related to their inability to replicate in a vaccinated person, thus eliminating the potential for vaccine-induced infection. Several early vaccines used this technology, especially before detection and isolation of specific microbial antigens that stimulate a protective immune response. Even with advances delineating specific microbial component antigens responsible for inducing immunity, many viral vaccines still use this approach. As shown in Table 7-5, inactivated vaccines can be effective yet also have several possible disadvantages. One of the latter, in particular, must be mentioned: the importance of being certain the treated microorganisms are killed or inactivated. A few years after the release and dramatic success of the IPV developed by Dr. Jonas Salk and his co-workers at the University of Pittsburgh, a serious problem arose from the lack of complete inactivation of one vaccine batch. Some wild-type polio viruses were not destroyed, and these were injected into children during routine vaccination. Subsequently, several children who received the preparation containing both inactivated and viable viruses developed polio. Stricter quality control measures were put into place, and no further such incidents have been detected with this class of vaccine.

Live, Attenuated Vaccines

Many live, attenuated vaccines are thought to provide lifelong protection to a person who responds to the immunization regimen (i.e., measles, mumps, rubella). These vaccines are prepared by prolonged growth and passage of the microbial pathogen primarily in cell cultures. During the multiple passages, the virulent wild-type organism loses much of its pathogenicity but continues to replicate in vitro. Multiple mechanisms are probably responsible, including induction of mutations in critical microbial genes. The final vaccine can survive and replicate in host cells, and spread to and infect other cells for weeks, but does not cause the natural disease. The result is that replication of attenuated microorganisms in a vaccinated person provides much more antigenic stimulation than that seen with inactivated vaccines, and the host can develop very high levels of immunity that can last many years without booster doses. As noted in Table 7-6, however, this class of vaccine is not generally recommended for persons who are immune compromised. A major concern is that the individual's immune system might not be able to limit replication of attenuated organisms. In some cases, for example, immune-compromised infants who received the OPV developed vaccine-associated poliomyelitis. In addition, severely immune-compromised adults who had close contact with infants who received the OPV have a risk of infection from possible oral exposure to virus-laden fecal material. In a strong precautionary move to further minimize any vaccine risks, the CDC Advisory Committee on Immunization Practices changed the childhood polio recommendations in 2000, replacing the highly successful OPV with the IPV preparation.

Another issue common to all attenuated vaccines is the potential for the weakened microbial strain to eventually revert back to a virulent, disease-causing form. This has been addressed for most live vaccines by deletion of an

---

TABLE 7-6 Characteristics of Attenuated Vaccines

Advantages
- weakened form (attenuated) of wild-type viruses or bacteria
- must replicate in vaccinated host to be effective
- provide long-term protection
- requires only limited number of vaccination doses—usually effective with one dose
- immune response similar to that after natural infection

Disadvantages
- can infect and cause disease in certain recipients, particularly immune-compromised persons
- interference from circulating antibodies
- can spread to people who are not targeted for immunization
- risk of microbial reversion to virulent, disease-causing organisms
- unstable—sensitive to heat and light

TABLE 7-7 Characteristics of Component (Subunit) Vaccines

Advantages
- use primary microbial antigen(s) for stimulating immune protection
- nontoxic
- noninfectious
- provide known available antigen concentration

Disadvantages
- requires antigen purification—increases expense
- some component preparations less immunogenic than others (i.e., polysaccharide capsules versus surface proteins)
- vaccines limited to pathogens for which immune response to a single homogeneous component can protect vaccinated host
- may require boosters to maintain protection

TABLE 7-8 Characteristics of Product Vaccines

Advantages
- purified antigen from microbial culture
- no infection risk
- provide known antigen concentration
- no risk to immune-compromised people

Disadvantages
- require booster doses for continued immunity
- most currently available vaccines limited to exotoxin-mediated diseases

essential gene required for microbial virulence during attenuation procedures.

Component (Subunit) Vaccines

Immunity against microbial infections is often induced by some **component** or **subunit** of the etiologic microorganism (Table 7-7). Major emphasis is given to determining the antigen responsible for stimulating a protective immune response. Most of the available vaccines in this class use surface components isolated from bacteria or viruses as the antigen. Proteins are regarded as the best antigens in part because of their large size (i.e., high molecular weight) and stable primary, secondary, and tertiary structure, which allows efficient activation of immune lymphoid cells. Important examples are hepatitis B surface protein and proteins purified from cultures of *Bordetella pertussis*. Several component vaccines use capsules, because these are often the bacterial antigens that stimulate immunity. Because these cell components are primarily polysaccharide in structure, they are less immunogenic than protein antigens. Nonetheless, capsular polysaccharide vaccines are important in controlling numerous childhood and adult bacterial infections.

Microbial Product Vaccines

These vaccines have many features in common with several microbial component immunizing antigens (Table 7-8). **Product vaccines**, such as those that protect against tetanus and diphtheria, were among the first to purify the protein antigens from microbial cultures. Isolation of purified tetanus and diphtheria exotoxins from cultures of *Clostridium tetani* and *Corynebacterium diphtheriae* provided scientists with the factor responsible for disease pathogenesis. Before being tested as a vaccine candidate, the exotoxin must first be detoxified by treating it with formaldehyde. The product from such processing is called a toxoid, and it differs from the isolated toxin in

that toxoids are now nontoxic to the vaccinated host and retain most of the antigenicity of the parent molecule. Unfortunately, with the exception of the above-mentioned vaccines and the anthrax toxoid, development of this class of vaccine has been limited to those diseases that have exotoxin-mediated manifestations.

IMMUNIZATIONS FOR DENTAL HEALTHCARE PERSONNEL

Dental Healthcare Personnel (DHCP) are at particular risk for several vaccine-preventable diseases. Responsible professional organizations are obligated to educate, continuously inform, and provide balanced assessments of benefits, costs, and risks on the antigens that are recommended routinely for the immunization of healthcare personnel. Infection control programs in dentistry are to be designed to assess and minimize communicable disease risk in the dental environment. Immunizations and other prophylaxis against preventable diseases should be made available to all DHCP. At the time of employment, each person should be asked to provide documentation of previous immunizations. A review of this documentation will indicate which immunizations are needed, saving valuable time and emotional stress in the event that exposure occurs on the job. The following recommendations, developed to help prevent illness among DHCP and patients, cover immunizations in three areas of concern:

1. immunizations recommended at the time of employment for susceptible DHCP;
2. immunization regimens that require booster doses; and
3. immunizations and chemotherapeutic agents administered only in the event of inadvertent exposure to a communicable disease.

Immunization History

A history of immunization should be obtained carefully from DHCP at the time of initial employment. This history should be updated periodically. The most reliable way to determine the immunization history is to obtain the information from a record kept by the employees or their physicians. Age also may provide valuable clues to the likelihood of vaccination. People who were 10 years of age or older when the measles, mumps, and rubella vaccines were licensed (1963, 1967, 1969, respectively) are less likely to have received these vaccines than people who were younger or born since then. All states now require children entering or attending school to be immunized against certain infectious diseases; however, there are variations in state laws and their enforcement. If there is doubt about previous immunizations, it is best to assume that the person is nonimmunized.

Vaccine Administration

The recommended route of administration and dosages for each vaccine are specified on the package insert. Most vaccines for adults are given by intramuscular or subcutaneous injection. These injections usually are given in the deltoid muscle. Studies with hepatitis B vaccine in adults have shown that its immunogenicity is significantly lower when injections are given in the buttocks. The higher concentration of fat cells in this region can absorb and prevent some of the vaccine protein from getting into the circulation to sufficiently induce an immune response. This observation may apply to other vaccines, and the buttock is not recommended as a site of routine vaccination for adults.

Recording Immunizations

Each time a dental healthcare provider receives a dose of vaccine, a notation should be made in the medical record on a special immunization form. The information recorded should include the type of vaccine; the dose, route, and site of administration; the name of the person who gave the vaccine; the date the vaccine was given; the manufacturer and lot number; and the date the next dose is due. The National Childhood Vaccine Injury Act of 1986 mandates that healthcare providers who administer vaccines record this information, and the requirements apply to all patients, including adults.

Specific Vaccine Recommendations

The most recent immunization recommendations for DHCP were published in the CDC "Guidelines for Infection Control in Dental Health-care Settings–2003." These are summarized in Table 7-9. Additional clinically relevant information is discussed in the following sections.

Rubella (German Measles)

Universal immunization against the rubella virus generally is recommended for all healthcare providers, but particularly for previously nonimmunized women of childbearing age who do not have laboratory evidence of immunity. Not only are susceptible healthcare providers at risk of acquiring rubella, but they may transmit the disease to associates and patients, some of whom might be pregnant. Fetal infection can occur in as many as 80% of fetuses during the first trimester of pregnancy and to some extent in the second trimester, and it may produce serious birth defects.

The rubella vaccine contains live attenuated rubella virus that is prepared in human cell cultures. Women should receive the vaccine only if they are not pregnant and must be counseled not to become pregnant for 3 months after immunization because of the potential risk of infecting the fetus in utero with the vaccine virus. Adverse reactions to the vaccine are infrequent in healthy people. The most common complication is joint pain, usually of the small distal joints, reported by as many as 40% of adult vaccine recipients. Rarely, arthralgias may occur 3 to 25 days after vaccination and persist for as long as 10 days. As with all live attenuated virus vaccines, the rubella vaccine should not be given to immune-compromised patients.

Rubeola (Measles)

Universal immunization against rubeola is recommended for all young adults, particularly healthcare providers born after 1956, unless there is a physician-documented history of infection or vaccination after the age of 1 year or laboratory evidence of immunity. Those vaccinated between 1963 and 1967 with inactivated rubeola vaccine should be revaccinated to prevent severe atypical measles. It is safe to give rubeola vaccine to a person who is already immune either from natural infection or previous vaccination. Nonpregnant, susceptible people exposed to the rubeola virus may receive protection if immunized within 72 hours after exposure.

The rubeola vaccine contains live attenuated measles virus that is prepared in cell cultures made from chick embryos; however, the chance of allergic reactions occurring in people allergic to eggs, chickens, or feathers is low. Because the rubeola vaccine contains live attenuated virus, it should not be given to immune-compromised or pregnant patients. Rubeola may be prevented or modified in susceptible pregnant personnel by administration of immune globulin within 6 days after exposure. In approximately 5% to 15% of vaccine recipients, symptoms of attenuated measles, characterized by fever, begin to develop 5 to 12 days after vaccination. A transient rash may occur in approximately 5% of vaccinated patients.

Mumps

Healthcare workers are likely to be exposed to mumps and experience the consequences of infection, characterized

TABLE 7-9 Recommended Vaccines for Healthcare Personnel

Immunizations Strongly Recommended for Healthcare Personnel				
Vaccine	Dose Schedule	Indications	Major Precautions and Contraindications	Special Considerations
Hepatitis B recombinant vaccine*	Three-dose schedule administered intramuscularly in the deltoid; 0, 1, 6; second dose administered 1 month after first dose; third dose administered 4 months after second dose. Booster doses are not necessary for persons who have developed adequate antibodies to hepatitis B surface antigen.	HCP at risk for exposure to blood and body fluids.	History of anaphylactic reaction to common baker's yeast. Pregnancy is not a contraindication.	No therapeutic or adverse effects on HBV-infected persons; cost-effectiveness of prevaccination screening for susceptibility to HBV depends on costs of vaccination and antibody testing and prevalence of immunity in the group of potential vaccines; HCP who have ongoing contact with patients or blood should be tested 1–2 months after completing the vaccination series to determine serologic response. If vaccination does not induce adequate antibodies to hepatitis B surface antigen (>10mlU/mL), a second vaccine series should be administered.
Influenza vaccine (inactivated)[¶]	Annual single-dose vaccination intramuscularly with current vaccine.	HCP who have contact with patients at high risk or who work in chronic-care facilities; HCP aged ≥50 years or who have high-risk medical conditions.	History of anaphylactic hypersensitivity to eggs or to other components of the vaccine.	Recommended for women who will be in the second or third trimesters of pregnancy during the influenza season and women in any state of pregnancy who have chronic medical conditions that are associated with an increased risk of influenza.[§]
Measles live-virus vaccine	One dose administered subcutaneously (SC); second dose ≥4 weeks later.	HCP who were born during or after 1957 without documentation of (i) receipt of two doses of live vaccine on or after their first birthday, (ii) physician-diagnosed measles, or (iii) laboratory evidence of immunity. Vaccine should also be considered for all HCP who have no proof of immunity, including those born before 1957.	Pregnancy; immunocompromised[†] state (including human immunodeficiency virus-infected persons with severe immunosuppression); history of anaphylactic reactions after gelatin ingestion or receipt of neomycin; or recent receipt of antibody-containing blood products.	Measles, mumps, rubella (MMR) is the recommended vaccine if recipients are also likely to be susceptible to rubella or mumps; persons vaccinated between 1963 and 1967 with (i) measles killed-virus vaccine alone, (ii) killed-virus vaccine followed by live-virus vaccine, or (iii) vaccine of unknown type, should be revaccinated with two doses of live-virus measles vaccine.
Mumps live-virus vaccine	One dose SC; no booster.	HCP believed susceptible can be vaccinated; adults born before 1957 can be considered immune.	Pregnancy; immunocompromised[†] state; history of anaphylactic reaction after gelatin ingestion or receipt of neomycin.	MMR is the recommended vaccine.
Rubella live-virus vaccine	One dose SC; no booster.	HCP, both male and female, who lack documentation of receipt of live vaccine on or after their first birthday, or lack laboratory evidence of immunity can be vaccinated. Adults born before 1957 can be considered immune, except women of childbearing age.	Pregnancy; immunocompromised[†] state; history of anaphylactic reaction after receipt of neomycin.	Women pregnant when vaccinated or who become pregnant with 4 weeks of vaccination should be counseled regarding theoretic risks to the fetus; however, the risk of rubella vaccine-associated malformations among these women is negligible. MMR is the recommended vaccine.

(continued)

TABLE 7-9 Recommended Vaccines for Healthcare Personnel *(continued)*

Immunizations Strongly Recommended for Healthcare Personnel				
Vaccine	Dose Schedule	Indications	Major Precautions and Contraindications	Special Considerations
Varicella-zoster live-virus vaccine	Two 0.5-mL doses SC 4–8 weeks apart if aged ≥13 years.	HCP without reliable history of varicella or laboratory evidence of varicella immunity.	Pregnancy; immunocompromised[†] state; history of anaphylactic reaction after receipt of neomycin or gelatin; recent receipt of antibody-containing blood products; salicylate use should be avoided for 6 weeks after vaccination.	Because 71% to 93% of U.S.-born persons without a history of varicella are immune, serologic testing before vaccination might be cost-effective.

Adapted from Bolyard EA, Hospital Infection Control Practices Advisory Committee. Guidelines for infection control in healthcare personnel, 1998. Am J Infect Control 1998;26:289–354; CDC. Immunization of healthcare workers: recommendations of the Advisory Committee on Immunization Practices (ACIP) and the Hospital Infection Control Practices Advisory Committee (HICPAC). MMWR 1997;46(No. RR-18); CDC. Prevention and control of influenza: recommendations of the Advisory Committee on Immunization Practices (ACIP). MMWR 2003;52:1–34; CDC. Using live, attenuated influenza vaccine for prevention and control of influenza: supplemental recommendations of the Advisory Committee on Immunization Practices (ACIP). MMWR 2003;52(No. RR-13).

[*]A federal standard issued in December 1991 under the Occupational Safety and Health Act mandates that hepatitis B vaccine be made available at the employer's expense to all HCP occupationally exposed to blood or other potentially infectious materials. The Occupational Safety and Health Administration requires that employers make available hepatitis B vaccinations, evaluations, and follow-up procedures in accordance with current CDC recommendations.

[†]Persons immunocompromised because of immune deficiencies, human immunodeficiency virus infection, leukemia, lymphoma, generalized malignancy; persons receiving immunosuppressive therapy with corticosteroids, alkylating drugs, antimetabolites; or persons receiving radiation.

[§]Vaccination of pregnant women after the first trimester might be preferred to avoid coincidental association with spontaneous abortions, which are most common during the first trimester. However, no adverse fetal effects have been associated with influenza vaccination.

[¶]A live attenuated influenza virus (LAIV) is Food and Drug Administration approved for healthy persons aged 5–49 years. Because of the possibility of transmission of vaccine viruses from recipients of LAIV to other persons and in the absence of data on the risk of illness and among immunocompromised persons infected with LAIV viruses, the inactivated influenza vaccine is preferred for HCP who have close contact with immunocompromised persons.

by the involvement of major salivary glands, possibly meningitis, and, in men, painful swelling of the testicles or orchitis. The vaccine contains live attenuated mumps virus grown in chick embryo cell cultures. Reactions to the vaccine are rare; however, people with a history of anaphylactic reaction after eating eggs should not be vaccinated. Boosters are not required.

Hepatitis B

A more detailed discussion of hepatitis B vaccination can be found in Chapter 2. Primary immunization with hepatitis B vaccine consists of three intramuscular doses of 1.0 mL each. The second and third doses should be given 1 and 6 months, respectively, after the first. The deltoid muscle is the preferred site because injections given into the buttocks were found to yield a lower seroconversion rate than expected. Because the vaccine contains only noninfectious hepatitis B surface antigen particles, there should be no risk to the fetus. In contrast, HBV infection in a pregnant woman may result in severe disease for the mother and chronic infection for the newborn. Pregnancy should not be considered a contraindication to the use of this vaccine for people who are otherwise eligible. Soreness at the site of the injection is the most common adverse effect associated with the hepatitis B vaccine.

Influenza

Influenza vaccination is strongly recommended for DHCP and other healthcare providers. Not only will vaccination reduce time lost from work but also will minimize the transmission of influenza from healthcare providers to patients. Annual immunization is recommended, particularly for healthcare providers with diabetes and other metabolic diseases; providers with severe anemia, hemoglobinopathies, or immunosuppression; providers with chronic pulmonary, cardiovascular, or renal disease; providers older than 65 years of age; and all other health providers who may have contact with high-risk patients.

Adult immunization with the influenza virus vaccine consists of one 0.5-mL intramuscular dose of vaccine. The most common associated side effect of the vaccine is local tenderness for 1 to 2 days at the injection site; this occurs in less than one third of recipients. Malaise and low-grade fever for as long as 48 hours are infrequent, and hypersensitivity reactions are rare.

The viruses contained in the influenza vaccine are grown in chick embryo cultures and inactivated with formalin to minimize the amount of residual egg protein in the vaccine. After viral inactivation, the intact virus is split into its components before administration. Thus influenza vaccination cannot cause influenza in a vaccinated individual. Although allergic reactions are rare, people who have had signs and symptoms of an anaphylactic reaction to eggs should not receive the vaccine.

The virus content of the vaccine is revised each year to incorporate new strains that are expected to be prevalent for the upcoming influenza season. When the vaccine contains the prevalent strains of viral organisms in a given year, the incidence of influenza is reduced by as much as 90% in immunized people; however, the immunity produced by the vaccine is temporary, and annual reimmunization with the appropriate strains is necessary.

Varicella-Zoster

The varicella-zoster vaccine, called Varivax, was licensed for use in the United States in 1995 after extensive testing in Europe, Japan, and Korea. Varivax is an attenuated viral preparation using the Oka strain and is intended for nonimmune children and health professionals without a reliable history of chickenpox or serologic laboratory evidence of immunity against varicella. Transmission of varicella-zoster virus can occur via droplets before eruption of skin lesions. Both children and adults should receive two injections of the vaccine, which has been shown to stimulate immunity in more than 95% of recipients. The vaccine is immunogenic and has been highly effective in preventing disease. A minority of vaccine recipients may develop a mild case of chickenpox from the first vaccine dose. The vaccine is not recommended for pregnant women and immune-compromised individuals.

Tetanus-Diphtheria

Although not specifically discussed in the current CDC recommendations for DHCP, tetanus-diphtheria (Td) vaccination is routinely included in recommendations for all health professionals. Healthcare providers not previously immunized should receive a series of two doses of Td (adult) vaccine 4 to 8 weeks apart, followed by a booster 6 to 12 months later. Subsequent to the primary series of immunizations, a Td booster should be administered every 10 years.

Previously vaccinated healthcare providers with puncture wounds or lacerations should receive a Td booster if more than 10 years have elapsed since their last booster. Those with severe or heavily contaminated wounds may require adsorbed tetanus toxoid *and* human tetanus immune globulin if their history of previous primary tetanus immunizations is inadequate or not definite. If boosters are given too often, tetanus toxoid can cause severe local pain and swelling.

SUMMARY

DHCP are at risk for possible occupational infection by a variety of microorganisms. Several of these can be prevented by immunization. These vaccine-preventable diseases include hepatitis B, influenza, measles, mumps, rubella, and varicella. In one example of their efficacy, adherence to vaccine recommendations has been very successful in dramatically reducing the incidence of hepatitis B and other infections in healthcare professionals. The cost-effectiveness of disease prevention by immunization rather than by disease treatment should prompt an acute interest in the immunization status of DHCP.

Review Questions

1. _____ is credited with introducing the smallpox vaccine as an effective method of preventing disease epidemics.

   A. Jonas Salk

   B. Edward Jenner

   C. Joseph Lister

   D. Ignaz Semmelweis

2. Barriers to achieving high vaccination levels among adults include the following:

   A. Missed opportunities to vaccinate during contacts with healthcare providers for unrelated office visits.

   B. Lack of perceived risk to vaccine-preventable diseases.

   C. Mistaken perception that vaccine-preventable diseases have been virtually eliminated from many developed countries.

   D. Patient and provider fears concerning adverse events after vaccination.

   E. All of the above.

3. When an individual develops a symptomatic or asymptomatic infection and recovers with their immune system actively producing a protective immune response, this is an example of

   A. natural active immunity

   B. artificial passive immunity

   C. artificial active immunity

4. When an individual receives an injection of antibodies from an immune person to prevent the onset of infection, this is an example of

   A. natural active immunity

   B. artificial passive immunity

   C. artificial active immunity

5. Which of the following is NOT an example of a property or requirement of an ideal vaccine?

   A. safe

   B. provide lifelong immunity

   C. should be immunosuppressive

   D. should be nonallergenic

6. In general, immunizations with _____ virus vaccines should be avoided in immunocompromised patients.

   A. live

   B. egg

   C. inactivated

   D. standard

7. Which is NOT a major class of vaccine?

   A. inactivated

   B. attenuated

   C. product

   D. antigenic

8. The hepatitis B vaccine is an example of a(n) _____ vaccine.

   A. inactivated

   B. attenuated

   C. antigenic

   D. component

9. The tetanus vaccine is an example of a(n) _____ vaccine.

   A. inactivated

   B. attenuated

   C. product

   D. component

10. Which immunizations are strongly recommended for DHCP?

    A. hepatitis B

    B. influenza

    C. measles, mumps, rubella

    D. varicella-zoster

    E. all of the above

    F. both A and B only

Critical Thinking

1. What immunizations does your employer furnish to you? Do you have a checklist in your office for new employees?

SELECTED READINGS

CDC. Adult immunization: recommendations of the Immunization Practices Advisory Committee (ACIP). MMWR 1984;33:1S–68S.

CDC. Control and prevention of rubella: evaluation and management of suspected outbreaks, rubella in pregnant women, and surveillance for congenital rubella syndrome. MMWR 2001;50(RR-12):1–24.

CDC (Centers for Disease Control and Prevention). Epidemiology and Prevention of Vaccine-Preventable Diseases. 10th ed. Washington, DC: Public Health Foundation; 2007.

CDC. Guidelines for infection control in dental health-care settings, 2003. MMWR 2003;52(RR-17):1–66.

CDC. Immune globulins for protection against viral hepatitis. MMWR 1981;30:423–428, 433–435.

CDC. Immunization of healthcare workers: recommendations of the Advisory Committee on Immunization Practices (APIC) and the Hospital Infection Control Practices Advisory Committee (HICPAC). MMWR 1997;46(RR-18):1–42.

CDC. Prevention and control of influenza. Recommendations of the Advisory Committee on Immunization Practices (ACIP). MMWR 2007;56(RR06):1–54.

CDC. Prevention of varicella. Recommendations of the Advisory Committee on Immunization Practices (ACIP). MMWR 2007;56(RR04):1–40.

CDC. Recommendations for protection against viral hepatitis. MMWR 1985;34:313–324, 329–335.

CDC. Suboptimal response to hepatitis B vaccine given by injection into the buttock. MMWR 1985;34:105–108, 113.

CDC. Ten great public health achievements—United States, 1900–1999. MMWR 1999;48:241–243.

Gardner P, Schaffner W. Immunization of adults. N Engl J Med 1993;328:1252–1258.

Nichol KL, Lind A, Margolis KL, et al. The effectiveness of vaccination against influenza in healthy, working adults. N Engl J Med 1995;333:889–993.

Nichol KL, Lofgren RP, Gapinski J. Influenza vaccination: knowledge, attitudes, and behavior among high-risk outpatients. Arch Intern Med 1992;152:106–110.

Palenik CJ, Govoni M. An immunization program for dental practices. Compend Contin Educ Dent 2004;25 (1 Suppl):17–22.

Plotkin SA, Orenstein WA. Vaccines. 4th ed. Philadelphia, PA: WB Saunders; 2004.

Poland GA, Jacobson RM. Prevention of hepatitis B with the hepatitis B vaccine. N Engl J Med 2004;351:2832–2838.

8

Personal Protective Equipment

John A. Molinari

Jennifer A. Harte

LEARNING OBJECTIVES

After completion of this chapter individuals should be able to:

1 Discuss the purpose and importance of personal protective equipment (PPE).

2 Discuss indications for using gloves, masks, protective eyewear, and protective clothing.

3 Differentiate between examination, sterile, and utility gloves, and discuss indications for use.

4 Discuss procedures for donning and removing PPE.

5 Describe occupational reactions associated with glove usage.

KEY TERMS

Aerosol: particles of respirable size generated by both humans and environmental sources that can remain viable and airborne for extended periods in the indoor environment; commonly generated in dentistry during use of handpieces, ultrasonic scalers, and air/water syringes.

Allergic contact dermatitis (ACD): a type IV or delayed-hypersensitivity reaction resulting from contact with a chemical allergen (e.g., poison ivy, certain components of patient care gloves), generally localized to the contact area. Reactions occur slowly over 12–48 hours.

Anaphylaxis (immediate anaphylactic hypersensitivity): a severe and sometimes fatal type I reaction in a susceptible person after a second exposure to a specific antigen (e.g., food, pollen, proteins in latex gloves, or penicillin) after previous sensitization. Anaphylaxis is characterized commonly by respiratory symptoms, itching, hives, and rarely by shock and death (anaphylactic shock).

Droplet nuclei: particles 5 μm or less in diameter that are formed by dehydration of airborne droplets containing microorganisms that can remain suspended in the air for long periods of time.

Droplets: small particles of moisture (e.g., spatter) that may be generated when a person coughs or sneezes, or when water is converted to a fine mist by an aerator or shower head. Intermediate in size between drops and droplet nuclei, these particles tend to quickly settle out from the air, so even though they may still contain infectious microorganisms, any risk of disease transmission is generally limited to persons in close proximity to the droplet source.

Food and Drug Administration (FDA): the FDA promotes and protects the public health by helping safe and effective products reach the market in a timely way, monitors products for continued safety after they are in use, and helps the public get the accurate, science-based information needed to improve health.

Irritation contact dermatitis (ICD): the development of dry, itchy, irritated areas on the skin, which can result from frequent hand washing and gloving as well as exposure to chemicals. This condition is not an allergic reaction.

Latex: a milky white fluid extracted from the rubber tree *Hevea brasiliensis* that contains the rubber material cis-1,4 polyisoprene.

Latex allergy: a type I or immediate anaphylactic hypersensitivity reaction to the proteins found in natural rubber latex (NRL).

Mycobacterium tuberculosis (M. tuberculosis): the namesake member organism of the *M. tuberculosis* complex, and the most common causative infectious agent of

tuberculosis (TB) disease in humans. At times, the species name refers to the entire *M. tuberculosis* complex, which includes *M. bovis* and five other related species.

N-95 respirator: one of nine types of disposable particulate respirators. The "95" refers to the percentage of particles filtered (see "particulate respirator" below).

National Institute for Occupational Safety and Health (NIOSH): the federal agency responsible for conducting research and making recommendations for the prevention of work-related disease and injury. The institute is part of the Centers for Disease Control and Prevention (CDC).

Occupational Safety and Health Administration (OSHA): established in 1971, OSHA aims to ensure worker safety and health in the United States by working with employers and employees to create better working environments; setting and enforcing standards; providing training, outreach, and education; establishing partnerships; and encouraging continual improvements in workplace safety and health.

Oral surgical procedure: involves the incision, excision, or reflection of tissue that exposes normally sterile areas of the oral cavity. Examples include biopsy, periodontal surgery, apical surgery, implant surgery, and surgical extractions of teeth (e.g., removal of erupted or nonerupted tooth requiring elevation of the mucoperiosteal flap, removal of bone or sectioning of teeth, and suturing if needed).

Other potentially infectious materials (OPIM): an OSHA term that refers to (a) the following human body fluids: semen, vaginal secretions, cerebrospinal fluid, synovial fluid, pleural fluid, pericardial fluid, peritoneal fluid, amniotic fluid, saliva in dental procedures, any body fluid that is visibly contaminated with blood, and all body fluids in situations where it is difficult or impossible to differentiate between body fluids; (b) any unfixed tissue or organ (other than intact skin) from a human (living or dead); and (c) HIV-containing cell or tissue cultures, organ cultures, and HIV- or HBV-containing culture medium or other solutions; and blood, organs, or other tissues from experimental animals infected with HIV or HBV.

Particulate respirator Mask (PRM): also known as an "air-purifying respirator" because it protects by filtering particles out of the air you breathe. Workers can wear any one of the available particulate respirator masks (PRMs) for protection against diseases that are spread through the air, if they are NIOSH-approved and they have been properly fit-tested and maintained. NIOSH-approved disposable respirators are marked with the manufacturer's name, the part number (P/N), the protection provided by the filter (e.g., N-95), and the word NIOSH. The "95" refers to the percentage of particles filtered.

Personal protective equipment (PPE): specialized clothing or equipment worn by an employee for protection against a hazard (e.g., gloves, masks, protective eyewear, and gowns). General work clothes (e.g., uniforms, pants, shirts, and blouses) not intended to function as protection against a hazard are not considered to be PPE.

Standard precautions: universal precautions were based on the concept that all blood and all body fluids that might be contaminated with blood should be treated as infectious because patients with bloodborne infections can be asymptomatic or unaware they are infected. The relevance of universal precautions to other aspects of disease transmission was recognized, and in 1996 the CDC expanded the concept and changed the term to "standard precautions." Standard precautions integrate and expand the elements of universal precautions into a standard of care designed to protect healthcare personnel (HCP) and patients from pathogens that can be spread by blood or any other body fluid, excretion, or secretion. Standard precautions apply to contact with (a) blood; (b) all body fluids, secretions, and excretions (except sweat), regardless of whether they contain blood; (c) nonintact skin; and (d) mucous membranes. Saliva has always been considered a potentially infectious material in dental infection control; thus, no operational difference exists in clinical dental practice between universal precautions and standard precautions.

Wicking: absorption of a liquid by capillary action along a thread or through material (e.g., the enhanced penetration of liquids through undetected holes in a glove).

Dental healthcare personnel (DHCP) and their patients can be exposed to a variety of microorganisms via blood or oral and respiratory secretions. These microorganisms may include numerous pathogenic bacteria, viruses, and fungi, such as hepatitis B virus (HBV), hepatitis C virus (HCV), human immunodeficiency virus (HIV), herpes simplex viruses, influenza viruses, *Candida albicans*, *M. tuberculosis*, cytomegalovirus, staphylococci, and streptococci. Infections can be transmitted within dental healthcare settings in several ways. These include direct contact with blood, saliva, and other secretions; indirect contact with contaminated instruments, operatory equipment, and environmental surfaces; contact of conjunctival, nasal, or oral mucosa with **droplets** (e.g., spatter) containing microorganisms generated from an infected person and propelled a short distance, such as by coughing, sneezing, or talking; and inhalation of airborne microorganisms that are able to remain suspended in the air for long periods. Infection via these routes requires a susceptible host; a pathogen with sufficient infectivity and numbers to cause infection; a reservoir or source that allows the pathogen to survive and multiply, such as blood; a mode of transmission from the source to the host; and a portal through which the pathogen may enter the host. Appropriate interaction of these factors is commonly referred to as the chain of infection.

Standard precautions must be observed routinely in the care of all dental patients, because not all infected patients can be identified by medical history, physical examination, or laboratory tests. In addition, specific precautions must be taken to reduce the risk of *M. tuberculosis* and other airborne microbial transmissions. Techniques used to interfere with this initial step in the infectious disease process are called barrier precautions. The implementation and appropriate use of personal barriers have changed the face of infectious disease risk for all healthcare professionals by providing physical barriers between the body and source of contamination, and reducing the exposure to exogenous potential pathogens, thereby assisting host immune defenses to resist infection.

This chapter concentrates on **personal protective equipment (PPE)** used to protect the skin and the mucous membranes of the eyes, nose, and mouth of DHCP from exposure to blood or **other potentially infectious materials (OPIM)**. The primary PPE used in dental healthcare settings includes gloves, surgical masks, protective eyewear with solid side shields, face shields, and protective clothing (e.g., gowns and jackets). Shoe and head covers are less frequently used types of PPE. Wearing gloves, surgical masks, protective eyewear, and protective clothing in specified circumstances to reduce the risk of exposures to bloodborne pathogens is mandated by the **Occupational Safety and Health Administration (OSHA)**. With normal use, PPE material should prevent the passage of fluids to skin, undergarments, or mucous membranes of the eyes, nose, or mouth. These important protective measures have been stressed by all federal and state OSHA regulations, in that they require an employer to provide appropriate PPE in appropriate sizes for all employees who will be using them. Selecting PPE is based on the type of dental procedure and/or the likely mode(s) of transmission. As will also be discussed below, all PPE should be removed before DHCP leave patient-care areas.

GLOVES

When minor trauma occurs to the hands, visual inspection cannot disclose every break in the epidermis. Any abrasion, cut, or minor trauma can compromise the integrity of the skin, and minor traumata can be portals for a variety of viral and bacterial organisms found in a patient's oral cavity. Dental professionals who were previously trained using "wet finger dentistry" can readily identify with the possible ramifications of the above statements. Instances of herpetic whitlow and staphylococcal pyoderma were not uncommon when bare hands were used to treat patients (Fig. I-14). Fortunately, the routine use of gloves when providing care has caused these and many other occupational infections to become historical examples that document the increased safety of today's dental care. In addition to helping to reduce exposure to HBV, the incidence of many other occupational infections has shown a dramatic decline. For the protection of DHCP and the patient, medical gloves always must be worn when there is a potential for contacting blood, blood–contaminated saliva, or mucous membranes. Several types of gloves and a variety of materials are available, including **latex**, vinyl, nitrile, and chloroprene, with latex still used as the gold standard for glove material. The selection of gloves should be based on multiple use factors, including the type of procedure to be performed, anticipated contact with chemicals, latex sensitivity, and sizing.

The effectiveness of intact gloves in preventing the penetration of microorganisms into the skin does not diminish the necessity for hand washing or other hand hygiene procedures when changing gloves. Remember, *wearing gloves does not replace routine hand hygiene practices*. Hands must be washed before gloving and after removing gloves. Hand washing immediately following glove removal ensures the removal of potentially infectious material that might have penetrated the glove via unrecognized tears or from improper glove removal. This keeps the level of skin bacteria to a minimum and reduces the irritating buildup of microorganisms that can multiply in the moist, warm environment that is created under the gloves.

Quality control regarding the manufacture and labeling of gloves has also improved over the years to assist clinicians in glove selection, such that gloves currently manufactured for healthcare purposes are subject to **Food and Drug Administration (FDA)** evaluation and clearance (Table 8-1). Even though the FDA has identified levels of maximum defects allowed for glove manufacturers, intact gloves eventually fail with exposure to mechanical (e.g., sharps, fingernails, or jewelry) and chemical (e.g., dimethyacrylates) hazards over time. Medical gloves are manufactured as single-use disposable items to be used on one patient and then discarded appropriately. The reuse of contaminated gloves increases infection risks to both dental personnel and their patients. For example, microorganisms from the first patient may enter inherent pinholes or tears. They may begin to multiply under the gloves or enter small cuts or

abrasions on the skin. As glove material becomes less effective with prolonged use, washing, and exposure to body fluids, accumulating organisms on hands may also exit through increasingly larger defects into the next patient's mouth. Washing of gloves may cause "**wicking**" (penetration of liquids through undetected holes in the gloves) and is not recommended. Furthermore, microorganisms cannot be removed reliably from glove surfaces, and deterioration of gloves can occur by exposure to disinfectants, oils, certain oil-based lotions, and heat treatments, such as autoclaving. If an alcohol-based hand rub is used, the hands should be thoroughly dried before gloving, because hands still wet with an alcohol-based product can increase the risk of glove perforation. OSHA regulations also mandate that when gloves are torn, cut, or punctured, they should be removed as soon as patient safety permits. DHCP then should wash their hands thoroughly and reglove to complete the dental procedure.

Leakage rates vary by glove material (e.g., latex, vinyl, and nitrile), duration of use, and type of procedure performed, as well as by manufacturer. Studies have shown that vinyl gloves have higher failure rates than latex or nitrile gloves when tested under simulated and actual clinical conditions. The real and perceived implications of these observations must be considered in the light of occupational infection risks. Newer generations of vinyl gloves are far superior to earlier ones with regard to fit, elasticity, and in-use life expectancy. Health professionals should be assured that as long as they use vinyl or any other patient-care gloves appropriately, the potential for occupational infection from bacterial, viral, and mycotic pathogens will be greatly reduced. To additionally optimize glove performance, it is important to maintain short fingernails, minimize or eliminate hand jewelry, and use engineering and work-practice controls to avoid injuries with sharps. Because of the diverse selection of dental materials on the market, dental practitioners also should consult glove manufacturers regarding the chemical compatibility of glove materials. Disinfectants, composite resins, and bonding agents are just several examples of chemicals and materials routinely used in dental settings that can compromise the integrity of latex, vinyl, nitrile, and other synthetic glove materials.

Patient Examination Gloves

The least expensive type of glove is the nonsterile, disposable patient-examination glove that fits both hands and comes in a variety of sizes (e.g., extra small, small, medium, and large). The disadvantage of these gloves is that the fit can be too tight or too loose. Fitted or hand-specific (i.e., right/left) disposable nonsterile gloves are available and may provide a better fit and cause less hand fatigue. Nonsterile disposable gloves are appropriate for examinations and other nonsurgical procedures.

TABLE 8-1 Types of Gloves

Glove Type	Indications	Comments	Commercially Available Glove Materials*	Attributes[†]
Patient examination gloves[§]	Patient care, examinations, other nonsurgical procedures involving contact with mucous membranes, and laboratory procedures	Nonsterile and sterile single-use disposable; use for one patient and discard appropriately	• NRL • Nitrile • Nitrile and chloroprene (neoprene) blends • Nitrile and NRL blends • Butadiene methyl methacrylate • Polyvinyl chloride (PVC, vinyl) • Polyurethane • Styrene-based copolymer	1, 2 2, 3 2, 3 1, 2, 3 2, 3 4 4 4, 5
Surgeon's gloves[§]	Surgical procedures	Sterile single-use disposable; use for one patient and discard appropriately	• NRL • Nitrile • Chloroprene (neoprene) • NRL and nitrile or chloroprene blends • Synthetic polyisoprene • Styrene-based copolymer • Polyurethane	1, 2 2, 3 2, 3 2, 3 2 4, 5 4
Nonmedical gloves (Commonly referred to as utility, industrial, or general-purpose gloves. Should be puncture- or chemical-resistant, depending on the task. Latex gloves do not provide adequate chemical protection.)	• Housekeeping procedures (e.g., cleaning and disinfection) • Handling contaminated sharps or chemicals • Not for use during patient care	Sanitize after use.	• NRL and nitrile or chloroprene blends • Chloroprene (neoprene) • Nitrile • Butyl rubber • Fluoroelastomer • Polyethylene and ethylene vinyl alcohol copolymer	2, 3 2, 3 2, 3 2, 3 3, 4, 6 3, 4, 6

Adapted from CDC. Guidelines for infection control in dental health-care settings–2003. MMWR 2003;52(RR-17):18.

*Physical properties can vary by material, manufacturer, and protein and chemical composition.

[†] 1–Contains allergenic NRL proteins.

  2–Vulcanized rubber, contains allergenic rubber-processing chemicals.

  3–Likely to have enhanced chemical and/or puncture resistance.

  4–Nonvulcanized and does not contain rubber-processing chemicals.

  5–Inappropriate for use with methacrylates.

  6–Resistant to most methacrylates.

[§]Medical or dental gloves include patient examination gloves and surgeons' (i.e., surgical) gloves, and are medical devices regulated by the FDA. Only FDA-cleared medical or dental patient examination gloves and surgical gloves can be used for patient care.

Sterile Surgeon's Gloves

The most expensive type of gloves are sterile surgeon's gloves, but their cost is minor compared with the protection provided. Sterile surgeon's gloves should be used when performing **oral surgical procedures**. Sterile gloves provide excellent tactility, comfort, and dexterity, and are available as right- and left-handed fitted items. Sterile gloves minimize transmission of microorganisms from the hands of surgical DHCP to patients, and prevent contamination of the hands with the patient's blood and body fluids. Additionally, sterile surgeon's gloves are more rigorously regulated by the FDA for sterility assurance and are less likely than patient-examination gloves to harbor pathogens that could potentially contaminate an operative wound. Also, they may provide an increased level of

protection for DHCP if exposure to blood is likely. Additional protection may also be obtained by wearing two pairs of surgical gloves. It is important to note that the effectiveness of wearing two pairs of gloves in preventing disease transmission has not been demonstrated; however, the majority of studies among healthcare personnel (HCP) and DHCP have demonstrated a lower frequency of inner glove perforation and visible blood on the surgeon's hands when double gloves are worn.

Nonmedical Gloves

Nonmedical utility gloves, such as neoprene or polynitrile gloves, are too thick and bulky for intraoral use, but their puncture resistance makes them excellent for handling contaminated instruments and cleaning contaminated surfaces. Utility gloves can be washed or disinfected for reuse, unlike gloves used during patient-care activities; however, they should be routinely inspected and replaced if tears, cracks, or other signs of deterioration occur.

DERMATITIS CONDITIONS ASSOCIATED WITH GLOVE USAGE

The increased use of gloves has been accompanied by increased reports of occupation-related allergic and non-allergic reactions to NRL among HCP, DHCP, and patients. Also, reports of occupation-related irritant and allergic dermatitis from frequent and repeated use of hand-hygiene products and exposure to chemical disinfectants have become increasingly common. Three types of reactions are associated with latex products: irritation reactions, Type I (immediate) hypersensitivity, and Type IV (delayed) hypersensitivity reactions (Table 8-2). As a general introduction to a discussion of these adverse conditions, any individual experiencing symptoms or problems should be evaluated by a qualified healthcare professional. The common practice of changing to a "new" brand of latex gloves and using creams or other "self-cures" is not recommended. Obtaining an accurate diagnosis through medical history, physical examination, and diagnostic tests can be challenging, but is key to managing occupational allergies. In addition, DHCP should be familiar with the signs and symptoms of latex sensitivity, and procedures should be in place for minimizing latex-related health problems among DHCP and patients while protecting them from infectious materials. These procedures should include (a) reducing exposures to latex-containing materials by using appropriate work practices, (b) training and educating DHCP, (c) monitoring symptoms, and (d) substituting nonlatex products when appropriate.

Nonspecific Irritation Dermatitis (Irritation Contact Dermatitis)

Nonspecific irritation dermatitis, or **irritation contact dermatitis (ICD)**, is a nonallergic process that damages superficial layers of the skin. Also termed irritation dermatitis, it is primarily caused by a variety of contact challenges with chemicals to the integrity of the skin. Damage to epithelial tissues develops as dry, itchy, irritated areas on the skin around the area of contact (Fig. I-15). Symptoms usually develop gradually over a period of days to weeks and are localized to the areas of exposure. The prevalence of nonspecific irritation dermatitis in DHCP was previously reported to range from 12% to 67%. Skin irritation may be caused by soaps, frequent hand washing, inadequate hand drying, and mechanical irrita-

tion, such as sweating inside gloves. Since the primary defense against infection and transmission of pathogens is healthy, unbroken skin, it is imperative for DHCP to reduce or avoid exposure to the irritant after an irritant is identified. Several approaches are available to assist in prevention of dermatitis. Basic hand hygiene principles should be reviewed, including hand washing techniques and appropriate use of lotions. The potential of detergents to cause skin irritation varies considerably, but can be reduced by adding emollients. Lotions are often recommended to ease the dryness resulting from frequent hand washing and to prevent dermatitis from glove use. However, petroleum-based lotion formulations can cause breakdown of latex gloves. For that reason, lotions that contain petroleum or other oil emollients may affect the integrity of gloves and should only be used at the end of the workday. Be sure to verify with the manufacturer that the lotion is compatible with latex. Other items to review for exclusion may include disinfectant products used in the office.

Type I Natural Latex Hypersensitivity

Latex hypersensitivity is a well-recognized harmful immune response to NRL products. Most commonly these include gloves, condoms, balloons, prophylaxis cups, dental dam, orthodontic elastics, and tourniquets. Latex also can be found in many household products, such as toys, pacifiers, sports racquet handles, rubber shoes, elastic in clothing, and stretch textiles. Like other forms of type I hypersensitivity, allergic manifestations can develop as either localized or systemic reactions. Symptoms usually occur within minutes of exposure (i.e., immediate) and can include urticaria, pruritis, rhinitis, conjunctivitis, laryngeal edema, bronchospasm, asthma, angioedema, **anaphylaxis**, and death.

Type I allergies result from synthesis of IgE antibodies to specific latex allergens. NRL is obtained from the outdoor tropical rubber tree, *Hevea brasiliensis*. Latex sap from this tree contains over 250 proteins, of which only those few having molecular weights ranging from 14 to 200 Kd are responsible for induction of IgE. These proteins comprise about 3% of NRL. Individuals with a cutaneous type I allergy to latex often find that their hands begin to burn and itch soon after they don gloves. They may also notice the rapid appearance of hives and localized edema following challenge with latex proteins (Fig. I-16). Itching of hands and urticaria may also extend beyond the site of exposure. Patients allergic to NRL may also experience similar symptoms during intraoral examination or after placement of a latex dam. Sneezing, conjunctivitis, cough, wheezing, shortness of breath, hypotension, dizziness, loss of consciousness, anaphylaxis, and shock all can develop as presenting symptoms. Systemic respiratory symptoms are more likely to occur with mucous membrane exposure to latex. This is the

TABLE 8-2 Key Characteristics of Occupation-Related Allergies in Dentistry

Characteristic	Type of Occupation-Related Allergy or Dermatitis		
	Type I (Immediate) Allergy to NRL*	Type IV (Delayed) Allergy or ACD	Irritant Contact Dermatitis
Immune System Involvement	Systemic; immunoglobulin E-mediated reactions	Localized; T-cell mediated	Localized inflammation; no immune system involvement
Location of Reaction	Over entire body, because of circulating antibodies	On skin; usually confined to contact area†	On skin; confined to contact area
Sources of Potential Allergens or Irritants In Dentistry	Plant-based proteins in NRL products	Chemicals such as natural and synthetic rubber processing chemicals, glutaraldehyde, methacrylates; some small proteins	Chemicals such as detergents, acids, alkalies, oils, and solvents; continual work in abrasive, caustic or wet environments
Potential Risk Factors	• Allergic reactions to kiwis, bananas, avocados, chestnuts, tomatoes and potatoes, as well as timothy grass, birch tree, and weed pollens • Allergic reactions to latex balloons, condoms, gloves, and natural rubber products • History of allergies (atopy), skin reactions, or eczema • History of myelomeningocele (spina bifida) or multiple childhood surgeries • Regular and repeated occupational or recreational exposure to latex products	History of allergies (atopy), skin reactions, eczema, or dermatitis	• History of allergies (atopy), skin reactions, eczema, or dermatitis • Female sex • Age • Ethnicity
Exposure	Skin, mouth, nose, lungs, intravenous, or surgical sites	Skin or mucosal contact	Skin or mucosal contact
Initiation of Symptoms	Within minutes or hours of contact	Within hours or days of contact	Within minutes or hours of contact
Cessation of Symptoms	After a few hours of contact	After a few weeks of contact	Soon after irritant is removed
Symptoms	**Skin:** Hives, swelling, burning, tightness, itching, redness, tingling **Lungs:** Asthma, wheezing, bronchospasm, coughing, sneezing, rhinitis, angioedema **Other:** Nausea, vomiting, diarrhea, cramps, hypotension, tachycardia, anaphylactic shock	**Skin:** Soreness, itching, cracking, peeling, scabbing, crusting, papules, drying, swelling, thickening, redness, scaling, vesicles†	**Skin:** Soreness, burning, stinging, redness, swelling, blisters

Reprinted with permission from Hamann CP, DePaola LG, Rodgers PA. Occupation-related allergies in dentistry. J Am Dent Assoc 2005;136:501. Copyright 2005 American Dental Association. All rights reserved. Reproduced by permission.

*NRL: natural rubber latex.

†Although less common, respiratory symptoms may occur if the allergen is inhaled.

case with patients undergoing dental procedures. Exposure can occur from the gloves or from NRL-containing dental materials (i.e., rubber dams, prophylaxis cups, or orthodontic elastics). Generalized or systemic anaphylaxis symptoms can range from mild respiratory distress to life-threatening respiratory collapse. Edema can develop around the site of an injection along with difficulty in breathing and swallowing. The latter manifestations result from bronchial constriction and laryngeal edema. Shock may follow because of sudden peripheral capillary permeability, vasodilation, and a rapid decline in the challenged person's blood pressure. Anaphylactic death in extremely sensitized individuals can occur very rapidly despite initiation of emergency resuscitation procedures. Fortunately, the overwhelming majority of affected people survive episodes of type I allergic reactions, and recovery is usually complete within an hour.

A high latex allergen count in the ambient air also can result in symptoms of NRL hypersensitivity in an allergic person. This usually occurs in areas where powdered latex gloves are used repeatedly. In this case, latex proteins can adhere onto cornstarch powder particles during manufacturing processes. Cornstarch powder in latex gloves is rarely an allergen; however, it may contain varying concentrations of latex allergens absorbed from gloves. As the gloves are removed from boxes, aerosolized proteins bound to the powder can become suspended in the air and remain so for prolonged periods. The presence of excessive powder on latex gloves, along with frequent removal from boxes during the day, can cause substantial particle aerosolization in the immediate vicinity and can contaminate other nonlatex products. Subsequent respiratory and conjunctival exposure of sensitized persons to the offending proteins can stimulate symptom onset. Coughing, wheezing, shortness of breath, and/or respiratory distress may develop, with the severity dependent on the extent of a person's sensitization.

Diagnosis of type I latex hypersensitivity should include an occupational and clinical history. As of yet, there is no standardized commercially available skin test for **latex allergy** in the United States. There are, however, commercially available extracts in Europe. All testing done in the United States with the different latex extracts remains experimental, and they are used mainly for research. A commercially available radioallergosorbent (RAST) blood test for latex recently became available. It should be noted that even with more sensitive serologic assays, a negative result does not exclude the presence of hypersensitivity in a high-risk person.

People with a high exposure to latex products, including DHCP, are at increased risk for latex hypersensitivity. The risk for sensitization appears to increase with greater exposure. Thus, repeated oral and mucosal exposure to gloves, NRL prophylaxis cups, NRL dental dams, and NRL orthodontic elastics in dental settings setting may result in NRL hypersensitivity in susceptible patients. A history of atopy or surgery, especially during childhood, is an additional, important risk factor. Patients with genitourinary anomalies, spina bifida (neural tube defects), or other disorders necessitating repeated urinary catheterization also are at an increased risk for latex allergy. Cross-reacting allergies to NRL also may be more likely to develop in people with certain fruit and nut allergies. Banana, avocado, kiwi, and chestnut allergies are among the most commonly reported in this latter category.

The American Dental Association (ADA) began investigating the prevalence of type I latex hypersensitivity among DHCP at the ADA annual meeting in 1994. In 1994 and 1995 approximately 2,000 dentists, hygienists, and assistants volunteered for skin-prick testing. Results demonstrated that 6.2% of those tested were positive for type I latex hypersensitivity. Data from the subsequent 5 years of this ongoing cross-sectional study indicated a decline in prevalence from 8.5% to 4.3%. Another major study from the Mayo Clinic (Rochester, MN) found a substantial decrease in the incidence of latex allergies since 1993. This downward trend is similar to that reported by other studies and may be related to the use of latex gloves with lower allergen content and less powder.

Reinforcement for this conclusion has come from clinical investigations indicating that work areas where only powder-free, low-allergen latex gloves were used demonstrated low or undetectable amounts of latex allergy-causing proteins and fewer symptoms among HCP related to NRL allergy. Because of the role of glove powder in exposure to latex protein, the **National Institute for Occupational Safety and Health (NIOSH)** recommends that if latex gloves are chosen, HCP should be provided with reduced-protein, powder-free gloves. Nonlatex (e.g., nitrile or vinyl), powder-free, and low-protein gloves are also available. Although they are rare, potentially life-threatening anaphylactic reactions to latex can occur, and dental practices should be appropriately equipped and have procedures in place to respond to such emergencies.

DHCP and dental patients with latex allergy should avoid direct contact with latex-containing materials and be in a latex-safe environment with all latex-containing products removed from their vicinity. Dental patients with histories of latex allergy can be at risk from dental products (e.g., prophylaxis cups, dental [rubber] dams, orthodontic elastics, and medication vials). Furthermore, any latex-containing devices that cannot be removed from the treatment area should be adequately covered or isolated. Individuals might also be allergic to chemicals used in the manufacture of NRL and synthetic rubber gloves as well as metals, plastics, or other materials used in dental care; therefore, taking thorough health histories for both patients and DHCP, followed by avoidance of contact with potential allergens, can minimize the possibility of adverse reactions. Table 8-3 offers some precautions that should be considered to ensure safe treatment for patients who have possible or documented latex allergy.

Allergic Contact Dermatitis

In contrast to ICD, **allergic contact dermatitis (ACD)** or Type IV delayed-type hypersensitivity is the most common immunologic reaction to gloves, accounting for as many as 33% of allergy-tested DHCP. In contrast to Type I allergies directed against latex protein components, the etiologies of ACD are chemicals used in the glove manufacturing process (i.e., accelerators, antioxidants, and thiurams) and not the latex itself. Other chemicals used in

TABLE 8-3 Considerations in Providing Safe Treatment for Patients with Possible or Documented Latex Allergy

- Screen all patients for latex allergy (e.g., health history, medical consultation when latex allergy is suspected).

- Educate all DHCP on the different types of reactions to latex (i.e., ICD, ACD, and latex allergy) and the risks that these pose for patient and staff.

- Consider sources of latex other than gloves. Dental patients with latex allergy histories may be at risk from a variety of dental products, including (but not limited to) prophylaxis cups, dental (rubber) dams, and orthodontic elastics.

- Use only non–latex-containing materials in the treatment environment as alternatives. Ensure a latex-safe environment or one in which no personnel use latex gloves and no patient contact occurs with other latex devices, materials, and products.

- Remove all latex-containing products from the patient's vicinity. Adequately cover/isolate any latex containing devices that cannot be removed from the treatment environment.

- Be aware that latent allergens in the ambient air can cause respiratory and or anaphylactic symptoms in people with latex hypersensitivity. It may be advisable to schedule patients with latex allergy as the first appointment of the day to minimize inadvertent exposure to airborne latex particles.

- Frequently clean all working areas contaminated with latex powder/dust.

- Frequently change ventilation filters and vacuum bags used in latex-contaminated areas.

- Have latex-free kits (e.g., dental treatment and emergency) available at all times.

- Be aware that allergic reactions can be provoked from indirect contact as well as direct contact (e.g., being touched by someone who has worn latex gloves). Hand hygiene, therefore, is essential.

- Communicate latex allergy (e.g., verbal instructions, written protocols, posted signage) to other personnel to prevent them from bringing latex-containing materials into the treatment area.

- If latex-related complications occur during or after the procedure, manage the reaction and seek emergency assistance as indicated. Follow current medical emergency response recommendations for management of anaphylaxis.

the manufacture of gloves may also account for some reactions. ACD forms slowly, with a several-hour delay, and is manifested as a rash that reaches maximal appearance 24–48 hours after challenge. Lesions are usually confined to the area of contact (Fig. I-17). This chronic inflammatory reaction is well demarcated on the skin and is surrounded by localized edema. The onset of Type IV allergic symptoms is prolonged to allow sufficient numbers of lymphocytes to migrate to challenge sites, with the resultant secretion of cytokines attracting other inflammatory cells, such as macrophages and neutrophils. ACD can take a minimum of 4 days to heal, with necrosis, scabbing, and sloughing of affected epithelium. It is also important to realize that other chemicals found in the dental setting, such as methacrylates and glutaraldehydes (Fig. I-18), can cause ACD. Avoidance is key when managing Type I and/or Type IV allergies, because each exposure may lead to increased sensitization and a more severe reaction. For example, DHCP with ACD to methacrylates must avoid contact with dental bonding agents, such as by developing "no-touch" techniques. DHCP who are allergic to thiurams or carbamates should avoid products containing either of these chemicals. Multiple alternative commercial choices are becoming more available, including

gloves and other products (e.g., dental dams) made of polyvinyl chloride (PVC or vinyl), polyurethane (polyisocyanates), or styrene-base copolymers.

Among DHCP, an awareness of the existence of latex hypersensitivity (Table 8-2) can significantly reduce the risk to providers and their patients, especially in view of the concern raised about the possibility of progression of Type IV (delayed) latex hypersensitivity to Type I (immediate) hypersensitivity. In addition, clinicians can expect to treat an increasing number of allergic patients in their facilities. DHCP should be knowledgeable in recognizing early signs and symptoms of patient allergic reactions to latex and be prepared to provide appropriate care when needed (Table 8-4).

MASKS

When a tooth is cut with a high-speed turbine handpiece or cleaned with an ultrasonic scaler, blood, saliva, and other debris are atomized and expelled from the mouth. Dental **aerosols**, therefore, can be defined as solid or liquid airborne particles that are a source of microorganisms capable of inducing illness. Particles larger than 50 μm in diameter have inertial forces greater than the

---

TABLE 8-4 Latex Allergy: Summary and Recommendations

- Healthcare personnel should be familiar with the different types of latex hypersensitivities, immediate and delayed, and the risks they pose to them and their patients.

- Hand washing after glove use may reduce future development of latex hypersensitivity in DHCP.

- All people with immediate-type allergy symptoms (e.g., eye symptoms, nasal symptoms, cough, wheezing, decreased blood pressure, dizziness) developing within minutes of latex exposure should avoid any contact with latex products.

- Latex allergens in the ambient air can cause respiratory and/or anaphylactic symptoms in a susceptible person.

- Inadvertent exposure to latex may cause reactions that should be treated aggressively, especially when anaphylaxis is involved.

- Oral healthcare providers with hand dermatitis are advised to use hypoallergenic gloves that are free of the offending chemicals.

- Dental patients may be at risk for development of reactions to latex gloves, dental (rubber) dams, prophy cups, or orthodontic elastics during a dental procedure.

- It is advisable that all patients with spina bifida have latex-free dental and medical procedures. This is recommended because of the especially high incidence of life-threatening reactions to latex products in such patients.

- People with immediate-type symptoms are advised to wear an allergy alert label and to carry medication to be used in emergency situations, as explained by the appropriate medical personnel.

- Latex allergies should be documented in medical/dental records and given similar importance as other drug- or local anesthetic-related hypersensitivities.

- Identification of latex-containing devices in oral healthcare settings and substitution with latex-free dental products is vital.

- Product labels may not clearly state the latex content; therefore, extra caution is warranted.

- Latex-free kits and gloves should be available in all dental offices and clinics, and should be used instead of latex-containing ones in high-risk people.

---

frictional force of air and are ballistic in nature. The highest concentration of microorganisms is found 2 feet in front of the patient, where oral healthcare providers usually are positioned. When the droplets that contain organisms evaporate, residual **droplet nuclei** form and remain in the operatory. These aerosol particles are usually smaller than 10 μm in diameter and cannot be seen.

Infectious aerosols are composed of dust or droplet nuclei. The dustborne aerosols can be removed from the air by sedimentation, but droplet nuclei remain suspended in the air for a long time. Droplet nuclei settle slowly and are spread through the operatory by air currents, contaminating the atmosphere. Ninety-five percent of dental aerosols are 5 μm or less in diameter. It has been shown that when an isolated tooth was contaminated with a tracer organism, *Serratia marcescens,* 60% of the generated aerosols contained viable particles capable of direct penetration into the alveoli. Large droplets and debris (50–100 μm in diameter) will fall to the floor and mix with dust within a 2-foot range. Activity in the operatory disturbs settled, contaminated dust, and airborne particles settle on skin and clothing, releasing as many as 1,000 particles per minute.

Bacterial counts of one viable particle (VP) per cubic foot of air are considered acceptable in surgical operating rooms. During the use of high-speed turbines, bacterial counts may reach 109 to 300 VPs per cubic foot of air, and a 250% increase over background counts can be measured 35 minutes after a 1.5- to 50.0-minute operative procedure. Thirty minutes after instrumentation with an ultrasonic scaler, 5,000 VPs per cubic foot of air were found, representing a 3,000% increase in the bacterial count. Ninety percent of the bacterial shower released by ultrasonic scalers has been associated with alpha hemolytic streptococci, which can remain airborne and viable for as long as 24 hours. Other microorganisms discovered in dental aerosols include staphylococci, diphtheroids, pneumococci, tubercle bacilli, influenza virus, hepatitis viruses, rhinoviruses, and herpesviruses.

Masks that cover the mouth and nose can effectively reduce inhalation of potentially infectious aerosol particles. They also protect the mucous membranes of the mouth and nose from direct contamination via spatter, splashes, or sprays of blood or OPIM. Their importance requires that clinicians consider the properties of an ideal face mask when selecting one for their own use. They should ensure that it (a) does not come into contact with the nostrils or lips; (b) has a high bacterial filtration efficiency (BFE) rate; (c) fits snugly around the entire periphery of the mask; (d) does not cause fogging of eyewear; (e) is easy to put on and remove; (f) is made of a fabric that does not irritate the skin or induce allergic reactions; and (g) is made of a fabric that does not collapse during wear or when wet.

Masks are now designed to meet almost any condition routinely encountered in dentistry. They must be worn whenever aerosols or spatter may be generated, and as such their use remains a standard of practice. If a mask is worn longer than 20 minutes in an aerosol environment, however, the outside surface of the mask becomes a nidus of pathogenic bacteria rather than a barrier. Also, the outer surface of the mask can become contaminated if it is touched with contaminated fingers. It is recommended that a new mask be worn for each patient, and that masks be changed routinely at least once every hour and more often in the presence of heavy aerosol contamination.

The reemergence of TB as a major public-health and health-professional infection of concern also triggered a reevaluation of TB preventive measures and equipment (refer to Chapter 4). When a person shares air space with a patient who has infectious TB, standard surgical masks may not be effective in preventing the inhalation of droplet nuclei containing tubercle bacilli in sufficient numbers to provide protection against the transmission of TB. A better alternative is the disposable **particulate respirator mask (PRM)**, which was designed to provide a tight face seal and was originally developed to protect workers in industrial settings. PRMs may be most useful when appropriate ventilation is not available and signs and symptoms suggest a high potential for infectiousness, and when the patient is potentially infectious and is undergoing a procedure likely to produce either droplet spatter or aerosols of oral and respiratory fluids, regardless of the presence of appropriate ventilation. HCP can wear any one of the particulate respirators available for protection against diseases that are spread through the air if they are approved by NIOSH, and if they have been properly fit-tested and maintained. NIOSH-approved disposable respirators are marked with the manufacturer's name, the part number (P/N), the protection provided by the filter (e.g., **N-95**), and the word NIOSH. The number "95," for example, refers to the percentage of particles filtered.

Comfort influences the acceptability of PRMs. Generally, the more efficient the PRMs, the more difficult it is to breathe through them, and the greater the perceived discomfort. A proper fit is imperative to protect against inhalation of droplet nuclei. When gaps are present, the PRM will function more like a funnel and provide virtually no protection. PRMs should be provided by oral healthcare facilities and worn by DHCP who are in the same setting with a patient whose signs and symptoms suggest a high potential for infectiousness, and who will be performing procedures that are likely to produce droplet nuclei and spatter of oral and respiratory fluids. DHCP should be trained adequately in the use and

disposal of PRMs and should follow manufacturers' instructions carefully.

As with any technique that requires full compliance to achieve maximum benefits, errors in mask usage can cause problems. The first issue relates to instances in which DHCP do not change masks between patient treatments. As mentioned above, these barriers can lose filtration capabilities rapidly when exposed to high concentrations of aerosolized spatter. A second common error occurs when a DHCP does not wear the mask properly and the mask does not cover the nostrils. To demonstrate the problem here, Figure I-19 uses the "red saliva" model described in Chapter 1 to demonstrate the extent of respiratory airborne exposure that can occur when a dental hygienist does not wear a mask properly during an a periodontal procedure using an ultrasonic scaling device.

PROTECTIVE EYEWEAR

During dental procedures, large particles of debris and saliva can be ejected toward the oral-healthcare provider's face. These particles can contain large concentrations of bacteria and can physically damage the eyes. Protective eyewear is indicated to prevent both physical injury and infection from aerosolized oral microbes. Of particular concern are the herpes simplex viruses and *Staphylococcus aureus* (Fig. I-20); however, most members of the normal oral flora must also be considered ocular opportunistic pathogens. The eyewear that gives the best protection has side shields and is large enough to adequately cover and protect the wearer's eyes from macroscopic and microscopic injury (Fig. I-21). Some models are made to fit over regular corrective glasses. Personal eyeglasses are not considered to be PPE. A surgical mask and protective eyewear with solid side shields are adequate for procedures in which small amounts of spatter or splashes are likely. Adding a clear plastic disposable or nondisposable face shield may be useful when more protection is desired. When wearing a face shield, DHCP should also wear a mask. Face shields can extend from the chin to the crown, and some even wrap around the sides of the head, offering side protection. Safety, or protective, eyeglasses for the patient also should be considered for protection from accidentally dropped instruments, chemical splashes, and other foreign-object injuries. Contaminated reusable protective eyewear, such as clinician and patient protective eyewear, should be washed thoroughly with soap and water, rinsed well, and, when visibly soiled, disinfected between patients according to the manufacturer's instructions.

PROTECTIVE CLOTHING

Protective clothing, such as reusable or disposable gowns, laboratory coats, jackets, and uniforms, should be worn when clothing or exposed skin is likely to be soiled with blood or other body fluids. The OSHA bloodborne pathogens standard requires sleeves to be long enough to protect the forearms when the gown is worn as PPE (i.e., when spattering and spraying of blood, saliva, or OPIM to the forearms are anticipated). PPE does not have to be fluid-impervious to meet OSHA standards, but must prevent contamination of skin and underlying clothing. Cotton or cotton/polyester fabrics are acceptable as PPE if the sleeve length is long. DHCP should change protective clothing when it becomes visibly soiled, and as soon as feasible if it has been penetrated by blood or other potentially infectious fluids. Protective garments should be removed before DHCP leave areas of the dental healthcare facility used for laboratory, instrument processing, or patient-care activities. OSHA prohibits home laundering of items considered to be PPE; the employer is required to launder or clean any reusable PPE contaminated with blood, saliva, or other infectious material. This can be done in the office or contracted through a commercial laundry service. As an alternative, the office may choose to use disposable protective clothing. Appropriate PPE (e.g., gloves) should be used when handling contaminated laundry. Contaminated reusable PPE should be placed in red bags or appropriately labeled containers.

HEAD AND SHOE COVERS

Head and shoe covers are less frequently used types of PPE, but should be considered if contamination is likely.

OSHA does not mandate the use of shoe and head covers in dentistry. DHCP may want to consider using shoe covers when contamination of footwear is anticipated, such as during surgical procedures where unusually heavy bleeding may be anticipated (e.g., maxillofacial reconstructive surgery and trauma surgery). Head covers are optional but may be useful in decreasing contamination of DHCP during ultrasonic scaling, surgical procedures using rotary or ultrasonic instrumentation, and manual decontamination of dental instruments, where spraying and spattering of blood and OPIM may be generated. Head covers also provide maximum protection to patients during surgical procedures.

DENTAL (RUBBER) DAMS

It has been demonstrated that the use of a dental, or rubber, dam consistently reduces bacterial counts with or without an air-water spray combination. The dental dam is most effective in reducing bacterial counts when water spray and high-velocity air evacuation are used. Water reduces the number of microorganisms in aerosols when a spray is used, and proper patient positioning should further minimize the formation of droplets, spatter, and aerosols during treatment. Although the dental dam and high-velocity air evacuation can be considered engineering controls to minimize the spread of droplets, spatter, and aerosols, DHCP must still use gloves, masks, protective eyewear, and protective clothing during patient treatment.

TABLE 8-5 Suggested Sequence for Donning and Removing PPE*

Donning PPE	Removing PPE
Protective Clothing • Select appropriate type and size • Fasten all snaps, buttons, or ties **Mask** • Place over the nose, mouth, and chin • Adjust the flexible nose piece over the nose bridge • Secure on the head with ties or elastic **Protective Eyewear** • Position protective eyewear over eyes and secure to the head using the ear pieces or headband **Gloves** • Don gloves last (after hand washing) • Select correct type and size • Insert hands into gloves • Extend gloves over protective clothing cuffs	**Gloves** • Grasp outside edge near wrist and peel away from hand, turning glove inside out • Hold in opposite gloved hand • Slide ungloved finger under the wrist of the remaining glove • Peel off from inside, creating a bag for both gloves • Discard appropriately **Protective Eyewear** • Grasp ear or head pieces with ungloved hands and lift away from face • Set aside for cleaning/disinfection or dispose of appropriately **Protective Clothing** • Unfasten snaps, buttons, or ties • Remove protective clothing away from the body • Discard if disposable; if reusable place in appropriate laundry container **Mask** • Remove from face by only touching the ties or elastic bands • Discard appropriately • Wash your hands

*The type of PPE used will vary based on the dental procedure. The combination of PPE selected will affect the sequence of donning and removal. Areas of PPE that have or are likely to have become contaminated, or have been in contact with contaminated materials or environmental surfaces, are on the outside and front. The inside, outside back, and ties on the head and back are areas of PPE that are not likely to have become contaminated.

Table 8-6 Safe Work Practices to Protect Yourself and Limit the Spread of Contamination
• Keep gloved hands away from the face.
• Avoid touching or adjusting other PPE.
• Limit surfaces and items touched.
• Change gloves when torn or heavily contaminated; wash hands before donning new gloves.
• Wash your hands.

DONNING AND REMOVING PERSONAL PROTECTIVE EQUIPMENT

The type of PPE used will vary based on the dental procedure. Also, the combination of PPE selected will affect the sequence of donning and removal. PPE is available to protect you from exposure to infectious agents; therefore, it is important to put on and take off PPE in a manner that minimizes further spread of contamination (Table 8-5). Hand washing immediately after removing PPE is key. If your hands become visibly contaminated during PPE removal, wash them before continuing to remove the PPE. Table 8-6 describes suggestions for limiting cross contamination in the dental operatory.

SUMMARY

The barrier techniques of using gloves, masks, protective eyewear, and protective clothing protect the skin and mucous membranes of the eyes, nose, and mouth of DHCP from exposure to blood and OPIM during dental procedures. They interfere with the initial step (exposure) in the development of an infectious disease. The increased use of gloves has been accompanied by increased reports of occupationally-related allergic and irritant dermatitis reactions to NRL among HCP, DHCP, and patients. DHCP should be familiar with the signs and symptoms of latex sensitivity and procedures should be in place to minimize latex-related health problems among DHCP and patients while protecting them from infectious materials.

✓ Practical Dental Infection Control Checklist

General Considerations
❑ Is PPE available in a variety of types and sizes?
❑ Is PPE donned and removed in a manner that minimizes further spread of contamination?

❑ Is contaminated laundry (e.g., reusable PPE) placed in an appropriately marked container according to local policy?
❑ Is PPE removed before leaving the work area?

Masks, Protective Eyewear, and Face Shields
❑ Do DHCP wear eye protection with solid side shields and a surgical mask, or a face shield and a surgical mask, to protect mucous membranes of the eyes, nose, and mouth during procedures likely to generate splashing or spattering of blood or other body fluids?
  ❑ Is a NIOSH-approved, disposable PRM worn when airborne isolation precautions are required (e.g., for protection against diseases that are spread through the air, such as tuberculosis)?
❑ Do DHCP always wear a mask when wearing a face shield?
❑ Do DHCP change masks between patients or during patient treatment if the mask becomes wet?
❑ Is reusable facial protective equipment (e.g., clinician and patient protective eyewear or face shields) cleaned with soap and water, or if visibly soiled, cleaned and disinfected between patients?

Protective Clothing
❑ Do DHCP wear protective clothing (e.g., a long-sleeved reusable or disposable gown, laboratory coat, or uniform) that covers personal clothing and skin (e.g., forearms) likely to be soiled with blood, saliva, or OPIM?
❑ Do DHCP change protective clothing if it is visibly soiled?
❑ Do DHCP change protective clothing immediately or as soon as feasible if it is penetrated by blood or other potentially infectious fluids?
❑ Do DHCP remove barrier protection, including gloves, mask, eyewear, and gown before departing work area (e.g., dental patient care, instrument processing, or laboratory area)?

Gloves
❑ Does the dental office/clinic ensure that appropriate gloves in the correct size are readily accessible?
❑ Do DHCP wear medical gloves when a potential exists for contacting blood, saliva, OPIM, or mucous membranes?
❑ Do DHCP wear a new pair of medical gloves for each patient, remove them promptly after use, and wash hands immediately to avoid transfering of microorganisms to other patients or environments?
❑ Do DHCP remove gloves that are torn, cut, or punctured as soon as feasible and wash hands before regloving?

❑ Are appropriate gloves (e.g., puncture- and chemical-resistant utility gloves) used when cleaning instruments and performing housekeeping tasks involving contact with blood or OPIM?

❑ Does the dental office/clinic consult with glove manufacturers regarding the chemical compatibility of glove material and dental materials used?

Sterile Surgeon's Gloves and Double Gloving during Oral Surgical Procedures

❑ Are sterile surgeon's gloves worn when performing oral surgical procedures?

Head and Shoe Covers

❑ Are head and shoe covers available if personnel request them?

❑ Are head and shoe covers worn if contamination is likely?

Contact Dermatitis and Latex Hypersensitivity

❑ Does the dental office/clinic have policies and procedures for evaluation, diagnosis, and management of DHCP with suspected or known occupational contact dermatitis?

  ❑ Does the dental office/clinic seek a definitive diagnosis by a qualified healthcare professional for any DHCP with suspected latex allergy to carefully determine its specific etiology and appropriate treatment as well as work restrictions and accommodations?

❑ Are DHCP educated regarding the signs, symptoms, and diagnoses of skin reactions associated with frequent hand hygiene and glove use?

❑ Are all patients screened for latex allergy (e.g., take health history and refer for medical consultation when latex allergy is suspected)?

❑ Is a latex-safe environment available for patients and DHCP with latex allergy?

❑ Are emergency treatment kits with latex-free products available at all times?

Review Questions

1. PPE is used to protect the skin and the mucous membranes of the eyes, nose, and mouth of DHCP from exposure to blood or OPIM.

A. True

B. False

2. Which of the following is not considered PPE?

A. Gloves

B. Protective eyewear

C. Long-sleeved jacket

D. Short-sleeved top

E. Mask

3. Wearing gloves does not replace hand washing. Hands must be washed before donning gloves, but not after removing gloves.

A. The first statement is true. The second statement is false.

B. The first statement is false. The second statement is true.

C. Both statements are true.

D. Both statements are false.

4. Gloves must be worn when there is the potential for contacting

A. Mucous membranes

B. Saliva

C. Blood

D. Intact skin during an extraoral exam

E. A, B, and C

F. All of the above

5. This type of glove is worn during oral surgical procedures.

A. Patient examination gloves

B. Sterile surgeon's gloves

C. Utility gloves that are puncture- and chemical-resistant

D. None of the above

6. A mask should be changed

A. Once a day

B. After each patient

C. Only if it is wet

D. Every 20 minutes

7. Which of the following statements about protective eyewear is false?

A. Protective eyewear is indicated not only to prevent physical injury, but also to prevent infection.

B. Personal eyeglasses can substitute for protective eyewear.

C. Contaminated reusable protective eyewear should be washed thoroughly with soap and water, rinsed well, and when visibly soiled, disinfected between patients, according to the manufacturer's directions.

D. Protective eyewear must contain side shields.

8. A face shield and mask may be worn when additional protection is desired from spray and spatter generated during dental procedures.

A. True

B. False

9. Which of the following statements about protective clothing is false?

A. Protective clothing should be changed when it becomes visibly soiled and as soon as feasible if penetrated by blood or other potentially infectious fluids.

B. Protective clothing must prevent contamination of skin and underlying clothing.

C. It is permissible to allow employees to launder protective clothing at home as long as there is just a small amount of contamination.

D. Gloves and other PPE should be used when handling contaminated laundry.

10. The following reactions are considered to be allergic reactions.

A. Irritant contact dermatitis

B. ACD

C. Type I latex hypersensitivity

D. A, B, C

E. A and C

F. B and C

11. NRL _____ attached to glove powder are responsible for latex allergy.

A. Aerosols

B. Allergens

C. Proteins

12. Latent allergens in the ambient air can cause respiratory and or anaphylactic symptoms in people with latex hypersensitivity.

A. True

B. False

Critical Thinking

1. A coworker develops the symptoms of dry, itchy, irritated skin on her hands. What are the possible causes of this dermatitis? Could it be caused from a product used outside of the dental office/clinic?

2. When reviewing your patient's health history, you notice that she indicated that she is allergic to latex. When discussing this with you, the patient reports that she has been evaluated and diagnosed by her allergist. What are some items you would take into consideration when providing dental care to this patient?

3. What types of PPE are provided in your office/clinic? Where is the PPE kept? Are there a variety of sizes available?

4. Place samples of the PPE available in your office/clinic in front of you.

a. What PPE would you wear if performing or assisting with a(n)

i. Dental prophylaxis?

ii. Periodontal surgery?

iii. Amalgam restoration?

iv. Dental examination?

b. Arrange the PPE in order of donning it and removing it for the above procedures.

SELECTED READINGS

Abel LC, Miller RL, Micik RE, et al. Studies on dental aerobiology: IV. Bacterial contamination of water delivered by dental units. J Dent Res 1971;50:1567–1579.

Allergic reactions to latex-containing medical devices. FDA medical alert. MDA 1991;21:2–3.

Allmers H, Brehler R, Chen Z, et al. Reduction of latex aeroallergens and latex-specific IgE antibodies in sensitized workers after removal of powdered natural rubber latex gloves in a hospital. Allergy Clin Immunol 1998;102:841–846.

American Dental Association Council on Scientific Affairs. The dental team and latex hypersensitivity. J Am Dent Assoc 1999;130:257–264.

Avery CM, Hjort A, Walsh S, et al. Glove perforation during surgical extraction of wisdom teeth. Oral Surg Oral Med Oral Pathol Oral Radiol Endodont 1998;86:23–25.

Bagga BSR, Murphy RA, Anderson AW, et al. Contamination of dental unit cooling water with oral micro-organisms and its prevention. J Am Dent Assoc 1984;109:712–716.

Baur X, Chen Z, Allmers H. Can a threshold limit value for natural rubber latex airborne allergens be defined? J Allergy Clin Immunol 1998;101:24–27.

Baur X, Jager D. Airborne antigens from latex gloves. Lancet 1990;335:912.

Belting CM, Haberfelde GC, Juhl LK. Spread of organisms from dental air rotor. J Am Dent Assoc 1964;68:648–651.

Berky ZT, Luciano WJ, James WD. Latex glove allergy: a survey of the U.S. Army Dental Corps. JAMA 1992;268:2695–2697.

Berndt U, Wigger-Alberti W, Gabard B, et al. Efficacy of a barrier cream and its vehicle as protective measures against occupational irritant contact dermatitis. Contact Dermatitis 2000;42:77–80.

Blinkhorn AS, Leggate EM. An allergic reaction to rubber dam. Br Dent J 1984;156:402–403.

Bolyard EA, Tablan OC, Williams WW, et al. Hospital Infection Control Practices Advisory Committee. Guideline for infection control in healthcare personnel, 1998. Am J Infect Control 1998;26:289–354.

Bond WW, Petersen NJ, Favero MS, et al. Transmission of type B viral hepatitis via eye inoculation of a chimpanzee. J Clin Microbiol 1982;15:533–534.

Brown RV. Bacterial aerosols generated by ultra-high speed cutting instruments. J Dent Child 1965;32:112–117.

Bubak ME, Reed CE, Fransway AF, et al. Allergic reactions to latex among healthcare workers. Mayo Clin Proc 1992;67:1075–1079.

Burke FJ, Baggett FJ, Lomax AM. Assessment of the risk of glove puncture during oral surgery procedures. Oral Surg Oral Med Oral Pathol Oral Radiol Endodont 1996;82:18–21.

CDC. Guideline for hand hygiene in healthcare settings: recommendations of the Healthcare Infection Control Practices Advisory Committee and the HICPAC/SHEA/APIC/IDSA Hand Hygiene Task Force. MMWR 2002;51(RR-16):1–45.

CDC. Guidelines for infection control in dental health-care settings, 2003. MMWR 2003;52(RR-17):1–66.

CDC. Guidelines for preventing the transmission of tuberculosis in health-care settings, with special focus on HIV-related issues. MMWR 1990;39(RR-17):1–29.

CDC. Guidelines for prevention of transmission of human immunodeficiency virus and hepatitis B virus to health-care and public-safety workers. MMWR 1989;38(Suppl S-6):1–37.

CDC. Hepatitis B virus: a comprehensive strategy for eliminating transmission in the United States through universal childhood vaccination. MMWR 1991;40(RR-13):1–25.

CDC. National Institute for Occupational Safety and Health. NIOSH alert: preventing allergic reactions to natural rubber latex in the workplace. Cincinnati, OH: U.S. Department of Health and Human Services, Public Health Service, CDC, National Institute for Occupational Safety and Health; 1997.

CDC. Personal protective equipment (PPE) in healthcare settings. Available at http://www.cdc.gov/ncidod/dhqp/ppe.html. Accessed August 2007.

CDC. Protection against viral hepatitis: recommendations of the Immunization Practices Advisory Committee (ACIP). MMWR 1990;39(RR-2):2–5.

CDC. Public Health Service statement on management of occupational exposure to human immunodeficiency virus, including considerations regarding zidovudine post-exposure use. MMWR 1990;39(RR-1):1–14.

CDC. Recommendations for preventing transmission of human immunodeficiency virus and hepatitis B virus during exposure-prone invasive procedures. MMWR 1991;40(RR-8):1–9.

CDC. Recommendations for prevention of HIV in health-care settings. MMWR 1987;36(2S):1–16.

CDC. Recommended infection-control practices for dentistry. MMWR 1986;35:237–242.

CDC. Update: universal precautions for prevention of transmission of human immuno-deficiency virus, hepatitis B virus, and other bloodborne pathogens in healthcare settings. MMWR 1988;37:377–382, 387–388.

Davies PA. Please wash your hands. Arch Dis Child 1982;57:647–648.

Fernandez de Corres L, Moneo I, Munoz D, et al. Sensitization from chestnuts and bananas in patients with urticaria and anaphylaxis from contact with latex. Ann Allergy 1993;70:35–39.

Fisher AA. Allergic contact reactions in health personnel. J Allergy Clin Immunol 1992;90:729–738.

Gani JS, Anseline PF, Bissett RL. Efficacy of double versus single gloving in protecting the operating team. Aust N Z J Surg 1990;60:171–175.

Garner JS, Favero MS. Guideline for handwashing and hospital environmental control. Publication no. 99–1117. Atlanta, GA: CDC; 1985.

Hamann CP, DePaola LG, Rodgers PA. Occupation-related allergies in dentistry. J Am Dent Assoc 2005;136:500–510.

Hamann CP, Rodgers PA, Sullivan K. Allergic contact dermatitis in dental professionals: effective diagnosis and treatment. J Am Dent Assoc 2003;134:185–194.

Hamann CP, Rodgers PA, Sullivan KM. Occupational allergens in dentistry. Curr Opin Allergy Clin Immunol 2004;4:403–409.

Hamann CP, Turjanmaa K, Rietschel R, et al. Natural rubber latex hypersensitivity: incidence and prevalence of type I allergy in the dental professional. J Am Dent Assoc 1998;129:43–54.

Heilman DK, Jones RT, Swanson MC, et al. A prospective, controlled study showing that rubber gloves are the major contributor to latex aeroallergen levels in the operating room. J Allergy Clin Immunol 1996;98:325–330.

Hermesch CB, Spackman GK, Dodge WW, et al. Effect of powder-free latex examination glove use on airborne powder levels in a dental school clinic. J Dent Educ 1999;63:814–820.

Hunt LW, Fransway AF, Reed CE, et al. An epidemic of occupational allergy to latex involving healthcare workers. J Occup Environ Med 1995;37:1204–1209.

Hunt LW, Kelkar P, Reed CE, et al. Management of occupational allergy to natural rubber latex in a medical center: the importance of quantitative latex allergen measurement and objective follow-up. J Allergy Clin Immunol 2002;110(suppl 2):S96–S106.

Jaeger D, Kleinhans D, Czuppon AB, et al. Latex-specific proteins causing immediate-type cutaneous, nasal, bronchial, and systemic reactions. J Allergy Clin Immunol 1992;89:759–768.

Kelly KJ, Kurup V, Zacharisen M, et al. Skin and serologic testing in the diagnosis of latex allergy. J Allergy Clin Immunol 1993;91:1140–1145.

Kelso JM, Sodhi N, Gosselin VA, et al. Diagnostic performance characteristics of the standard Phadebas RAST, modified RAST, and Pharmacia CAP system versus skin testing. Ann Allergy 1991;67:511–514.

Klein RC, Party E, Gershey EL. Virus penetration of examination gloves. Biotechniques 1990;9:196–199.

Korniewicz DM, El-Masri M, Broyles JM, et al. Performance of latex and nonlatex medical examination gloves during simulated use. Am J Infect Control 2002;30:133–138.

Korniewicz DM, Kirwin M, Cresci K, et al. Leakage of latex and vinyl exam gloves in high- and low-risk clinical settings. Am Ind Hyg Assoc J 1993;54:22–26.

Korniewicz DM, Laughon BE, Cyr WH, et al. Leakage of virus through used vinyl and latex examination gloves. J Clin Microbiol 1990;28:787–788.

Korniewicz DM, Laughon BE, Butz A, et al. Integrity of vinyl and latex procedure gloves. Nurs Res 1989;38:144–146.

Kotilainen HR, Brinker JP, Avato JL, et al. Latex and vinyl examination gloves. Quality control procedures and implications for healthcare workers. Arch Intern Med 1989;149:2749–2753.

Langmuir AD. Contact and airborne infections. In: Maxcy KE, Rosenau, MJ, eds. Preventive Medicine and Public Health. 10th ed. New York: Appleton-Century-Crofts; 1973:248.

Leger RR, Meeropol E. Children at risk: latex allergy and spina bifida. J Pediatr Nurs 1992;7:371–376.

Lu DP, Zambito RF. Aerosols and cross-infection in the dental practice: a historic view. Gen Dent 1981;29:136–143.

Madden RM, Hausler WJ, Leaverton PE. Study of some factors contributing to aerosol production by the air turbine handpiece. J Dent Res 1969;48:341–345.

McCormick RD, Buchman TL, Maki DG. Double-blind, randomized trial of scheduled use of a novel barrier cream and an oil-containing lotion for protecting the hands of healthcare workers. Am J Infect Control 2000;28:302–310.

Merchant VA, Molinari JA, Pickett T. Microbial penetration of gloves following usage in routine dental procedures. Am J Dent 1992;5:95–96.

Micik RE, Miller RL, Mazzarella MA, et al. Studies on dental aerobiology: I. Bacterial aerosols generated during dental procedures. J Dent Res 1969;48:49–56.

Molinari JA, Harte JA. Dental services. APIC Text of Infection Control and Epidemiology: Principles and Practice. 2nd ed. Washington, DC: APIC; 2005:51-1–51-23.

M'Raihi L, Charpin D, Pons A, et al. Cross-reactivity between latex and banana. J Allergy Clin Immunol 1991;87:129–130.

Nutter AF. Contact urticaria to rubber. Br J Dermatol 1979;101:597–598.

Oei HD, Tijook SB, Chang KC. Anaphylaxis due to latex allergy. Allergy Proc 1992;13:121–122.

Otis LL, Cottone JA. Prevalence of perforations in disposable latex gloves during routine dental treatment. J Am Dent Assoc 1989;118:321–324.

Ownby DR, Tomlanovich M, Sammons N, et al. Anaphylaxis associated with latex allergy during barium enema examinations. AJR Am J Roentgenol 1991;156:903–908.

Palenik MS, Miller CH. Approaches to preventing disease transmission in the dental office. Dent Asepsis Rev 1984;5:1–2.

Patton LL, Campbell TL, Evers SP. Prevalence of glove perforations during double-gloving for dental procedures. Gen Dent 1995;43:22–26.

Petersen NM, Bond WW, Favero MS. Air sampling for hepatitis B surface antigen in a dental operatory. J Am Dent Assoc 1979;99:465–467.

Pippin DJ, Verderame RA, Weber KK. Efficacy of face masks in preventing inhalation of airborne contaminants. J Oral Maxillofac Surg 1987;45:319–323.

Pistocco LR, Bowers GM. Demonstration of an aerosol produced by air-water spray and air-turbine pieces. US Navy Med 1962;40:24.

Pitten FA, Herdemann G, Kramer A. The integrity of latex gloves in clinical dental practice. Infection 2000;28:388–392.

Pokowitiz WM, Hoffman H. Dental aerobiology. NY J Dent 1971;37:337–351.

Primeau MN, Adkinson Jr NF, Hamilton RG. Natural rubber pharmaceutical vial closures release latex allergens that produce skin reactions. J Allergy Clin Immunol 2001;107:958–962.

Rankin KV, Jones DL, Rees TD. Latex glove reactions found in a dental school. J Am Dent Assoc 1993;124:67–71.

Register-General of Great Britain. Death from Respiratory Tuberculosis. London: HM Printing Office; 1931.

Rego A, Roley L. In-use barrier integrity of gloves: latex and nitrile superior to vinyl. Am J Infect Control 1999;27:405–410.

Rodriguez M, Vega F, Garcia MT, et al. Hypersensitivity to latex, chestnut, and banana. Ann Allergy 1993,70:31–34.

Saary MJ, Kanani A, Alghadeer H, et al. Changes in rates of natural rubber latex sensitivity among dental school students and staff members after changes in latex gloves. J Allergy Clin Immunol 2002;109:131–135.

Schwimmer A, Massoumi M, Barr CE. Efficacy of double gloving to prevent inner glove perforation during outpatient oral surgical procedures. J Am Dent Assoc 1994;125:196–198.

Short LJ, Bell DM. Risk of occupational infection with bloodborne pathogens in operating and delivery room settings. Am J Infect Control 1993;21:343–350.

Siegel JD, Rhinehart E, Jackson M, et al. Guideline for isolation precautions: preventing transmission of infectious agents in healthcare settings. CDC 2007:1–219.

Siew C, Hamann C, Gruninger SE, et al. Type I latex allergic reactions among dental professionals, 1996–2001. J Dent Res 2003;82(Special Issue):1718.

Slater JE. Allergic reactions to natural rubber. Ann Allergy 1992;68:203–209.

Slater JE, Mostello LA, Shaer C, et al. Type I hypersensitivity to rubber. Ann Allergy 1990;65:411–414.

Smart ER, Macleod RI, Lawrence CM. Allergic reactions to rubber gloves in dental patients: report of three cases. Br Dent J 1992;172:445–447.

Spendlove JC, Fannin KF. Source, significance, and control of indoor microbial aerosols: human health aspects. Public Health Rep 1983;98:229–244.

Stevens RE. Preliminary study: air contamination with micro-organisms during use of air turbine handpieces. J Am Dent Assoc 1963;66:237–239.

Tarlo SM, Sussman G, Contala A, et al. Control of airborne latex by use of powder-free latex gloves. J Allergy Clin Immunol 1994;93:985–989.

Themido R, Brandao FM. Contact allergy to thiurams. Contact Dermatitis 1984;10:251.

Tokars JI, Culver DH, Mendelson MH, et al. Skin and mucous membrane contacts with blood during surgical procedures: risk and prevention. Infect Control Hosp Epidemiol 1995;16:703–711.

Tomazic VJ, Shampaine EL, Lamanna A, et al. Cornstarch powder on latex products is an allergen carrier. J Allergy Clin Immunol 1994;93:751–758.

Trape M, Schenck P, Warren A. Latex gloves use and symptoms in healthcare workers 1 year after implementation of a policy restricting the use of powdered gloves. Am J Infec Control 2000;28:352–358.

Turjanmaa K. Incidence of immediate allergy to latex gloves in hospital personnel. Contact Dermatitis 1987;17:270–275.

Turjanmaa K, Kanto M, Kautiainen H, et al. Long-term outcome of 160 adult patients with natural rubber latex allergy. J Allergy Clin Immunol 2002;110(suppl 2):S70–S74.

Turjanmaa K, Reunala T, Alenius H, et al. Allergens in latex surgical gloves and glove powder. Lancet 1990;336:1588.

Underhill TE, Terezhalmy GT. Epidemiologic aspects of infectious diseases important to dentists. Comp Cont Edu Dent 1986;7:48–57.

Underhill TE, Terezhalmy GT, Cottone JA. Prevention of cross-infections in the dental environment. Comp Cont Educ Dent 1986;7:260–269.

U.S. Department of Labor, Occupational Safety and Health Administration. 29 CFR Part 1910.1030. Occupational exposure to bloodborne pathogens; needlesticks and other sharps injuries; final rule. Fed Regist 2001;66: 5317–5325. [As amended from and includes 29 CFR Part 1910.1030. Occupational exposure to bloodborne pathogens; final rule. Fed Regist 1991;56:64174–64182.]

Van Ketel WG. Contact urticaria from rubber gloves after dermatitis from thiurams. Contact Dermatitis 1984;11:323–324.

Warpinski JR, Folger J, Cohen M, et al. Allergic reaction to latex: a risk factor for unsuspected anaphylaxis. Allergy Proc 199112:95–102.

Wyss M, Elsner P, Wuthrich B, et al. Allergic contact dermatitis from natural latex without contact urticaria. Contact Dermatitis 1993;28:154–156.

Yassin MS, Lierl MB, Fischer TJ, et al. Latex allergy in hospital employees. Ann Allergy 1994;72:245–249.

Yunginger JW, Jones RT, Fransway AF, et al. Extractable latex allergens and proteins in disposable medical gloves and other rubber products. J Allergy Clin Immunol 1994;93:836–842.

Zaza S, Reeder JM, Charles LE, et al. Latex sensitivity among perioperative nurses. AORN J 1994;60:806–812.

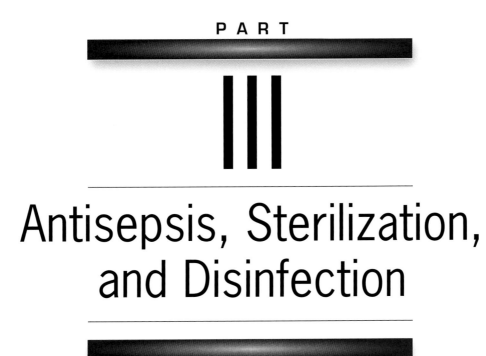

III

Antisepsis, Sterilization, and Disinfection

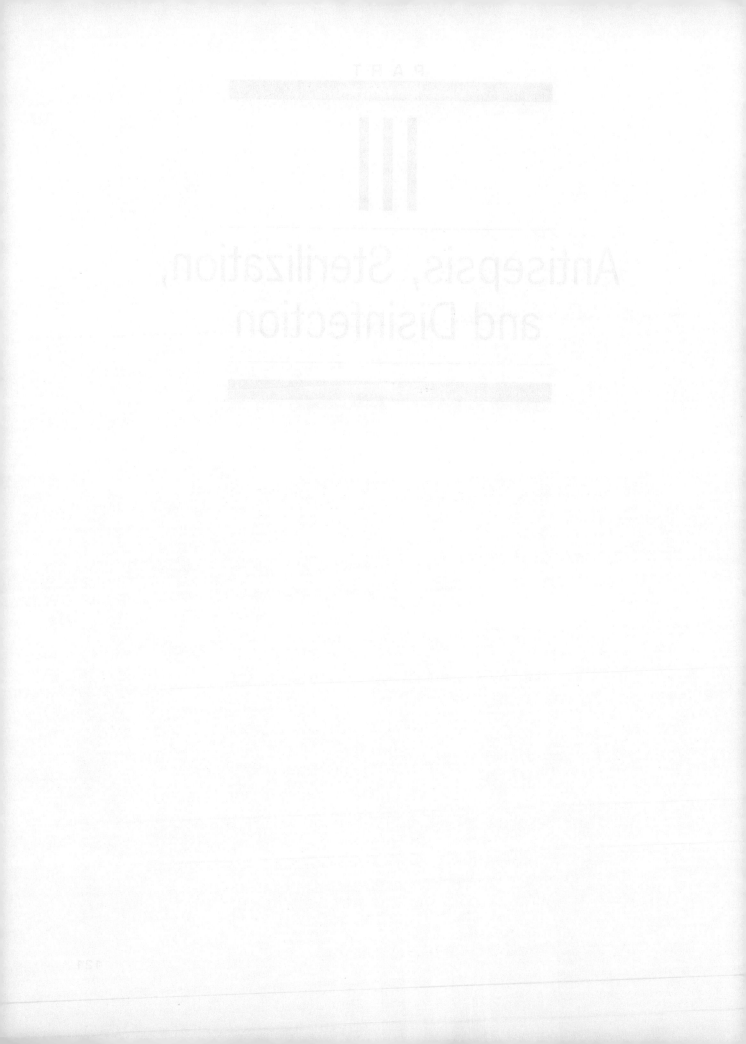

PART

III

Antisepsis, Sterilization,
and Disinfection

9

Antisepsis and Hand Hygiene

Nancy Andrews

Eve Cuny

John A. Molinari

Jennifer A. Harte

LEARNING OBJECTIVES

After completion of this chapter individuals should be able to:

1 Understand the role of healthcare workers' hands in the transmission of infections in healthcare settings.

2 Discuss the difference between transient and resident flora and their relationship to hand-hygiene practices and disease transmission.

3 Identify reasons for hand-hygiene failure in healthcare settings.

4 Identify the appropriate hand-hygiene method and product for routine (nonsurgical) and oral surgical dental procedures.

5 Understand the difference between plain soap, antimicrobial soap, and alcohol-based hand hygiene agents.

6 Identify desirable characteristics of hand hygiene products.

7 Discuss the various active ingredients in hand hygiene products.

KEY TERMS

Alcohol-based hand rub: an alcohol-containing preparation designed for application to the hands to reduce the number of viable microorganisms on the hands. In the United States, such preparations usually contain 60% to 95% ethanol or isopropanol. These are waterless antiseptic agents that do not require the use of exogenous water. After such an agent is applied, the hands are rubbed together until the agent has dried.

Antimicrobial soap: a soap (i.e., detergent) containing an antiseptic agent.

Antiseptic: a germicide that is used on skin or living tissue for the purpose of inhibiting or destroying microorganisms. Examples include alcohols, chlorhexidine, chlorine, hexachlorophene, iodine, chloroxylenol (PCMX), quaternary ammonium compounds, and triclosan.

Antiseptic hand rub: the process of applying an antiseptic hand-rub product to all surfaces of the hands to reduce the number of microorganisms present.

Antiseptic hand wash: washing hands with water and soap or detergents containing an antiseptic agent.

Artificial fingernails: substances or devices applied or added to the natural nails to augment or enhance the wearer's own nails. They include, but are not limited to, bondings, tips, wrappings, and tapes.

Detergents: compounds that possess a cleaning action and have hydrophilic and lipophilic parts. Although products used for hand washing or antiseptic hand wash in a healthcare setting represent various types of detergents, the term "soap" is used to refer to such detergents in this book. Detergents make no antimicrobial claims on the label.

Emollients (humectants): ingredients in hand-hygiene and hand-care products that add moisture to skin and reduce skin dryness.

Food and Drug Administration (FDA): the FDA promotes and protects the public health by helping safe and effective products reach the market in a timely way; monitors products for continued safety after they are in use; and helps the public get the accurate, science-based information needed to improve health.

Hand hygiene: a general term that applies to hand washing, antiseptic hand wash, antiseptic hand rub, and surgical hand antisepsis.

Hand washing: washing hands with plain (i.e., nonantimicrobial) soap and water.

Irritation contact dermatitis (ICD): the development of dry, itchy, irritated areas on the skin, which can result from frequent hand washing and gloving as well as exposure to chemicals. This condition is not an allergic reaction.

Multiresistant organisms: microorganisms that demonstrate resistance to multiple antibiotic medications.

Oral surgical procedure: involves the incision, excision, or reflection of tissue that exposes normally sterile areas of the oral cavity. Examples include biopsy, periodontal surgery, apical surgery, implant surgery, and surgical extractions of teeth (e.g., removal of erupted or nonerupted tooth requiring elevation of mucoperiosteal flap, removal of bone or sectioning of tooth, and suturing if needed).

Persistent activity: prolonged or extended activity that prevents or inhibits the proliferation or survival of microorganisms after application of the product. This activity may be demonstrated by sampling a site several minutes or hours after application and demonstrating bacterial antimicrobial effectiveness when compared with a baseline level. In the past, this property was also called "residual activity." Both substantive and nonsubstantive active ingredients can show a persistent antimicrobial effect if they lower the number of bacteria significantly during the hand-washing period. Substantivity is an attribute of certain active ingredients that adhere to the stratum corneum (i.e., remain on the skin after rinsing or drying) to provide an inhibitory effect on the growth of bacteria remaining on the skin.

Plain soap: soaps or detergents that do not contain antimicrobial agents or contain very low concentrations of such agents that are effective solely as preservatives; also referred to as nonantimicrobial soap.

Resident flora: species of microorganisms that are always present on or in the body and are not easily removed by mechanical friction.

Substantivity: see "persistent activity."

Surfactants: surface-active agents that reduce surface tension. They help cleaning by loosening, emulsifying, and holding soil in suspension, which can then be more readily rinsed away.

Surgical hand scrub: an antiseptic-containing preparation that substantially reduces the number of microorganisms on intact skin; it is broad-spectrum, fast-acting, and persistent.

Transient flora: microorganisms that may be present in or on the body under certain conditions and for certain lengths of time; they are easier to remove by mechanical friction than resident flora.

Hand washing is the single most important measure healthcare personnel (HCP) can take to prevent the transmission of infectious diseases in healthcare settings. Organisms on the hands of HCP are responsible for many of the over 2 million healthcare-associated (previously termed *nosocomial*) infections each year in the United States. Most of the documented infections in the scientific literature occur in in-patient settings, such as hospitals and long-term care facilities. Numerous studies over the past century and a half have also shown that proper hand antisepsis decreases infection rates among patients in hospital settings. The recommendations regarding techniques and products have been periodically modified as the understanding of cross infection has increased, along with the development of new antimicrobial agents used in hand-hygiene preparations.

Hand hygiene is equally important in dental treatment settings, affording protection for both the patient and the dental professional. This statement is appropriate despite a lack of published epidemiologic studies linking hand contamination and infection in dental healthcare settings. In the absence of investigations specific to traditional dental office settings, it is important to understand the results of studies conducted in the acute care arena. Many of the infection-control recommendations concerning dental professional and patient risks are based on epidemiological, clinical, and scientific knowledge obtained from medical studies. In this regard, the scientific literature strongly supports a connection between improved hand-hygiene practices and reduction of infections among patients. The Centers for Disease Control and Prevention (CDC) periodically issues specific guidelines for hand hygiene. The most recent update is the 2002 *Guideline for Hand Hygiene in Health-care Settings*, and it applies to all workers in all healthcare settings.

Organisms on a clinician's hands may be transferred to the patient's mucous membranes or into the patient's bloodstream via injection sites and openings in gingival tissue during dental treatment. Similarly, workers who touch objects, tissue, or body fluids contaminated with microorganisms may transfer infectious agents to themselves when touching their mouth, nose, eyes, or cuts and scrapes on otherwise intact skin. Effective hand-hygiene practices, combined with the proper wearing of gloves, are equally essential elements of infection control. Just as washing one's hands is not a substitute for wearing gloves, wearing gloves is not a substitute for hand washing.

HISTORICAL BACKGROUND

In 1847 Ignaz Semmelweis instituted the first known hand-hygiene program at the First Clinic in the General Hospital of Vienna. After noticing that maternal infection rates were much higher among women delivering babies in the clinic operated by physicians and medical students than the infection rate among women giving birth in the midwives' clinic, Semmelweis determined the cause was cross contamination. Physicians and students would go directly to the maternity ward to deliver babies after performing cadaver dissections. Semmelweis concluded that cadaver material present on the physicians' hands was the cause of the infections among the mothers. He further surmised that there was no cross contamination between the anatomy laboratory and the midwives' clinic. Semmelweis subsequently began a campaign to have HCP perform hand-hygiene procedures when treating patients.

Around the same time in England, Oliver Wendell Holmes determined that infections could spread by the unclean hands of HCP, and he subsequently recommended the use of an **antiseptic** hand-cleaning agent between patient contacts. Although this had little impact on improving the aseptic practices of HCP of his time, his early studies along with those of Semmelweis provided the core concept that hand hygiene is a fundamental component of healthcare infection-control programs.

Accumulated documentation in the scientific literature strongly supports a connection between improved hand-hygiene practices and reduced infections among patients. The 2002 CDC guideline for hand hygiene cites prolific published evidence that hand antisepsis is likely the most important aspect of preventing the spread of infectious diseases in healthcare settings. Despite this, improving hand-hygiene compliance in healthcare facilities continues to be a major ongoing task for infection-control practitioners.

TRANSMISSION OF DISEASES VIA HANDS

Much of the science regarding transmission of diseases on the contaminated hands of HCP appears in the medical literature and related documentation of healthcare-associated infections. This provides a model for making recommendations in all healthcare settings, including dentistry. Understanding the method of disease transmission from workers' hands provides the basis for recommendations for hand-hygiene practices. Multiple studies document that contamination on a nurse's hands can result from seemingly innocuous patient contacts, including taking a patient's pulse, blood pressure, or oral temperature; touching a patient's hand; and other activities that do not involve direct contact with a wound or body fluids. It is also common to transfer organisms from environmental surfaces to a worker's hands. If the organisms are capable of survival and a worker fails to perform proper hand hygiene, there is a potential for transmission of organisms to another patient, an environmental surface that will come into direct contact with another patient, or unprotected areas on the worker's skin.

TYPES OF FLORA FOUND ON SKIN

The types of microorganisms found on an individual's hands fall into two categories: **resident flora** and **transient flora**. Resident flora are those organisms that normally reside on a person's body. Organisms found on the skin are located in the deeper layers of skin and provide the body with innate immune protection against disease-causing organisms. These resident microorganisms, such as coagulase-negative staphylococci, micrococci, and diphtheroids, are not commonly associated with healthcare-associated infections. If disrupted (for instance, by hand washing), resident flora reestablish themselves at the same site in the skin. However, hands may also be persistently colonized with potentially pathogenic flora such as *Staphylococcus aureus*, Gram-negative bacilli, or yeasts. These transient flora are organisms that reside on the outer skin surfaces and are acquired by direct contact with patients or contaminated items. Potential pathogens present in blood, saliva, and dental plaque can contaminate the hands of dental personnel. These microbial forms are able to infect a host by passing through dermal defects, and also can contaminate instruments, dental equipment, and environmental surfaces. Although they are more likely to be associated with healthcare-associated infections, transient flora are also more easily removed or inactivated with proper hand-hygiene practices than resident flora. Both the clinical studies by Semmelweis described above and later investigations by Joseph Lister a few years later implied that the hands of medical personnel were sources of pathogenic (i.e., transient) bacteria. Despite subsequent evidence to support this conclusion, many health practitioners refused to consider their hands as potential threats to the well-being of their patients. Even fewer clinicians considered that their patients might be infecting them.

GENERAL HAND WASHING AND HYGIENE CONSIDERATIONS

All infection-control recommendations stress the importance and clinical impact of hand washing. Its primary purpose is the mechanical removal of transient microorganisms from the skin, preventing cross contamination and cross infection from contaminated hands. Even with the availability of multiple water-based and waterless preparations, there are several important areas HCP should consider when selecting products for their facilities (Table 9-1).

ADHERENCE TO RECOMMENDED HAND-HYGIENE PROCEDURES

Many people take it for granted that HCP routinely wash their hands before having contact with patients or equipment that will contact a patient in a hospital, clinic, or any

TABLE 9-1 Hand-Hygiene Considerations

1. Consider skin sensitivities and allergies of personnel when selecting preparations.

2. The initial procedure at the beginning of the day should include a thorough hand wash.

3. Use appropriate hand washing and rinsing techniques, with particular attention to thumbs and fingertips.

4. Subsequent hand-hygiene procedures should last approximately 15 seconds or the time recommended for the specific preparation.

5. Do not wear jewelry or long nails.

6. Clean thoroughly under nails.

7. When washing hands, rinse with cool or tepid water and dry completely before donning gloves.

8. Keep epithelial integrity intact.

other healthcare setting. However, research has shown that high numbers of healthcare-associated infections, including the spread of **multiresistant organisms**, result from poor compliance with hand-hygiene practices. Adherence of HCP to recommended hand-hygiene procedures has historically been poor, with an overall average rate of only 40% in hospital settings. Even when HCP wash their hands they sometimes fail to follow proper procedures, such as removing jewelry, covering all areas of the hands with the cleaning agent, and using a proper length of time for effective hand hygiene. Self-reported reasons for lack of compliance frequently include the following:

- Lack of awareness of basic hand-hygiene principles;
- Understaffing and insufficient time;
- Hand-washing agents cause skin irritation and dryness (via frequent use of soap and water);
- Inconvenient location/lack of sinks;
- Lack of soap and paper towels;
- Wearing gloves as substitute for hand washing;
- Hands don't look dirty; and
- Perceived low risk of cross-infection.

Before 2002, the recommended routine hand-hygiene procedures included washing with soap and water, but did not include the use of alcohol-based hand products unless hand-washing facilities were unavailable. **Alcohol-based hand rubs** are alcohol-containing preparations (e.g., gels, foams, rinses) designed to reduce the number of viable microorganisms on the hands. In the United States, these preparations usually contain 60% to 95% ethanol or isopropanol. These waterless antiseptic agents do not require the use of exogenous water. After such an agent is applied, the hands are rubbed together until the agent has dried. Alcohol or antimicrobial impregnated towelettes also may be considered as a possible alternative to washing hands with **plain soap** and water. These towelettes are not as effective as either alcohol-based hand rubs or washing with **antimicrobial soap** and water because of the small amount of alcohol contained in a towelette.

Several clinical investigations have shown that the incidence of healthcare-associated infections decreased as the adherence of HCP to recommended hand-hygiene practices improved. Several reports also documented that hand-hygiene compliance increased with use of alcohol-based rubs. Accumulated data show that alcohol hand-hygiene preparations are rapidly effective against most skin organisms, are easy and fast to use, and do not require the presence of sinks. Since hand washing is effective and important to remove debris and organisms from hands, but suffers when it is the only protocol because of lack of compliance, the 2002 CDC hand-hygiene recommendations advocated a combined protocol of hand washing and alcohol-based hand rubs for routine hand antisepsis.

HAND HYGIENE FOR NONSURGICAL DENTAL PROCEDURES

There are several acceptable choices for nonsurgical dental procedures, such as dental examinations, preventive procedures, restorative dentistry, and endodontic procedures. Either plain soap or antimicrobial soap and water can be used. If hands are not visibly soiled, the choice of an alcohol-based hand rub is also acceptable. Several factors must be considered when making the decision regarding which approach is best for a given situation. Personnel in the office should consider the type of procedures, degree of contamination likely, and the need for persistent antimicrobial activity. Additional factors to consider when deciding which products to use include the accessibility of hand-washing facilities, chemical sensitivities to antimicrobial agents in the hand preparations, and personal preferences. Indications for hand hygiene can be reviewed in Table 9-2.

Hand-Washing Techniques for Nonsurgical Procedures

Dental healthcare personnel (DHCP) should wash hands with either plain soap or an antimicrobial hand-wash agent and water at the beginning of the work day. Since pathogenic organisms have been found on or around bar soap during and after use, liquid preparations are preferable (Fig. 9-1). An additional recommendation includes the use of hand-free controls whenever possible. Following the initial procedure, an alcohol-based hand

rub is an acceptable hand-hygiene choice if the hands are not visibly soiled. Numerous studies have compared the efficacy of plain or antimicrobial soaps with that of alcohol-based hand rubs in reducing counts of viable bacteria on hands, and the overwhelming majority found that the latter reduced bacterial counts on hands more than washing hands with soaps or **detergents** containing a variety of antimicrobial products. For soiled hands, however, it is necessary to use soap or a hand antiseptic with water to remove debris and clean. Alcohols do not remove bioburden from contaminated skin or environmental surfaces. Instead, they act on proteinaceous material by dehydration and denaturation.

Adherence to each step in the hand-washing procedure is necessary to effectively remove microorganisms (see Table 9-2). For the most effective hand hygiene, remove jewelry and do not wear long, false, or ornamented fingernails. Smooth any rough areas of sharp fingernails. Avoid hot and very cold water, as temperature extremes can increase the risk of dermatitis and discourage adequate rinsing. Disposable towels are preferable to multiple-use cloth towels, which may harbor microorganisms and contaminate hands when drying. Care must also be taken so as not to recontaminate the hands after cleaning them. Finally, a disposable towel should be used to turn off manual faucets. When hand lotion is used, a water-based lotion should be chosen instead of a petroleum-containing product, because petroleum-based ingredients can compromise latex glove integrity.

When using an alcohol-based hand rub (see Table 9-2), apply an adequate amount to the palm of one hand and rub the hands together, covering all surfaces of the hands and fingers, until the hands are dry. Follow the manufacturer's recommendations regarding the volume of product to use. If the hands feel dry after they are rubbed together for 10–15 seconds, an insufficient volume of product likely was applied (Fig. 9-2). The drying effect of alcohol can be reduced or eliminated by choosing a product with 1% to 3% glycerol or other skin-conditioning agents. It is acceptable to apply waterless hand rubs repeatedly without washing hands with soap and water. Personnel then may feel a "build-up" of **emollients** on their hands after repeated use of these products, and thus washing the hands with soap and water after 5 to 10 applications of the waterless product is recommended. One should also consider potential problems when using powdered gloves after applying alcohol hand-rubs. Residual powder left on the hands by powdered gloves will not be removed as well, and may interfere with the antimicrobial action of the alcohol-based products. For this reason, DCHP may want to consider wearing powderless gloves when using this class of hand-hygiene agents.

Waterless products (e.g., alcohol-based hand rubs) are especially useful when water facilities are unavailable (e.g., during dental screenings in schools) or during boil-water advisories. As mentioned above, alcohol-based

TABLE 9-2 Types of Hand Hygiene

Methods	Agent	Purpose	Technique	Duration (minimum)	Indications
Routine Hand wash	Water and non-antimicrobial soap (i.e., plain soap)*	Remove soil and transient microorganisms	• Wet hands and wrists under cool running water • Dispense hand-washing agent sufficient to cover hands and wrists • Rub the agent into all areas, with particular emphasis around nails and between fingers • Rinse thoroughly with cool water • Dry hands completely with a disposable towel before donning gloves • Use a towel to turn off the faucet if automatic controls are not available	15 seconds	• Before and after treating each patient (e.g., before glove placement and after glove removal). • After barehanded touching of inanimate objects likely to be contaminated by blood or saliva. • Before leaving the dental operatory or the dental laboratory. • When visibly soiled.[†] • Before regloving after removing gloves that are torn, cut, or punctured.
Antiseptic Hand wash	Water and antimicrobial soap (e.g., chlorhexidine, iodine and iodophors, chloroxylenol [PCMX], triclosan)	Remove or destroy transient microorganisms and reduce resident flora (persistent activity)		15 seconds	
Antiseptic Hand Rub	Alcohol-based hand rub[†]	Remove or destroy transient microorganisms and reduce resident flora (persistent activity)	• Apply the product to palm of one hand • Rub hands together, covering all surfaces of hands and fingers, until hands are dry[†] • Allow hands to dry completely before donning gloves • Follow manufacturer's recommendations regarding volume of product to use	Rub hands until the agent is dry[†]	
Surgical Antisepsis	Water and antimicrobial soap (e.g., chlorhexidine, iodine and iodophors, chloroxylenol [PCMX], triclosan)	Remove or destroy transient microorganisms and reduce resident flora (persistent activity)	• Remove rings, watches, and bracelets before beginning • Remove debris from underneath fingernails using a nail cleaner under running water • Wet hands and wrists under cool running water • Using an antimicrobial agent scrub hands and forearms for the length of time recommended by the manufacturer's instructions before rinsing with cool water • Dry hands completely (use of a sterile towel is ideal) before donning sterile surgeon's gloves	2–6 minutes (longer scrub times are generally not indicated)	• Before donning sterile surgeon's gloves for oral surgical procedures
	Water and non-antimicrobial soap (i.e., plain soap)* followed by an alcohol-based surgical hand-scrub product with persistent activity		• Prewash hands and forearms with non-antimicrobial (plain) soap* and water • Thoroughly rinse and dry hands and forearms • Follow the manufacturer's instructions for the surgical hand-scrub product with persistent activity • Allow hands to dry completely before donning sterile surgeon's gloves	Follow manufacturer's instructions for surgical hand scrub product with persistent activity	

Adapted from: CDC. Guidelines for infection control in dental health-care settings—2003. MMWR 2003;52(RR-17):15; USAF guidelines for infection control in dentistry (https://decs.nhgl.med.navy.mil); accessed July 2008.

*Pathogenic organisms have been found on or around bar soap during and after use. Use of liquid soap with hands-free dispensing controls is preferable.

[†]60% to 95% ethanol or isopropanol. Alcohol-based hand rubs should *not* be used in the presence of visible soil or organic material. If using an alcohol-based hand rub, apply adequate amount to palm of one hand and rub hands together, covering all surfaces of the hands and fingers, until hands are dry. Follow manufacturer's recommendations regarding the volume of product to use. If hands feel dry after rubbing hands together for 10–15 seconds, an insufficient volume of product likely was applied. The drying effect of alcohol can be reduced or eliminated by adding 1% to 3% glycerol or other skin-conditioning agents.

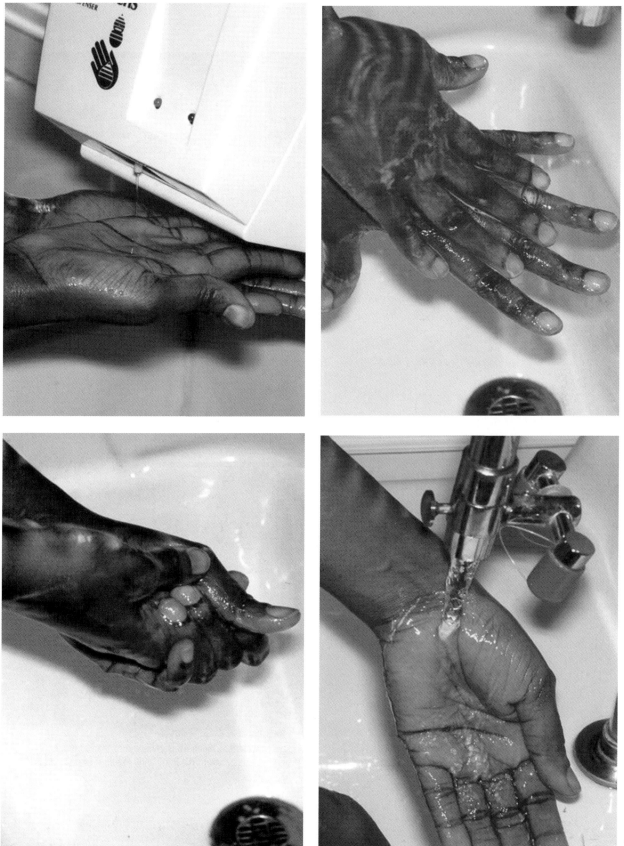

FIGURE 9-1 Routine hand-washing technique when using soap or an antimicrobial antiseptic with water. **(A)** After first wetting hands with water, apply plain or antimicrobial agent. **(B)** Rub hands together vigorously for at least 15 seconds, being careful to clean all areas of the hands and fingers. Special attention should be paid to thumbs, between fingers, and fingertips. **(C)** Be certain to clean both hands equally, because in some instances the dominant hand may do most of the work, while the recessive hand receives most of the benefit. **(D)** Completely rinse soap off hands using cool or tepid water. *(continued)*

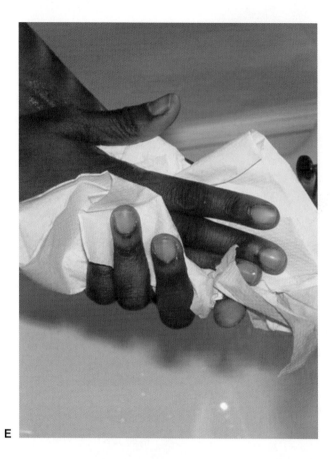

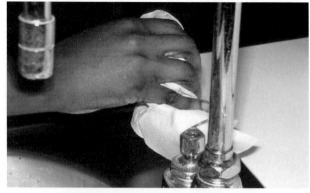

F

E

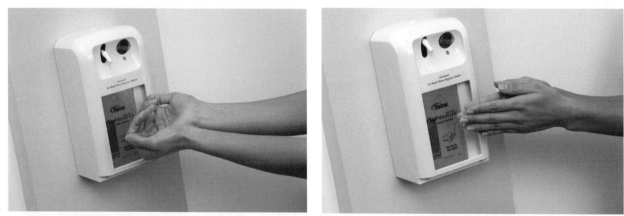

FIGURE 9-1 *(Continued)* **(E)** Dry hands thoroughly with a disposable towel. **(F)** When washing hands using a manually operated faucet, use the towel to turn water off.

A

B

FIGURE 9-2 Hand-hygiene procedure using an automatically dispensed waterless alcohol-based hand rub. **(A)** Place hands in appropriate position in front of automatic dispenser to apply sufficient waterless agent. **(B)** Rub hands together to cover all surfaces of hands and fingers with the antiseptic. *(continued)*

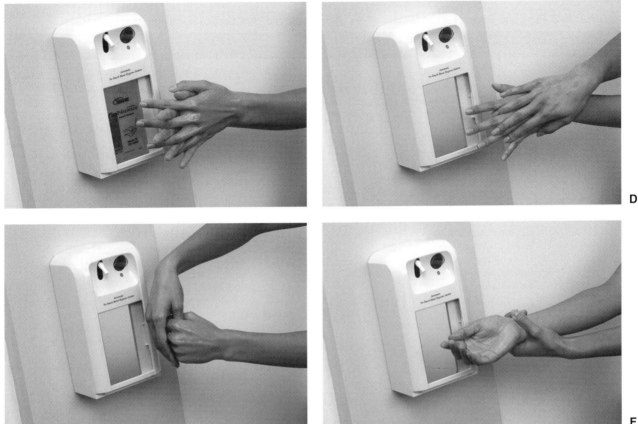

FIGURE 9-2 *(Continued)* **(C–F)** Continue to rub all areas of hands until dry. For most alcohol-based hand-hygiene agents a 15-second minimum exposure on skin is required.

hand rubs should not be used in the presence of visible soil or organic material. Table 9-3 compares the pros and cons of traditional hand-washing techniques with alcohol-based hand rubs.

HAND HYGIENE FOR ORAL SURGICAL PROCEDURES

The purpose of surgical hand antisepsis is to eliminate transient flora and to reduce resident flora for the duration of the procedure to prevent the introduction of organisms into the operative site in the event of breaks in gloves. The invasive nature of **oral surgical procedures** (i.e., biopsy, periodontal surgery, apical surgery, implant surgery, and surgical extraction of teeth) indicates a need for a heightened level of hand hygiene. Skin bacteria can multiply rapidly under surgical gloves and might contaminate a surgical site if gloves become punctured or torn. Since surgical procedures also tend to be longer than restorative or preventive procedures, selection of an antimicrobial agent with residual activity rather than plain soap and water or alcohol-based hand rubs alone is indicated.

Hand-Washing Technique for Oral Surgical Procedures

It is important to use a combination of surgical hand antisepsis and sterile surgeon's gloves for oral surgical procedures (see Table 9-2). While plain soap and water are acceptable for routine dental procedures, recommendations for oral surgery personnel include the use of antimicrobial soap and water, or plain soap and water followed by an alcohol hand rub that contains an antimicrobial agent with **persistent activity**. Skin bacteria can rapidly multiply under surgical gloves if hands are washed with soap that is not antimicrobial. Surgical antimicrobial agents should, therefore, effectively reduce microorganisms on intact skin, be nonirritating, and have a broad spectrum of activity and a persistent antimicrobial effect.

Traditionally, long (10-minute) scrub times were recommended. This practice can lead to skin damage. Studies have demonstrated that shorter scrub times reduce bacterial counts as effectively as a 10-minute scrub; therefore, the current recommendation is to follow the manufacturer's instructions, which usually include a

TABLE 9-3 Pros and Cons of Hand Washing* vs. Alcohol-Based (Antiseptic) Hand Rubs†

Technique	Pros (+)	Cons (−)
Hand Washing	+ Can use plain or antimicrobial soaps + Effective antimicrobial activity with antimicrobial soaps + Effectiveness only minimally affected by organic matter + Sinks readily available and accessible in most dental settings + Familiar technique + Allergic reactions to antimicrobial active ingredients are rare + Irritation dermatitis related to hand washing may be solved by relatively simple techniques or changes	− Frequent hand washing may cause skin dryness, chapping, and irritation − Compliance with recommended hand-washing protocol is traditionally low − Takes more time than antiseptic hand rubs − Requires sink and water and paper towels or air dryers − Personal habits and preferred products such as hand lotions may undermine professional training − Strong fragrances and other ingredients may be poorly tolerated by sensitive people − Water alone may be a skin irritant − Time and technique are critical
Alcohol-Based (Antiseptic) Hand Rub	+ Provides more effective antiseptic action on visibly clean hands than hand washing with plain or antimicrobial soaps + Faster protocol than hand washing + Reduced skin irritation and dryness compared to hand washing + May be used in absence of sinks and water, and during boil-water notices + Allergic reactions to alcohol or additives are rare + Reduces use of paper towels, waste	− Not indicated for use when hands are visibly dirty or contaminated − Dispensing proper amount is critical − Hands must be dry before agent is applied − Frequent use may cause skin dryness or irritation if product lacks effective emollients/skin conditioners − Agent may temporarily sting compromised skin − Strong fragrances and other ingredients may be poorly tolerated by sensitive people − Alcohol products are flammable, should be stored away from flames − Residual powder may interfere with effectiveness or comfort of antiseptic rub − Hand-washing stations must still be accessible for times when waterless sanitizers are inappropriate

Adapted with permission from the Organization for Safety and Asepsis Procedures. From Policy to Practice: OSAP's Guide to the Guidelines. Washington, DC: OSAP, 2004:23.
*Hand washing performed according to recommended protocol, as outlined in this chapter.
†Antiseptic hand rubs meet recommended product selection criteria as defined in this chapter.

2- to 6-minute scrub. Another change is that using a scrub brush is no longer recommended.

Most alcohol sanitizers do not provide the residual activity needed for surgical hand antisepsis if used alone. Therefore, if an alcohol-based product is used for surgical hand antisepsis, several steps must be taken (see Table 9-2). First, choose an alcohol-based surgical hand-scrub product with persistent activity and follow the manufacturer's instructions. Before applying the alcohol solution, pre-wash the hands and forearms with plain or non-antimicrobial soap, rinse, and dry the hands and forearms completely. After application of the alcohol-based product, allow the hands and forearms to dry thoroughly before donning sterile gloves.

DESIRABLE FEATURES OF HAND-HYGIENE AGENTS

Hand-hygiene agents should be selected based on the kind of procedure being done and the level of exposure anticipated. Features of the products, active ingredients, and practical use characteristics influence product selection, as well as meeting the needs of the protocol.

Products that are not well accepted by HCP can be a deterrent to hand washing. Therefore, it is important to solicit input from all users when evaluating or selecting new hand-hygiene products for the dental office. Key considerations in selecting hand-hygiene products are effectiveness, potential irritants and allergens in the active ingredients, skin integrity after repeated use, compatibility with any lotions used in the dental office, scent and other personal preferences, dispensing/delivery systems, staff acceptance, and cost per use.

PREPARATIONS USED FOR HAND HYGIENE
Plain or Nonantimicrobial Soaps

Soaps and synthetic anionic detergents are examples of anionic preparations. Soaps are salts of long aliphatic carboxylic acids of animal and plant fats. Most synthetic anionic detergents contain alkali and/or aryl sulfates or sulfonates. The alkali and sodium salt allow soaps to kill streptococci, treponemes, pneumococci, gonococci, and influenza viruses. These effects not withstanding, the primary value of anionic detergents appears to be primarily in their mechanical cleansing action, which results in the removal of dirt, soil, and various organic substances from hands. Plain soap is adequate when the purpose of washing is to remove skin debris and microbes. Since intact skin is the most important barrier to infection, nonantimicrobial soaps should have ingredients to prevent skin irritation, dryness, and damage to help preserve skin integrity. Nonantimicrobial soaps can be associated with skin irritation and dryness; however, the addition of emollients to these products can reduce such effects.

Active Ingredients in Antimicrobial Hand-Hygiene Agents

The U.S. **Food and Drug Administration's (FDA)** Division of Over-the-Counter Drug Products regulates **antiseptic hand wash** products intended for used by HCP. Testing requirements for HCP hand-wash products and **surgical hand scrubs** are outlined by the FDA, and products intended for use as HCP hand washes are evaluated using a standardized method. Optimal antisepsis agents are broad-spectrum, have persistence, and are fast acting. A brief review of common antimicrobial agents used in hand-hygiene products follows (Table 9-4).

Chlorhexidine Gluconate

Chlorhexidine gluconate (CHG) is a cationic bisbiguanide. Antimicrobial activity appears to result from its attachment to and disruption of microbial cytoplasmic membranes. Resultant cell death occurs from precipitation of cellular contents. CHG remains significantly effective in the presence of organic material, including blood. Another important feature of this important antimicrobial antiseptic relates to its persistence during use. Although they significantly lower the concentration of microorganisms on the skin with a single application, CHG hand antiseptics necessitate repeated washings throughout the day to attain maximal effectiveness. The active form of the chemical accumulates and remains in the epithelial tissues for prolonged periods, thus leaving a residual effect after each wash procedure. The property is called **substantivity** and fosters the build-up of an antimicrobial "barrier" against many common transient skin contaminants. Natural soaps, inorganic anions, nonionic **surfactants**, and anionic emulsifying agents in some hand creams may inactivate CHG, however. Products containing 2% CHG are slightly less effective than those with 4%. Although its immediate antimicrobial activity is slower than that of alcohol, concentrations of CHG in the 0.5% to 1% range added to alcohol sanitizers provide significantly greater residual activity than alcohol alone. Little if any skin absorption of CHG occurs and true allergic reactions are uncommon, but contact with eyes may cause conjunctivitis, and skin irritation related to concentration and frequency of use may occur.

TABLE 9-4 Antimicrobial Spectrum and Characteristics of Hand-Hygiene Antiseptic Agents*

Group	Gram-positive bacteria	Gram-negative bacteria	Mycobacteria	Fungi	Viruses	Speed of Action	Comments
Alcohols	+++	+++	+++	+++	+++	Fast	Optimum concentration 60% to 95%; no persistent activity
Chlorhexidine (2% and 4% aqueous)	+++	++	+	+	+++	Intermediate	Persistent activity; rare allergic reactions
Iodine compounds	+++	+++	+++	++	+++	Intermediate	Causes skin burns; usually too irritating for hand hygiene
Iodophors	+++	+++	+	++	++	Intermediate	Less irritating than iodine; acceptance varies
Phenol derivatives	+++	+	+	+	+	Intermediate	Activity neutralized by nonionic surfactants
Triclosan	+++	++	+	−	+++	Intermediate	Acceptability on hands varies
Quaternary ammonium compounds	+	++	−	−	+	Slow	Used only in combination with alcohols; ecological concerns

Adapted from CDC. Guideline for hand hygiene in health-care settings: recommendations of the Health-care Infection Control Practices Advisory Committee and the HICPAC/SHEA/APIC/IDSA Hand Hygiene Task Force. MMWR 2002;51[RR-16]:45.

+++, excellent; ++, good, but does not include the entire bacterial spectrum; +, fair; −, no activity or not sufficient.

*Hexachlorophene is not included because it is no longer an accepted ingredient of hand disinfectants.

Iodine and Iodophors

Iodine is one of the oldest antiseptic classes used for application onto skin, mucous membranes, abrasions, and other wounds. The high reactivity of this halogen with its target substrate provides it with potent germicidal effects. It rapidly penetrates cell walls and acts by iodination of proteins and subsequent formation of protein salts. Target microbial cells lyse as a result of impaired protein synthesis and cell membrane alteration. Because iodine is insoluble in water, traditionally it was prepared as a tincture, with the iodide salt being dissolved in alcohol. Iodine in this form continues to be an effective, broad-spectrum antiseptic, as shown by the fact that, at different concentrations, tinctures of iodine are cytotoxic for Gram-positive and Gram-negative bacteria, tubercle bacilli, fungi, and most viruses. This form of iodine has some serious drawbacks, however. It is irritating to wounded skin and allergenic. Hypersensitivity reactions to iodine also have been commonly noted, with tissue manifestations ranging from mild to severe in allergic persons.

Iodophors have largely replaced iodine as the active ingredient in currently available antiseptics. Iodophors are compounds of elemental iodine, iodide, or triiodide, and a polymer carrier. The amount of "free" iodine present determines the iodophor level of antimicrobial activity. Combining iodine with various polymers increases iodine solubility, promotes sustained release of iodine, and reduces skin irritation. The carriers themselves are surfactants that are water-soluble and react with epithelial areas to increase tissue permeability. Thus, the active iodine that is released is better absorbed. In addition, the pH, temperature, exposure time, concentration of total available iodine, and the amount and type of organic and inorganic compounds present affect the antimicrobial activity of iodine. Iodine and iodophors have significantly reduced efficacy in the presence of organic substances such as blood or sputum. Although a residual antimicrobial effect has been observed after hand washing, it has not been precisely established. While some research has shown activity for up to 1 hour on ungloved hands after hand washing, other research shows poor residual activity under gloves. With regard to their adverse effects, iodophors are less irritating to skin and allergenic than iodine, but cause more irritation contact dermatitis (ICD) than other commonly used antiseptics.

Chloroxylenol Parachlorometaxylenol (PCMX)

Parachlorometaxylenol (PCMX), or chloroxylenol, is a halogen-substituted phenolic compound that has been widely used in the United States since the 1950s as a preservative in various products, such as cosmetics, and as an antimicrobial agent in soaps. Antimicrobial activity appears to occur because of inactivation of bacterial enzymes and alteration of cell walls. Its antimicrobial

spectrum includes good activity against Gram-positive bacteria, but only fair effectiveness against Gram-negative microbes, mycobacteria, and certain viruses. Adding ethylene-diaminetetraacetic acid (EDTA) increases the effectiveness of PCMX solutions against *Pseudomonas spp.* and other pathogens. The reports of the relative efficacy of PCMX compared to other hand-hygiene preparations are inconsistent, partly because of variations in concentrations and the presence of EDTA. PCMX is less rapidly active than CHG or iodophors and has less residual activity. Organic matter only minimally affects PCMX, but it is neutralized by nonionic surfactants. PCMX is absorbed through the skin, but it appears to be safe and generally well tolerated, and is not usually allergenic. PCMX concentrations in available antimicrobial soaps range from 0.3% to 3.75%.

Quaternary Ammoniums

Quaternary ammonium preparations represent examples of cationic surface-active detergents. They are a varied group of chemical compounds made up of a nitrogen atom directly linked to four alkyl groups. Alkyl benzalkonium chlorides are the most widely used type in antiseptics. First used in 1935 for preoperative cleaning of surgeons' hands, the antimicrobial activity appears to occur because of adsorption into the cytoplasmic membrane causing leakage of cytoplasmic constituents. Gram-positive bacteria are the most susceptible microbial forms. Unfortunately, variable antimicrobial activity has been observed for many Gram-negative bacteria. Thus, these agents are prone to contamination by Gram-negative bacteria, and have little or no destructive effects against many fungi and viruses. In addition, organic material and anionic detergents adversely affect antimicrobial activity. Over the last 15–20 years, new formulations have attempted to address this potential for contamination, and benzalkonium chloride and benzethonium chloride are being reintroduced in hand-hygiene preparations as alcohol-free alternatives to the majority of available products.

Triclosan

Triclosan is added to soaps and other consumer products in concentrations between 0.2% and 2% for antimicrobial activity. This nonionic, colorless substance enters bacterial cells, acting on the cytoplasmic membrane and synthesis of RNA, fatty acids, and proteins by binding to the carrier protein reductase. Triclosan tends to be bacteriostatic for a broad range of microbes at concentrations of 0.1–10 μg/mL, or bactericidal at concentrations of 25–500 μg/mL. Triclosan (0.1% after a 1-minute hand wash) reduces bacterial counts on hands less effectively than CHG, iodophors, or alcohol-based products. Although triclosan-containing preparations demonstrate persistent activity, the pH; presence of surfactants, emollients, or humectants; and ionic nature of a formulation all may affect efficacy. Although surfactants may inhibit antimicrobial activity, the presence of organic material, such as blood, will not inhibit activity. People are usually able to tolerate products with concentrations of less than 2%, and there are no widespread reports of allergenic reactions. Reports indicate that product contamination is possible, resulting in a lack of activity against Gram-negative bacilli. Bacteria also have demonstrated resistance to triclosan through the development of a triclosan-resistant enzyme, apparently more readily than to other antiseptic agents. This continues to be an area of active investigation regarding the continued use of triclosan as a hand-hygiene antiseptic. Of particular concern is the selection for mutant bacteria that are resistant to multiple antibiotics, including fluoroquinolones, through exposure to triclosan.

Alcohols

Ethanol and isopropanol have been used for many years as skin antiseptics and surface disinfectants. As a result, historically they have been considered to be widely beneficial agents for effective antisepsis. In the United States, currently available hand-hygiene preparations usually contain 60% to 95% ethanol or isopropanol. Both of these chemicals are effective protein denaturants and lipid solvents. The latter property probably enhances their antimicrobial range because of the cidal effect on *Mycobacterium tuberculosis* and enveloped viruses, such as herpes simplex viruses. In general, alcohols exhibit a fairly broad spectrum of activity under certain conditions, are fast acting in destroying microorganisms on skin, and cause less skin irritation. Even though numerous studies have documented that alcohol-based antiseptics effectively reduce bacterial counts on hands, it is important to note that waterless rubs and sprays should also contain additional antimicrobial ingredients, such as CHG, quaternary ammonium compounds, octenidine, or triclosan, to achieve persistent activity on the skin. This helps to reduce the proliferation of microbes under gloves as well as to counteract potential contamination in the case of breaks in the gloves. Additionally, the product should contain emollients to prevent skin drying and dermatitis. The emollient should be oil-free and petroleum-free to avoid compromising glove barriers.

Variables that affect the efficacy of alcohol-based products include the type, concentration, and volume of alcohol used; the contact time; and whether the hands are wet when the alcohol is applied. Small volumes of alcohol are less effective than washing with soap and water. The CDC has promoted this class of antiseptics in recent years as a means to improve clinical compliance with hand hygiene, and data collected over the last few years suggest a decrease in hospital-acquired infections, attributable in part to improved hand hygiene by HCP.

IRRITATION DERMATITIS RELATED TO HAND HYGIENE

Healthy, intact skin is the primary barrier against infection. Skin damage changes the skin flora, resulting in more frequent colonization by staphylococci and Gram-negative bacilli. Frequent repeated use of hand-hygiene agents, especially soaps and detergents, has been associated with **irritation contact dermatitis (ICD)** among HCP, most frequently those reporting a history of skin problems. Detergents damage skin by denaturing the stratum corneum proteins, changing intercellular lipids, and decreasing corneocyte water-binding capacity. This non-immunological condition is the most common form of adverse occupational skin reaction. In affected persons the epithelium typically becomes reddened because of acute inflammation, as well as dry, irritated, and even cracked in some severe cases (Fig. 9-3). Virtually all symptoms stop at the boundary of the glove cuff with skin. In addition to frequent hand washing and use of harsh chemical agents, failure to completely rinse off chemical agents, irritation from cornstarch powder in gloves, excessive perspiration on hands while wearing gloves, improper hand washing techniques, and failure to dry hands thoroughly after rinsing are common factors that can initiate and aggravate irritant dermatitis. Other contributing factors to dermatitis include using hot water for hand washing, low humidity, failure to use supplementary hand lotion, and the quality of paper towels.

The degree of skin irritation varies considerably and can be lessened by choosing products with emollients and humectants. Antimicrobial agents (e.g., PCMX, CHG, iodophors, and iodine) or other ingredients in the formulation may also cause irritant contact dermatitis. Alcohol sanitizers are among the safest antiseptics, but can still cause dryness and skin irritation. However, studies have shown that alcohol-based hand rubs containing emollients were less irritating to the skin than the soaps or detergents tested.

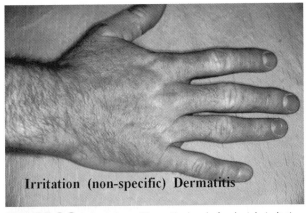

FIGURE 9-3 Irritant dermatitis on the hand of a dental student.

SKIN CARE

For optimal skin care, use the least irritating hand-hygiene product appropriate for the procedure and rinse the soap completely off of the hands and dry thoroughly. Lotions are often recommended to ease the dryness resulting from frequent hand washing and to prevent dermatitis from glove use. However, petroleum-based lotion formulations can weaken latex gloves and increase permeability. For that reason, lotions that contain petroleum or other oil emollients should only be used at the end of the work day. When selecting hand lotions, it is important to consider the interaction between lotions, gloves, dental materials, and antimicrobial products.

STORAGE AND DISPENSING OF HAND-CARE PRODUCTS

Hand-washing products, including plain or nonantimicrobial soap, and antiseptic products can become contaminated or support the growth of microorganisms. Liquid products should be stored in closed containers and dispensed from either disposable containers or containers that are washed and dried thoroughly before refilling. Soap should not be added to a partially empty dispenser, because the practice of topping off might lead to contamination. Signs of contamination include the product becoming discolored or cloudy, or developing an unusual odor. Always store and dispense products according to the manufacturer's directions.

FINGERNAILS AND JEWELRY

Microbial counts on hands are highest under and around the fingernails. **Artificial fingernails** and nail extensions are likely to harbor more Gram-negative organisms than natural nails. They have also been associated with multiple outbreaks of fungal and bacterial infections in hospitals. Fingernails should be short enough to allow DHCP to thoroughly clean underneath them and prevent glove tears. Sharp nail edges or broken nails are also likely to increase glove failure. Long artificial or natural nails can make donning gloves more difficult and can cause gloves to tear more readily. Freshly applied nail polish on natural nails does not appear to increase microbial loads if the nails are short, but chipped nail polish can harbor microorganisms.

It is unknown whether wearing jewelry increases the likelihood of transmitting pathogens, but some investigations have shown that skin under rings is more heavily colonized (particularly with Gram-negative bacilli, *Staphylococcus aureus,* or dermatomycotic fungi) than fingers without rings. Jewelry may interfere with effective rinsing during hand washing, allowing build-up of soaps and other irritants. Over time, difficult-to-dry areas under rings may develop dermatitis or even a chronic dermato-

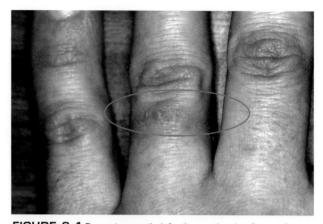

FIGURE 9-4 Dermatomycotic infection on the ring finger of a dental assistant. This person routinely wore her ring while working in a dental facility. She did not properly dry her hands after washing. Over a period of time the epithelial integrity under the ring was compromised and became secondarily infected with environmental fungi.

mycotic infection (i.e., "athlete's foot of the finger") (Fig. 9-4). Hand jewelry also can interfere with glove use by making it difficult to don the gloves or wear the correct size, and by tearing the gloves.

FLAMMABILITY AND ALCOHOL-BASED HAND RUBS

In Europe, where alcohol-based hand rubs have been used extensively for years, the incidence of fires associated with such products has been low. The results of a recent survey in the U.S. also support this. However, since alcohols are flammable, precautions should be taken to minimize any potential fire risk. The National Fire Protection Association (NFPA) has published guidelines allowing alcohol-based hand rubs in healthcare facilities if several safety conditions are met:

- The egress corridor width is 6 feet or greater and dispensers are separated at least 4 feet apart.

- The maximum individual dispenser fluid capacity is 1.2 liters for dispensers in rooms, corridors, and areas open to corridors, and 2.0 liters for dispensers in suites of rooms.

- If using wall-mounted dispensers, do not install over or directly adjacent to electrical outlets and switches.

- In locations with carpeted floor coverings, dispensers installed directly over carpeted surfaces are permitted only in areas with sprinklers.

- Each smoke compartment may contain a maximum aggregate of 10 gallons of alcohol-based hand-rub solution in dispensers and a maximum of 5 gallons in storage.

EDUCATIONAL AND MOTIVATIONAL PROGRAMS

Educational programs should address the impact of improved hand hygiene on disease transmission rates, awareness of hand-hygiene guidelines, knowledge about the low adherence rate to hand hygiene, and information about the use of hand-hygiene and skin-care protection products. Making a change, such as introducing alcohol-based hand rubs, without providing ongoing education and motivation may only result in a temporary improvement in hand-hygiene practices. Ongoing educational and motivational activities may be needed for long-lasting compliance and improvement in hand-hygiene practices.

SUMMARY

Hand hygiene is the most important aseptic procedure in the prevention of healthcare-associated infections. Hand hygiene significantly reduces microbes on the hands and protects both patients and the dental staff. Hand-washing products include plain soap and agents with antimicrobial activity. Educating all members of the dental team on the importance of proper hand washing is critical to the success of the office infection-control program.

✔ Practical Dental Infection Control Checklist

General Considerations

❑ Do DHCP perform hand hygiene
  ❑ when hands are visibly contaminated with blood or OPIM?
  ❑ after barehanded touching of inanimate objects likely to be contaminated by blood, saliva, or respiratory secretions?
  ❑ before and after treating each patient?
  ❑ before donning gloves?
  ❑ immediately after removing gloves?
❑ Do DHCP perform hand hygiene with either non-antimicrobial or antimicrobial soap and water when hands are visibly dirty or contaminated with blood or OPIM?
❑ If hands are not visibly soiled, do DHCP use an alcohol-based hand rub according to the manufacturer's instructions?
❑ Before performing oral surgical procedures, do DHCP perform surgical hand antisepsis before donning sterile surgeon's gloves, following the manufacturer's instructions by using antimicrobial soap and water?
  ❑ If an alcohol-based surgical hand-scrub product with persistent activity is used, are hands cleaned with soap and water and dried before applying the waterless product?

❑ Are liquid hand-care products stored in either disposable closed containers or closed containers that can be washed and dried before refilling?
  ❑ Are reusable dispensers or containers for soap or lotion washed and dried before refilling?

Special Considerations for Hand Hygiene and Glove Use

❑ Are hand lotions used to prevent skin dryness associated with hand washing?
❑ Is the compatibility of lotion and antiseptic products considered?
❑ Is the effect of petroleum or other oil emollients on the integrity of gloves considered during product selection and glove use?
❑ Do DHCP keep fingernails short with smooth, filed edges to allow thorough cleaning and prevent glove tears?
❑ Are DCHP discouraged from using artificial fingernails?
❑ If hand or nail jewelry is worn, is it removed if it makes donning gloves more difficult or compromises the fit and integrity of the glove?

Review Questions

1. Hand hygiene refers to:

   A. Hand washing with plain soap and water.

   B. Using an antiseptic hand rub (e.g., alcohol, chlorhexidene)

   C. Hand washing with an antimicrobial soap and water.

   D. All of the above.

2. Which of the following statements about transient flora is true?

   A. They are attached to deeper layers of the skin.

   B. They colonize superficial layers of the skin.

   C. They are more easily removed by routine hand washing.

   D. They are acquired by HCP during direct contact with patients or contaminated environmental surfaces.

   E. A, C, D

   F. B, C, D

   G. All of the above

3. Each of the following statements regarding hand hygiene is true except:

   A. Overall adherence among healthcare personnel is approximately 40%.

   B. Cleaning your hands before and after patient contact is one of the most important measures for preventing the spread of microorganisms in healthcare settings.

C. Hand hygiene is not necessary if gloves are worn.

D. Studies have shown an increased recovery of Gram-negative bacteria from personnel wearing artificial nails.

4. When using plain or antimicrobial soap, hands should be rubbed for at least _____ with particular emphasis around the nails and between the fingers.

A. 10 seconds

B. 15 seconds

C. 1 minute

D. 2 minutes

5. Each of the following statements regarding alcohol-based hand rubs is true except:

A. Alcohol-based hand rubs reduce bacterial counts on the hands of HCP more effectively than plain soaps.

B. Alcohol-based hand rubs can be made more accessible than sinks or other hand-washing facilities.

C. Alcohol-based hand rubs require less time to use than traditional hand washing.

D. Alcohol-based hand rubs have been demonstrated to cause less skin irritation and dryness than hand washing using soap and water.

E. Alcohol-based hand rubs are only effective if they are applied for >60 seconds.

6. Ensure that the alcohol-based hand rub has completely dried before putting on gloves. If you feel a "build-up" on your hands after five to 10 uses of an alcohol based-hand rub, wash your hands with soap and water.

A. The first statement is true. The second statement is false.

B. The first statement is false. The second statement is true.

C. Both statements are true.

D. Both statements are false.

7. Each of the following statements regarding surgical hand hygiene is true except:

A. When performing a surgical hand scrub, an antimicrobial soap must be used.

B. When performing a surgical hand scrub, hands and forearms should be scrubbed for 6–12 minutes.

C. If an alcohol-based hand rub is used, the hands must first be washed with soap and water.

D. A surgical hand scrub is indicated before biopsy procedures, periodontal and implant surgery, and surgical extractions of teeth.

8. Alcohol-based hand rubs have the potential to increase compliance with hand washing in health-care facilities. Alcohol-based rubs can be used if hands are visibly soiled.

A. The first statement is true. The second statement is false.

B. The first statement is false. The second statement is true.

C. Both statements are true.

D. Both statements are false.

9. Alcohol-based hand rub products are flammable; therefore:

A. They should be stored away from high temperatures or flames.

B. Dispensers should be wall-mounted near electrical outlets.

C. Users should be aware of NFPA guidance.

D. A and C

E. A, B, and C

10. The following should be considered when choosing hand-hygiene products for your facility:

A. Efficacy against various pathogens

B. Acceptance of the product by HCP

C. Dispenser systems

D. All of the above

Critical Thinking

1. Before beginning dental treatment, you use an alcohol-based hand rub instead of soap and water before putting on your gloves. A patient asks you why you didn't "wash" your hands. How do you respond?

2. A new employee brings in a bottle of hand lotion to the dental office/clinic. You look at the label and see that it contains petroleum. How do you explain to her that she cannot use this in the dental office? Can she continue to use it at home?

3. A new employee comes into work with artificial fingernails. How do you explain to her that she should keep her nails short?

4. What types of hand-hygiene preparations do you use in the dental office/clinic? Can you identify the main ingredients from the label?

5. Go to one of the office's dental operatories. Take turns demonstrating the correct procedures for

   a. routine hand washing;

   b. using an alcohol-based hand rub;

   c. surgical hand scrub using antimicrobial soap and water.

SELECTED READINGS

Archibald LK, Corl A, Shah B, et al. *Serratia marcescens* outbreak associated with extrinsic contamination of 1% chlorxylenol soap. Infect Control Hosp Epidemiol 1997;18:704–709.

Baumgardner CA, Maragos CS, Walz J, et al. Effects of nail polish on microbial growth of fingernails: dispelling sacred cows. AORN J 1993;58:84–88.

Berndt U, Wigger-Alberti W, Gabard B, et al. Efficacy of a barrier cream and its vehicle as protective measures against occupational irritant contact dermatitis. Contact Dermatitis 2000;42:77–80.

Boyce JM, Pearson ML. Low frequency of fires from alcohol-based hand rub dispensers in healthcare facilities. Infect Control Hosp Epidemiol 2003;24:618–619.

Casewell M, Phillips I. Hands as route of transmission for *Klebsiella* species. Br Med J 1977;2:1315–1317.

CDC. Guideline for hand hygiene in health-care settings: recommendations of the Health-care Infection Control Practices Advisory Committee and the HICPAAC/SHEA/APIC/IDSA Hand Hygiene Task Force. MMWR 2002;51(RR-16):1–46.

CDC. Guidelines for infection control in dental health-care settings–2003. MMWR 2003;52(RR-17):1–66.

Cuny E. Current concepts in hand hygiene. Compend Contin Educ Dent 2004;25(1 Suppl):11–16.

Dewar NE, Gravens DL. Effectiveness of septisol antiseptic foam as a surgical scrub agent. Appl Microbiol 1973;26:544–549.

Doebbeling BN, Pfaller MA, Houston AK, et al. Removal of nosocomial pathogens from the contaminated glove. Ann Intern Med 1988;109:394–398.

Faoagali J, Fong J, George N, et al. Comparison of the immediate, residual, and cumulative antibacterial effects of Novaderm R,* Novascrub R,* Betadine Surgical Scrub, Hibiclens, and liquid soap. Am J Infect Control 1995;23:337–343.

Field EA, McGowan P, Pearce PK, et al. Rings and watches: should they be removed prior to operative dental procedures? J Dent 1996;24:65–69.

Foca M, Jakob K, Whittier S, et al. Endemic *Pseudomonas aeruginosa* infection in a neonatal intensive care unit. N Engl J Med 2000;343:695–700.

Grohskopf LA, Roth VR, Feikin DR, et al. *Serratia liquefaciens* bloodstream infections from contamination of epoetin alfa at a hemodialysis center. N Engl J Med 2001;344:1491–1497.

Gupta A, Della-Latta P, Todd B, et al. Outbreak of extended-spectrum beta-lactamase—producing *Klebsiella peneumoniae* in a neonatal intensive care unit linked to artificial nails. Infect Control Hosp Epidemiol 2004;25:210–215.

Hedderwick SA, McNeil SA, Lyons MJ, et al. Pathogenic organisms associated with artificial fingernails worn by healthcare workers. Infect Control Hosp Epidemiol 2000;21:505–509.

Hobson DW, Woller W, Anderson L, et al. Development and evaluation of a new alcohol-based surgical hand scrub formulation with persistent antimicrobial characteristics and brushless application. Am J Infect Control 1998;26:507–512.

Hoffman PN, Cooke EM, McCarville MR, et al. Microorganisms isolated from skin under wedding rings worn by hospital staff. Br Med J 1985;290:206–207.

Jacobson G, Thiele JE, McCune JH, et al. Handwashing: ring-wearing and number of micro-organisms. Nurs Res 1985;34:186–188.

Kabara JJ, Brady MB. Contamination of bar soaps under "in-use" conditions. J Environ Pathol Toxicol Oncol 1984;5:1–14.

Larson E. A causal link between handwashing and risk of infection? Examination of the evidence. Infection Control 1988;9:28–36.

Larson E. Handwashing: it's essential—even when you use gloves. Am J Nurs 1989;89:934–939.

Larson E, Killien M. Factors influencing handwashing behavior of patient care personnel. Am J Infect Control 1982;10:93–99.

Larson E, Anderson JK, Baxendale L, et al. Effects of a protective foam on scrubbing and gloving. Am J Infect Control 1993;21:297–301.

Larson EL, Butz AM, Gullette DL, et al. Alcohol for surgical scrubbing? Infect Control Hosp Epidemiol 1990;11:139–143.

Larson EL, Early E, Cloonan P, et al. An organizational climate intervention associated with increased handwashing and decreased nosocomial infections. Behav Med 2000;26:14–22.

Larson E, Leyden JJ, McGinley KJ, et al. Physiologic and microbiologic changes in skin related to frequent handwashing. Infect Control 1986;7:59–63.

Larson EL, Norton Hughes CA, Pyrak JD, et al. Changes in bacterial flora associated with skin damage on hands of healthcare personnel. Am J Infect Control 1998;26:513–521.

Lowbury EJ. Aseptic methods in the operating suite. Lancet 1968;1:705–709.

Lowbury EJ, Lilly HA. Disinfection of the hands of surgeons and nurses. Br Med J 1960;1445–1450.

Mayer JA, Dubbert PM, Miller M, et al. Increasing hand-washing in an intensive care unit. Infect Control 1986;7:259–262.

McCormick RD, Buchman TL, Maki DG. Double-blind, randomized trial of scheduled use of a novel barrier cream and an oil-containing lotion for protecting the hands of healthcare workers. Am J Infect Control 2000;28:302–310.

McGinley KJ, Larson EL, Leyden JJ. Composition and density of microflora in the subungual space of the hand. J Clin Microbiol 1988;26:950–953.

McNeil SA, Foster CL, Hedderwick SA, et al. Effect of hand cleansing with antimicrobial soap or alcohol-based gel on microbial colonization of artificial fingernails worn by healthcare workers. Clin Infect Dis 2001;32:367–372.

Molinari JA. Clinic experiences with waterless alcohol-based hand hygiene antiseptics. Compend Contin Educ Dent 2006;27:84–86.

Molinari JA. Practical infection control for the 1990s: applying science to government regulations. J Am Dent Assoc 1994;127:1189-1197.

Moolenaar RL, Crutcher M, San Joaquin VH, et al. A prolonged outbreak of *Pseudomonas aeruginosa* in a neonatal intensive care unit: did staff fingernails play a role in disease transmission? Infect Control Hosp Epidemiol 2000;21:80–85.

Myers R, Larson E, Cheng B, et al. Hand hygiene among general practice dentists: a survey of knowledge, attitudes and practices. J Am Dent Assoc 2008;139:948–957.

Ojajärvi J. The importance of soap selection for routine hand hygiene in hospital. J Hyg (Lond) 1981;86:275–283.

Ojajärvi J, Mäkelä P, Rantasalo I. Failure of hand disinfection with frequent hand washing: a need for prolonged field studies. J Hyg (Lond) 1977;79:107–119.

Parry MF, Grant B, Yukna M, et al. Candida osteomyelitis and diskitis after spinal surgery: an outbreak that implicates artificial nail use. Clin Infect Dis 2001;32:352–357.

Passaro DJ, Waring L, Armstrong R, et al. Postoperative *Serratia marcescens* wound infections traced to an out-of-hospital source. J Infect Dis 1997;175:992–995.

Pittet D. Improving compliance with hand hygiene in hospitals. Infect Control Hosp Epidemiol 2000;21:381–386.

Pittet D, Hugonnet S, Harbarth S, et al. Effectiveness of a hospital-wide programme to improve compliance with hand hygiene. Lancet 2000;356:1307–1312.

Pottinger J, Burns S, Manske C. Bacterial carriage by artificial versus natural nails. Am J Infect Control 1989;17:340–344.

Price PB. New studies in surgical bacteriology and surgical technique. JAMA 1938;111:1993–1996.

Rotter M. Hand washing and hand disinfection. In: Mayhall CG, ed. Hospital Epidemiology and Infection Control. 2nd ed. Philadelphia: Lippincott Williams & Wilkins; 1999:1339–1355.

Rubin DM. Prosthetic fingernails in the OR: a research study. AORN J 1988;47:944–945.

Salisbury DM, Hutfilz P, Treen LM, et al. The effect of rings on microbial load of healthcare workers' hands. Am J Infec Control 1997;25:24–27.

Steere AC, Mallison GF. Handwashing practices for the prevention of nosocomial infections. Ann Intern Med 1975;83:683–690.

Trick WE, Vernon MO, Hayes RA, et al. Impact of ring wearing on hand contamination and comparison of hand hygiene agents in a hospital. Clin Infect Dis 2003;36:1383–1390.

U.S. Department of Health and Human Services, Centers for Medicare and Medicaid Services. 42 CFR Parts 403, 416, 418, 460, 482, 483, and 485. Fire safety requirements for certain healthcare facilities; final rule. Fed Regist 2006;71:55326–55341.

U.S. Department of Health and Human Services, Food and Drug Administration. Tentative final monograph for healthcare antiseptic drug products; proposed rule. Fed Regist 1994;59:31441–31452.

Widmer AF. Replace hand washing with use of a waterless alcohol hand rub? Clin Infect Dis 2000;31:136–143.

Wisniewski MF, Kim S, Trick WE, et al. Chicago Antimicrobial Resistance Project. Effect of education on hand hygiene beliefs and practices: a 5-year program. Infect Control Hosp Epidemiol 2007;28:88–91.

Wynd CA, Samstag DE, Lapp AM. Bacterial carriage on the fingernails of OR nurses. AORN J 1994;60:796, 799–805.

Zimakoff J, Kjelsberg AB, Larson SO, et al. A multicenter questionnaire investigation of attitudes toward hand hygiene, assessed by the staff in fifteen hospitals in Denmark and Norway. Am J Infec Control 1992;20:58–64.

10

Antimicrobial Preprocedural Mouth Rinses

Gail Molinari

LEARNING OBJECTIVES

After completion of this chapter individuals should be able to:

1 Describe the ideal properties for an antimicrobial mouth rinse.

2 Identify properties of chemical classes considered as antimicrobial rinse agents.

3 Describe the effects of preprocedural rinsing on salivary microbial populations.

4 Comprehend the potential benefits of preprocedural mouth rinses as chemical barriers to microbial cross-contamination and cross-infection during dental treatment.

5 Use accumulated scientific and clinical evidence to make informed decisions regarding implementation of preprocedural mouth rinses as a component of a comprehensive infection-control program.

INTRODUCTION AND RATIONALE FOR ANTIMICROBIAL ORAL RINSES

The use of antimicrobial chemical agents in medicine and dentistry dates back to the pioneering work of Dr. Joseph Lister in the 1860s. He was the first to advocate and use carbolic acid, a simple phenol, as an all-purpose handwash agent, a wound antiseptic for surgical sites, and a sterilant for contaminated instruments. Later generations of phenolics and other chemicals have proven to be extremely useful as antiseptics, antibiotics, and environmental surface disinfectants. A wide variety of microorganisms are often found in the form of **spatter** or **aerosols**, which may contaminate equipment and treatment area environmental surfaces, and potentially infect exposed respiratory tissues of dental care providers. The application of antimicrobial chemicals to the oral mucous membranes was introduced in the 1950s as an infection-control measure. Since then, the continued evolution of this non-barrier technique using later generations of chemicals has helped to minimize potential cross-contamination between patients and dental healthcare personnel (DHCP). However, the science is unclear concerning the incidence and nature of bacteremias from oral procedures, the relationship of these bacteremias to disease, and the preventive benefit of antimicrobial rinses.

ORAL MICROFLORA, SPATTER, AND AEROSOLS

The oral cavity provides a rich environment for growth of microbial life forms relating to conditions of oxygen, temperature, and nutrients. These provide ideal incubators for the growth of many microbial forms. Most microbial forms are harmless saprophytic bacteria, yet opportunist and even outright pathogens also can be routinely isolated. In addition to harboring numerous species of aerobic, facultative, and anaerobic bacteria, many adults have been infected with and can shed multiple viruses, including herpesviruses (i.e., herpes simplex viruses (HSVs), Epstein-Barr viruses, and cytomegaloviruses) and respiratory viruses (i.e., influenza, enteroviruses, and rhinoviruses).

While the tissues of the oral cavity are known to have a high natural resistance to infection, aerosolization of microbes during many dental procedures can present as sources for cross-contamination and possible cross-infection, which can affect both DCHP and their patients. In addition, concerns about occupational exposure of DHCP to bloodborne agents (i.e., HBV, HCV, and HIV) have included the delineation of possible risks from generating blood-containing aerosols. Although current data do not support a documented risk for DHCP, concerns remain and need to be addressed. This includes accomplishing a fundamental infection control goal: lowering the potential for exposure by reducing the concentrations of aerosolized microorganisms. This was recognized early on by investigators, as exemplified by Rubbo in 1960 when he advocated that "dentists should aim at standards of asepsis consistent with a sound surgical technique and a sensible appreciation of the possible infectious sequelae." Proposed methods include many of the infection-control practices routinely used in today's dental practices, along with the use of **preprocedural mouth rinsing**.

Spatter and aerosols may be produced by many dental instruments, including high- and low-speed handpieces and ultrasonic scaling devices. Airborne biological debris originating from a patient's oral cavity can settle on surfaces more than 3 feet away. Aerosols, which are air-suspended liquid or solid particles measuring less than 10 μm in diameter, can contain high concentrations of airborne bacteria, including *Mycobacterium tuberculosis* and *Legionella pneumophila*, as well as numerous respiratory viruses, such as influenza and rhinoviruses. It is important to remember that the transmission route for these various infectious organisms is typically through inhalation.

Dispersed airborne droplets measuring less than 10 μm can also be inhaled and can penetrate alveoli, particularly when DHCP do not wear a protective face mask. This was discussed in Chapter 1, with aerosolization of microorganisms included as one of the three major routes of infectious disease transmission for DHCP. Even though advances in protective measures associated with dental infection control (i.e., hand hygiene, personal protective equipment [PPE], vaccines, heat sterilizers, and disinfectants) have proven effective in lowering many occupational risks, the patient's mouth remains the major source of potential cross-infection between clinician and patient. Although DHCP routinely wear masks during patient treatment, microbial-laden aerosols can remain airborne in the vicinity of DHCP for extended intervals when masks are removed after completion of treatment procedures.

Multiple studies have shown that the use of an antimicrobial mouth rinse prior to dental procedures can significantly reduce both aerobic and anaerobic bacterial levels in saliva and aerosolized bacterial concentrations for up to 40–60 minutes after rinsing. Despite accumulated data from numerous investigations supporting this conclusion, there is presently no scientific evidence available to indicate that preprocedural mouth rinsing with an antimicrobial rinse prevents clinical infection for those who are in the direct path of aerosols, dentists, dental hygienists, and dental assistants. Conversely, there are also no data to indicate that DHCP are becoming sick from these aerosols or spatter.

ANTIMICROBIAL MOUTH RINSES

Properties of an Ideal Agent

It is imperative that possible applications and limitations must first be compared with the characteristics of an ideal agent when chemical preparations are considered for clinical use. Suggested properties for an ideal antimicrobial preprocedural mouth rinse are presented in Table 10-1. When reviewing these features, it is important to note that a desired efficacy against a broad range of microorganisms must be tempered with host tolerance considerations. For example, while a broad spectrum of antimicrobial activity is desirable, the active chemical component should possess a range of activity appropriate for the intraoral site of application. Thus, it is not necessary for an oral rinse to inactivate spores or other highly resistant vegetative microbes. In addition, while numerous antimicrobials have the capability to destroy high concentrations of bacteria, viruses, and fungi, there are important tissue-compatibility issues that also must be considered during evaluation of products as possible antiseptics. These include an agent's potential toxicity for oral soft and hard tissues, the allergenic potential of any of its components, and the possibility of disruption and alteration of the normal oral microflora with repeated use. Consideration should also be given to inclusion of alcohols as an emulsification ingredient. Although they are safe for use by the vast majority of the population, rinses containing significant amounts of alcohol are poorly tolerated by patients with mucositis or those undergoing head and neck radiation. Patients also should not be exposed to alcohol if they are pregnant, nursing, or being treated for alcoholism. Individuals may also be resistant to using mouth rinses with higher ethanol concentrations

TABLE 10-1 Properties of an Ideal Antimicrobial Mouth Rinse

1 Broad spectrum (antibacterial, antiviral, antifungal)
2 Prolonged residual (i.e., substantivity) activity after each use
3 Not inactivated by bacteria or host
4 Low allergenic potential with repeated usage
5 Easy to use (i.e., pleasant flavor, short duration of exposure necessary)
6 Lack of development of resistant microbial strains
7 Nontoxic/noncarcinogenic to oral tissues
8 Nontoxic/noncarcinogenic if systemically absorbed
9 Nonalcoholic
10 Clinically significant desired effect
11 Causes minimal disruption to the normal oral flora
12 Reasonable cost for routine use

because of personal preference, given the observation that formulations containing high concentrations of ethanol can cause more discomfort and pain than rinses with lower alcohol content.

Various antimicrobial agents have been suggested as possible candidates for the purpose of reducing the bacterial load of aerosols/spatter generated during dental treatment. Published studies indicate that several have been used in clinical settings. One investigation surveyed antiseptic mouth rinse use in Army dental clinics. Over 84% of the respondents used preprocedural rinses in their practices. Their stated purpose was to either prevent possible disease transmission to DHCP or decrease the chances of postoperative infection. The most commonly used rinses were chlorhexidine gluconate (CHG) and phenol-based essential oil preparations. Although no commercially available preparation meets all of the criteria for an ideal agent, a variety of chemical agents have been studied and used in attempts to reduce concentrations of oral microflora. Representative chemical classes are summarized in Table 10-2.

EVIDENCE CONSIDERING INFECTION CONTROL RATIONALE FOR PREPROCEDURAL MOUTH RINSES

Preparation of intraoral mucosal tissues with topical antiseptics prior to the injection of local anesthesia was introduced in the 1950s. It was found that when a topical

TABLE 10-2 Characteristics of Representative Antimicrobial Mouth Rinses

Chemical Class	Mechanism of Action	Clinical Considerations
Phenolic-Related Essential Oils	• Alters bacterial cell wall • Possible interference with coaggregation, recolonization, and subsequent growth of microorganisms • Extraction of endotoxin from oral Gram-negative bacteria • Inhibition of prostaglandins (antiinflammatory activity)	• Broad spectrum • Low substantivity (1st generation) • Some can have objectionable taste • No extrinsic staining • No loss of taste perception • No increased calculus formation
Bis-biguanides	• Binds to bacteria cell membrane to increase permeability and allow leakage of cytoplasmic contents • Adsorption, damage to permeability barriers, and precipitation of the cytoplasm	• Broad spectrum; effective against many Gram-positive and Gram-negative bacteria, aerobes, facultatives, strict anaerobes, yeasts, and fungi, and many viruses, including HSV and HIV-1 • Prolonged in vivo activity (substantivity) • Development of extrinsic yellow-brown stain • Promotes supragingival calculus formation • Potential aftertaste and/or disturbed taste sensation • Transient swelling of salivary glands
Quaternary ammonium compounds	• Increases permeability of cell membrane, leading to cell lysis • Decreases cell metabolism	• Active primarily against gram positive bacteria • Inactivated by the presence of organic matter, low pH, anionic compounds • Limited capacity to stay in contact with tissues • Occasionally incur oral ulceration and discomfort, and a mild burning of the tongue
Oxygenating agents	• Inhibit anaerobic bacteria • Release molecular oxygen • Foaming action may produce a transient mechanical debridement	• Rapid breakdown in the presence of organic material and bacterial catalase • Occasional oral ulceration after frequent (3×/day) use • Should not be swallowed
Halogens	• Oxidation of amino (NH^-), thiol (SH^-), and phenolic hydroxyl (OH^-) groups in amino acids and nucleotides • Interaction with unsaturated fatty acids in cell walls and membranes • For povidone iodine: irreversible iodination of bacterial proteins and oxidation • For oxychlorosene and chloramines-T: liberate free chlorine	• Microbiocidal for Gram-positive and Gram-negative bacteria, fungi, mycobacteria, viruses, and protozoans • Disagreeable taste • May stain teeth and tongue • Lack substantivity • Rapidly inactivated in the presence of organic matter

antiseptic was not applied prior to local anesthesia administration, a large number of oral flora could become implanted in the tissues at each injection site. Potential infection was shown to be reliably controlled by the application of CHG or povidone-iodine for 15 seconds prior to needle insertion.

The use of antimicrobial rinses prior to dental appointments also has been well documented to reduce the concentrations of microorganisms that can be released in treatment aerosols or spatter. With regard to possible application as a recommended infection-control practice, a brief description of representative research in this area is necessary, illustrating the ability of mouth rinses to reduce occupational, airborne, microbial contamination.

In one investigation, the effect of preprocedural rinsing with 0.12% CHG on the intraoral bacterial load was studied in patients with moderate to advanced periodontitis. Forty patients underwent scaling and root planing proce-

dures. One group was given dual rinses of CHG 1 minute apart prior to the dental treatment. Salivary samples were collected 30 minutes later and again either at 60 minutes or after treatment was completed. Control patients rinsed only with sterile water. When the 19 patients in the experimental group were compared with those in the control group, it was found that repeated use of CHG resulted in a significant reduction in the salivary bacterial load (97% over baseline levels). At 30 and 60 minutes postrinse assay intervals, the aerobic bacteria were reduced 77% in the CHG group compared to control subjects and 96% compared to baseline concentrations. It was concluded that "preprocedural rinsing with CHX has a profound and sustained effect on the aerobic and facultative flora of the oral cavity."

CHG also has been shown to be an effective virucidal agent, with in vitro activity demonstrated against HSV, cytomegalovirus, influenza viruses, parainfluenza virus, and hepatitis B virus (HBV) within a 30-second exposure. Other in vivo investigations in animals suggested that when 0.2% CHG was applied topically to HSV-infected tissues of mice, a reduction was demonstrated in the subsequent development of viral lesions and anti-HSV titers. It was thus suggested that a CHG rinse could be beneficial in controlling intraoral HSV infection. These data were expanded in a report published in 2000 indicating that both a 0.12% CHG formulation and a phenolic essential-oil mouth rinse were able to completely inhibit HIV-1 growth in tissue culture monolayers with a 30-second exposure.

The efficacy of preprocedural rinsing with a commercially available phenolic essential-oil preparation prior to the use of an ultrasonic scaling device has been reported. A 94.1% reduction in recoverable colony forming units (CFU) from aerosols was noted following a 30-second rinse, with the essential-oil product used in combination with a subsequent 10-minute ultrasonic scaling procedure. These data were significant compared to a 33.9% reduction in CFU following the use of a 5% hydroalcohol control rinse with the ultrasonic procedure. The observed reduction in bacterial level was maintained for 40 minutes, an interval analogous to the duration of many typical dental appointments. A similar reduction of 60% to 65% of viable bacteria in saliva samples was noted after rinsing with the phenolic essential-oil antiseptic. This was manifested by decreases of approximately 50% in streptococci and aerobic and anaerobic flora for 30–60 minutes after rinsing. Conversely, a control rinse procedure resulted in a 10% to 20% decrease in total flora. A later investigation compared bacteremias following a preprocedural phenol essential-oil rinse with that after a control rinse, when the rinse procedures were conducted in conjunction with subgingival irrigation. Overall, the use of the antiseptic mouth rinse resulted in aerobic and anaerobic bacterial counts in blood samples that were 92.3% and 87.8% lower, respectively, than those found for the control group.

Recommending organizations, such as the American Heart Association (AHA), Centers for Disease Control and Prevention (CDC), and American Dental Association (ADA), have offered limited support for the efficacy of preprocedural mouth rinsing. The 1985 guidelines issued by the ADA's Council on Dental Therapeutics and the Council on Prosthetic Services and Dental Laboratory Relations stated that "patients should rinse with a mouth wash before beginning an examination or treatment to reduce risks." In 1997, the AHA recommendations regarding the prevention of bacterial endocarditis following dental treatment included comments addressing preprocedural mouth rinsing with an antimicrobial solution. This procedure was advocated as a potential method for reducing the incidence or magnitude of bacteremia in patients at risk of developing endocarditis following bacteremia-inducing dental procedures. The CDC

"Guidelines for Infection Control in Dental Health-care Settings–2003" also included a section on antimicrobial preprocedural mouth rinses. In that section it was noted that there was inconclusive scientific evidence that these mouth rinses prevented infections in DHCP or patients.

The most recent AHA recommendations regarding infective endocarditis, published in 2007, reviewed the scientific evidence relating to endocarditis prophylaxis and concluded that the "results are contradictory with regard to the efficacy of the use of topical antiseptics in reducing the frequency of bacteremia associated with dental procedures, but the preponderance of evidence suggests that there is no clear benefit." The authors also concluded that "it is unlikely that topical antiseptics are effective to significantly reduce the frequency, magnitude, and duration of bacteremia associated with a dental procedure."

However, numerous published studies had demonstrated that a preprocedural rinse with an antimicrobial product is able to reduce concentrations of microorganisms in aerosols and spatter generated during dental procedures that use rotary instruments. The CDC stated that "preprocedural mouth rinses can be most beneficial before a procedure that requires using a prophylaxis cup or ultrasonic scaler because rubber dams cannot be used to minimize aerosol and spatter generation and, unless the provider has an assistant, high-volume evacuation is not commonly used." However, the CDC concluded that there were insufficient data to recommend preprocedural mouth rinses to prevent clinical infections in patients or DHCP, and considered this an unresolved issue.

SUMMARY

No specific guidelines exist for the routine use of a preprocedural mouth rinse as a component of a comprehensive infection-control program. A review of the literature regarding preprocedural mouth rinses reveals that the results are equivocal concerning the preventive benefit of antimicrobial rinses with respect to the nature and incidence of bacteremias from invasive dental procedures. Inconsistent study designs, small sample sizes, randomization, and examiner blinding are just a few variables that make these investigations challenging. There are also no data to support the notion that preprocedural mouth rinses prevent infection in DHCP.

The evidence does support the use of preprocedural mouth rinses to reduce the number of microorganisms the patient might release in the form of aerosols or spatter that subsequently can contaminate DHCP and equipment operatory surfaces. The choice is not a simple one, but a careful examination of accumulated evidence will better prepare DHCP to make an informed decision when making appropriate choices regarding which patients should use a preprocedural mouth rinse and which preparation should be used (Table 10-3).

TABLE 10-3 Clinical Procedure for the Use of an Antimicrobial Preprocedural Mouth Rinse

Who	Although not mandated, the use of an antimicrobial mouth rinse may be beneficial for all dental patients to produce a transient reduction in the overall numbers of microorganisms in the oral cavity that a patient might release in the form of aerosols or spatter, which subsequently can contaminate DHCP and equipment operatory surfaces.
What	An antimicrobial preparation with substantivity.
When	Immediately before a dental procedure likely to release aerosols or spatter in which a rubber dam and high-volume evacuation are not used.
Where	In the dental operatory after the patient is seated in the dental chair.
How	The appropriate dose is given to the patient in a disposable cup; the patient is instructed to rinse for 30–60 seconds and then expectorate into a cup or the chairside suction.

2. Rinsing with an antimicrobial preprocedural mouth rinse prevents clinical infection in dental healthcare personnel.

A. True

B. False

3. Studies have demonstrated that an antimicrobial preprocedural mouth rinse can produce a transient reduction in the level of oral microorganisms in aerosols and spatter generated during routine dental procedures with rotary instruments.

A. True

B. False

4. Having patients use a preprocedural mouth rinse may be most be beneficial before:

A. Procedures using a prophylaxis cup.

B. Procedures using an ultrasonic scaler.

C. Dental extractions using rotary instruments.

D. All of the above.

If a practitioner does decide to use a preprocedural mouth rinse, he or she should first consider the patient's medical status, oral hygiene/oral health, and ability to rinse and expectorate. For example, young children who are less than 5–6 years of age generally do not possess the neuromuscular control to be able to rinse and expectorate without swallowing a mouth rinse. The same is true for many adult patients who are elderly or compromised by a stroke or other neuromuscular condition.

✔ Practical Dental Infection Control Checklist

❑ Are preprocedural mouth rinses considered as a means to reduce the level of oral microorganisms in aerosols and spatter generated during routine dental procedures?

Review Questions

1. A preprocedural mouth rinse is often used by patients before a dental procedure to:

A. Reduce the number of microorganisms released from the oral cavity during dental procedures.

B. Eliminate the need to disinfect environmental surfaces following dental procedures.

C. Eliminate the need to use a rubber dam during dental procedures.

D. A and B

E. All of the above.

Critical Thinking

1. Does your dental office/clinic offer preprocedural mouth rinses to your patients? If yes, what product do you use?

2. A new patient asks you why you are having him rinse before he gets his teeth cleaned. How do you respond?

SELECTED READINGS

ADA Councils on Dental Therapeutics and Prosthetic Services and Dental Laboratory Relations. Guidelines for infection control in the dental office and the commercial dental laboratory. J Am Dent Assoc 1985:110:969–972.

Baqui AAMA, Kelley JI, Jabra-Rizk MA, et al. In vitro effect of oral antiseptics on human immunodeficiency virus-1 and herpes simplex virus type 1. J Clin Periodontol 2001;28:610–616.

Bernstein D, Schiff G, Echler G, et al. In vitro virucidal effectiveness of a 0.12% chlorhexidine gluconate mouthrinse. J Dent Res 1990;69:874–876.

Bolanowski SJ, Gesheider, GA, Sutton SV. Relationship between oral pain and ethanol concentration in mouthrinses. J Periodont Res 1995;30:192–197.

Bonine L. Effect of chlorhexidine rinse on the incidence of dry socket in impacted mandibular third molar extraction sites. Oral Surg Oral Med Oral Pathol 1995;79: 154–158.

Briner WW, Buckner RY, Rebitski GF. Effect of chlorhexidine gluconate mouthrinse on plaque bacteria. J Periodont Res 1986;21:44–52.

Brown AR, Papasian CJ, Shultz P, et al. Bacteremia and intraoral suture removal: can an antimicrobial rinse help? J Am Dent Assoc 1998;129:1455–1461.

Buckner RY, Kayrouz GA, Briner W. Reduction of oral microbes by a single chlorhexidine rinse. Compend Contin Educ Dent 1994;15:512–520.

Cawson RA, Curson I. The effectiveness of some antiseptics on the oral mucous membrane. Br Dent J 1959;117:208–211.

CDC. Guidelines for infection control in dental health-care settings, 2003. MMWR 2003;52(RR-17):1–66.

Ciancio S. Expanded and future uses of mouthrinses. J Am Dent Assoc 1994;125:29S–32S.

Dajani AS, Taubert KA, Wilson W, et al. Prevention of bacterial endocarditis: recommendations by the American Heart Association. J Am Med Assoc 1997;129: 1794–1801.

DePaola L, Minah GE, Overholser CD, et al. Effect of an antiseptic mouthrinse on salivary microbiota. Am J Dent 1996;9:93–95.

Fine DH, Meddieta C, Barnett ML, et al. Efficacy of preprocedural rinsing with an antiseptic in reducing viable bacteria in dental aerosols. J Periodontol 1992;63:821–824.

Fine DH, Yip J, Furgang D, et al. Reducing bacteria in dental aerosols: preprocedural use of an antiseptic mouthrinse. J Am Dent Assoc 1993;124:56–58.

Harrel SK, Molinari J. Aerosols and spatter in dentistry. A brief review of the literature and infection control implications. J Am Dent Assoc 2004;135:429–437.

Hennessy B, Joyce A. A survey of preprocedural antiseptic mouth rinse use in Army dental clinics. Military Med 2004;169:600–603.

Klyn SL, Cummings DE, Richardson BW, et al. Reduction of bacteria-containing spray produced during ultrasonic scaling. Gen Dent 2001;49:648–652.

Larsen PE. The effect of a chlorhexidine rinse on the incidence of alveolar osteitis following the surgical removal of impacted mandibular third molars. J Oral Maxillo Surg 1991;49:932–937.

Litsky BY, Mascis JD, Litsky W. Use of an antimicrobial mouthwash to minimize the bacterial aerosol contamination generated by the high-speed drill. Oral Surg Oral Med Oral Pathol 1970;29:25–30.

Lockhart PB. An analysis of bacteremias during dental extractions. A double-blind, placebo-controlled study of chlorhexidine. Arch Intern Med 1996;156:513–520.

Miller RL, Micik RE, Abel C, et al. Studies on dental aerobiology. II. Microbial splatter discharged from the oral cavity of dental patients. J Dent Res 1971;50:621–625.

Molinari JA, Molinari G. Is mouthrinsing before dental procedures worthwhile? J Am Dent Assoc 1992;123:75–80.

Overholser CD, Meiller TF, DePaola LG, et al. Comparative effects of 2 chemotherapeutic mouthrinses on the development of supragingival dental plaque and gingivitis. J Clin Periodontol 1990;17:575–579.

Rahn R. Preventing post-treatment bacteremia. J Am Dent Assoc 1995;126:1145–1149.

Riep BG, Bernimoulin JP, Barnett ML. Comparative antiplaque effectiveness of an essential oil and an amine fluoride/stannous fluoride mouthrinse. J Clin Periodontol 1990;26:164–168.

Rubbo SD. Asepsis and antisepsis in dentistry. Austral Dent J 1960;5;61–69.

Veksler AE, Kayrouz GA, Newman MG. Reduction of salivary bacteria by preprocedural rinses with chlorhexidine 0.12%. J Periodontol 1991;62:649–651.

Wilson W, Taubert KA, Gewitz M, et al. Prevention of infective endocarditis: guidelines from the American Heart Association: a guideline from the American Heart Association Rheumatic Fever, Endocarditis, and Kawasaki Disease Committee, Council on Cardiovascular Disease in the Young, and the Council on Clinical Cardiology, Council on Cardiovascular Surgery and Anesthesia, and the Quality of Care and Outcomes Research Interdisciplinary Working Group. Circulation 2007;116:1736–1754.

Wilson W, Taubert KA, Gewitz M, et al. Prevention of infective endocarditis: guidelines from the American Heart Association: a guideline from the American Heart Association Rheumatic Fever, Endocarditis and Kawasaki Disease Committee, Council on Cardiovascular Disease in the Young, and the Council on Clinical Cardiology, Council on Cardiovascular Surgery and Anesthesia, and the Quality of Care and Outcomes Research Interdisciplinary Working Group. J Am Dent Assoc 2007;138:739–760.

Wyler D, Miller RL, Micik RE. Efficacy of self-administered preoperative oral hygiene procedures in reducing the concentration of bacteria in aerosols generated during dental procedures. J Dent Res 1971;50:509.

11

Sterilization Procedures and Monitoring

Jennifer A. Harte

John A. Molinari

LEARNING OBJECTIVES

After completion of this chapter individuals should be able to:

1 Differentiate between disinfection and sterilization.

2 Discuss categories of patient-care items as they relate to disinfection and sterilization.

3 Describe the three most commonly used heat sterilization methods: steam under pressure (autoclaving), dry heat, and unsaturated chemical vapor.

4 Describe the advantages and disadvantages of the three most common methods of heat sterilization.

5 Describe special considerations in sterilization: flash sterilization (unwrapped instruments), dental handpieces, and heat-sensitive instruments.

6 Describe sterilization monitoring recommendations and other elements of a sterility assurance program.

KEY TERMS

Air removal test: a diagnostic test for prevacuum steam sterilizers that checks for the sterilizer's ability to remove air from the chamber.

Autoclave: an instrument for sterilization that uses moist heat under pressure.

Bead sterilizer (endodontic dry-heat sterilizer): a device that uses small glass beads (1.2–1.5 mm in diameter) and high temperature (217–232°C/423–450°F) for brief exposures (e.g., 45 seconds) to inactivate microorganisms. The term is a misnomer because the device has not been cleared by the FDA as a sterilizer.

Biological indicator (BI): a device to monitor the sterilization process that consists of a standardized population of bacterial spores known to be resistant to the mode of sterilization being monitored. BIs indicate whether all the parameters necessary for sterilization were present.

Chemical indicator: a device to monitor the sterilization process that changes color or form with exposure to one or more of the physical conditions within the sterilizing chamber (e.g., temperature, steam). Chemical indicators are intended to detect potential sterilization failures that could result from incorrect packaging, incorrect loading of the sterilizer, or malfunctions of the sterilizer. A "pass" response does not verify that the items are sterile.

Chemical sterilant: chemicals used for the purpose of destroying all forms of microbial life, including bacterial spores.

Chemical vapor sterilizer (Chemiclave): an instrument for sterilization that uses hot formaldehyde vapors under pressure.

Control biological indicator: a BI from the same lot as a test indicator that is left unexposed to the sterilization cycle and then incubated to verify the viability of the test indicator. The control indicator should yield positive results for bacterial growth.

Critical: the category of medical devices or instruments that are introduced directly into the human body, either into or in contact with the bloodstream or normally sterile areas of the body (e.g., surgical instruments and scalpel). These items are so called because of the substantial risk of acquiring infection if the item is contaminated with microorganisms at the time of use.

Disinfectant: a chemical agent used on inanimate (i.e., nonliving) objects (e.g., floors, walls, and sinks) to destroy virtually all recognized pathogenic microorganisms, but not necessarily all microbial forms (e.g., bacterial endospores). The EPA groups disinfectants according to whether the

product label claims they are "limited," "general," or "hospital" disinfectants.

Disinfection: the destruction of pathogenic and other kinds of microorganisms by physical or chemical means. Disinfection is less lethal than sterilization because it destroys most recognized pathogenic microorganisms, but not necessarily all microbial forms, such as bacterial spores. Disinfection does not ensure the margin of safety associated with sterilization processes.

Dry heat: used to sterilize materials that might be damaged in the presence of water vapor.

Dry-heat sterilizer: an instrument for sterilization that uses heated air; dry-heat sterilizers used in dentistry include static-air and forced-air types.

Exposure time: period of time during a sterilization or disinfection process in which items are exposed to the sterilant or disinfectant at the parameters specified by the manufacturer (e.g., time, concentration, temperature, and pressure).

Flash sterilization: a process designed for the steam sterilization of unwrapped patient-care items for immediate use. Currently, the time required for flash sterilization depends on the type of sterilizer and the type of item (i.e., porous vs. nonporous items). This process is usually only used in emergency situations (e.g., when a short turnaround time is needed).

Food and Drug Administration (FDA): the FDA promotes and protects the public health by helping safe and effective products reach the market in a timely way; monitors products for continued safety after they are in use; and helps the public get the accurate, science-based information needed to improve health.

Gravity displacement sterilizer: a type of steam sterilizer in which incoming steam displaces residual air through a port or drain in or near the bottom (usually) of the sterilizer chamber.

High-level disinfectant: a liquid chemical germicide registered by the FDA and used in the disinfection process for critical and semicritical patient-care devices. It inactivates vegetative bacteria, mycobacteria, fungi, and viruses, but not necessarily high numbers of bacterial spores. The FDA further defines a high-level disinfectant as a sterilant used under the same contact conditions except for a shorter contact time.

Implantable device: according to the FDA, a "device that is placed into a surgically or naturally formed cavity of the human body if it is intended to remain there for a period of 30 days or more" [21 CFR 812.3(d)].

Mechanical indicator: devices (e.g., gauges, meters, displays, and printouts) that display an element of the sterilization process (e.g., time, temperature, and pressure).

Noncritical: the category of medical items or surfaces that carry the least risk of disease transmission. This category has been expanded to include not only noncritical medical devices but also environmental surfaces. Noncritical medical devices touch only unbroken (nonintact) skin (e.g., a blood pressure cuff). Noncritical environmental surfaces can be further divided into clinical contact surfaces (e.g., a light handle) and housekeeping surfaces (e.g., floors and countertops).

Prevaccum steam sterilizer: a type of steam sterilizer in which air is removed from the chamber and the load by means of pressure and vacuum excursions at the beginning of the cycle.

Semicritical: the category of medical devices or instruments (e.g., mouth mirror and amalgam condenser) that come into contact with mucous membranes and do not ordinarily penetrate them.

Spaulding classification: a strategy for sterilizing or disinfecting inanimate objects and surfaces based on the degree of risk involved in their use. The three categories are: critical, semicritical, and noncritical. The system also

establishes three levels of germicidal activity for disinfection (high, intermediate, and low).

Spore test: see "biological indicator."

Steam sterilization: a sterilization process that uses saturated steam under pressure for a specified exposure time and at a specified temperature as the sterilizing agent.

Sterilant: a liquid chemical germicide that destroys all forms of microbiological life, including high numbers of resistant bacterial spores.

Sterile/sterility: state of being free from all living microorganisms. In practice, it is usually described as a probability function (e.g., the probability of a surviving microorganism being 1 in 1,000,000).

Sterilization: the destruction or removal of all forms of life, with particular reference to microbial organisms. The limiting factor and requirement for sterilization is the destruction of heat-resistant bacterial and mycotic spores.

Tabletop steam sterilizer: a compact steam sterilizer that has a chamber volume of not more than 2 cubic feet and generates its own steam when distilled or deionized water is added by the user.

Unsaturated chemical vapor sterilization: a sterilization process that uses hot formaldehyde vapors under pressure.

Sterilization is the most important component of an infection-control program. Following the basic rule "Do not disinfect when you can sterilize" provides the highest level of patient protection. A basic understanding of the difference between sterilization and disinfection is essential. **Sterilization** is a procedure that destroys all microorganisms, including large numbers of resistant bacterial spores, which are the most difficult microorganisms to kill. **Disinfection** destroys microorganisms by physical or chemical means and is less lethal than sterilization. Spores are not killed during disinfection procedures. As a result, disinfection does not ensure the degree of safety associated with sterilization processes. Generally, the term disinfection is reserved for chemicals applied to inanimate surfaces.

This chapter describes the three most commonly used heat sterilization methods in dentistry: steam under pressure (autoclaving), dry heat, and unsaturated chemical vapor. Instrument-processing procedures, including cleaning, packaging, sterilization, and storage, will be discussed in Chapter 16. A brief discussion of less common methods used to sterilize or perform high-level disinfection of heat-sensitive instruments, including the use of ethylene oxide and liquid chemical germicides, is also included. A later portion of the chapter discusses the

importance of a sterility assurance program and sterilization monitoring procedures.

STERILIZATION OVERVIEW

The use of heat to sterilize items dates back hundreds of years and has been recognized as the most efficient and reliable method of sterilization. In both medical and dental settings, the historical practice of immersing items in liquid chemical germicides (i.e., "cold" sterilization) to sterilize patient-care instruments between patients should be limited in use and is recommended only when a heat-tolerant or disposable instrument is not available. Infection-control guidelines and recommendations from the American Dental Association (ADA) and Centers for Disease Control and Prevention (CDC) have addressed proper infection-control procedures, including instrument-processing strategies. These recommendations recognize heat sterilization of patient-care items as the standard of care. In the opinion of the authors, heat sterilization is *required* for all instruments and items that go into a patient's mouth and can withstand repeated exposure to high temperatures.

Table 11-1 presents a classification scheme used by the CDC for categorizing patient-care items (e.g., dental

	TABLE 11-1 Categories of Patient-Care Items		
Category	**Definition**	**Examples in Dentistry**	**Comments**
Critical	Penetrate soft tissue, contact bone, enter into or contact the bloodstream or other normally sterile tissue.	Surgical instruments, periodontal scalers, scalpels, surgical dental burs	Have the greatest risk of transmitting infection—clean and heat sterilize.
Semicritical	Contact mucous membranes or nonintact skin, but will not penetrate soft tissue, contact bone, or enter into or contact the bloodstream or other normally sterile tissue.	Dental mouth mirror, amalgam condenser, reusable dental impression trays, dental handpieces.*	Have a lower risk of transmission—clean and heat sterilize. If a semicritical item is heat-sensitive, it should, at a minimum, be processed with high-level disinfection.
Noncritical	Contact with intact skin.	Radiograph head/cone, blood pressure cuff, facebow, pulse oximeter.	Pose the least risk of transmission of infection—clean and disinfect or use disposable barrier protection.

*Although dental handpieces are "by definition" considered a semicritical item, they should always be heat-sterilized between uses and not high-level disinfected.
Adapted from CDC. Guidelines for infection control in dental health-care settings–2003. MMWR 2003;52(RR-17):20.

instruments, devices, and equipment) depending on the potential risk of transmitting infection if the item becomes contaminated during use. These categories (i.e., critical, semicritical, and noncritical) were first used by Spaulding in 1968 when he discussed strategies for disinfecting and sterilizing medical and surgical instruments, and is sometimes referred to as the **Spaulding classification**. This system, or variations of it, has been used in infection control recommendations and guidelines over the years including the recent CDC "Guidelines for Infection Control in Dental Health-Care Settings—2003."

Critical items such as surgical instruments and scalpels used to penetrate soft tissue or bone have the greatest risk of transmitting infection and should be cleaned and sterilized by heat. Needles and scalpel blades are examples of critical items that come in **sterile** packaging and are considered single-use disposable. These items must be used for only one patient and then discarded appropriately. They are not intended to be cleaned and reprocessed for use on another patient. **Semicritical** items touch mucous membranes or nonintact skin and have a lower risk of transmission, but because most semicritical items in dentistry are heat-tolerant, they also should be sterilized by using heat. If a semicritical item is heat-sensitive, it should, at a minimum, be processed with a **high-level disinfectant**.

Noncritical patient-care items pose the least risk of transmission of infection, contacting only intact skin. In most cases, cleaning, or if the item is visibly soiled, cleaning followed by disinfection with an Environmental Protection Agency (EPA)-registered hospital **disinfectant** is adequate. If the item is visibly contaminated with blood, an EPA-registered hospital disinfectant with a tuberculocidal claim (i.e., intermediate-level disinfectant) should be used. Environmental surface disinfection and products are discussed in Chapters 12 and 13.

STERILIZATION METHODS

All medical devices sold in the United States must first be cleared by the **Food and Drug Administration (FDA)**, including sterilization equipment. The manufacturer submits documentation describing the device, the manufacturing facilities, and results of studies conducted to support any claims of effectiveness and safety made for the device. The use of commercially available ovens used for cooking is not a substitute for a tested and approved sterilizer. The insulation requirements, temperature criteria, and testing methods for the former are not as stringent as the requirements for FDA-cleared medical devices.

In dentistry, heat-tolerant instruments are usually sterilized by steam under pressure (autoclaving), dry heat, or unsaturated chemical vapor. The method chosen must be compatible with the items to be sterilized and the sterilization wrapping materials or containers, such as cassettes. For example, some items that can tolerate steam under pressure may be destroyed by the high temperatures used with dry-heat sterilizers. Characteristics of the three most commonly used heat sterilization methods can be found in Table 11-2.

Steam Sterilization

The steam sterilizer, or **autoclave**, is the most commonly used form of heat sterilization in healthcare facilities for items that are not sensitive to heat and moisture, because it is a dependable and cost-effective process. Steam sterilizers use moist heat at higher temperatures in the form of saturated steam under pressure. As the steam fills the sterilizer chamber, cooler air is pushed out via an escape valve, which then closes and slows a build-up of pressure. **Steam sterilization** requires exposure of each item to direct steam contact at a

TABLE 11-2 Characteristics of Commonly Used Heat Sterilization Methods in Dentistry

Method	Process Overview	Cycle time and temperature*	Packaging Material Requirements†	Advantages	Disadvantages	Biological Monitoring
Steam Gravity displacement	Moist heat at higher temperatures in the form of saturated steam under pressure	15–30 min at 250°F/121°C	Must allow steam to penetrate • *Acceptable:* wrapped perforated metal trays/cassettes, paper, plastic, cloth, paper/plastic peel pouches • *Unacceptable:* closed metal and glass containers	• Time-efficient • Good penetration • Can be used with packaged items • Ability to process wide range of materials without destruction	• Corrosion of non-stainless-steel metal items • Do not use closed containers • Possible deposits from using hard water • May leave instruments wet at end of cycle • May damage heat-sensitive plastics and rubber items • May dull certain sharp items	*Geobacillus stearothermophilus* (formerly known as *Bacillus stearothermophilus*) Incubation temperature range: 55–60°C (131–140°F)¶
Prevacuum		3.5–10 min at 270°F/132°C				
Dry Heat Static Air	Hot air rises inside the chamber through natural convection	60–120 min at 320°F/160°C	Must not insulate items from heat and must not be destroyed by the temperature used. • *Acceptable:* wrapped perforated metal trays/cassettes, paper bags, aluminum foil, polyfilm plastic tubing • *Unacceptable:* plastic and paper bags that cannot withstand dry-heat temperatures	• No corrosion or rust • Does not dull cutting edges • Items dry after cycle • Closed containers may be used if a spore test is used to confirm appropriate kill	• May damage heat-sensitive plastic and rubber items • Items must be thoroughly dried before processing • Long cycle time • May not be appropriate for handpieces§	*Bacillus atrophaeus* (formerly known as *Bacillus subtilis*) Incubation temperature: 30–37°C¶ (86–98.6°F)
Forced Air	Heated air is circulated throughout the chamber at a high velocity	12 min at 375°F/190°C		• Time-efficient • No corrosion or rust • Does not dull cutting edges • Items dry after cycle	• May damage plastic and rubber items • Items must be thoroughly dried before processing • May damage heat-sensitive items • May not be appropriate for handpieces§	
Unsaturated Chemical Vapor	Hot formaldehyde vapors under pressure	20 min at 270°F/132°C	Vapors must be allowed to precipitate on contents and must not react with packaging material. Plastics should not contact sides of the sterilizer. • *Acceptable:* wrapped perforated metal trays/cassettes, paper, or paper plastic peel pouches. • *Unacceptable:* closed metal trays and sealed glass jars.	• Time-efficient • No corrosion or rust • Items dry after cycle	• Special solutions required • Ventilation must be adequate • Items must be thoroughly dried before processing • May damage heat-sensitive plastics • Do not used closed containers • Do not use thick wrapping materials • May not be appropriate for handpieces§	*Geobacillus stearothermophilus* (formerly known as *Bacillus stearothermophilus*) Incubation temperature range: 55–60°C (131–140°F)¶

*Cycle times do not include warm-up times and may vary with the brand of sterilizer; follow the manufacturer's instructions for sterilizing conditions.

† Use only materials approved by the sterilizer manufacturer.

§ Consult handpiece manufacturer.

¶ Follow the manufacturer's instructions for incubation time/temperature.

required temperature and pressure for a specified time to kill microorganisms. The items in the sterilizer chamber absorb heat as the saturated steam condenses. Steam sterilizers are available in a range of sizes, from smaller tabletop models (Fig. 11-1) to large, floor-standing units (Fig. 11-2). It is the heat, not the pressure inside a steam sterilizer, that actually kills the microorganisms.

Sources of steam include admission through steam lines, a steam generator, or self-generation of steam within the chamber. A **tabletop steam sterilizer** generates its own steam when distilled or deionized water is added by the user. Larger sterilizers, which are typically used in hospitals and dental schools, can be connected directly to a steam line or to a water line that allows them to generate their own steam. Two common operating temperatures and times are 250°F (121°C) for 15–30 minutes or 270°F (132°C) for 3–10 minutes. These times do not include sterilizer warm-up or cool-down periods. Also, sterilization intervals may vary with the load size, the use of different instrument wraps, and the nature of the materials to be sterilized. Most surgical wrapping materials, commercial sterilization bags, and pouches will allow the steam to penetrate sufficiently to kill all microbial forms.

A

B

C

FIGURE 11-1 **(A,B)** Examples of tabletop steam sterilizers. **(C)** Example of a tabletop sterilizer with the door open, showing a typical chamber size.

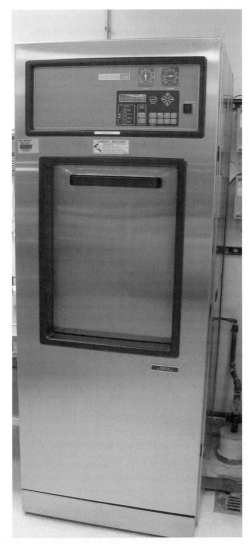

FIGURE 11-2 Example of a hospital steam sterilizer.

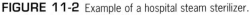

Even when thick wrapping materials are used, a maximal sterilization period of 30 minutes usually suffices. In addition, advances in sterilizer technology have allowed the application of higher temperatures and pressures for shorter cycle intervals in newer equipment. The importance of following the manufacturer's instructions when operating and maintaining sterilization equipment cannot be emphasized enough.

Gravity Displacement vs. Prevacuum Steam Sterilizers

The two basic types of steam sterilizers are the gravity displacement sterilizer and the prevacuum sterilizer. Until recently, gravity displacement sterilizers constituted the majority of sterilizers used in dentistry. Although prevacuum sterilizers with large chamber sizes have been available for many years in hospitals, dental schools, and large clinics, only recently have smaller tabletop versions been developed and made available in the United States.

Most tabletop sterilizers currently in use in dental practices are **gravity displacement sterilizers**, in which the steam is self-generated within the chamber or created by a steam generator that is a part of the sterilizer. The steam enters at the top or the sides of the sterilizer, and because the steam is lighter than air, unsaturated air is pushed out of the chamber through a drain or escape valve. Of concern during this process is the formation of cool air pockets within the chamber resulting in extended penetration times for porous items. Also, because these air pockets do not reach the required temperatures for sterilization, a sterilization failure may occur that might not be detected via routine sterilization monitoring. As a result, some sterilizers use pressure-pulsing techniques along with gravity displacement techniques to help remove the air from the chamber before the sterilization cycle. Also, some steam sterilizers now have a prevacuum cycle that removes air from the chamber before the steam enters.

In contrast to gravity displacement sterilizers, **prevacuum steam sterilizers** are fitted with a pump that creates a vacuum in the chamber to ensure air is removed from the sterilizing chamber before the steam enters. Compared to gravity displacement, this procedure allows faster and more thorough steam penetration throughout the entire load. These prevacuum units also have a poststerilization vacuum cycle that facilitates drying, providing dry instrument packs at the end of the sterilization process. If a vacuum drying cycle is not available, other methods for drying packs include using an automatic open-door drying cycle or having the sterilizer pull in fresh air through filters. If these options are not available, it is necessary to manually open the sterilizer door to allow moisture to escape. Regardless of the drying method used, before removing and handling packages, it is critical to allow packages to dry and cool inside the sterilizer chamber to maintain sterility. Packs should not be touched until they are cool and dry because hot packs act as wicks, absorbing moisture and hence bacteria from hands and the environment. Also, wet packs can tear easily.

To ensure that prevacuum sterilizers are working as intended, they should be tested periodically for adequate air removal and air leaks. Air removal testing cannot be performed on gravity displacement equipment and therefore does not apply. In larger floor-standing prevacuum sterilizers, the **air removal test** is generally performed in an empty chamber at the beginning of each day before the first processed load. A commercially prepared test pack is usually placed near the door and over the drain. If the test pack indicates that the sterilizer failed the air removal test, the sterilizer should not be used until it is inspected by sterilizer maintenance personnel and then passes the air removal test. Air removal testing should also be performed during initial sterilizer installation, following sterilization failures (i.e., a positive **biological indicator (BI)**), and after sterilizer relocation, malfunction, or repair. Daily testing may not be indicated for some of the newer tabletop prevacuum steam sterilizers because of built-in tests or alarm systems and design differences. As always, it is recommended that users follow the sterilizer manufacturer's directions regarding frequency and use of air removal tests.

Corrosion or accumulation of rust on metallic instruments, orthodontic pliers, and scissors may be a problem when using steam sterilization. Also, sharp instruments may become dull over time. Even the most efficient autoclaves contain sufficient oxygen to cause corrosion or dulling of cutting instruments. One way to reduce corrosion is to apply rust inhibitors that contain sodium nitrite to the instruments before steam sterilization. This preventive coating uses chemicals that vaporize in the autoclave and protect metal from oxidation by hydrolysis. Also, to minimize these and other unit problems, users should follow the sterilizer manufacturer's recommended preventive maintenance schedule.

Dry Heat

Dry heat is used to sterilize materials that might be damaged in the presence of water vapor, such as burs and certain orthodontic instruments. Although dry heat has the advantages of having a low operating cost and being noncorrosive, it is a prolonged process and the high temperatures required are not suitable for certain patient-care items and devices. Also, instruments must be dry before the sterilization process is performed. Dry-heat sterilization is accomplished by the transfer of heat energy to objects upon contact. Microorganisms are destroyed via dehydration. As proteins dehydrate and dry, their resistance to denaturation increases. Thus, at a given temperature, dry heat sterilizes much less efficiently than moist heat. Because dry air is not as efficient a heat conductor as moist heat at the same temperature, a much higher temperature is required for a dry-heat unit to accomplish sterilization. Common operating temperatures are 320°F to 375°F (160°C to 190°C). These temperatures are suitable for sterilizing metal instruments, which are resistant to high temperatures and can rust or dull in the presence of water vapor. Consequently, many dental healthcare personnel (DHCP) prefer to use **dry-heat sterilizers** in their offices because sharp cutting edges are preserved on surgical instruments; however, these high temperatures will destroy many rubber- and plastic-based materials, melt the solder of most impression trays, weaken some fabrics, and destroy paper materials. Also, certain internal components of dental handpieces cannot withstand the high temperatures reached in dry-heat units. While older models of dry-heat sterilization equipment may not tolerate packaged instruments, as new equipment is purchased it should be checked to see if it can accommodate packaging materials. The manufacturer's instructions should always be consulted to ensure that dry-heat sterilization is appropriate.

Static-Air and Forced-Air Dry-Heat Sterilizers

Dry-heat sterilizers used in dentistry include static-air and forced-air types. The static-air type or oven-type sterilizer has heating coils in the bottom or sides of the unit that cause hot air to rise inside the chamber through natural convection. Once the sterilizer is preheated to the desired temperature, the instruments are placed in the heated chamber and heated for the recommended time period, and the instruments are removed and allowed to cool naturally. Heat-up times can range from 15 to 30 minutes and the sterilization cycle is typically 1 to 2 hours at 320°F (160°C). Thus, the long cycle time with this type of unit is a disadvantage because it can slow the flow of instrument recirculation.

The forced-air dry-heat sterilizer or rapid heat-transfer sterilizer circulates heated air through the chamber at a high velocity, permitting a more rapid transfer of energy from the air to the instruments, thereby reducing the time needed for sterilization. After the sterilizing temperature of 375°F (190°C) has been reached, **exposure times** range from 6 minutes for unpackaged items to 12 minutes for packaged items. Some units use continuous heating, while others begin heating from room temperature.

With the continuous-heating unit, a load is placed into the heated chamber and an exposure time is selected. The chamber temperature decreases because of the cool load. The load and chamber are heated to the selected temperature and the exposure time begins once the chamber temperature returns to its preestablished level. At the end of the exposure period, the load is removed from the chamber and allowed to cool. With the other type of unit, the load is placed in a room-temperature or cold chamber. The processing conditions are selected and the cycle is started. Simultaneous heating of the chamber and the load occurs. Exposure time begins when the selected chamber temperature is reached. At the end of the exposure time, the load is allowed to cool in the chamber.

A common problem when using dry-heat sterilizers is the failure of users to properly time the sterilization interval. Because penetration of dry heat into the center of an instrument pack is low and depends on both the size of the packages and the type of wrapping material used, users must be certain that the chamber is preheated appropriately before beginning the sterilization cycle. A common misuse of this equipment occurs when the chamber door is opened and an instrument pack is removed or quickly added during the timed cycle. This interrupts the cycle, and thus timing must begin all over again because the temperature drops when the door is opened. Additionally, it is important to maintain adequate space between instrument packs when loading them into a dry-heat sterilizer. Because air does not circulate well in this equipment, failure to ensure uniform hot air distribution during the cycle may cause some packages to become sterilized while others in the same load are not. Placing packages on their edges, as opposed to stacking them, allows proper separation. Thick wrappings and larger-than-normal packages also can significantly increase the time required for sterilization. As with any sterilization method, it is important to follow the manufacturer's instructions for loading, compatibility of packaging materials, and other operating parameters.

Unsaturated Chemical Vapor

Unsaturated chemical vapor sterilizers are sometimes referred to as a Harvey sterilizer or Chemiclave. The principle of operation of **unsaturated chemical vapor sterilization** is similar to that of steam sterilizers, but there are several important differences. Instead of using distilled or deionized water, the process involves heating a premixed chemical solution (purchased from the manufacturer) of various alcohols, water, and a small percentage (0.23%) of formaldehyde in a closed pressurized chamber that produces the sterilizing vapor. The temperature and pressure required for chemical vapor sterilizers are greater than those for the autoclave. The sterilization cycle is typically 20 minutes at the exposure temperature of 270°F (132°C). With this method, packages must be wrapped loosely to allow the chemical vapors to condense on the instrument surfaces during the cycle. Thick, tightly wrapped items will require longer exposure times because of the inability of the unsaturated chemical vapors to penetrate as well as saturated steam under pressure (i.e., autoclave).

A major advantage of using unsaturated chemical vapor sterilizers is the short cycle time, which is similar to that of the autoclave. Because of the low level of water present during the cycle, there is decreased corrosion and rusting of instruments such as orthodontic pliers, wires, bands, and carbon steel dental burs. Another advantage is that dry instruments can be removed at the end of the cycle. Instruments need to be dry before sterilization. If metal instruments are not completely dry, chemicals can accumulate on the wet surfaces, resulting in corrosion. Linens, liquids, items in dense packages, nylon tubing, closed containers, or items that cannot withstand high temperatures should not be sterilized with this method.

Of concern is the release of residual chemical vapors containing formaldehyde and methyl alcohol when the chamber door is opened at the end of the cycle. These can leave an unpleasant odor in the area. Adequate ventilation is required. Additionally, formaldehyde has been identified as a carcinogen; therefore, as with any chemical in the dental office, users should consult the manufacturer Material Safety Data Sheet (MSDS) regarding correct procedures for handling or working with hazardous chemicals. The current OSHA occupational exposure limit (29 CFR 1910.1048) for formaldehyde is 0.75 ppm as a time-weighted average (TWA). Recent technological advances include postprocess purge cycles (approximately 7 minutes) and filters to decrease residual vapors in the chamber and limit environmental exposure. This also helps minimize the smell from the chemicals when opening the sterilizer door. Finally, state and local authorities should be consulted regarding hazardous waste disposal requirements for the sterilizing solution.

SPECIAL CONSIDERATIONS

Flash Sterilization/Unwrapped Instruments

"Flash" or "fast" steam sterilization is defined as a process designed for the steam sterilization of patient-care items for immediate use. Currently, the time required for **flash sterilization** depends on the type of sterilizer and the type of item involved (i.e., porous or nonporous). A flash sterilization cycle usually operates at higher temperatures for shorter times. The flash sterilization cycle is preprogrammed to a specific time and temperature setting established by the manufacturer based on the type of sterilizer control (e.g., gravity displacement or prevacuum). To allow immediate contact with the steam in the short cycle, the instrument is usually unwrapped. However, if the manufacturer's instructions allow, special types of packaging materials may be used. If critical instruments, such as surgical instruments intended for immediate use, are flash-sterilized, they must be handled aseptically during removal from the

sterilizer and transport to the point of use (e.g., transported in a sterile covered container). Flash sterilization should not be used for reasons of convenience, as an alternative to purchasing additional instrument sets, or to save time. Flash sterilization should be used only in carefully selected clinical situations when certain conditions are met (Table 11-3).

Processing Heat-Sensitive Items

There are very few items that cannot be heat sterilized between patients. It cannot be overemphasized that heat-tolerant or disposable alternatives are available for the majority of items used in dentistry. The CDC emphasizes that heat sterilization is the method of choice when sterilizing dental instruments and devices, and that if an item is heat-sensitive, a heat-stable alternative or disposable item is preferred. If heat-sensitive items must be used, they can be sterilized using a low-temperature sterilization method, such as ethylene oxide gas (ETO), or by immersing them in a liquid chemical germicide registered by the FDA as a **sterilant**.

ETO has been used extensively in larger healthcare facilities. Its primary advantage is its ability to sterilize heat- and moisture-sensitive patient-care items with reduced harmful effects. However, extended sterilization times of 10 to 48 hours, and potential hazards to patients and DHCP that necessitate stringent health and safety requirements, make this method impractical for private-practice settings. Also, dental handpieces cannot be effectively sterilized with this method because of decreased penetration of ETO gas flow through the small lumens in the handpiece. Other types of low-temperature sterilization (e.g., hydrogen peroxide gas plasma) exist but are currently not practical for dental offices.

If heat-stable or disposable alternatives are not available, heat-sensitive critical and semicritical instruments

TABLE 11-3 Flash Sterilization: Do's and Don'ts	
Do	**Don't**
• Clean and dry instruments before the flash sterilization cycle. • Use mechanical and chemical indicators for each flash sterilization cycle. • To avoid contamination and thermal injury, allow instruments to dry and cool in the sterilizer before they are handled.	• Do not use flash sterilization for reasons of convenience, as an alternative to purchasing additional instrument sets, or to save time. • Do not package or wrap instruments used during flash sterilization unless the sterilizer is specifically designed and labeled for this use. • Do not flash-sterilize implantable devices.

Courtesy of the USAF Dental Evaluation and Consultation Service.

and devices can be processed by immersing them in liquid chemical germicides (e.g., hydrogen peroxide-based products, peracetic acid, or glutaraldehyde) registered by the FDA as sterilants. Sterilizing instruments using **chemical sterilants** may require up to 12 hours of complete immersion, whereas high-level disinfection for semicritical instruments requires shorter immersion times (12–90 minutes). When a liquid chemical germicide is used for sterilization, certain poststerilization procedures are essential. Items need to be (a) rinsed with sterile water after removal to remove toxic or irritating residues, (b) handled using sterile gloves and dried with sterile towels, and (c) delivered to the point of use in an aseptic manner. If it is necessary to store the instrument before use, the instrument should not be considered sterile and should be sterilized again just before use. In addition, the sterilization process with liquid chemical sterilants cannot be verified with BIs (i.e., spore tests).

Because of the limitations for sterilization using liquid chemical germicides, they are almost never used to sterilize instruments. Rather, these chemicals are more often used for high-level disinfection of semicritical items. These chemicals are highly toxic. Eye irritation, respiratory effects, and skin sensitization have been reported. The manufacturer's instructions regarding dilution, immersion time, temperature, and safety precautions for using chemical sterilants/high-level disinfectants must be followed precisely. Because of their lack of chemical resistance to glutaraldehydes, medical gloves are not an effective barrier. When using glutaraldehydes, other factors might apply, such as room exhaust ventilation of 10 air exchanges/hour to ensure safe conditions for personnel working in the area. A common misuse is to use these high-level disinfectants as an environmental surface disinfectant or instrument-holding solution. These chemicals should not be used for applications other than those indicated in their label instructions. The manufacturer's instructions must be followed closely to ensure the effectiveness of the process and the safety of DHCP.

When using appropriate precautions, such as closed containers to limit vapor release, chemically resistant gloves and aprons, goggles, and face shields, glutaraldehyde-based products can be used without tissue irritation or adverse health effects. However, because of the numerous limitations (Table 11-4), the use of heat-sensitive semicritical items that must be processed with liquid chemical germicides is strongly discouraged; heat-tolerant or disposable alternatives are available for almost all such items.

Bead Sterilizers

Bead sterilizers have been used in dentistry to sterilize endodontic files, broaches, rotary instrument tips, and other metallic instrument tips. The FDA has determined

TABLE 11-4 Liquid Chemical Germicides Used for Chemical Sterilization or High-Level Disinfection

Advantages	Disadvantages
+ Can sterilize items that would be damaged by heat	− Less reliable than heat methods − Very time-consuming − Has a limited use-life − Is expensive in the long run − Cannot be spore-tested for effectiveness − Toxic fumes may require special ventilation − Personal protective equipment required during use − Cannot be used with packaged items − Items must be rinsed off with sterile water − May rust or corrode instruments

Courtesy of the USAF Dental Evaluation and Consultation Service.

that a risk of infection exists with these devices because of their potential failure to sterilize dental instruments. If a bead sterilizer is used, DHCP assume the risk of employing a dental device that the FDA has deemed neither safe nor effective. Bead sterilizers must never be used to sterilize devices for reuse on another patient.

Dental Handpieces

Multiple semicritical dental devices that touch mucous membranes are attached to the air or waterlines of the dental unit. These devices include high- and low-speed handpieces, prophylaxis angles, ultrasonic and sonic scaling tips, air abrasion devices, and air and water syringe tips. During treatment, the internal portions of handpieces and other devices attached to the air and waterlines may become contaminated with patient saliva, blood, and other oral debris. Although no epidemiologic evidence implicates these instruments in disease transmission, studies of high-speed handpieces using dye expulsion have confirmed the potential for retracting oral fluids into internal compartments of the device. This determination indicates that retained patient material can be expelled intraorally during subsequent uses. Studies have shown that the internal portions of some low-speed handpiece motors have the potential to become contaminated when used with both disposable and reusable prophylaxis angles, and there is the potential for internal contamination to be released through the prophylaxis angle into the mouth of a patient during subsequent uses. Because of this, any dental device connected to the dental air/water system that enters the patient's mouth should be run to discharge water, air, or a combination thereof for a minimum of 20–30 seconds after each patient. This procedure is intended to help physically flush out patient material that might have entered the turbine and air and waterlines.

Heat sterilization is required between patients for all dental handpieces or other intraoral devices that can be removed from the dental unit air or waterlines. This includes all handpiece attachments, such as nose cones, prophylaxis angles, and motors. Surface disinfection or immersion in chemical germicides is not an acceptable reprocessing method. Ethylene oxide gas cannot adequately sterilize internal components of handpieces. In clinical evaluations of high-speed handpieces, cleaning and lubrication were the most critical factors in determining performance and durability.

Table 11-5 provides a summary of the steps involved in handpiece asepsis. This protocol should not be used in place of the manufacturer's instructions. A variety of systems to help with handpiece maintenance before heat sterilization are commercially available. The products range from manually-operated purging stations to automated equipment that cleans, lubricates, and purges multiple handpieces (Fig. 11-3). With automatic maintenance systems, the handpieces are simply snapped onto the appropriate coupler, the door is closed, and after the start button is pushed, all processes

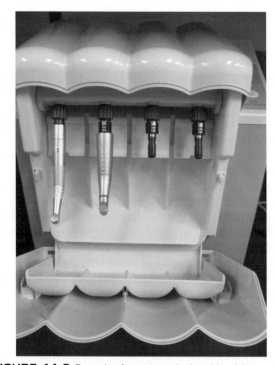

FIGURE 11-3 Example of an automatic dental handpiece maintenance unit that cleans, lubricates, and purges multiple handpieces. After the process is complete, the handpieces can be packaged and heat-sterilized.

occur automatically. At the completion of the cycle, the handpieces are ready for packaging and heat sterilization. Automated maintenance systems have the potential to save time, provide consistency to the overall handpiece maintenance process, and reduce repair costs. The manufacturer's instructions for cleaning, lubrication, and sterilization should be followed closely to ensure both the effectiveness of the process and the longevity of handpieces.

Some components of dental instruments are permanently attached to dental unit waterlines, and although they do not enter the patient's oral cavity, they are likely to become contaminated with oral fluids during treatment procedures. Handles or dental unit attachments of saliva ejectors, high-speed air evacuators, and air/water syringes should be covered with impervious barriers that are changed after each use (Fig. 11-4). If the item becomes visibly contaminated during use, DHCP should clean and disinfect with an EPA-registered hospital disinfectant with intermediate-level activity before using it on the next patient.

STERILIZATION MONITORING

Sterilization procedures are routinely monitored using a combination of mechanical, chemical, and BIs (Table 11-6). These indicators evaluate the sterilizing conditions and the procedure's effectiveness. The indicator

---

TABLE 11-5 Dental Handpiece Asepsis Summary*

Using appropriate personal protective equipment:

1. Remove all visible debris and flush handpiece water and/or air lines for 20–30 seconds with the bur in place.

2. Remove the bur from the handpiece. Clean and thoroughly dry the handpiece according to the manufacturer's instructions—most manufacturers do not recommend ultrasonic cleaning or soaking the handpiece.

3. Apply the handpiece cleaner and/or lubricant—some manufacturers have combined the lubricant with the cleaner. Do not overlubricate.

4. Attach to an air/water system and expel (with the bur or a bur blank in place) excess lubricants. This step is critical because it distributes lubricant to the air turbine assembly and expels any excess. Failure to do this may result in excess lubricant accumulation in the working assembly and "gumming" of the excess in the rotating assemblies during heat sterilization.

5. Clean the fiberoptics (at both ends of the handpiece) with a damp cotton swab according to the manufacturer's instructions.

6. Package the handpiece and any accessories and heat sterilize. Follow the manufacturer's recommendations regarding the type of heat sterilizer.

7. If poststerilization lubrication is required, handle the handpiece aseptically. To minimize cross-contamination, try to do this as close to the time of actual use as possible, and by opening just the end of the bag and spraying the lubricant into the handpiece.

*Note: This protocol should not be used in place of the manufacturer's instructions. The most important factor in handpiece maintenance is to follow the manufacturer's instructions.

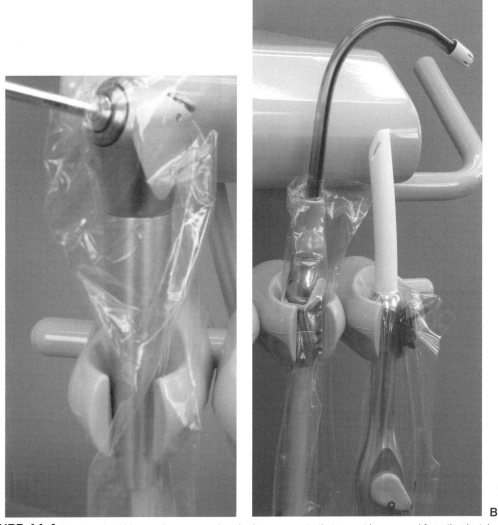

A   B

FIGURE 11-4 Barriers should be used to protect dental-unit components that cannot be removed from the dental unit waterlines. Barriers should be placed on the **(A)** air and water syringe handle and **(B)** the saliva ejector and high-speed air evacuator handles, and changed between patients.

must be appropriate for the sterilization process being used (e.g., steam autoclave, dry heat, or unsaturated chemical vapor) and always used according to the manufacturer's instructions (e.g., proper location in the sterilizer). Initial and recurrent training, staff supervision, maintenance and calibration of equipment, and recordkeeping are also important elements of a sterility assurance program.

Mechanical Monitoring

Mechanical indicators evaluate cycle time, temperature, and pressure by observing the gauges or displays on the sterilizer and noting these parameters for each load (Fig. 11-5). Large hospital-type sterilizers have recording devices that print out these parameters. If a tabletop sterilizer does not have a recording device, a printing

device can usually be purchased and retrofitted to the sterilizer. Because this technique detects conditions only in the sterilizer chamber, not conditions within the packages being processed, it is important to note that mechanical monitoring may not detect procedural problems, such as improperly loading the sterilizer, or problems arising from using incorrect packaging materials. Even though correct readings do not ensure sterilization, incorrect readings can be the first indication of a problem with the sterilization cycle.

Chemical Monitoring

Chemical indicators, internal and external, use sensitive chemicals to assess physical conditions (e.g., time and temperature) during the sterilization process. Common forms of these indicators include paper strips,

TABLE 11-6 Sterilization Monitoring Summary

	Mechanical	Chemical	Biological (i.e., spore tests)
How?	Assessment of cycle time, pressure, and temperature by examining the record chart/computer printout (or if not available, by visually observing the gauges). *Note:* The sterilizer gauges indicate conditions in the sterilizer chamber, not conditions within the packages being processed.	Heat-sensitive inks that change color when exposed to heat, heat and time, or heat, time, and steam.	Commercially prepared preparations containing live bacterial spores that are known to be resistant to the mode of sterilization being monitored. *Note:* • Always use a matching control (i.e., BI and control from the same lot number)—this is not placed in the sterilizer, but is incubated along with the spore test. • Incubation times can vary from 1 to 7 days depending on the type of BI.
When?	Every cycle	Internal chemical indicator: inside every package External chemical indicator: on the outside of the package when the internal indicator is not visible	At least once a week and in every load containing implantable devices.
Why?	• Incorrect readings could be the first indication of problem with the sterilizer.	• Indicator test results are received immediately upon completion of the sterilization cycle and could provide an early indication of a potential problem. • External indicators provide a quick, easy way to visually identify whether the package was processed through a sterilizer • Internal indicators provide verification that the sterilant (e.g., steam) reached the instruments inside the package.	• The sterilization process is directly assessed using the most resistant microorganisms (e.g., *Geobacillus stearothermophilus* [steam or chemical vapor] or *Bacillus atrophaeus* [dry heat]); the most valid method for monitoring the effectiveness of the sterilization process and sterility of processed items.

Courtesy of the USAF Dental Evaluation and Consultation Service.
Note: The indicator must be appropriate for the sterilization process being used (e.g., steam autoclave, dry heat, unsaturated chemical vapor) and used according to the manufacturer's instructions (e.g., proper location in the sterilizer or in the package).

labels, and steam pattern cards (Fig. 11-6). Because chemical indicators do not contain microbial spores, they cannot prove that sterilization has been achieved; however, they allow detection of certain equipment malfunctions and can help identify procedural errors. External indicators applied to the outside of a package, such as chemical indicator tape or special markings, change color rapidly when a specific parameter is reached, and they verify that the package has been exposed to the sterilization process. Some external indicators change color long before appropriate sterilization conditions are even met. "Autoclave" tape is an example of an external indicator that can be problematic at times because it often changes to show the striped pattern following a brief exposure to steam. External indicators do not guarantee that sterilization has been achieved or even that a complete sterilization cycle has occurred. External indicators are primarily used to identify packages that have been processed through a heat sterilizer, thus preventing the accidental use of unprocessed items (Fig. 11-7).

It is recommended to place a chemical indicator on the inside of each package to evaluate whether the instruments were exposed to the sterilization conditions. In other words, internal chemical indicators should be used inside each package to ensure that the sterilizing agent has penetrated the packaging material and actually reached the instruments inside (Fig. 11-8). If the internal indicator is not visible from the outside, also place an external chemical indicator on the package. Internal chemical indicators are sometimes referred to as multiparameter indicators if they are designed to react to two or more parameters (e.g., time and temperature; or time, temperature, and the presence of steam). A multiparameter internal chemical indicator can provide a more reliable indication that sterilization conditions have been met. Presently, multiparameter internal indicators are available only for steam sterilizers (i.e., autoclaves). Because chemical indicator test results are received when the sterilization cycle is complete, they can provide an early indication of a problem and where in the process the problem might exist. If either mechanical indicators or internal or external chemical indicators indicate inadequate processing, items in the load should not be used until reprocessed.

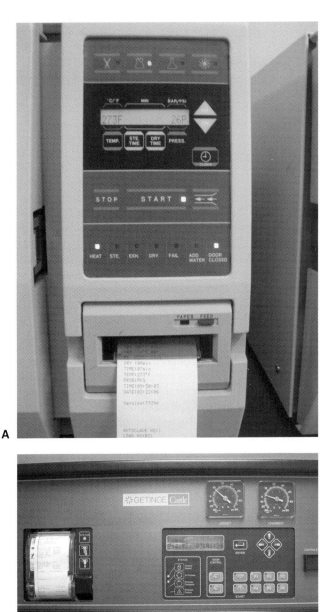

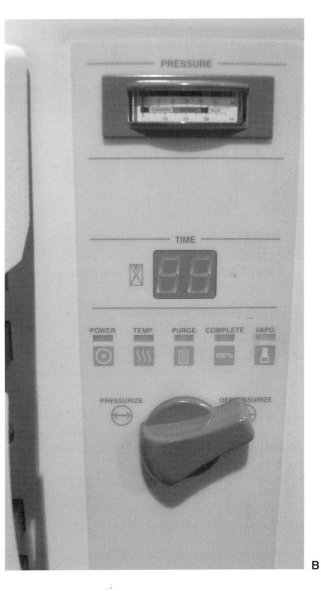

FIGURE 11-5 Examples of recording devices on **(A,B)** a table-top steam sterilizer and **(C)** a hospital steam sterilizer used to assess cycle time, temperature, and pressure during the sterilization cycle.

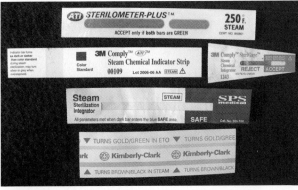

FIGURE 11-6 Examples of internal chemical indicators.

Biological Monitoring

Even when sterilizer gauges display correct values for internal conditions, and chemical indicators indicate that appropriate chamber conditions have been reached to achieve sterilization, the use of calibrated BIs is considered the main guarantee of sterilization. BIs (i.e., **spore tests**) are the most accepted method for monitoring the sterilization process because they assess it directly by killing known highly resistant microorganisms (e.g., *Geobacillus* or *Bacillus* species), rather than merely testing the physical and chemical conditions necessary for sterilization. These preparations contain bacterial spores, which are more resistant

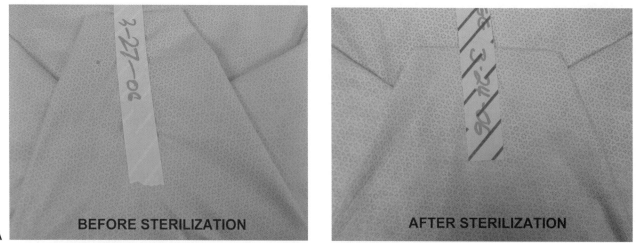

A   BEFORE STERILIZATION   AFTER STERILIZATION   B

FIGURE 11-7 External chemical indicators are used to identify packages that have been processed through the sterilizer. The photos show **(A)** a package before sterilization and **(B)** a package that has been through the sterilization cycle, as illustrated by the pattern on the external indicator tape.

to heat than viruses and vegetative bacteria. Because spores used in BIs are more resistant and present in greater numbers than the common microbial contaminants found on patient-care equipment, an inactivated BI indicates that other potential pathogens in the load have been killed. BIs are available in the form of either self-contained vials containing spore suspensions or bacterial spore-impregnated paper strips in glassine envelopes (Fig. 11-9). The test medium contained in the vials or used to incubate test strips includes a pH indicator. A color change occurs when spores germinate and produce acids, providing a visual display of sterilization cycle success or failure. The manufacturer's directions should determine the placement and location of BIs in the sterilizer, as well as appropriate incubation times and temperatures. A **control BI**, from the same lot as the test indicator and not processed through the

sterilizer, should be incubated with the test BI; the control BI should yield positive results for bacterial growth.

It is important to understand that the indicator must be appropriate for the sterilization process being used (e.g., steam autoclave, dry heat, or unsaturated chemical vapor). In other words, a spore test designed for one sterilization method is not necessarily the appropriate mode to use for other procedures. The organisms used are calibrated concentrations of either *Geobacillus stearothermophilus* or *Bacillus atrophaeus* spores. *G. stearothermophilus* is the appropriate biological for monitoring steam sterilizers and unsaturated chemical vapor sterilizers, while *B. atrophaeus* preparations provide a more rigorous challenge for dry-heat sterilizers. Both types of spores may be present in a single vial so that it can be used to test any of the sterilization modes. This is referred to as a dual-species BI and is common with

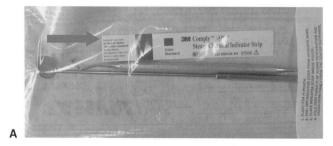

A

FIGURE 11-8 Chemical indicators placed inside packages identify that items inside the package have been exposed to the sterilizing agent.

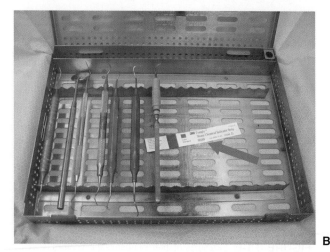

B

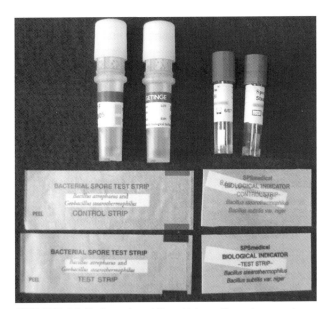

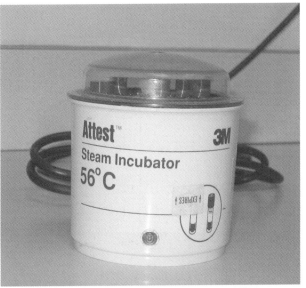

A

FIGURE 11-9 Examples of BIs, which are the main guarantee of sterilization because they contain spores of highly resistant microorganisms.

spore strips. Proof of destruction of these heat-resistant forms after exposure to the sterilization cycle is used to infer that all microorganisms exposed to the same conditions have been destroyed, and represents the most sensitive check of sterilizer efficacy. Items labeled with the statement "equivalent to biological indicators" (or similar wording), enzyme tablets, or integrating indicators that do not contain spores are not acceptable methods of biological monitoring.

In-office biological monitoring is available (Fig. 11-10) or mail-in sterilization monitoring services (e.g., from private companies or dental schools) can be used to test both the BI and the control (Fig. 11-11). Although some DHCP have expressed concern that delays caused by mailing specimens might cause false-negatives, studies have determined that mail delays have no substantial effect on final test results. BIs usually require 1–7 days of incubation to detect viable spores. BIs are available that can provide results in as little as 1–3 hours for gravity or vacuum steam sterilizers when incubated in a special auto-reader incubator. In contrast to enzyme tablets or integrating indicators, the rapid-readout BIs contain spores. The rapid-readout indicator is usually used in hospital settings with operating rooms where instruments are frequently quarantined until the results of the BI are available. Additional information about these special indicators can be obtained from the Association for the Advancement of Medical Instrumentation (AAMI).

The CDC recommends that correct functioning of sterilization cycles should be verified for each sterilizer using a BI and control at least once a week. Other suggestions regarding the frequency of biological monitor-

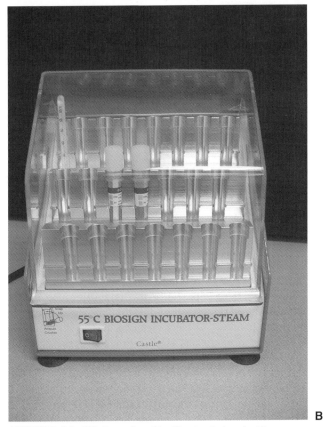

B

FIGURE 11-10 Examples of in-office incubators for BIs.

ing are listed in Table 11-7. Readers should also consult state laws regarding requirements for using BIs. Every load containing **implantable devices** should be monitored with mechanical, chemical, and BIs, and the items quarantined until BI results are known. However, in an

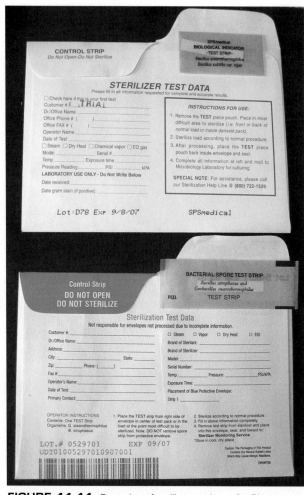

FIGURE 11-11 Examples of mailing envelopes for BI test strips sent to a private company or dental school for incubation.

TABLE 11-7 Spore Testing of Small Office Sterilizers

When	Why
Once per week, PLUS	To verify proper use and functioning.
Whenever a new type of packaging material or tray is used	To ensure that the sterilizing agent is getting inside to the surface of the instruments.
After training of new sterilization personnel	To verify proper use of the sterilizer.
During initial uses of a new sterilizer	To ensure unfamiliar operation instructions are being followed.
First run after repair of a sterilizer	To ensure sterilizer is functioning properly.
With every implantable device and hold device until results of the test are known	Extra precautions for items implanted in tissue.
After any other change in sterilizing procedures.	To ensure change does not interfere with sterilization.

Reprinted with permission from Miller CH, Palenik CJ. Sterilization, disinfection, and asepsis in dentistry. In: Block SS, ed. Disinfection, Sterilization, and Preservation. 5th ed. Philadelphia, PA: Lippincott Williams & Wilkins; 2001:1054.

emergency, placing implantable items in quarantine until spore tests are known to be negative might be impossible. The importance of the routine use of BIs cannot be overemphasized. Instrument processing is a complex process. Correct cleaning, packaging, sterilizer loading procedures, sterilization methods, or high-level disinfection methods are essential to ensure that an instrument is adequately processed and safe for reuse on patients. BIs can ascertain the effectiveness of many of the tasks inherent in instrument processing (Table 11-8).

A variety of factors may diminish the effectiveness of an autoclave, dry-heat, or unsaturated chemical vapor sterilizer. Common problems that apply to all sterilization methods are presented in Table 11-9. Cleaning (discussed in Chapter 16) is the most critical step in instrument processing because it involves the removal of debris and organic contamination from an instrument or device. If blood, saliva, and other contamination are not

removed, these materials can shield underlying microorganisms and potentially compromise the sterilization process. If the packaging material is not compatible with the method of sterilization (e.g., closed container in a steam sterilizer) or excessive material is used, the sterilizing agent may not adequately contact the instrument surface resulting in a sterilization failure. If the material chosen cannot tolerate high temperatures, such as with dry-heat sterilizers, it may melt. Overloading the sterilizer chamber can increase sterilizer warm-up times and may prevent thorough contact of the sterilizing agent with all items in the sterilizer. Racks and trays are usually provided with the sterilization equipment, or can be purchased separately, to help users with proper loading procedures. Insufficient time at the proper temperature can result from human error when the sterilizer

TABLE 11-8 Biological indicator tests (Spore Tests)

- Packaging material
- Packaging procedure
- Sterilizer loading
- Sterilizer use
- Sterilizer functioning

TABLE 11-9 Common Errors That Can Result in Sterilization Failure

- Improper precleaning of instruments

- Improper packaging (e.g., wrong packaging material for the method of sterilization, too many instruments per package, excessive packaging material)

- Overloading the sterilizer (e.g., packages not spaced adequately)

- Inappropriate sterilization time, temperature, and/or pressure (e.g., inadequate or excessive temperature, inadequate time, interrupted sterilization cycle)

- Inadequate maintenance of sterilization equipment (e.g., faulty or worn seals, gaskets, heating coils)

- Use of inappropriate equipment (e.g., household ovens, toaster ovens)

TABLE 11-11 Recommendations in the Event of a Positive Spore Test

1. Remove the sterilizer from service and review sterilization procedures (e.g., work practices and use of mechanical and chemical indicators) to determine whether operator error could be responsible.

2. Retest the sterilizer by using biological, mechanical, and chemical indicators after correcting any identified procedural problems.

3. If the repeat spore test is negative, and mechanical and chemical indicators are within normal limits, put the sterilizer back in service.

The following are recommended if the repeat spore test is positive:

1. Do not use the sterilizer until it has been inspected or repaired, or the exact reason for the positive test has been determined.

2. Recall, to the extent possible, and reprocess all items processed since the last negative spore test.

3. Before placing the sterilizer back in service, rechallenge the sterilizer with BI tests in three consecutive empty chamber sterilization cycles (or in three consecutive fully loaded chamber sterilization cycles if using a tabletop sterilizer) after the cause of the sterilizer failure has been determined and corrected.

door is open during the cycle or timers are set incorrectly. This will ultimately lead to incomplete sterilization. Routine maintenance of sterilization equipment is critical because defective control gauges may not reflect actual conditions inside the sterilizer, door gaskets and seals can become worn, variations in temperature can occur, and other sterilizer malfunctions are possible (Table 11-10).

Although sterilization failures are not common, they do occur (about 1% of the time for steam). Studies show that failures usually occur because of operator error, not because of a true sterilizer mechanical malfunction. If a BI is positive, it means that the spores were not killed. The sterilizer producing the positive spore test must be immediately taken out of service to prevent further use

TABLE 11-10 Examples of Sterilizer Preventive Maintenance

1. Read, reread, and use the instruction manual.

2. If using steam autoclaves, use only the type of water recommended by the manufacturer (e.g., distilled, deionized).

Perform the following according to the manufacturer's written instructions:

3. Drain and flush the reservoir.

4. Check the door gaskets.

5. Check chamber vents and drain screens.

6. Clean the internal chamber and external surfaces.

7. Check recording charts/printers.

until circumstances surrounding the event have been thoroughly investigated. A positive BI is a serious event and the sterilizer must not be used until it has been inspected and/or repaired. The CDC-recommended procedures to follow when the sterilizer fails a spore test are presented in Table 11-11.

If the mechanical (e.g., time, temperature, and pressure) and chemical (i.e., internal or external) indicators demonstrate that the sterilizer is functioning correctly, a single positive spore test probably does not indicate sterilizer malfunction. Items other than implantable devices do not necessarily need to be recalled; however, the spore test should be repeated immediately after correctly loading the sterilizer and using the same cycle that produced the failure. The sterilizer should be removed from service, and all records reviewed of chemical and mechanical monitoring since the last negative BI test. Also, sterilizer operating procedures should be reviewed, including packaging, loading, and spore testing, with all persons who work with the sterilizer to determine whether operator error could be responsible (Table 11-12). Overloading, failure to provide adequate package separation, and incorrect or excessive packaging material are all common reasons for a positive BI in the absence of mechanical failure of the sterilizer unit. A second monitored sterilizer in the office can be used or a loaner from a sales or repair company can be obtained to minimize office disruption while waiting for the repeat BI.

TABLE 11-12 Items to Review after a Positive Spore Test

• Past sterilization records (e.g., mechanical, chemical, and biological monitoring)

• Sterilizer operating procedures, including compliance with recommendations

Ask the following questions:
• Were there any changes in packaging or loading procedures?

• Were the time and temperature controls set correctly?

• Was a new staff member involved with processing instruments?

• Were the proper spore tests used and were the manufacturer's instructions followed (e.g., proper incubation time/temperature, same lot number, used before expiration, stored correctly)?

If the repeat test is negative and chemical and mechanical monitoring indicates adequate processing, the sterilizer can be put back into service. If the repeat BI test is positive, and packaging, loading, and operating procedures have been confirmed as performing correctly, the sterilizer should remain out of service until it has been inspected, repaired, and rechallenged with BI tests in three consecutive empty chamber sterilization cycles. If using a tabletop sterilizer, it is recommended to rechallenge the sterilizer in three consecutive fully loaded chamber sterilization cycles if using a tabletop sterilizer. When possible, items from suspect loads dating back to the last negative BI should be recalled, rewrapped, and resterilized.

Sterilization Records

Maintaining records of mechanical, chemical, and biological monitoring is an important part of a dental infection-control program. Examples of other useful items to

TABLE 11-13 Examples of Items to Maintain in a Sterilization Log

• Date and time of cycle

• Mechanical, chemical, and biological monitoring results, including the results of the control spore test

• Sterilizer identification number (if more than one sterilizer is used in the office)

• The individual conducting the test

• Nature and date of any malfunctions or repairs

Courtesy of the USAF Dental Evaluation and Consultation Service.

maintain in the office sterilization log are listed in Table 11-13. This not only establishes accountability and documents that procedures have been completed, but accurate and complete records can be useful in investigating equipment malfunctions and helping to determine whether a recall is necessary, and the extent of the recall. These records should be retained long enough to comply with state and local regulations.

SUMMARY

Sterilization is the most important component of an infection-control program and is a complex process requiring specialized equipment, adequate space, qualified DHCP, and routine monitoring for quality assurance. Instrument processing (cleaning, packaging, sterilization, and storage) requires multiple steps, with sterilization being just one part of the process. Heat-sterilizing dental instruments between patients is the standard of care. Users have several choices when selecting equipment to use in their practice: steam under pressure (autoclaving), dry heat, and unsaturated chemical vapor. Following the basic rule "Do not disinfect when you can sterilize" provides the highest level of patient protection.

✓ Practical Dental Infection Control Checklist

General Considerations

❏ Are FDA-cleared medical devices used for sterilization and are the manufacturer's instructions followed for correct use and maintenance?

❏ Are reusable critical and semicritical dental instruments cleaned and heat-sterilized before each use?

❏ Are packages allowed to dry in the sterilizer before they are handled to avoid contamination?

❏ If available, are heat-stable semicritical alternatives used?

❏ Have heat-sensitive semicritical instruments been replaced with heat-tolerant or disposable versions?

  ❏ If heat-stable alternatives are not available, are heat-ensitive critical and semicritical instruments reprocessed by using FDA-cleared sterilant/high-level disinfectants or an FDA-cleared low-temperature sterilization method (e.g., ethylene oxide)?

    ❏ Are the manufacturer's instructions followed for use of chemical sterilants/high-level disinfectants?

  ❏ If single-use disposable instruments are used, are they used only once and disposed of correctly?

❏ Are noncritical patient-care items barrier-protected or cleaned, or, if visibly soiled, cleaned and disinfected after each use with an EPA-registered hospital disinfectant?

❑ If an item is visibly contaminated with blood, is an EPA-registered hospital disinfectant with a tuberculocidal claim (i.e., intermediate level) used?

❑ Are DHCP aware of all OSHA guidelines for exposure to chemical agents used for disinfection and sterilization?

Sterilization of Unwrapped Instruments

❑ Although not recommended as a routine practice, if instruments are sterilized unwrapped is there a written policy for how these instruments will be labeled and stored?

❑ Are instruments cleaned and dried before the unwrapped sterilization cycle?

❑ Are mechanical and chemical indicators used for each unwrapped sterilization cycle (i.e., is an internal chemical indicator placed among the instruments or items to be sterilized)?

❑ Are unwrapped instruments allowed to dry and cool in the sterilizer before they are handled, to avoid contamination and thermal injury?

❑ Are semicritical instruments that are sterilized unwrapped and will be used immediately or within a short time handled aseptically during removal from the sterilizer and transport to the point of use?

❑ Are critical instruments that are sterilized unwrapped intended for immediate reuse removed from the sterilizer and transported to the point of use in a manner that maintains sterility (e.g., transported in a sterile covered container)?

❑ When storing critical items, are they always wrapped before sterilization?

Implantable Devices

❑ Are implantable devices always wrapped before sterilization?

❑ Is a BI used for every sterilizer load that contains an implantable device?

❑ When sterilizing an implantable device are results verified before using the implantable device, whenever possible?

Dental Handpieces and Other Devices Attached to Air and Waterlines

❑ Are handpieces and other intraoral instruments that can be removed from the air and waterlines of dental units cleaned and heat-sterilized between patients?

❑ Are the manufacturer's instructions followed for cleaning, lubrication, and sterilization of handpieces and other intraoral instruments that can be removed from the air and waterlines of dental units?

❑ Are patients advised not to close their lips tightly around the tip of the saliva ejector to evacuate oral fluids?

Sterilization Monitoring

❑ Are mechanical, chemical, and biological monitors used according to the manufacturer's instructions to ensure the effectiveness of the sterilization process?

❑ Is each load monitored with mechanical (e.g., time, temperature, and pressure) and chemical indicators?

❑ Are the chemical indicators designed for the sterilization process being used (i.e., steam, dry heat, or chemical vapor)?

❑ Is a chemical indicator placed on the inside of each package?

❑ Is an external indicator also used if the internal indicator cannot be seen from outside the package?

❑ Are items/packages placed correctly and loosely into the sterilizer so as not to impede penetration of the sterilant?

❑ Are instrument packages only used if mechanical or chemical indicators indicate adequate processing?

❑ Are sterilizers monitored at least weekly by using a BI (i.e., spore test) with a matching control (i.e., the BI and control are from same lot number)?

❑ Is the spore test designed for the type of sterilizer being used (i.e., steam, dry heat, or chemical vapor)?

❑ In addition to at least weekly spore testing, is the sterilizer tested

❑ whenever a new type of packaging material or tray is used?

❑ after new sterilization personnel are trained?

❑ during initial uses of a new sterilizer?

❑ during the first run after repair of a sterilizer?

❑ with every implantable device, and are devices withheld from use until results of the test are known?

❑ after any other change in sterilizing procedures?

❑ If a prevacuum steam autoclave is used, is air removal testing performed daily or according to the manufacturer's instructions?

❑ Does the dental office/clinic have a written protocol to manage a sterilizer failure (i.e., positive spore test)?

❑ After a positive spore test:

❑ Is the sterilizer removed from service and are sterilization procedures reviewed (e.g., work practices and use of mechanical and chemical indicators) to determine whether operator error could be responsible?

❑ Is the sterilizer retested by using biological, mechanical, and chemical indicators after correcting any identified procedural problems?

❑ If the repeat spore test is negative, and mechanical and chemical indicators are within normal limits, is the sterilizer returned to service?

❑ If the repeat spore test is positive:

❑ Is the sterilizer removed from service until it has been inspected or repaired, or the exact reason for the positive test has been determined?

❑ To the extent possible, have all items that have been processed since the last negative spore test been recalled and reprocessed?

❑ Before placing the sterilizer back in service, is the sterilizer rechallenged with BI tests in three consecutive empty chamber sterilization cycles (or three fully loaded chamber sterilization cycles if using a tabletop sterilizer) after the cause of the sterilizer failure has been determined and corrected?

❑ Are sterilization records (i.e., mechanical, chemical, and biological) maintained in compliance with state and local regulations?

Review Questions

1. The three most common methods used to sterilize dental instruments are:

A. steam, dry heat, and flash sterilization

B. steam, unsaturated chemical vapor, and liquid chemical germicides

C. steam, dry heat, and unsaturated chemical vapor

D. dry heat, unsaturated chemical vapor, and liquid chemical germicides

2. According to the CDC, heat-tolerant critical and semi-critical patient-care items should be sterilized by:

A. liquid chemical germicides

B. heat

C. heat, only if contaminated with blood

D. intermediate-level disinfectants

3. Which statement is true regarding sterilization?

A. Sterilization is less lethal than disinfection.

B. Sterilization is not as safe as disinfection.

C. Sterilization using liquid chemical germicides is the most commonly used method for dental instruments.

D. Sterilization is a procedure that uses a physical or chemical procedure to destroy all microorganisms, including substantial numbers of resistant bacterial spores, which are the most difficult microorganisms to kill.

4. Following the sterilization cycle with _____ wet packages is a common occurrence.

A. dry heat

B. unsaturated chemical vapor

C. steam

5. These types of sterilizers minimize corrosion and rust on carbon-steel instruments:

A. steam and dry heat

B. dry heat and unsaturated chemical vapor

C. steam and unsaturated chemical vapor

6. Which of the following is false regarding wet instrument packages?

A. It is critical to allow packages to dry and cool inside the sterilizer chamber to maintain sterility.

B. Packages should not be touched until they are cool and dry because hot packs act as wicks, absorbing moisture and hence bacteria from hands.

C. If packages are not completely dry following the sterilization cycle, they should be removed and placed near a fan to complete the drying process.

D. Paper packaging materials may become torn if wet packages are handled.

7. Sterilization procedures are routinely monitored using a combination of

A. mechanical, standard, and biological indicators.

B. mechanical, chemical, and biological indicators.

C. chemical and biological indicators.

D. mechanical, autoclave, and standard indicators.

8. A _____ indicator is placed inside every package to verify that the sterilant reached the instruments inside the package.

A. mechanical

B. chemical

C. biological

D. chemical and biological

9. If either mechanical indicators or internal or external chemical indicators indicate inadequate processing, items in the load should not be used until reprocessed.

A. True

B. False

10. The CDC recommends using BIs (i.e., spore tests) at least _____.

A. daily

B. weekly

C. monthly

D. yearly

Critical Thinking

1. What are three main types of sterilizers used in dentistry? What are some advantages and disadvantages of each type? What type of sterilizer do you have in your dental office/clinic? Is the manufacturer's instruction manual kept by the sterilizer?

2. You have a new employee in the dental office/clinic and she wants to use a glutaraldehyde solution to soak instruments instead of heat-sterilizing them. She claims that it is quicker, less expensive, and works just as well. How would explain to her that heat sterilization is the standard of care for dental instruments and you don't use liquid chemical sterilants (e.g., glutaraldehydes) in your dental office/clinic?

3. You're training a new employee to work in your instrument processing area. How do you explain the importance and rationale for performing mechanical, chemical, and biological monitoring?

4. You're setting up for your next patient and after opening the package you notice that the internal chemical indicator has not changed color. What should you do? What could be the cause? Would you use the instruments for your patient? Why or why not?

5. Place your sterilization monitoring log book in front of you. How often do you perform biological monitoring (i.e., spore testing)? Do you always use a control BI? Do you also record the results of the mechanical and chemical monitoring? Is the log book complete or is some information missing?

6. You receive an e-mail from your spore-testing service telling you that the BI (i.e., spore test) is positive. Do you have a written protocol in your office addressing what steps to take in the event of a positive spore test? What is the first thing you should do and why? What are some items you would review after a positive spore test?

7. What are some common errors that lead to a sterilization failure?

SELECTED READINGS

AAMI, American National Standards Institute. Chemical sterilants and high level disinfectants: a guide to selection and use. AAMI TIR7:1999. Arlington, VA: AAMI; 2000.

AAMI, American National Standards Institute. Comprehensive guide to steam sterilization and sterility assurance in health care facilities. ANSI/AAMI ST79:2006. Arlington, VA: Association for the Advancement of Medical Instrumentation, 2006.

AAMI, American National Standards Institute. Dry heat (heated air) sterilizers. ANSI/AAMI ST50:2002. Arlington, VA: AAMI; 2004.

AAMI, American National Standards Institute. Safe use and handling of glutaraldehyde-based products in health-care facilities. ANSI/AAMI ST58-1996. Arlington, VA: AAMI; 1996.

AAMI, American National Standards Institute. Steam sterilization and sterility assurance using table-top sterilizers in office-based, ambulatory-care medical, surgical, and dental facilities. ANSI/AAMI ST40-1998. Arlington, VA: AAMI; 1998.

AAMI, American National Standards Institute. Table-top dry heat (heated air) sterilization and sterility assurance in healthcare facilities. ANSI/AAMI ST40:2004. Arlington, VA: AAMI 2005.

American Dental Association. ADA statement on infection control in dentistry. Available at: http://www.ada.org/prof/resources/positions/statements/infectioncontrol.asp. Accessed July 2008.

Andersen HK, Fiehn NE, Larsen T. Effect of steam sterilization inside the turbine chambers of dental turbines. Oral Surg Oral Med Oral Pathol Oral Radiol Endod 1999;87:184–188.

Andres MT, Tejerina JM, Fierro JF. Reliability of biologic indicators in a mail-return sterilization-monitoring service: a review of 3 years. Quintessence Int 1995;26:865–870.

CDC. Guidelines for environmental infection control in health-care facilities: recommendations of CDC and the Healthcare Infection Control Practices Advisory Committee (HICPAC). MMWR 2003;52(RR-10).

CDC. Guidelines for infection control in dental health-care settings–2003. MMWR 2003;52(RR-17):1–66.

CDC. National Institute for Occupational Safety and Health. Glutaraldehyde: occupational hazards in hospitals. Cincinnati, OH: U.S. Department of Health and Human Services, Public Health Service, CDC, National Institute for Occupational Safety and Health, 2001. DHHS publication (NIOSH) 2001–2115.

Checchi L, Montebugnoli L, Samaritani S. Contamination of the turbine air chamber: a risk of cross-infection. J Clin Periodontol 1998;25:607–611.

Chin JR, Miller CH, Palenik CJ. Internal contamination of air-driven low-speed handpieces and attached prophy angles. J Am Dent Assoc 2006;137:1275–1280.

Crawford JJ. Clinical asepsis in dentistry. Mesquite TX: Oral Medicine Press; 1987.

Crawford JJ, Broderius C. Control of cross-infection risks in the dental operatory: prevention of water retraction by bur cooling spray systems. J Am Dent Assoc 1988;116:685–687.

Epstein JB, Rea G, Sibau L, et al. Assessing viral retention and elimination in rotary dental instruments. J Am Dent Assoc 1995;126:87–92.

Food and Drug Administration. Dental handpiece sterilization [Letter]. Rockville, MD: U.S. Department of Health and Human Services, Food and Drug Administration; 1992.

Gooch B, Marianos D, Ciesielski C, et al. Lack of evidence for patient-to-patient transmission of HIV in a dental practice. J Am Dent Assoc 1993;124:38–44.

Hamann CP, DePaola LG, Rodgers PA. Occupation-related allergies in dentistry. J Am Dent Assoc 2005;136:500–510.

Hamann CP, Rodgers PA, Sullivan K. Allergic contact dermatitis in dental professionals: effective diagnosis and treatment. J Am Dent Assoc 2003;134:185–194.

Hamann CP, Rodgers PA, Sullivan KM. Occupational allergens in dentistry. Curr Opin Allergy Clin Immunol 2004;4:403–409.

Harte JA. Advances in steam sterilizers: an assessment of new pre- and postvacuum technology for dental offices. Dent Pract Rep 2005;(Suppl 1):1–7.

Harte JA, Miller CH. Sterilization update 2003. Compend Contin Educ Dent 2004;25(1 Suppl):24–29.

Hastreiter RJ, Molinari JA, Falken MC, et al. Effectiveness of dental office instrument sterilization procedures. J Am Dent Assoc 1991;122:51–56.

Herd S, Chin J, Palenik CJ, et al. The in vivo contamination of air-driven low-speed handpieces with prophylaxis angles. J Am Dent Assoc 2007;138:1360–1365.

Joslyn LJ. Sterilization by heat. In: Block SS, ed. Disinfection, Sterilization, and Preservation. 5th ed. Philadelphia, PA: Lippincott Williams & Wilkins; 2001:695–728.

Kolstad RA. How well does the chemiclave sterilize handpieces? J Am Dent Assoc 1998;129:985–991.

Kuehne JS, Cohen ME, Monroe SB. Performance and durability of autoclavable high-speed dental handpieces. NDRI-PR 92-03. Bethesda, MD: Naval Dental Research Institute; 1992.

Leonard DL, Charlton DG. Performance of high-speed dental handpieces subjected to simulated clinical use and sterilization. J Am Dent Assoc 1999;130: 1301–1311.

Lewis DL, Arens M, Appleton SS, et al. Cross-contamination potential with dental equipment. Lancet 1992;340:1252–1254.

Lewis DL, Boe RK. Cross-infection risks associated with current procedures for using high-speed dental handpieces. J Clin Microbiol 1992;30:401–406.

Parker IV HH, Johnson RB. Effectiveness of ethylene oxide for sterilization of dental handpieces. J Dent 1995;23:113–115.

Pratt LH, Smith DG, Thornton RH, et al. The effectiveness of two sterilization methods when different precleaning techniques are employed. J Dent 1999;27:247–248.

Miller CH, Palenik CJ. Instrument processing. In: Miller CH, Palenik DJ, eds. Infection control and management of hazardous materials for the dental team. 3rd ed. St. Louis: Mosby; 2005:191–241.

Miller CH, Palenik CJ. Sterilization, disinfection, and asepsis in dentistry. In: Block SS, ed. Disinfection, sterilization, and preservation. 5th ed. Philadelphia, PA: Lippincott Williams & Wilkins; 2001:1049–1068.

Miller CH, Sheldrake MA. The ability of biological indicators to detect sterilization failures. Am J Dent 1994;7:95–97.

Mills SE, Kuehne JC, Bradley Jr DV. Bacteriological analysis of high-speed handpiece turbines. J Am Dent Assoc 1993;124:59–62.

Molinari JA, Harte JA. Dental services. In: APIC Text of Infection Control and Epidemiology. 2nd ed. Washington, DC: APIC 2005;51-1–51-23.

Molinari JA, Gleason MJ, Merchant VA. Sixteen years of experience with sterilization monitoring. Compend Contin Educ Dent 1994;15:1422–1432.

Occupational Safety and Health Administration. Formaldehyde standard. Washington, DC: OSHA 29 CFR Part 1910.1048.

Ravis SM, Shaffer MP, Shaffer CL, et al. Glutaraldehyde-induced and formaldehyde-induced allergic contact dermatitis among dental hygienists and assistants. J Am Dent Assoc 2003;134:1072–1078.

Spaulding EH. Chemical disinfection of medical and surgical materials. In: Lawrence CA, Block SS, eds. Disinfection, Sterilization, and Preservation. Philadelphia, PA: Lea & Febiger; 1968:517–531.

U.S. Department of Health and Human Services, Food and Drug Administration. 21 CFR Part 872.6730. Dental devices; endodontic dry heat sterilizer; final rule. Fed Regist 1997;62:2903.

U.S. Department of Health and Human Services. Infection control file: practical infection control in the dental office. Atlanta, GA/Rockville, MD: CDC/FDA; 1993.

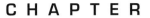

CHAPTER

12

Environmental Surface Infection Control: Disposable Barriers and Chemical Disinfection

John A. Molinari

Jennifer A. Harte

LEARNING OBJECTIVES

After completion of this chapter individuals should be able to:

1 Describe intermediate-, low-, and high-level disinfectants and indications when each should be used.

2 Discuss the potential for contaminated environmental surfaces to transmit infectious pathogens.

3 List categories of contaminated environmental surfaces.

4 Describe the Spaulding classification for chemical sterilants and disinfectants.

5 Explain the necessity for cleaning before subsequent disinfection of environmental surfaces.

6 Consider the use of disposable covers to assist in achieving infection-control goals.

7 Describe ideal properties for chemical disinfectants and government requirements for regulated, available products.

8 Discuss and compare the properties of the various classes of environmental surface cleaners and disinfectants.

KEY TERMS

Chemical sterilant: chemicals used for the purpose of destroying all forms of microbial life including bacterial spores.

Cleaning: the removal of visible soil and organic debris, either manually or mechanically, which results in a reduction in the number of microorganisms and the removal of organic matter, such as blood, tissue, and other biological material that may interfere with sterilization and disinfection. Cleaning is the first step in any sterilization or disinfection process.

Clinical contact surface: a surface contaminated from patient materials either by direct spray or spatter generated during dental procedures or by contact with dental healthcare personnel's gloved hands. These surfaces can subsequently contaminate other instruments, devices, hands, or gloves. Examples of such surfaces include light handles, switches, dental radiograph equipment, dental chairside computers, reusable containers of dental materials, drawer handles, faucet handles, countertops, pens, telephones, and doorknobs.

Decontamination: a process or treatment that renders a medical device, instrument, or environmental surface safe to handle. According to the Occupational Safety and Health Administration (OSHA), "the use of physical or chemical means to remove, inactivate, or destroy bloodborne pathogens on a surface or item to the point where they are no longer capable of transmitting infectious particles and the surface or item is rendered safe for handling, use, or disposal" [29 CFR 1910.1030].

Detergents: compounds that possess a cleaning action and have hydrophilic and lipophilic parts. Although products used for hand washing or antiseptic hand wash in a healthcare setting represent various types of detergents, the term "soap" is used to refer to such detergents in this book. Detergents make no antimicrobial claims on the label.

Disinfectant: a chemical agent used on inanimate (i.e., nonliving) objects (e.g., floors, walls, and sinks) to destroy virtually all recognized pathogenic microorganisms, but not necessarily all microbial forms (e.g., bacterial endospores). The Environmental Protection Agency (EPA) groups disinfectants on whether the product label claims to be a "limited," "general," or "hospital" disinfectant.

Disinfection: the destruction of pathogenic and other kinds of microorganisms by physical or chemical means. Disinfection is less lethal than sterilization because it destroys most recognized pathogenic microorganisms, but not necessarily all microbial forms, such as bacterial spores. Disinfection does not ensure the margin of safety associated with sterilization processes.

Environmental Protection Agency (EPA): the mission of the EPA is to protect human health and the environment; the EPA works to develop and enforce regulations that implement environmental laws enacted by Congress.

Food and Drug Administration (FDA): the FDA promotes and protects the public health by helping safe and effective products reach the market in a timely way; monitors products for continued safety after they are in use; and helps the public get the accurate, science-based information needed to improve health.

High-level disinfectant: a liquid chemical germicide registered by the FDA used in the disinfection process for critical and semicritical patient-care devices that inactivates vegetative bacteria, mycobacteria, fungi, and viruses but not necessarily high numbers of bacterial spores. The FDA further defines a high-level disinfectant as a sterilant used under the same contact conditions except for a longer contact time.

Hospital disinfectant: a germicide that is registered by the EPA for use on inanimate objects in hospitals, clinics, dental offices, or any other medical-related facility. Efficacy is demonstrated against *Salmonella enterica* (formerly *Salmonella choleraesuis*), *Staphylococcus aureus*, and *Pseudomonas aeruginosa*.

Housekeeping surface: environmental surfaces (e.g., floors, walls, ceilings, and tabletops) that are not involved in direct delivery of patient care in healthcare facilities.

Intermediate-level disinfectant: a liquid chemical germicide registered by the EPA as a hospital disinfectant and with a label claim of potency as a tuberculocidal. Intermediate-level disinfection is a process that inactivates most vegetative bacteria, most fungi, and some viruses, but cannot be relied on to inactivate resistant microorganisms, such as mycobacteria or bacterial spores.

Low-level disinfectant: a liquid chemical germicide registered by the EPA as a hospital disinfectant. OSHA requires low-level disinfectants also to have a label claim for potency against human immunodeficiency virus (HIV) and hepatitis B virus (HBV) if used for disinfecting clinical contact surfaces. Low-level disinfection is a process that will inactivate most vegetative bacteria, some fungi, and some viruses but cannot be relied on to inactivate resistant microorganisms (e.g., mycobacteria or bacterial spores).

Spaulding classification: a strategy for sterilization or disinfection of inanimate objects and surfaces based on the degree of risk involved in their use. The three categories are: critical, semicritical, and noncritical. The system also established three levels of germicidal activity for disinfection (high, intermediate, and low).

Surface barrier: material that prevents the penetration of microorganisms, particulates, and fluids. Barrier choices range from inexpensive plastic food wrap to commercially available custom-made covers.

Published guidelines for infection control include the use of **chemical sterilants** and **disinfectants** when it is not possible to heat sterilize or dispose of items that become contaminated during treatment. In addition, numerous environmental surfaces routinely become contaminated with saliva, blood, and exudate (i.e., bioburden) during provision of care and require surface **cleaning** and disinfection or placement of disposable covers between patients. These inanimate items include dental equipment, light handles, counter surfaces, doorknobs, reusable medical containers, and dental unit hose lines. Cleaning and **decontamination** processes before subsequent patient treatment remain important, yet often misunderstood, components of an effective infection-control program. Although the introduction of multiple classes of disinfectant products and types of disposable barriers have assisted practitioners in implementing recommended protocols that address surface contamination, some clinicians still remain confused regarding potential hazards and recommendations for prevention of cross-infection.

A variety of commercial products are available as disposable covers and disinfectants. It is important to recognize at the outset that the effectiveness of any surface disinfectant depends on several factors, including the following: (a) the concentration and nature of contaminant microorganisms, (b) the concentration of chemical, (c) the exposure time, and (d) the amount of accumulated bioburden. **Disinfection** is defined as the destruction of pathogenic microorganisms on inanimate surfaces. When used as disinfectants, chemicals are not effective against highly resistant forms such as bacterial and mycotic spores. The use of these chemicals thus represents a compromise from the guideline: *Do not disinfect when you can sterilize.* Available product formulations include environmental surface solutions, sprays, foams, and wipes, each having a specific rationale for use.

CLASSIFICATION OF CONTAMINATED PATIENT-CARE ITEMS AND ENVIRONMENTAL SURFACES

Chemical germicides manufactured for environmental surface disinfection are regulated and registered by the **Environmental Protection Agency (EPA)**, in contrast to products marketed as antiseptics, which are formulated for use on living tissues and regulated by the **Food and Drug Administration (FDA)**. It is important to realize that these two agencies use different procedures and criteria for product approval. Thus one should not attempt to interchange the use of disinfectants and antiseptics. Unfortunately, misuse of products remains, leading to tissue toxicity reactions and equipment failures.

Choosing appropriate surface disinfectants also has become confusing because of exaggerated manufacturer claims and misleading assays reported in the literature. Therefore, the actual performance capabilities of individual agents may be obscured. Confusion also arises when dentists and other treatment providers are not aware of guidelines that assist in the selection of appropriate chemicals. In the area of surface disinfection, this can be alleviated initially by comparing the efficacy of available agents with published criteria for an *ideal* surface disinfectant (Table 12-1). As shown here, properties to be considered include penetration and activity in the presence of bioburden, a broad antimicrobial spectrum, residual activity that becomes reactivated when surfaces are moistened, minimal toxicity, and compatibility with disinfected surfaces. The most desirable disinfectant also would be tuberculocidal and virucidal. None of the available products fulfill all of these criteria. This statement will be explored further when properties of available classes of chemicals are compared with the features of an ideal agent in later sections.

A standard system of classification for chemical sterilants and disinfectants was proposed by Spaulding in 1972. The **Spaulding classification** was developed

---

TABLE 12-1 Properties of an Ideal Disinfectant*

Broad spectrum
   Should always have the widest possible antimicrobial spectrum

Fast-acting
   Should always have a rapidly lethal action on all vegetative forms of bacteria, fungi, and viruses

Not affected by physical factors
   Active in the presence of organic matter, such as blood, sputum, and feces

Nontoxic

Nonallergenic

Surface compatibility
   Should not compromise integrity of dental equipment and metallic surfaces
   Should not cause the disintegration of cloth, rubber, plastics, or other materials

Residual effect on treated surfaces

Easy to use

Odorless
   An inoffensive odor would facilitate its routine use

Economical
   Cost should not be prohibitively high

*A product with all of these features does not exist.
Adapted from Molinari JA, Campbell MD, York J. Minimizing potential infections in dental practice. J Mich Dent Assoc 1982;64:411–416.

TABLE 12-2 Summary of Methods for Decontamination in the Dental Office

Item Category	Item Definition	Is Item Used in the Mouth?	Potential Risk of Disease Transmission*	Method of Decontamination
Critical	Penetrate soft tissue, contact bone, enter into or contact the bloodstream, or other normally sterile tissue	Yes	Very high to high	Sterilization
Semicritical	Contact mucous membranes or nonintact skin, but will not penetrate soft tissue, contact bone, enter into or contact the bloodstream, or other normally sterile tissue	Yes	Moderate	Sterilization or high-level disinfection†
Noncritical items‡	Contact with intact skin	No	Low to none	Intermediate- to low-level disinfection or simple cleaning§

*Depends on the nature and amount of contamination and how the item or surface is used.
†Depends on whether the instruments are damaged by heat. The majority of semicritical items in dentistry are heat tolerant and therefore should be sterilized with heat.
‡Includes environmental surfaces, which carry an even lower risk of disease transmission than medical instruments.
§Depends on whether the items are contaminated visibly by blood. If an item is visibly contaminated with blood, use an intermediate-level disinfectant.

originally for classifying hospital instruments according to their use and degree of contamination, but also can be adapted to include dental instruments and equipment. A modification of Spaulding's original scheme was published in 1991. The major emphasis of this expanded classification designation is aimed at differentiating the infection risks from contaminated medical instruments compared with those from other medically related devices or environmental surfaces. Patient-care items and equipment are placed into one of three categories: critical, semicritical, and noncritical (Table 12-2). In addition, classes for chemical germicide use are related to their sterilization or disinfection capabilities (Table 12-3). These include the efficacy against vegetative bacteria, tubercle bacilli, fungal spores, lipid- and nonlipid-containing viruses, and bacterial endospores (Fig. 12-1).

High-level disinfectants are analogous to EPA-registered sporicides because they are capable of inactivating resistant bacterial spores and all other microbial forms. The ability to kill bacterial spores is an essential criterion for inclusion of a chemical into the sterilant and high-level disinfectant categories. Examples of these chemical sterilants include ethylene oxide gas, immersion glutaraldehyde solutions, peracetic acid, and certain hydrogen peroxide preparations. These have been useful for sterilizing materials that cannot withstand heat sterilization procedures. However, a prolonged immersion time of up 12 hours is required to achieve sterilization with glutaraldehydes and a 16- to 24-hour requirement for ethylene oxide gas sterilization. The interval can be even longer under conditions of heavy contamination. Although high-level disinfectants are capable of sterilizing immersed items, these chemicals often are misused.

Instead of immersing items in an activated glutaraldehyde solution for the required interval, personnel may use only a 20- to 30-minute exposure and rinse the "sterilized" materials in nonsterile, sanitized water. These items are, at best, disinfected (sometimes the phrase "relatively sterile" is even used). Use of these "cold sterilization" procedures represents one of the most abused aspects of infection control. Because the solutions routinely used under the above conditions cannot guarantee destruction of all microbial forms present and cannot be

TABLE 12-3 Class of Chemicals to Use for Each Disinfection Process*

For This Process	Use This Class of Chemical
Sterilization	Sterilant/disinfectant (with prolonged contact time)
High-level disinfection	Sterilant/disinfectant (with a short contact time)
Intermediate-level disinfection	Hospital disinfectant with a tuberculocidal claim
Low-level disinfection	Hospital disinfectant without a tuberculocidal claim

*The names of these classes of chemicals are controlled by law. The manufacturer of a disinfectant cannot use these terms without federal approval. These terms will appear on the label of the chemical. The U.S. EPA and FDA regulate chemical germicides used in healthcare settings. The FDA regulates chemical sterilants used on critical and semicritical medical devices, and the EPA regulates gaseous sterilants and liquid chemical disinfectants used on noncritical surfaces.

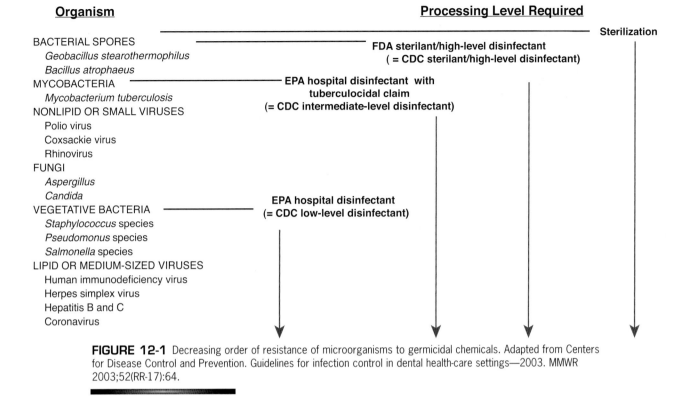

FIGURE 12-1 Decreasing order of resistance of microorganisms to germicidal chemicals. Adapted from Centers for Disease Control and Prevention. Guidelines for infection control in dental health-care settings—2003. MMWR 2003;52(RR-17):64.

biologically monitored using calibrated bacterial spore-containing vehicles, cold sterilization is actually a misnomer. This procedure should not be confused with accepted methods of sterilization. In addition, as mentioned in Chapter 11, this type of infection-control practice has little, if any, use in dentistry.

Intermediate-level disinfectants may not inactivate bacterial endospores but do kill other microbial forms, especially tubercle bacilli. *Mycobacterium tuberculosis* presents a severe challenge to chemical disinfectants because of its outer cellular wax and lipid layers. Therefore, it is considered to be among the more resistant microorganisms after bacterial endospores. Chlorine compounds, iodophors, alcohols, and many phenolic disinfectants are included in this class. It should be remembered that there can be differences between intermediate-level disinfectants with regard to their ability to inactivate small, nonlipid (hydrophilic) viruses, which are much more resistant than medium-sized, lipid-coated (lipophilic) viruses (Table 12-4). Thus, the ability to destroy *M. tuberculosis* does not necessarily signify that a chemical solution is able to inactivate all viruses. When an intermediate-level disinfectant is selected for use in dentistry, it should be EPA registered as a tuberculocidal hospital disinfectant, with appropriate virucidal activity. The designation "**hospital disinfectant**" is given by the EPA to products that are documented to kill three species of basic test bacteria: *S. aureus, S. enterica* (for-

merly *S. choleraesuis*), and *P. aeruginosa.* Separate test data, obtained with EPA-recognized assays, must be submitted by the manufacturers and approved by the EPA to allow inclusion of a "tuberculocidal" claim on product labels and literature.

Chemical agents with the narrowest antimicrobial range are classified as **low-level disinfectants**. Examples of common disinfectants in this group include simple quaternary ammonium compounds, simple phenolics, and detergents. They are suitable for cleaning environmental surfaces and disinfecting those surfaces that are not contaminated with potentially infectious material but are unacceptable otherwise. Although low-level disinfectants may inactivate certain viruses and vegetative bacteria, they can have irregular cidal activity against

TABLE 12-4 Major Virus Categories

Hydrophilic Viruses	Lipophilic Viruses
Rotavirus WA	Herpes simplex-1
Rotavirus SA 11	Herpes simplex-2
Poliovirus type 2	Influenza
HBV	HIV

resistant Gram-negative bacteria, such as *Pseudomonas sp.*, and will not kill tubercle bacilli or nonlipid viruses.

ENVIRONMENTAL SURFACES AS SOURCES OF CROSS-INFECTION

Treatment areas typically become contaminated with blood, saliva, and other body fluids during patient care, yet at the present time there are no data to confirm cross-infection to dental professionals or their patients. It must be remembered that certain bacteria, viruses, and fungi are able to survive on environmental surfaces for extended periods. These, like other microbes that are able to persist outside a host, may possibly remain infectious for prolonged intervals and may require more extensive disinfection procedures.

An unfortunate reminder of the ability of certain pathogens to remain viable outside of a host was recently published in May of 2007. It involved patient-to-patient transmission of HBV in an oral surgery practice. The Centers for Disease Control and Prevention (CDC) was unable to determine the mechanism of viral cross-infection and could only speculate in the absence of definitive evidence. HBV is a very hardy hydrophilic virus and can persist in dried blood for 7 days on inanimate surfaces. Infectious virions can remain on surfaces even in the absence of visible blood. One possibility for HBV transmission proposed by the CDC was that cross-infection in this instance occurred from environmental surfaces contaminated with blood from the source patient.

In a similar manner as with other infection-control issues, much of the evidence addressing cross-infection from environmental surfaces has come from medical outbreaks and look-back investigations. Included are numerous instances of hospital-acquired infections involving bacterial pathogens. A major emerging environmental problem is associated with methicillin-resistant *S. aureus*. *S. aureus* is among the most adaptable microorganisms and is able to remain viable in dried blood and exudate on environmental surfaces for weeks. Cross-infection usually occurs person to person via colonized or contaminated hands, but most staphylococcal strains have been shown to survive for weeks to months on contaminated inanimate surfaces. The presence of many of the virulent strains has also been confirmed during disease outbreaks in hospitals and other clinical settings. Another Gram-positive coccus, *Enterobacter faecium,* is also a common, serious microbial contaminant of medical equipment and environmental surfaces. These bacteria are relatively hardy in the environment and can be detected for up to 7 days on electronic thermometers, countertops, bedrails, and linens.

With regard to the potential for viruses to survive on inanimate surfaces, several microbes tend to remain recoverable because of their minimal metabolic activity and relatively resistant structural components. In addition to HBV discussed above, readily transmissible viruses such as influenza and rhinoviruses can also survive for hours or even days after cross-contamination from nasal secretions onto items such as handkerchiefs, pens, doorknobs, and countertops. For additional documentation of survival studies for human pathogenic viruses, the reader is referred to an excellent review by Assar and Block.

CLASSIFICATION OF ENVIRONMENTAL SURFACES AND DISINFECTION STRATEGIES

Environmental surfaces are classified as noncritical items in the Spaulding classification and can be divided into **clinical contact** and **housekeeping surfaces** (Table 12-5). These designations represent the most recent modification of the Spaulding classification system. Environmental surfaces in the dental operatory are surfaces or equipment that do not directly contact the patient. As mentioned in the above section, these surfaces frequently become contaminated during patient care and can serve as reservoirs for microbial cross-contamination. Implicit in the definition of housekeeping environmental surfaces is the suggestion of a very small potential for cross-infection during treatment. The lack of evidence suggesting a risk to dental care providers or their patients represents the basis for recommendations in this area. Thus the 2003

TABLE 12-5 Categories of Environmental Surfaces

Type of Surface	Definition	Examples
Clinical Contact	Surfaces that are frequently touched or that become contaminated and subsequently contact instruments, devices, hands, or gloves	Light handles, switches, dental x-ray equipment, chairside computers, drawer handles, faucet handles, countertops, pen, telephone handle, doorknob
Housekeeping	Surfaces that do not come into contact with patients or devices used in dental procedures	Floors, walls, sinks

Courtesy of the USAF Dental Evaluation and Consultation service.

CDC infection-control guidelines for dentistry recommend that most housekeeping environmental surfaces need to be cleaned with only soap and water or an EPA-registered detergent/low-level disinfectant. The nature and type of surface and extent of contamination are determining factors for the level of chemical exposure. Preparation of clinical contact surfaces between patients also provides reasonable choices. One is the use of impermeable disposable barriers for those surfaces that cannot withstand exposure to chemical disinfectants. For those surfaces that are not visibly contaminated with blood, saliva, or other body fluids and can tolerate chemical disinfection, an alternative recommendation is to clean and subsequently disinfect them using either an EPA-registered low-level disinfectant with an HBV and HIV inactivation claim or an intermediate-level (i.e., tuberculocidal) hospital disinfectant. If visibly contaminated with blood, these environmental surfaces must then be disinfected with an EPA-registered intermediate-level disinfectant. This designation indicates that a disinfectant is capable of killing *M. tuberculosis, S. aureus, P. aeruginosa, S. enterica* (formerly *S. choleraesuis*), *S. choleraesuis, Escherichia coli,* representative fungi, hydrophilic viruses, and lipophilic viruses.

SURFACE BARRIER COVERS

There are two effective approaches to reduce the potential for cross-contamination and cross-infection from dental environmental surfaces. These involve either the use of **surface barrier** covers to prevent the surface or item from becoming contaminated or cleaning and disinfecting the surface after contamination occurs. Usually a combination of both approaches is used in dental settings to effectively manage environmental surfaces.

Surface barriers include a variety of single-use disposable covers, including clear plastic wrap, bags, sheets, tubing, plastic-backed paper and other materials that are impervious to moisture. Using barriers to protect surfaces and equipment is useful, especially if the surfaces are (a) touched frequently by gloved hands during patient care, (b) likely to be contaminated with blood or other potentially infectious materials, or (c) difficult to clean (e.g., chair control panels, air/water syringe buttons, and light handles). Adaptation of certain surface covers will depend on the evaluation of potential advantages and disadvantages for their inclusion in an overall infection-control program (Table 12-6).

A long-standing infection-control recommendation in this area states that disposable barriers should be removed and discarded between patients while dental personnel are still wearing gloves, because these items can become contaminated during patient care. In addition, it is not necessary to clean and disinfect a properly covered surface unless the barrier fails or the surface becomes accidentally contaminated during treatment.

TABLE 12-6 Factors to Consider for Use of Surface Disposable Covers

Advantages	Disadvantages
1. Prevent cross-contamination	1. Need a variety of sizes and types of covers
2. Protect difficult-to-clean surfaces	2. Many plastics items are non-biodegradable
3. Less time-consuming than cleaning and disinfection	3. Undesirable aesthetic appearance
4. Reduces use of potentially harmful chemicals	4. Additional costs over chemical sprays and wipes

MECHANISMS OF ANTIMICROBIAL CHEMICAL ACTION

Most chemical sterilants and disinfectants disrupt target cells by acting as cytoplasmic poisons. This general lack of specificity limits the usefulness of these agents to inanimate objects. Any part or all of four major portions of microbial cells can be affected: the cell wall, plasma membrane, cytoplasmic contents (particularly enzymes), and nuclear material. Resultant microbial destruction is accomplished by one of several possible reactions or a combination of multiple effects. These will be discussed further for each class of chemical disinfectant.

CHEMICAL DISINFECTANTS

Detergents (Surface-Active Substances)

Detergents are preparations that alter the nature of interfaces to lower surface tension and increase cleaning. The antimicrobial effect occurs primarily on the cell membrane by alteration of the osmotic barrier. This results in increased cell permeability, and target cells subsequently cannot maintain their integrity. Common surface-active agents are classified as nonionic, anionic, or cationic. Nonionic chemicals do not possess any antimicrobial properties. Synthetic anionic detergents and soaps are examples of anionic preparations. Soaps are salts of long-chain aliphatic carboxylic acids of animal and plant fats. Most synthetic anionic detergents contain alkyl and/or aryl sulfates or sulfonates. The alkali content and sodium salt allow soaps to kill streptococci, treponemes, pneumococci, gonococci, and influenza viruses. These effects notwithstanding, the primary value of anionic detergents seems to be in their mechanical cleansing action.

Quaternary ammonium preparations are examples of cationic surface-active disinfectants. These agents are germicidal in a much lower concentration than nonionic detergents and can remain bacteriostatic in relatively high dilutions. The most probable site of antimicrobial action for quaternary ammonium solutions is the cell membrane. Alteration of the membrane triggers the release of enzymes and cellular metabolites, with Gram-positive bacteria being most susceptible to destruction.

Three generations of quaternary ammoniums have been developed for use since 1915: simple benzalkonium chloride, substituted benzalkonium compounds, and dual quaternary ammonium compounds. The dual quats were first manufactured in 1955 and have the commercial use of the three types. Quaternary ammonium agents can be bactericidal in both acid and alkaline environments, and are bacteriostatic at lower concentrations. Unfortunately, variable antimicrobial activity has been observed with simple quaternary ammoniums against many Gram-negative bacteria, in addition to little or no destructive effects against bacterial spores, fungi, and most viruses. For example, several quaternary ammonium preparations can become contaminated easily by Gram-negative bacteria such as *Pseudomonas* species (Table 12-7). A substantial amount of scientific data demonstrated the ineffectiveness of early generations of these cationic agents against many pathogens that may be transmitted during the practice of dentistry. These include the etiologic agent for tuberculosis. Removing any doubt concerning the feasibility of quaternary ammonium preparations, the American Dental Association (ADA) Council on Dental Therapeutics eliminated them from the ADA Acceptance Program as disinfectants in 1978. Thus benzalkonium chloride, dibenzalkonium chloride, cetyldimethylethylammonium bro-

TABLE 12-8 Characteristics of Alcohol–Dual Quaternary Ammonium Compounds

Advantages	Disadvantages
1. EPA-registered intermediate-level disinfectants for environmental surfaces	1. Variable alcohol concentrations in different products can affect surface-cleaning capabilities
2. Broad antimicrobial spectrum	2. Possible rapid evaporation from surfaces with solutions with high alcohol concentrations
3. Rapidly tuberculocidal in 1–5 min	
4. Available as prepared disinfectants	

mide, and other similar chemicals are not recommended as a single agent for routine intermediate-level surface disinfection in dentistry. Quaternary ammonium solutions are good cleaning agents, however, and are marketed for health professions as disinfectant cleansers on the basis of this cleaning ability. More recently developed formulations incorporating alcohols with dual quaternary ammonium compounds have been approved by the EPA as demonstrating tuberculocidal activity (Table 12-8). The alcohol component of such products seems to be primarily responsible for the extended antimicrobial spectrum, with the quaternary ammonium portion serving as the surface cleaning agent.

Alcohols

Ethyl alcohol and isopropyl alcohol have been used extensively for many years as skin antiseptics and surface disinfectants. As a result, they have been considered historically as widely beneficial agents for effective antisepsis. Both of these agents are effective protein denaturants and lipid solvents. The latter property probably enhances their antimicrobial range because of the destructive effect on *M. tuberculosis* and enveloped lipophilic viruses, such as herpes simplex viruses. In general, alcohols exhibit a fairly broad antimicrobial spectrum of activity under certain conditions (Table 12-9).

Ethyl alcohol is relatively nontoxic, colorless, nearly odorless and tasteless, and readily evaporates without residue. Isopropyl alcohol is less corrosive than ethyl alcohol because it is not oxidized as rapidly to acetic acid and acetaldehyde. They are not recommended as single agents for use as environmental surface disinfectants, however, because of several serious problems inherent in their chemical actions. For example, they are not effective in the presence of tissue proteins and glycoproteins, such as those found in saliva and blood. Alcohols historically have been shown to be poor cleaning agents in the pres-

TABLE 12-7 Disinfectant Characteristics of Quaternary Ammonium Compounds (Alcohol-Free)

Advantages	Disadvantages
1. EPA registered as low-level disinfectants for noncritical surfaces	1. Not tuberculocidal, sporicidal, or virucidal against hydrophilic viruses
2. Cationic detergents—good surface cleaners	2. Inactivated by anionic detergents (i.e., soaps and hard water)
3. Bactericidal against Gram-positive bacteria, fungicidal, virucidal against lipophilic viruses	3. Inactivated by organic matter
4. Pleasant odor	4. Evidence suggesting variable activity against Gram-negative bacteria
5. Low tissue toxicity	

TABLE 12-9 Characteristics of Alcohols* as Surface Disinfectants

Advantages	Disadvantages
1. Rapidly bactericidal	1. Not sporicidal
2. Tuberculocidal and virucidal	2. Diminished activity with bioburden (i.e., unable to clean surfaces contaminated with body fluids)
3. Only slightly irritating	3. Damaging to certain materials, including rubber and plastics
4. Benefits from positive historic perception	4. Flammable
5. Economical	5. Rapid evaporation rate with diminished activity against viruses in dried blood, saliva, and other secretions on surfaces

*Applies to 70% isopropyl and 70% ethyl alcohol.

ence of bioburden. Exposure to alcohol denatures and dehydrates proteins, making them insoluble and tenaciously adherent to most surfaces. A coating of denatured bioburden can protect contaminant microorganisms from the destructive effects of alcohols for prolonged intervals. Rapid evaporation from treated environmental surfaces also limits alcohol activity on protein-coated bacteria and viruses, which are found commonly in the spatter generated during dental procedures. Other problems include the corrosiveness of alcohols on metal surfaces and destruction of certain materials (i.e., plastics and vinyl coverings).

Vegetative bacteria are killed by exposure to high concentrations of alcohol (70% optimum), the most notable pathogen being *M. tuberculosis*. The concentration of an alcohol preparation is critical to its antimicrobial effectiveness. When the 70% concentration is exceeded, the initial dehydration of microbial proteins allows these cell components to resist the subsequent detrimental denaturation effects. Therefore, the exposed microorganisms are able to remain viable for longer periods of time. In summary, alcohols are not regarded as effective surface cleansing agents, an important first step in the preparation for disinfection and sterilization procedures. For the reasons cited above, the CDC, ADA, and Organization for Safety and Asepsis Procedures do not recommend alcohol as an environmental surface disinfectant.

Iodine and Iodophors

Iodine is one of the oldest antiseptics for application onto skin, mucous membranes, abrasions, and other wounds. The high reactivity of this halogen with its target substrate gives it potent germicidal effects. It acts by iodination of proteins and subsequent formation of protein salts. Because iodine is insoluble in water, it has been prepared routinely as a tincture, with iodide salt being dissolved in alcohol. Iodine in this form continues to be an effective antiseptic, as shown by the fact that, at different concentrations, tinctures of iodine are toxic for Gram-positive and Gram-negative bacteria, tubercle bacilli, spores, fungi, and most viruses. This form of iodine has some serious drawbacks, however. It is irritating and allergenic, corrodes metals, and stains skin and clothing. Hypersensitivity reactions to tincture of iodine also have been common, with tissue manifestations ranging from mild to severe in allergic people.

Attempts to use the powerful germicidal action of iodine, while reducing its caustic and staining effects, led to the synthesis of later-generation iodine compounds. The basis for these formulations is the preparation of an agent in which iodine is held in dissociable complexes. These compounds, called iodophors, retain a similar broad antimicrobial spectrum compared with iodine tinctures but have the following added features: there is less irritation of tissues and they are significantly less allergenic, do not stain skin or clothing, and have prolonged activity after application (Table 12-10). Iodophors are prepared by combining iodine with a solubilizing agent or carrier. Common carriers include polyvinylpyrrolidone or ethoxylated nonionic detergents (poloxamers). These agents stabilize the iodine, minimize its

TABLE 12-10 Disinfectant Characteristics of Iodophors

Advantages	Disadvantages
1. EPA-registered intermediate-level surface disinfectant	1. Not a sterilant
2. Broad spectrum: Bactericidal, tuberculocidal, and virucidal against hydrophilic and lipophilic viruses	2. Unstable at high temperatures
3. Biocidal activity within 5–10 min	3. Dilution and contact time critical
4. Effective in dilute solution	4. Daily preparation necessary
5. Few adverse tissue reactions	5. Discoloration of some surfaces
6. Contain surfactant carrier that maintains surface moistness	6. Rust inhibitor necessary
7. Residual biocidal action	7. Inactivated by hard water (1:200)

toxicity, and slowly release the halogen to the tissues. The carriers themselves are surfactants that are water soluble and react with epithelial areas to increase tissue permeability. Thus the active iodine that is released is better absorbed.

Several iodophor preparations serve as disinfectants in hospitals, clinics, and other healthcare facilities. Their surfactant properties make them excellent cleaning agents before disinfection, and they have EPA-approved tuberculocidal activity within 5 to 10 minutes of exposure. Fresh solutions must be prepared daily because maximal tuberculocidal activity can be variable in solutions older than 24 hours. Diluting iodophor disinfectants in hard water also may cause rapid loss of antimicrobial activity; thus the general recommendation is to use distilled water to dilute iodophors and other similarly based disinfectants before use.

Chlorine-Containing Agents

The halogen chlorine primarily acts against microbial forms by oxidation, as hypochlorous acid, into which it is converted quickly by water. As a result, chlorine is more active in acid solutions. Elemental chlorine is a potent germicide, killing most bacteria in 15 to 30 seconds at concentrations of 0.10 to 0.25 ppm. Accepted chlorine-containing compounds in common use are hypochlorite solutions (Table 12-11). Diluted sodium

hypochlorite (1:10) in water was shown in the 1970s to be useful as a disinfectant, especially in hospital patient care areas considered to have been contaminated with hepatitis viruses. Because this chemical is unstable, fresh solutions must be prepared daily. Newer premixed sodium hypochlorite solutions also have appeared in the marketplace, which have resolved the 1-day reuse life problem observed in hypochlorite concentrates. Using a 1:100 dilution of sodium hypochlorite is an effective method to decontaminate a surface after a blood spill; however, using an EPA-registered sodium hypochlorite product is preferred. Despite its effectiveness as a disinfectant, this chlorine-releasing preparation has some obvious disadvantages. It can be corrosive to metals and irritating to skin and other tissues, and destroy many fabrics.

Phenols and Derivatives

The classic historical antimicrobial for surgical procedures was carbolic acid, first introduced into hospitals by Dr. Joseph Lister in the 1850s. This phenolic solution was used as an all-purpose surgical instrument immersion sterilant, hand-washing antiseptic, wound cleaner, and preparatory antimicrobial for surgical sites. The widespread effectiveness of these techniques in reducing the incidence of hospital-acquired infections was remarkable, and as a result, Lister has been called the "father of antisepsis" in many historic texts. It was first thought that postoperative infections would be virtually eradicated with widespread use of this phenol; however, because of severe tissue toxicity reported in people exposed to carbolic acid, its application was curtailed. Subsequent generations of phenolic compounds possessing different structures and properties have found useful roles as effective disinfectants and antiseptics. These agents act as cytoplasmic poisons by penetrating and disrupting microbial cell walls, leading to denaturation of intracellular proteins. The intense penetration capability of phenols is probably the major factor associated with their antimicrobial activity. Unfortunately, because of this property some preparations also can penetrate intact skin, causing local tissue damage and possible systemic complications. Thus, with the exception of the bisphenols, most phenolic derivatives are used primarily as disinfectants.

TABLE 12-11 Disinfectant Properties of Hypochlorites

Advantages	Disadvantages
1. EPA-registered intermediate-level surface disinfectant	1. Chemically unstable solution
2. Rapid antimicrobial action	2. Necessary to prepare diluted solutions fresh daily
3. Broad spectrum: bactericidal, tuberculocidal, and virucidal (also sporicidal under certain conditions)	3. Diminished activity by presence of organic matter
4. Effective in dilute solution	4. Unpleasant, persistent odor in high concentrations
5. Do not leave toxic residues	5. Irritating to skin and eyes
6. Low incidence of severe toxicity	6. Corrosive to metals
7. Unaffected by water hardness	7. Damaging to fabrics
8. Economical	8. Degrading to plastics and rubber

Complex (Synthetic) Phenols

In the mid-1980s, a new class of phenolic compounds was approved by the EPA as tuberculocidal surface disinfectants (Table 12-12). These contain more than one phenolic agent. Currently, most products contain two, but some formulations can have three phenols as the active com-

TABLE 12-12 Disinfectant Characteristics of Synthetic Phenols

Advantages	Disadvantages
1. EPA registered as intermediate-level surface disinfectant	1. Not sporicidal
2. Broad antimicrobial spectrum	2 Can degrade certain plastics and etch glass with prolonged exposure
3. Tuberculocidal	3. Difficult to rinse off certain materials
4. Useful on metal, glass, rubber, and plastic	4. Film accumulation on environmental surfaces
5. Residual biocidal action	5. Irritating to skin and eyes

pounds. Some products are ready to use, whereas others must be diluted with water. When used according to manufacturers' directions, complex phenolics offer a broad antimicrobial spectrum, including tuberculocidal activity. They also serve as good surface cleaners and are effective in the presence of detergents. Unfortunately, the penetration properties of phenols tend to cause epithelial toxicity in exposed tissues. To prevent this problem, appropriate utility gloves should be worn when these or any other disinfectant is handled. Several available synthetic phenolic disinfectants can also leave a film of residual dried solution on treated surfaces and discolor certain plastic items, such as dental light protective covers.

As might be expected with technologic advances in chemistry, disinfectants have been developed in recent years that contain combinations of phenol in an alcoholic base. These are available commercially as premixed spray preparations and are also EPA-approved as tuberculocidal, intermediate-level disinfectants. Because of their high concentration of alcohol, most of the formulations are only fair to poor in cleaning surfaces, the prerequisite step before environmental surface disinfection. Thus, when phenolic-alcohol disinfectants are selected for use, surface cleaning should be done initially with a water-based cleaning agent, such as soap and water.

Hydrogen Peroxide

The history of hydrogen peroxide use as an antimicrobial agent spans almost 200 years, with periodic applications for various products as disinfectants, antiseptics, or chemical sterilants. Some early preparations were found to be unstable and yielded only low levels of the chemi-

cal. This observation was partially responsible for the decline of hydrogen peroxide as a recommended antiseptic for wounds. Later formulations have attempted to correct previous problems with chemical stability and activity.

Hydrogen peroxide acts as an oxidant in tissues and microorganisms, yielding high concentrations of antimicrobial hydroxyl radicals. Accumulation of this anion is able to adversely affect multiple sites in bacterial cells, including membrane lipids, DNA, and other cell components. As a result, hydrogen peroxide is active against a wide range of microorganisms. It was marketed and used for many years as an antiseptic, where it served the dual purpose as an antimicrobial oxidant and a débriding agent for treating infection. Much of its clinical use in recent years has been as an effective chemical sterilant (6%), with an immersion time of 6 hours. Sporicidal activity can is attained at this high concentration with the extended immersion time. In recent years, accelerated and stabilized hydrogen peroxide formulations have been developed and found to be effective environmental surface cleaners and disinfectants (Table 12-13).

TABLE 12-13 Characteristics of Hydrogen Peroxides

Advantages	Disadvantages
1. EPA-registered high-level and intermediate-level disinfectant products available based on hydrogen peroxide concentrations	1. May compromise certain types of metals
2. Broad antimicrobial spectrum	2. Damage to ocular tissues with accidental exposure
3. Tuberculocidal	3. Few long-term use studies available
4. No activation required	
5. Good cleaner for removal of bioburden	
6. No odor or irritation issues for keratinized epithelial tissues with surface disinfectant formulations	
7. Stable and effective intermediate-level disinfectant on environmental surfaces	
8. Biodegradable—no environmental disposal concerns	

SUMMARY

Many commercial products are available for use as disinfectants or sterilants. Some of these are capable of surface cleaning and disinfection, some only disinfect, some sterilize with prolonged exposure intervals, some have an unpleasant odor, others stain or bleach surfaces, and some of the formulations are severe tissue irritants and corrosive to metallic surfaces. It is essential that before a surface disinfectant is purchased for routine use, the practitioner, dental hygienist, assistant, and laboratory technician obtain as much information as possible. This will allow subsequent decisions to be based on appropriate efficacy criteria and reduce the potential for product misuse. Certain products can be used for both surface cleaning and effective environmental surface disinfection, whereas others are useful disinfectants but require initial surface cleaning with another water-based solution. As healthcare professionals periodically evaluate available chemical classes and products, they must remember that they have choices. No single available product is the *only* one to use.

✔ Practical Dental Infection-Control Checklist

General Considerations

❏ Are manufacturer instructions followed for the correct use of cleaning and EPA-registered hospital disinfecting products?

❏ Are products only used that are intended for environmental surfaces (i.e., low- to intermediate-level disinfectant products)? Note: Liquid chemical sterilants and high-level disinfectants are not to be used for disinfection of environmental surfaces.

❏ Before disinfection, are surfaces cleaned according to manufacturer instructions?

❏ After cleaning, is the disinfectant allowed to remain on the treated surface for the longest recommended contact time on the product label?

❏ Do DCHP use PPE, as appropriate, when cleaning and disinfecting environmental surfaces?

❏ When considering dental office design and equipment selection, do DCHP evaluate dental equipment features from an infection-control perspective?

Clinical Contact Surfaces

❏ Are surface barriers used to protect clinical contact surfaces, particularly those that are difficult to clean (e.g., switches on dental equipment) and are the surface barriers changed between patients?

❏ Are clinical contact surfaces that are not barrier-protected cleaned and disinfected using an EPA-registered hospital disinfectant with a low-level (i.e., HIV and HBV label claims) to intermediate-level (i.e., tuberculocidal claim) activity after each patient?

❏ Is an intermediate-level disinfectant used if the surface is visibly contaminated with blood?

Housekeeping Surfaces

❏ Are housekeeping surfaces (e.g., floors, walls, and sinks) cleaned with a detergent and water or an EPA-registered hospital disinfectant/detergent on a routine basis (depending on the nature of the surface and type and degree of contamination) and as appropriate, based on the location in the facility, and when visibly soiled?

❏ Are mops and cloths cleaned after use and allowed to dry before reuse; or are single-use, disposable mop heads or cloths used?

❏ Are fresh cleaning or EPA-registered disinfecting solutions prepared daily and as instructed by the manufacturer?

❏ Are walls, blinds, and window curtains cleaned in patient-care areas when they are visibly dusty or soiled?

Review Questions

1. Environmental surface disinfectants must be registered with the
   A. FDA
   B. EPA
   C. OSHA
   D. CDC

2. The class of chemical that is classified as an anionic detergent is:
   A. sodium hypochlorite
   B. iodophor
   C. liquid soap
   D. quaternary ammonium solution
   E. complex phenol

3. Environmental surfaces that are not touched by contaminated hands, instruments, or other items during treatment are called _____ surfaces.
   A. housekeeping
   B. intraoperatory
   C. clinical contact
   D. superficial

4. Properties of iodophors as disinfectants include:
   A. stain skin easily

B. slow release of iodine for disinfection

C. destroy only Gram-positive bacteria

D. prepared as alcohol-based solutions for clinical use

5. Tuberculocidal activity has been demonstrated with active solutions of each of the following, except:

A. anionic detergents

B. 1:100 aqueous dilution of sodium hypochlorite

C. complex phenol disinfectants

D. alcohol-quaternary ammonium disinfectants

E. iodophor disinfectants

6. Which of the following microorganisms are readily killed by intermediate-level disinfection?

A. *S. aureus*

B. *M. tuberculosis*

C. HBV

D. HIV

E. All of the above

7. For a chemical to be classified as a "high-level disinfectant," it must be able to:

A. Inactivate hepatitis viruses within 10 minutes

B. Kill *M. tuberculosis* within 5 minutes of exposure time

C. Have a residual antimicrobial effect on treated surfaces

D. Destroy microbial spores with prolonged exposure

E. Be nontoxic on epithelial tissues

8. The use of disposable covers during patient care has which of the following features?

A. Less time-consuming than using disinfectants.

B. Purchase of fewer items.

C. Both A and B are correct.

D. Neither A nor B is correct.

Critical Thinking

1. Do you use protective surface barriers in your dental office/clinic? What items do you usually cover?

2. Go to one of the office's dental operatories. Demonstrate how you would take the protective surface barrier off to avoid contaminating the underlying surface(s).

SELECTED READINGS

ADA Council on Dental Therapeutics. Quaternary ammonium compounds not acceptable for disinfection of instruments and environmental surfaces in dentistry. J Am Dent Assoc 1978;97:855–856.

ADA Councils on Scientific Affairs and Dental Practice. Infection-control recommendations for the dental office and the dental laboratory. J Am Dent Assoc 1996;127:672–680.

Assar SK, Block SS. Survival of micro-organisms in the environment. In: Block SS, ed. Disinfection, Sterilization, and Preservation. 5th ed. Philadelphia, PA: Lippincott Williams & Wilkins; 2001:1221–1242.

Block SS. Peroxygen compounds. In: Block SS, ed. Disinfection, Sterilization, and Preservation. 5th ed. Philadelphia, PA: Lippincott Williams & Wilkins; 2001:185–204.

Bond WW, Favero MS, Petersen, NJ, et al. Inactivation of hepatitis B virus by intermediate to high-level disinfectant chemicals. J Clin Microbiol 1983;18:535–538.

Bond WW, Petersen NJ, Favero MS. Viral hepatitis B: aspects of environmental control. Health Lab Sci 1977;14:235–252.

CDC. Guidelines for infection control in dental health-care settings. MMWR 2003;51(RR-17):1–66.

Crawford JJ. State-of-the-art: practical infection control in dentistry. J Am Dent Assoc 1985;110:629–633.

Environmental Protection Agency. Advocacy of pesticide uses which do not appear on registered pesticide labels: amendment to the statement. Fed Regist 1986;51:19174–19175.

Favero MS, Bond WW. Chemical disinfection of medical and surgical materials. In: Block SS, ed. Disinfection, Sterilization, and Preservation. 5th ed. Philadelphia, PA: Lippincott Williams & Wilkins; 2001:881–917.

Favero MS, Bond WW. Sterilization, disinfection, and antisepsis in the hospital. In: Manual of Clinical Microbiology. 5th ed. Washington, DC: American Society for Microbiology; 1991:183–200.

Kobayashi H, Tsuzuki M, Koshimizu K, et al. Susceptibility of hepatitis B virus to disinfectants or heat. J Clin Microbiol 1984;20:214–216.

Lister J. On the antiseptic principle of the practice of surgery. Br Med J 1867;21:353–356.

Merianos JJ. Surface-active agents. In: Block SS, ed. Disinfection, Sterilization, and Preservation. 5th ed. Philadelphia, PA: Lippincott Williams & Wilkins; 2001:283–320.

Molinari JA. Surface disinfectants: read the labels. Compend Contin Ed Dent 2001;22:1086–1088.

Molinari JA, Harte JA. Dental services. In: APIC Text of Infection Control and Epidemiology. 2nd ed. Washington, DC: APIC Pub; 2005:51-1–51-23.

Molinari JA, Palenik CJ. Environmental surface infection control, 2003. Compend Contin Ed Dent 2004;25:30–37.

Molinari JA, Campbell MD, York J. Minimizing potential infections in dental practice. J Mich Dent Assoc 1982;64:411–416.

Molinari JA, Gleason MJ, Cottone JA, et al. Cleaning and disinfectant properties of dental surface disinfectants. J Am Dent Assoc 1988;117:179–182.

Molinari JA, Gleason MJ, Cottone JA, et al. Comparison of dental surface disinfectants. Gen Dent 1987;35:171–175.

Redd JT, Baumbach J, Kohn W, et al. Patient-to-patient transmission of hepatitis B virus associated with oral surgery. J Infect Dis 2007;195:1311–1314.

Runnells RR. Infection Control in the Former Wet Finger Environment. North Salt Lake, UT: IC Publications; 1987.

Rutala WA. 1994, 1995, and 1996 APIC Guidelines Committee. APIC guideline for selection and use of disinfectants. Association for Professionals in Infection Control and Epidemiology, Inc. Am J Infect Cont 1996;24:313–342.

Rutala WA, Cole EC. Ineffectiveness of hospital disinfectants against bacteria: a collaborative study. Infect Control 1987;8:501–506.

Rutala WA, Weber DJ. Cleaning, disinfection, and sterilization in healthcare facilities. In: APIC Infection Control and Applied Epidemiology: Principles and Practice. 2nd ed. Washington, DC: APIC Pub; 2005:21-1–21-11.

Sehulster LM, Chinn RYW, Arduino MJ, et al. Guidelines for environmental infection control in health-care facilities. Recommendations from CDC and the Healthcare Infection Control Practices Advisory Committee (HICPAC). Chicago, IL: American Society for Healthcare Engineering/American Hospital Association; 2004.

Spaulding EH. Chemical disinfection and antisepsis in the hospital. J Hosp Res 1972;9:5–31.

Spaulding EH. Chemical disinfection of medical and surgical materials. In: Lawrence CA, Block SS, eds. Disinfection, Preservation, and Sterilization. Philadelphia, PA: Lea & Febiger; 1968:517–531.

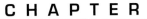

CHAPTER

13

How to Choose and Use Environmental Surface Disinfectants

John A. Molinari

Jennifer A. Harte

LEARNING OBJECTIVES

After completion of this chapter individuals should be able to:

1 Describe the importance of cleaning and disinfection procedures.

2 Describe how to select disinfectant products for use in the dental setting.

3 Describe how to clean and disinfect an environmental surface.

4 Describe possible misuse of disinfectant products along with potential adverse effects.

KEY TERMS

Cleaning: the removal of visible soil and organic debris, either manually or mechanically, that results in a reduction in the number of microorganisms and the removal or organic matter, such as blood, tissue, and other biological material that may interfere with sterilization and disinfection. Cleaning is the first step in any sterilization or disinfection process.

Disinfection: the destruction of pathogenic and other kinds of microorganisms by physical or chemical means. Disinfection is less lethal than sterilization, because it destroys most recognized pathogenic microorganisms, but not necessarily all microbial forms, such as bacterial spores. Disinfection does not ensure the margin of safety associated with sterilization processes.

Environmental Protection Agency (EPA): the mission of the EPA is to protect human health and the environment; the EPA works to develop and enforce regulations that implement environmental laws enacted by Congress.

Hospital disinfectant: a germicide that is registered by EPA for use on inanimate objects in hospitals, clinics, dental offices, or any other medical-related facility. Efficacy is demonstrated against *Salmonella enterica* (formerly *Salmonella choleraesuis*), *Staphylococcus aureus*, and *Pseudomonas aeruginosa*.

Intermediate-level disinfectant: a liquid chemical germicide registered by the EPA as a hospital disinfectant and with a label claim of potency as a tuberculocidal. Intermediate-level disinfection is a process that inactivates most vegetative bacteria, most fungi, and some viruses, but cannot be relied on to inactivate resistant microorganisms, such as mycobacteria or bacterial spores.

Low-level disinfectant: a liquid chemical germicide registered by the EPA as a hospital disinfectant. OSHA requires low-level disinfectants also to have a label claim for potency against HIV and HBV if used for disinfecting clinical contact surfaces. Low-level disinfection is a process that will inactivate most vegetative bacteria, some fungi, and some viruses but cannot be relied on to inactivate resistant microorganisms (e.g., mycobacteria or bacterial spores).

Other potentially infectious materials (OPIM): an OSHA term that refers to (a) the following human body fluids: semen, vaginal secretions, cerebrospinal fluid, synovial fluid, pleural fluid, pericardial fluid, peritoneal fluid, amniotic fluid, saliva in dental procedures, any body fluid that is visibly contaminated with blood, and all body fluids in situations where it is difficult or impossible to differentiate between body fluids; (b) any unfixed tissue or organ (other than intact skin) from a human (living or dead); and (c) HIV-containing cell or tissue cultures, organ cultures, HIV- or HBV-containing culture medium or other solutions, and blood, organs, or other tissues from experimental animals infected with HIV or HBV.

Spray-wipe-spray: disinfection of environmental surfaces using a two-step procedure. In the first step ("spray-wipe"), contaminated surfaces are precleaned by vigorously wiping the surface with a cleaning agent. The second step involves applying a disinfectant ("spray") over the entire precleaned surface and allowing it to remain moist for the contact time recommended by the manufacturer.

Wipe-discard-wipe: disinfection of environmental surfaces in a two-step procedure using disinfecting cloths or wipes. Two cloths must be used—one to clean and another to disinfect the surface.

In addition to recommending an increased use of disposable covers, infection-control guidelines routinely address the cleaning and disinfection of operatory surfaces that become contaminated with bioburden as a result of treatment procedures. The use of chemical disinfectants is warranted in certain instances because it is neither possible nor necessary to sterilize all contaminated items and surfaces. When one then considers the large number of operatory surfaces that may become coated with saliva, blood, or exudate (see Chapter 1), it becomes readily apparent that environmental surface disinfection constitutes a major portion of an effective asepsis program. This chapter will consider the rationale and procedures for surface disinfection by using information presented for chemical disinfectants in Chapter 12.

BASIC CRITERIA AND CONSIDERATIONS

The simplest way to approach the subject of environmental surface **disinfection** is to adhere to a basic premise of aseptic technique: *clean it first.* As straightforward and logical as this statement appears, operatory disinfection has continued to be a source of confusion for some dental professionals. Available chemical products include concentrates, premixed solutions, sprays, wipes, foams, and impregnated disposable wipes. Unfortunately, choosing an appropriate general-purpose surface cleaner and disinfectant may be difficult because of exaggerated claims by manufacturers and misleading assays reported in the literature. These analyses can obscure the actual performance capabilities of individual agents and also may yield information that is not clinically applicable or readily reproducible.

Each year additional surface disinfectant preparations appear in the marketplace. Yet, despite an increasingly crowded commercial arena, it is important for healthcare providers to realize that there is no single *best* product. Instead, there are choices of different, appropriate formulations, each of which has received **Environmental Protection Agency (EPA)** approval as a hospital-level disinfectant. If barriers are not used, surfaces should be cleaned and disinfected using an EPA-registered **hospital disinfectant** with a low-level (i.e., HIV and HBV label claims) to intermediate-level (i.e., tuberculocidal claim) activity after each patient. An **intermediate-level disinfectant** should be used when the surface is visibly contaminated with blood or **other potentially infectious materials (OPIM)**. The use of **low-level disinfectant** products with HIV and HBV label claims is supported by the scientific literature; however, selecting one appropriate product with a higher degree of potency (i.e., intermediate-level disinfectant) to cover all situations is more practical. Selection of a surface disinfectant for a practice or clinic also should include an evaluation of several determining factors (Table 13-1).

The importance of initial cleaning cannot be overemphasized and is included routinely in all infection-control recommendations. For example, the Centers for Disease Control and Prevention (CDC) regularly reinforces this concept in its published infection-control guidelines for all healthcare professionals. The American Dental Association also has stressed this repeatedly, as exemplified by the following section from the "Effective Infection Control" instructional program:

> **Cleaning** is the physical removal of debris. It has two major effects: First, it results in a reduction in the number of microorganisms present. Second, it removes organic matter, such as blood and tissue, and other debris that may interfere with sterilization and disinfection. In some instances, cleaning is all that is necessary. Most often, however, it is the preliminary step before sterilization or disinfection. In these instances it is referred to as precleaning. Precleaning is an essential step because sterilization and disinfection procedures may not be effective if items have not been cleaned first.

Initial cleaning and disinfection are important not only for aesthetic reasons, but also—and primarily—because together they minimize the potential for cross-infection from environmental surfaces. It also must be mentioned that manufacturers are required to state on the product label that the disinfectant should be used on precleaned surfaces. Although separate cleaners and disinfectants may be applied, chemical agents that accomplish both functions offer a more efficient approach. Thus a fundamental consideration for chemical selection should be the agent's ability to penetrate and preclean surfaces contaminated with saliva, blood, or exudate. EPA-approved sur-

---

TABLE 13-1 Decision Factors: Surface Cleaning and Disinfection

1. Efficacy:
   A. Assumptions:
      EPA registration
      Hospital-level disinfectant effective against:
      Staphylococcus aureus
      Salmonella enterica (formerly *Salmonella choleraesuis*)
      Pseudomonas aeruginosa
   B. Tuberculocidal: 10 minutes or less for visibly contaminated surfaces
   C. Virucidal:
      Lipophilic viruses (herpesviruses, HIV)
      Hydrophilic viruses (hepatitis B virus, poliovirus, coxsackievirus, rhinovirus)
      10 minutes or less
   D. Product efficacy verified by multiple studies, different investigators, agency recommendations

2. Choices:
   A. Cleaning ability: water-based (good) versus alcohol-based (usually poorer)
   B. Application method: pump spray versus aerosol spray or disposable disinfectant wipes
   C. Minimization of disadvantages of active agent(s) present in disinfectant preparations
      Chlorines—corrosive; damage clothes, plastics, rubber; usually prepared daily
      Iodophors—removable stains; prepared daily
      Synthetic phenols—film accumulation, damage plastics and rubber

3. Available products:
   A. Water-based:
      1. Pump spray:
         a. Concentrate
         b. Prediluted
      2. Aerosol spray
      3. Disposable wipes
   B. Alcohol-based:
      1. Pump spray
      2. Aerosol spray:
         a. Accusol aerosol
         b. Standard aerosol
      3. Disposable wipes

---

face disinfectants, such as iodophors, synthetic phenolics, chlorine compounds, and hydrogen peroxide products, among others, can both clean and disinfect.

It is also advisable to compare the products under consideration with the properties of an "ideal" disinfectant discussed in Chapter 12, and adhere to a series of other important guidelines outlined in Table 13-2. The criteria for effective disinfection call for the preparation and use of products according to their label directions, which have been approved by the EPA. Manufacturers' directions that call for dilution of disinfectants in water rather than alcohol must be followed, because otherwise the cleaning ability of the active agent will be impaired and the alcohol

---

TABLE 13-2 Guidelines for Selection of Liquid Disinfectants

The product must display an EPA number on its label.

Display of this number is proof that the product is registered with the EPA in compliance with federal law and that the product performs as claimed by the manufacturer. The EPA number also affords reasonable legal protection for the user in that only products in compliance with federal law are to be used in patient treatment.

The product must be used in strict compliance with the printed instructions on the labels.

Chemical and microbiologic considerations require use of the product in a disciplined manner to assure that the representations of the manufacturer will be accomplished. Ignoring instructions nearly always reduces microbial control.

For disinfection of contaminated surfaces, the product should state on the label that it kills *Mycobacterium tuberculosis*.*

The tubercle bacillus is a "benchmark" organism and is comparatively difficult to destroy. Tuberculocidal action assures that the product is an intermediate- or higher-level disinfectant and that it will destroy all pathogens that are potentially threatening in dentistry.

Adapted from R.R. Runnells: Dental infection control: update '88. Fruit Heights, UT: IC Publications; 1988.
*Surfaces can be cleaned and disinfected using an EPA-registered hospital disinfectant with a low-level (i.e., HIV and HBV label claims) to intermediate-level (i.e., tuberculocidal claim) activity after each patient. An intermediate-level disinfectant should be used when the surface is visibly contaminated with blood or OPIM. The use of low-level disinfecting products with HIV and HBV label claims is supported by the scientific literature; however, selecting one appropriate product with a higher degree of potency (i.e., intermediate-level disinfectant) to cover all situations might be more practical.

---

actually may increase the deleterious staining effects of some disinfectants, such as iodophors. Hands also should be protected with puncture-resistant utility gloves when cleaning and disinfecting items, and protective eyewear should be worn if the chemical might splash. It is also important to remember that to be effective, chemicals should remain in contact with the surface for the longest contact time indicated on the disinfectant label.

DISINFECTION PROCEDURES

Disinfection of environmental surfaces involves a two-step procedure, historically termed a **"spray-wipe-spray"** technique. As mentioned above, all surfaces to be disinfected must be precleaned before disinfection can occur. Water-based disinfectants, particularly those that contain a detergent, are effective in the initial precleaning step. For the most part, pump spray bottles are appropriate for cleaner/disinfectants, with a major exception being the application of hypochlorite solutions. When spray bottles are used, they provide the following advantages: (a) they allow active chemicals to better penetrate

equipment crevices; (b) they protect the germicide from being inactivated or absorbed by gauzes, paper towels, or sponges; and (c) they minimize the cost of gauze and other applicator materials. The prepared disinfectants should not be stored in containers with gauze because this may shorten the effective life of the disinfectant. A summary of some of the above statements, as well as other suggestions for surface disinfection, is presented in Table 13-3. Once a routine is established, a unit can be cleaned and the disinfectant applied in a few minutes. Traditionally, the time specified by most disinfectant manufacturers to keep surfaces wet after precleaning was 10 minutes; however, an increasing number of preparations with shorter mycobactericidal intervals are commercially available. Chemicals that require a 20-minute or longer tuberculocidal kill time are of limited value. Most disinfectants currently approved by the EPA were required to supply kill data of 5 minutes so that a 10-minute exposure interval could be recommended. This provides a 5-minute safety factor. Wetted, clean surfaces usually are ready to use by the time the patient is seated and prepared for treatment. Any excess disinfectant can be wiped away with a clean paper towel.

Disposable cloths or wipes presaturated with disinfectants are becoming more popular. If used correctly, cloth or paper disinfectant wipes are an effective choice for cleaning and disinfecting environmental surfaces. Because these products are saturated with chemical cleaners and antimicrobial agents, they decrease the amount of chemical sprayed in the environment. Most of the currently available disinfectant wipes contain a range of isopropanol concentrations in addition to other chemical agents that function primarily as surface cleaners. A commonly encountered problem when these products were first introduced was that they evaporated quickly and were not able to keep the surfaces wet for the required disinfection contact time. Several changes in the composition and thickness of the fabric and amount of liquid absorbed into the wipe have been implemented to address this concern. Also, to be effective, two cloths must be used—one to clean and another to disinfect the surface (also known as the **"wipe-discard-wipe"** technique). These disinfectant cloths may be a more convenient alternative to spraying chemicals to clean and disinfect surfaces; however, the product must meet all the requirements of a traditional liquid disinfectant (e.g., EPA registration) and the user is ultimately responsible for ensuring that the product is used correctly.

POTENTIAL FOR DISINFECTANT MISUSE

As with usage of any regulated chemical, problems may arise with environmental disinfectants when they are applied by spraying directly onto surfaces. Misuse or overuse of chemical preparations may arise in several ways. In addition to discoloring or compromising the

TABLE 13-3 Surface Disinfection Suggestions

1.	Surfaces that are difficult to disinfect (such as chair buttons, control buttons on the air-water syringe, switches on the unit, light handles, hoses, and hand-piece and air-water syringe holders) should be covered with plastic wrap, aluminum foil, or another material impervious to water. Covers should be replaced between each patient. It takes less time to replace a cover than to disinfect the uncovered surface between patients.
2.	Disinfecting electrical switches on the chair or unit may damage or cause a short in the switch. They should be covered!
3.	An EPA-registered hospital disinfectant should be used for both the cleaning step and the disinfecting step for uncovered surfaces. Using a water-based agent (e.g., iodophors, combination synthetic phenolics, or hydrogen peroxide) with both cleaning and disinfecting properties provides some protection during the cleaning step, helps sanitize any debris spattered by the cleaning procedure, and helps keep the number of different products that need to be ordered at a minimum.
4.	The primary difference between surface cleaners and disinfectants used in hospitals and surgery suites versus those used in dentistry is the ability to achieve a hydrophilic virus kill (rotavirus, poliovirus).
5.	Personnel must follow the manufacturer's directions on the disinfectant product label.
6.	Water, rather than alcohol, must be used to dilute agents that require dilution before use.
7.	One should use heavy, puncture-resistant nitrile rubber utility gloves during surface cleaning and disinfection to reduce chances of direct contamination of the hands.
8.	Protective eyeglasses must be used to protect eyes from splashes or spatter created when mixing solutions or cleaning surfaces with a brush.
9.	A mask must be used when cleaning and disinfecting to prevent inhalation or direct mucous-membrane contamination from spatter.
10.	Using separate cleaning and disinfectant products is acceptable; however, choosing a product that accomplishes both functions offers a more efficient approach.
11.	Using pump dispensers vs. aerosol sprays may decrease the amount of chemicals sprayed in the environment.
12.	Holding a paper towel behind the surface when spraying the disinfectant can reduce the excess spray.
13.	Keep countertops uncluttered by removing unnecessary items—this facilitates cleaning and disinfection procedures.
14.	Selecting one appropriate product with a higher degree of potency (i.e., intermediate-level disinfectant) to cover all situations might be more practical than maintaining both low- and intermediate-level disinfecting products in the dental office.

integrity of treated operatory surfaces, practice personnel can exhibit a variety of clinical manifestations. Respiratory problems such as wheezing or sneezing, development of allergies, ocular irritation, and headaches can occur from excessive spraying of a disinfectant. A review of protocols for environmental asepsis should be performed if personnel in a clinical facility develop these types of symptoms. Central to this reevaluation is the part that surface cleaning and disinfection play in overall infection-control goals. The objective is to destroy microorganisms, not to harm ourselves. Proper cleaning of equipment and counter surfaces can mechanically remove the overwhelming portion of microbe-laden bioburden, thereby making it unnecessary to subsequently spray clouds of aerosolized disinfection in treatment areas. If problems arise from spraying surfaces, certain questions need to be answered:

1. Do certain surfaces require cleaning only between patients, thus saving time and equipment integrity?

2. Can you find more of a role for disposable covers to lessen exposure to chemical?

By placing the principles of environmental cleaning and surface disinfection into perspective, such problems can be resolved in a healthier and less stressful manner for all personnel.

Infection Control of the Dental Unit

Each Morning before the First Patient of the Day

The CDC no longer recommends flushing dental unit waterlines at the beginning of the day because this practice does not affect biofilm in the waterlines or reliably improve the quality of water used during dental treatment. The spray-wipe-spray technique should be used on all nonsterilizable surfaces and equipment. First, clinical contact surfaces and items, such as the operatory cabinets, counters, sinks, bracket table, dental chair, chair

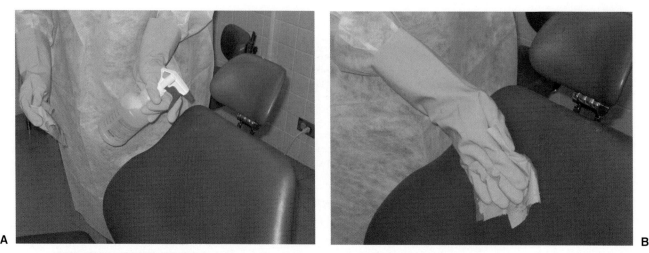

A

B

FIGURE 13-1 (A,B) Disinfecting nonsterilizable surface areas with the spray-wipe-spray technique.

control unit, air/water syringe, and light controls, should be cleaned (with an approved cleaner/disinfectant). After cleaning, these areas should be disinfected with an EPA-registered hospital disinfectant with an HIV, HBV claim (i.e., low-level disinfectant) or a tuberculocidal claim (i.e., intermediate-level disinfectant) that will kill hydrophilic and lipophilic viruses. An intermediate-level disinfectant should be used when the surface is visibly contaminated with blood or OPIM (Fig. 13-1). Alternatively, surface covers should be applied after cleaning.

Between Patients

Waterlines should be flushed for 20–30 seconds (Fig. 13-2). The handpieces (i.e., high- and low-speed handpieces, all handpiece attachments, and any other devices that

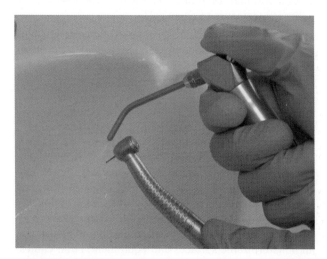

FIGURE 13-2 Flushing waterlines of the unit.

can be removed from the air and waterlines) and air-water syringe tip (if not disposable) should be sterilized. All clinical contact surfaces should be cleaned and disinfected with an approved surface cleaner/disinfectant. Alternatively, covers should be removed and discarded, and clean surface covers applied.

End of the Day

Personnel should clean and disinfect the floor around the dental chair and all countertops, dental unit surfaces, and clinical contact surfaces. A generous amount of cleansing solution should be evacuated through the evacuation lines (e.g., high-volume evacuator, low-volume suction lines) and the unit's solid waste filter trap should be cleaned or replaced.

Weekly

The main evacuation system trap and the inside and outside of drawers and cabinets should be cleaned and disinfected. In addition, as part of the routine asepsis protocol, the operatory and laboratory floors should be cleaned and disinfected thoroughly.

SUMMARY

Because it is not currently possible to provide absolute asepsis for all surfaces and objects during dental treatment, cleanup procedures should attempt to decontaminate those that are potential sources of cross-infection. It is not necessary to sterilize surfaces such as countertops, light handles, chair buttons, and unit controls because these are not considered "critical items" that require sterilization between each appointment. A thorough cleaning followed by appropriate disinfection according to chemical use instructions provides effective environmental surface disinfection. The most desirable disinfectants are virucidal, for both hydrophilic and lipophilic viruses, and tuberculocidal. Properties of the available classes of disinfectants, and the "how-to's" for their use, have been considered in this and previous chapters.

✔ Practical Dental Infection-Control Checklist

General Considerations

❑ Are the manufacturer's instructions followed for correct use of cleaning and EPA-registered hospital disinfecting products?

  ❑ Are only products that are intended for environmental surfaces (i.e., low- to intermediate-level disinfectant products) used? Note: liquid chemical sterilants and high-level disinfectants are not to be used for disinfection of environmental surfaces.

  ❑ Before disinfection, are surfaces cleaned according to the manufacturer's instructions?

  ❑ After cleaning, is the disinfectant allowed to remain on the treated surface for the longest recommended contact time on the product label?

❑ Do DHCP use PPE, as appropriate, when cleaning and disinfecting environmental surfaces?

❑ When considering dental office design and equipment selection, do DHCP evaluate dental equipment features from an infection-control perspective?

Clinical Contact Surfaces

❑ Are surface barriers used to protect clinical contact surfaces, particularly those that are difficult to clean (e.g., switches on dental equipment), and are the surface barriers changed between patients?

❑ Are clinical contact surfaces that are not barrier-protected cleaned and disinfected using an EPA-registered hospital disinfectant with a low-level (i.e., HIV and HBV label claims) to intermediate-level (i.e., tuberculocidal claim) activity after each patient?

  ❑ Is an intermediate-level disinfectant used if the surface is visibly contaminated with blood?

Housekeeping Surfaces

❑ Are housekeeping surfaces (e.g., floors, walls, and sinks) cleaned with a detergent and water or an EPA-registered hospital disinfectant/detergent on a routine basis (depending on the nature of the surface and type and degree of contamination) and as appropriate, based on the location in the facility, and when visibly soiled?

❑ Are mops and cloths cleaned after use and allowed to dry before reuse, or are single-use, disposable mop heads or cloths used?

❑ Are fresh cleaning or EPA-registered disinfecting solutions prepared daily and as instructed by the manufacturer?

❑ Are walls, blinds, and window curtains cleaned in patient-care areas when they are visibly dusty or soiled?

Dental Operatory Asepsis

At the beginning of the day before the first patient, do DHCP:

❑ perform initial handwashing of the day?

❑ don appropriate PPE and clean and disinfect operatory surfaces?

❑ turn on the dental unit and other equipment in the operatory?

❑ keep countertops uncluttered by removing unnecessary items?

❑ place disposable surface barriers on clinical contact surfaces?

During patient treatment, do DHCP minimize cross-contamination by:

❑ keeping their hands away from their face?

❑ limiting the surfaces touched?

❑ changing gloves when torn or heavily contaminated?

❑ using a dental (rubber) dam?

❑ using high-volume evacuation?

❑ using engineering and work practice controls to minimize injury with contaminated sharps?

❑ not touching or writing in the dental record while wearing gloves?

❑ not touching radiographs while wearing gloves?

❑ not picking up the telephone while wearing gloves?

❑ not touching non-barrier-protected computer equipment while wearing gloves?

❑ not using items dropped on the floor?

❑ not entering drawers/cabinets with contaminated gloves?

  ❑ If it is necessary to retrieve an item during treatment that is in a cabinet or drawer, is an aseptic technique used (e.g., using a sterile cotton forceps to retrieve the item, using an overglove, or removing gloves and washing hands)?

Between patients (operatory turnover), do DHCP:

❑ don appropriate PPE?.

❑ flush any device connected to the air/waterlines for a minimum of 20–30 seconds after each patient, including dental handpiece(s), air/water syringes, ultrasonic scalers, and Cavitron units?

❏ remove burs from dental handpieces and disconnect all devices from the dental unit?

❏ remove all surface barriers without touching the underlying surface and discard appropriately?

❏ clean and disinfect contaminated surfaces that were not barrier-protected, including patient safety glasses?

❏ remove PPE (clean and disinfect reusable PPE) and wash hands?

At the end of the day, do DHCP:

❏ don appropriate PPE?

❏ clean and disinfect clinical contact surfaces, dental unit surfaces, and countertops?

❏ clean the high-volume evacuator, low-volume suction lines, and suction/amalgam trap using an approved evacuation system cleaner according to the manufacturer's instructions?

❏ leave the dental operatory "clean and clear"?

Once a week do DHCP:

❏ clean and disinfect the main evacuation system trap?

❏ clean and disinfect the outside of drawers and cabinets?

❏ clean and disinfect operatory and laboratory floors?

Critical Thinking

1. Place the disinfectant you use in the dental office/clinic in front of you.

   a. What are the active agents/ingredients?

   b. Does it have an EPA number on the label?

   c. What classes of microorganisms are claimed to be killed?

   d. Is the disinfectant intermediate- or low-level? How can you tell?

   e. What is the recommended contact time?

2. One of your dental assistants comes back from an infection-control seminar and informs you that she wants the practice to switch to a completely new type of surface disinfectant. You have been using a spray product for years, but she is insisting that the speaker said that, "Only a wipe will provide the margin of safety for your office."

   a. What kinds of features should you look for when evaluating environmental surface disinfectants?

   b. How would use those desirable features to evaluate your current disinfectant as compared to the proposed wipe?

   c. What would be a few challenges the practice staff might face when moving to the new type of surface disinfectant?

---

3. Go to one of the office's dental operatories. Demonstrate how you would disinfect the dental operatory after the patient is dismissed.

Review Questions

1. Environmental surface disinfectants must be registered with the

   A. Food and Drug Administration (FDA).

   B. Environmental Protection Agency (EPA).

   C. Occupational Safety and Health Administration (OSHA)

   D. Centers for Disease Control and Prevention (CDC).

2. Which of the following statements about cleaning environmental surfaces is true?

   A. All surfaces to be disinfected must be precleaned before disinfection can occur.

   B. Cleaning is the chemical removal of debris.

   C. Cleaning results in a reduction of the number of microorganisms present.

   D. Cleaning removes organic matter, such as blood and tissue, that may interfere with disinfection.

   E. A, C, E

   F. All of the above.

3. If environmental surface barriers are not contaminated during treatment, they do not need to be changed between patients.

   A. True

   B. False

4. Surfaces that are difficult to clean and disinfect should be covered with environmental surface barriers. Examples include:

   A. Chair buttons

   B. Dental handpieces

   C. Handpiece hoses

   D. Light handles

   E. All of the above

   F. A, C, D

SELECTED READINGS

ADA. Effective Infection Control: A Training Program for Your Dental Office—Workbook. Chicago, IL: ADA 2004:30.

ADA Council on Scientific Affairs and Council on Dental Practice. Infection-control recommendations for the dental office and the dental laboratory. J Am Dent Assoc 1996;127:672–680.

CDC. Guidelines for infection control in dental health-care settings—2003. MMWR 2003;52(RR-17):1–66.

Cottone JA, Molinari JA. State-of-the-art infection control in dentistry. J Am Dent Assoc 1991;122:33–41.

Favero MS. Sterilization, disinfection, and antisepsis in the hospital. Manual of Clinical Microbiology. 5th ed. Washington, DC: American Society for Microbiology; 1991:183–200.

Favero MS, Bond WW. Chemical disinfection of medical and surgical material. In: Block SS, ed. Disinfection, Sterilization, and Preservation. 5th ed. Philadelphia, PA: Lippincott Williams & Wilkins; 2001:881–917.

Harte JA. Environmental asepsis. Cleaning and disinfecting clinical contact surfaces in the dental operatory. In Control Fact Sheet 2005:1–5.

Miller CH, Palenik CJ. Sterilization, disinfection, and asepsis in dentistry. In: Block SS, ed. Disinfection, Sterilization, and Preservation. 5th ed. Philadelphia, PA: Lippincott Williams & Wilkins; 2001:1049–1068.

Molinari JA. Update—disinfectant liquid sprays and wipes. Dental Advisor 2003:20;1–4.

Molinari JA, Gleason MJ, Cottone JA, et al. Cleaning and disinfectant properties of dental surface disinfectants. J Am Dent Assoc 1988;117:179–182.

Molinari JA, Gleason MJ, Cottone JA, et al. Comparison of dental surface disinfectants. Gen Dent 1987;35:171–175.

Molinari JA, Palenik CJ. Environmental surface infection control, 2003. Compend Contin Educ Dent 2004;25:30–37.

Runnells RR. Dental Infection Control: Update '88. Fruit Heights, UT: IC Publications; 1988.

Sehulster LM, Chinn RYW, Arduino MJ, et al. Guidelines for environmental infection control in health-care facilities. Recommendations from CDC and the Healthcare Infection Control Practices Advisory Committee (HICPAC). Chicago, IL: American Society for Healthcare Engineering/American Hospital Association; 2004.

14

Asepsis Considerations of Office Design and Equipment Selection

Nancy Andrews

Ross Andrews

LEARNING OBJECTIVES

After completion of this chapter individuals should be able to:

1 Understand the relative importance of input from the dental professional to the office design process.

2 Identify the key aspects of office design and equipment selection that impact asepsis in dental offices.

3 Evaluate dental equipment features and alternatives from an infection-control perspective.

4 Define and characterize infection-control zones in dental facilities.

5 Evaluate existing offices and/or equipment from an infection-control perspective.

KEY TERMS

American Society of Heating, Refrigerating and Air-Conditioning Engineers (ASHRAE): an international technical society organized to advance the arts and sciences of heating, ventilation, air-conditioning, and refrigeration. ASHRAE develops standards for refrigeration processes and the design and maintenance of indoor environments. It also publishes voluntary consensus standards, developed to define minimum values or acceptable performance. ASHRAE is accredited by the American National Standards Institute (ANSI) and follows ANSI's requirements for due process and standards development.

Aseptic technique: a procedure that breaks the cycle of cross-infection and ideally eliminates cross-contamination.

Building code: regulations established by a recognized agency that describe design loads, procedures, and construction details for structures. It usually applies to a designated political jurisdiction (e.g., city, county, or state).

Building systems: mechanical, electrical, plumbing, air-handling, and communication equipment and structures in buildings.

Clinical zone: office areas dedicated to patient treatment or direct support of patient treatment, including patient treatment rooms (operatories), dental laboratories, instrument-processing rooms/areas, radiography procedure and processing areas, and patient recovery areas. Clinical zones require the highest degree of infection control in dental settings. Aseptic technique and correct office and equipment design should contain and control contaminants within the clinical zone.

Commissioning: an inspection and evaluation process to verify and document that the facility and all of its systems and assemblies are planned, designed, installed, tested, operated, and maintained to meet the owner's project requirements. Commissioning is performed after construction and before occupation of a building.

Contiguous zones: rooms or areas located directly next to other areas in the same infection-control zones, allowing uninterrupted flow and use while applying a shared level of infection-control practices.

Employee zone: areas used primarily by dental workers for non–patient-treatment activities, including kitchens, lounges, closets and storage, private restrooms, and private offices. Correct office design and aseptic practices should protect the employee zone from contamination generated in other areas, and should not allow the transfer of potentially infectious or contaminated materials out of the area to other parts of the office.

Guidelines for the Design and Construction of Health Care Facilities: a joint publication of the American Institute of Architects (AIA), the Facility Guidelines Institute, and the U.S. Department of Health and Human Services. This publication attempts to address the specific requirements and best building practices for specialized clinical environments, and is often directly referenced by local and state building codes.

Heating, ventilation, and air conditioning (HVAC): a system that provides heating, ventilating, and/or cooling within or associated with a building.

Illumination Engineering Society of North America (IESNA): an organization that establishes and issues standards for building illumination.

Indoor air quality (IAQ): the quality of a facility's indoor air, including sensory comforts such as temperature, humidity, and air flow, or levels of contamination by chemicals, toxins, allergens, pathogens, and particulates.

Infection-control office zones: office areas grouped together by similar functions, resulting in zone-specific infection-control standards.

Public zone: areas of the office open to public access by patients, visitors, and nondental workers, including reception rooms, hallways, public restrooms, business offices, conference rooms, and utility rooms/areas. These areas should be clean and sanitary, but are not subject to the strict infection-control standards of the clinical zone.

Volatile organic compounds (VOCs): compounds that have a high vapor pressure and low water solubility. Many VOCs are human-made chemicals that are used and produced in the manufacture of paints, pharmaceuticals, refrigerants, and building materials.

It is important for dental professionals to understand the key aspects of office design and equipment selection relative to infection control, and to be able to work with designers, engineers, contractors, and vendors involved in creating, renovating, and maintaining office spaces. The topic of office design is so broad that only an overview of considerations related to infection control can be provided in this chapter. Along with aesthetics, cost, ergonomics, functionality, and efficiency, asepsis should be a fundamental consideration for initial dental office designs, as well as during periodic reevaluations and when renovating or upgrading spaces or equipment. Office design can and should communicate a practice's commitment to infection control. Areas dedicated to infection-control activities, such as instrument-processing areas, should be designed to support the size and type of the practice, current best practices, technology, and equipment. All other spaces and equipment should be selected and built with asepsis as an important criterion, even if their dedicated function is not limited to infection control. While the success of a facility's infection-control efforts requires training and application of safe practices, these can be undermined by poor space or equipment design. Conversely, the best facility with the most modern equipment can fail to control disease transmission when poor protocol is used. In brief, an office design that facilitates infection control makes safety protocols and **aseptic technique** applications easier to perform and more effective. Whenever possible, equipment should be selected to improve infection control rather than present infection-control challenges. Early adaptations to new technology must sometimes work with less than optimal infection-control considerations until further advancements can address such issues. Fortunately, as practitioners seek more aseptic alternatives, the industry has shown it can develop and provide them.

REGULATORY BACKGROUND

The design and construction of dental offices is typically regulated by local **building codes** that group them categorically with other professional office uses. For this reason, building codes typically do not address the specialized equipment, air quality, plumbing, electrical, and infection-control issues of dental facilities. It is common in the construction industry to reference more in-depth, nonmandated standards established by professional or industry organizations as a means of incorporating best-practice requirements into a building project.

Dental offices may be located in occupied homes, converted homes and shops, shopping malls, and mixed-use buildings that were designed and built for general use rather than to provide patient care. In such locations, **building systems** are unlikely to inherently support the variety of equipment, mechanical systems, chemicals, and airborne contaminants commonly found in dental facilities. Aerosolized contaminants and chemical fumes commonly generated during dental treatment may exceed the capabilities of air-handling systems that were designed for other uses. These problems are less severe in buildings designed specifically for medical/dental use. Air quality is best managed by well-designed structural **heating, ventilation, and air conditioning (HVAC)** systems that optimize air exchanges, filtration and purification, humidity control, and temperature. However, portable air filters, fans, exhaust systems, and scavengers are examples of temporary/immediate alternatives. These may be available through dental and dental laboratory equipment dealers.

Dental professionals should have an active role in the office design process along with architects, contractors, and building managers because they are uniquely qualified to contribute important information about the infection-control needs of dentistry at the appropriate time in the process of office design and equipment selection. It is important for the dental professional to have strong convictions about asepsis early in the design of the facility, since he/she will be held accountable to professional standards by agencies that oversee dental practice, such as the Occupational Safety and Health Administration (OSHA), health departments, and state boards of dental examiners.

How then should the dental professional identify the current accepted practices for dental office design? In the case of hospitals, clinics, and outpatient facilities, designers often consult the ***Guidelines for the Design and Construction of Health Care Facilities***, a joint publication of the American Institute of Architects (AIA), the Facility Guidelines Institute, and the U.S. Department of Health and Human Services. This publication attempts to address the specific requirements of specialized clinical environments and is often directly referenced by local and state building codes. While not mandated for dental office design, this resource is excellent for designing the more sensitive areas of the dental office.

OFFICE SPACE COMPONENTS AND INFECTION-CONTROL ZONES

The size and number of spatial components of a dental office may be primarily driven by (a) the size of the practice, (b) function and/or equipment, and/or (c) infection-control protocols. Public spaces and staff support areas are primarily determined by the size of the practice. In spaces that tend to be more modular and repeatable, such as treatment rooms, private offices, and clerical work stations, the size of a space may be a reflection of their function and the equipment needed. Recommended infection-control protocols can dictate a minimum acceptable space size for safety and to prevent cross contamination. Spaces in this category include the instrument-processing area, patient treatment rooms, radiography and other diagnostic/processing areas, laboratory areas, and other dedicated areas for specialized equipment and storage. The dental professional should identify those special components of the office that involve asepsis and confirm that they have ample space to meet the requirements for those protocols.

Room configuration may be just as important as the size of a space. If the space is not optimally configured, additional area or physical barriers may be required to achieve the recommended separations and relationships. This is especially applicable for utility areas, which are often relegated to leftover or oddly configured areas of the office plan, and where space deficiencies can result in serious infection-control compromises. For example, this type of error occurs when the suction-to-sewer plumbing connection is placed adjacent to the intake for the air compressor within the closed space of utility closets. The air gap at the plumbing connection allows potential contamination of the air intake to the air compressor. In a dental operatory where one or more assistants work with a clinician, the space must be laid out for all workers to have access to the patient, needed instruments, equipment, and supplies.

Infection-Control Zones

A useful way to approach the inherently different infection control needs of different office areas is to visualize three different **infection-control zones**: the clinical zone, the employee zone, and the public zone. These three zones are made up of rooms and areas grouped together by similar functions, resulting in zone-specific infection-control standards. The level of asepsis required for each zone should strongly influence how the space is designed and used, as well as the selection of furnishings and equipment. If each zone is designed properly, compliance with infection-control standards will be easier to achieve and more effective.

Leaving one zone and entering another may require the donning or removal of personal protective equipment (PPE), hand washing, or other appropriate activities. In addition to encouraging asepsis compliance, **contiguously located zones** enhance workplace efficiency. Transitional elements or features at the interface of two zones may facilitate compliance with appropriate infection-control standards. Boundaries between areas with different infection-control requirements can be made obvious with transitional elements, such as physical barriers (i.e., doors, walls, and signs) or indicated more subtly with changes in surfaces, materials, lighting, and finishes. Each zone has special considerations relative to a variety of design considerations, including space allocation and layout; worker traffic patterns, patient flow, building system considerations (i.e., plumbing, lighting, air management, and electrical systems, and surface materials and details), and specialized equipment (Fig. 14-1).

The **clinical zone** is the combined space dedicated to patient care, treatment items, and other objects directly involved with patient care. This zone requires the highest infection-control standards in the facility, since procedures performed in this zone are likely to generate potentially infectious fluids, materials, and aerosols, and contamination risks are most probable. The clinical zone includes the following office space components:

1. Patient treatment rooms

2. Instrument-processing area

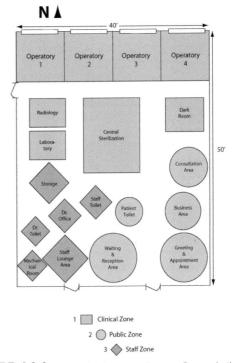

FIGURE 14-1 Three infection-control zones. Rooms in the same zones are located contiguously to improve asepsis and efficiency. (Courtesy of Mark Tholen, DDS, MBA.)

3. Dental laboratory

4. Radiography treatment, diagnostics, and processing

5. Patient recovery rooms/areas

Clinical zones require the use of barriers to protect surfaces, cleaning and disinfecting with chemical cleaners and disinfectants, use of PPE, hand washing, cleaning and sterilizing of instruments, and maintenance of equipment asepsis. To optimize asepsis in clinical zones, spaces should be large enough to perform separate tasks without causing cross-over to other work stations or interference with other workers, activities, or with patients. Aseptic technique is much more likely to be followed if the facility is designed for it and equipment encourages it. Work stations can be physically distanced or barriers can be built to separate spaces and activities. Staging and preparation areas, such as where instrument setups are assembled, should be protected from spray, splash, and aerosols, and sanitary storage should be easily accessible without cross-contamination.

In addition to doors and walls, pass-through cabinets are examples of physical barriers that reduce cross-contamination potential, especially if movable elements, such as doors and cabinets, open without hand contact (Fig. 14-2). When different activities must share the same space, the space should be cleaned

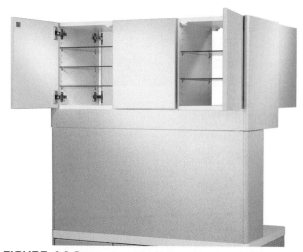

FIGURE 14-2 Pass-through cabinets act as physical barriers between areas while providing for movement of items through the barrier, as well as aseptic storage of instruments in closed cabinets. (Courtesy of Midmark Images.)

and disinfected, or barriers should be used to prevent surface contamination before the space is used for the next procedure. Current designs for clinics use materials and surfaces that should withstand these procedures. For example, intermediate- and low-level surface disinfectants are designed for use on hard, non-porous surfaces, so cloth upholstery and other porous surfaces are not recommended for clinical contact surfaces. Impervious barriers are recommended to cover dental chair upholstery, to reduce exposure to potentially damaging surface disinfectants. When the chair barriers are changed between patients, only exposed or contaminated clinical contact areas need to be cleaned and disinfected. Barriers can simply be replaced between patients using an aseptic technique, and chairs can be cleaned and disinfected as needed on a regular schedule.

Work stations, including equipment, should be organized to anticipate sequenced and/or shared work practices, thereby avoiding cross-contamination and inefficient flow patterns that might increase potential risks for occupational exposure. In clinical zones where patients enter, such as the operatory, patients must be kept separated from asepsis-sensitive equipment, materials, and items. Within such spaces, there should be a "patient zone" and a "clinician zone" with limited spots of shared space, such as the patient chair.

Clinical zones also should be designed to encourage containment of contamination generated during the use of the various spaces. Facilities to perform hand hygiene, don and remove PPE, clean and disinfect items entering and leaving clinic areas, and nontouch operating controls

of doors are examples of structural elements that encourage containment of contamination in an effort to control disease transmission (Fig. 14-3).

The **employee zone** is the combined area used by dental personnel for private activities. This area should be sanitary and protected from patient-related contamination. Workers should remove contaminated PPE before entering these areas and observe cleanliness procedures to avoid transferring contaminants from the employee zone to the clinical zone. The employee zone consists of:

1. Private offices
2. Private restrooms
3. Break room/lounge
4. Closets and personal storage areas

Giving employees a private entrance and immediate access to sinks, restrooms, and other areas without having to enter the clinical zone can help to enforce separation of the employee zone. In addition, space and layout for employee areas should reflect the number of workers and desired level of activities planned. Cleanable surfaces and materials make it easier to maintain asepsis, but textiles may be appropriate in nonclinical areas.

The **public zone** consists of areas open to patients, visitors, maintenance/repair persons, sales people, and employees. The level of infection control here is less controlled than that for both the employee and clinical zones, but the visibility and accessibility of this zone makes it important for establishing the perceived levels of cleanliness, asepsis, and safety for patients. A clean public zone is an indicator of a practice's commitment

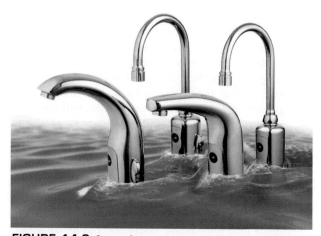

FIGURE 14-3 Sensor faucets, soap, and other hand-hygiene supply dispensers support asepsis. Sinks and other hand-hygiene equipment should be located to facilitate hand hygiene when leaving and entering clinical zones. (Courtesy of The Chicago Faucet Company.)

to a high standard of care, and is therefore a powerful internal and external marketing tool. Conversely, dirty, dark, dusty, or worn-out-appearing public areas can suggest low asepsis standards in other areas, even if this is not the case. Public areas should be spacious enough to allow comfortable distances between waiting or moving patients. The public zone consists of:

1. Reception area
2. Business areas, including the front desk, consultation room, separate appointment area, records and files, and business equipment areas
3. Hallways
4. Patient restrooms
5. Utility rooms/spaces (mechanical, electrical, plumbing, phone, and data areas)

The surfaces in public and employee areas are called "housekeeping surfaces"; they should be clean and sanitary, but are not subject to the strict infection-control standards of the clinical zone. The surface materials should, however, hold up to the use of surface disinfectants if they become contaminated with blood or other potentially infectious materials. It should be noted that patients may contaminate public surfaces with contaminated hands or body secretions, particularly after surgical procedures, making frequent cleaning and disinfection of room surfaces necessary. There are many textiles developed for hospitals and hospitality that have antimicrobial features, moisture resistance, excellent cleanability, and durability.

FLOW OF WORKERS, PATIENTS, AND/OR ITEMS OR CASES

A schematic or space plan of the facility establishes the relationships of the components (areas, rooms, and/or zones) and therefore the flow of patients and staff through the components. From an asepsis standpoint, it is generally considered good design to develop an organizational hierarchy of areas (zones) from the most public to the most aseptically sensitive, the goal being to minimize, if not completely eliminate, infectious exposure of patients and staff or cross-contamination of instruments, equipment, items, and supplies, especially as they are transported. Locating zones contiguously is most effective. Patient flow and worker flow patterns are designed around the equipment and work stations in clinical areas. Public areas need plenty of hall space and space around the business desk areas for people to move through without being cramped or interrupting employee movement. Having separate appointment areas and consultation rooms can avoid congestion and confusion, and provide privacy if needed. Workers should be able to enter employee areas and flow within them without entering the clinical zone or public zone.

BUILDING SYSTEM CONSIDERATIONS
Mechanical Systems

Indoor air quality (IAQ) applies to areas of sensory comfort, such as temperature, humidity, and air flow, that are managed by "air conditioning" systems, as well as to contamination levels of chemicals, toxins, allergens, pathogens, and particulates. Heating, ventilation, and air conditioning (HVAC) systems control temperature and humidity, and maintain clean air by controlling air flow (intake, exhaust, and exchange) and by such processes as filtration, trapping, detoxification, and irradiation of contaminants. Dental professionals can provide useful information about the challenges for mechanical systems in each area of the office, based on anticipated dental equipment, emissions, moisture generation, and the various uses of the spaces.

The use of ducts, rather than unducted air systems, to channel airflow provides superior air management and can be maintained over time. Rigid HVAC ductwork should be selected whenever possible. This duct material can promote air quality in several ways, including resistance to dust build-up, moisture condensation, microbial growth, insect and pest intrusion, and material degradation. If air flows through plenum spaces instead of ducts, these spaces should be (but rarely are) cleaned regularly, as dirt, dust, moisture, mold, pests and their droppings, and airborne irritants and allergens may build up. Filter replacement and duct cleaning exemplify maintenance protocols that benefit IAQ.

During office construction, patients, staff, and other building occupants should be protected from exposure to airborne contaminates, whether they are particulate or gaseous. New ductwork and equipment should be protected with barriers and seals to ensure that they are not compromised before being placed in service. Construction materials with inherently low levels of **volatile organic compounds (VOCs)** and other contaminants should be used. Before new spaces are occupied, adequate time should be allowed for materials such as adhesives, paints, and fabrics to off-gas.

In clinical zones, air-handling systems should be adequate to control the aerosolized particulates, moisture, and contamination. Air quality should be sustainable when equipment is being utilized at its maximum. As new equipment is added and the practice grows, air-handling systems and other utilities must be reevaluated, and upgraded as needed. Increased or specialized exhaust systems are appropriate for many items, including dust-producing equipment used in dental labs, lasers, and electrosurgery units. Mechanical engineers refer to the **American Society of Heating, Refrigerating and Air-Conditioning Engineers (ASHRAE)** for industry-wide standards and guidelines. Additional relevant recommendations are available through ASHRAE's *Special Project (SP) 91 Healthcare Facilities Design Guide.*

Electrical/Illumination Systems

Lighting in clinical zones should be sufficient to provide visibility for cleaning and disinfection. If lighting levels need to be restricted for patient comfort, computer screen visibility, etc., the use of dimming controls or separate switching should be mandated. Electrical engineers and lighting designers are guided by the recommendations of the **Illumination Engineering Society of North America (IESNA)** for appropriate lighting levels in various work environments. Standards more specific to the healthcare industry are available from various research papers, such as *Lighting for Hospitals and Health Care Facilities IESNA RP-29–95.*

Surface Materials Selection

Infection-control considerations for surface materials are cleanability, soil/stain resistance, porosity, durability, abrasion resistance, and tolerance to chemical cleaning. These, along with coloration, texture, and detailing considerations, are sometimes left to the later stages of design, but are of great importance to infection control. Clinical contact surface materials, details, and finishes should be designed to withstand frequently repeated cleaning and disinfection, and materials should be hard and nonporous whenever possible.

Housekeeping surfaces, such as floors, walls, and ceilings, should also be cleanable and show, rather than obscure, signs of contamination. While advances in the manufacture of carpeting have improved its cleanability and inherent antimicrobial properties, carpeting should be relegated to nonclinical areas. In clinical areas, flooring products that minimize joints and seams should be selected. Clinical-zone flooring material should be resilient, smooth, and nonpermeable, and able to be coved at the floor-wall intersection. Walls can be finished with durable, cleanable vinyl wall coverings, many of which are developed for the healthcare industry, or painted with a low-VOC commercial coating of sufficient sheen (semigloss/gloss) to resist frequent cleaning. Window coverings should be cleanable blinds or shades, rather than fabrics or other hard-to-clean materials. Ceilings, while not as likely to receive regular maintenance, should also be cleanable. Painted hard surfaces or acoustic materials designed for washability are appropriate. Ceiling accessories (i.e., grills, diffusers, light fixture trims, signaling devices, sprinkler heads) that resist particulate accumulation should be selected. Surface materials in employee and public zones, while not necessarily as critical as in the clinical zone, should be cleanable to encourage a high standard of cleanliness. Here textures and materials may be desired, but they should be chosen with maximum durability and resistance to dust and moisture penetration.

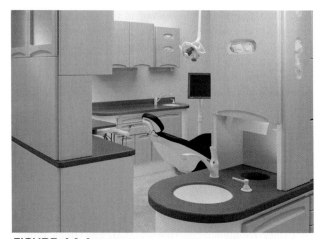

FIGURE 14-4 Built-in dispensers protect supplies and keep counters clear. Cabinet material is cleanable, whereas cardboard dispensers are not. (Courtesy of Midmark Images.)

Detail Considerations

Carefully consider finishes and details that directly impact the ability to maintain infection control. Single-use-item dispensers should be made of permanent materials, easily cleanable, and ideally wall-mounted or recessed in cabinetry (Figs. 14-4 and 14-5).

Complex shapes, joints, and grooves in surfaces should be avoided to minimize the opportunity for particulate and fluid retention or intrusion. Nontouch switches and controls, such as motion-sensing devices, can greatly reduce cross-contamination when using faucets, doors, cabinets, lights, equipment, and dispensers (Fig. 14-6). For operable cabinetry, such as drawers and doors, choose pulls with simple, smooth, easily cleanable, and/or coverable shapes.

COMMISSIONING AND MAINTENANCE PROTOCOLS

Commissioning should be performed after construction and before occupation of a new space. This inspection and evaluation process is used to verify and document that all systems and assemblies are operable and can be maintained. Over time, mechanical systems need to be maintained and serviced. The dental professional may be the only informational bridge to the team of individuals responsible for the ongoing operation, maintenance, and repair of these specialized devices and systems within the dental office. The dental professional should coordinate with the building manager to be sure that maintenance is performed. For example, in operatories, dental labs, and instrument-processing areas where equipment aerosolizes particulates, moisture, and infectious materials, air filters should be maintained carefully

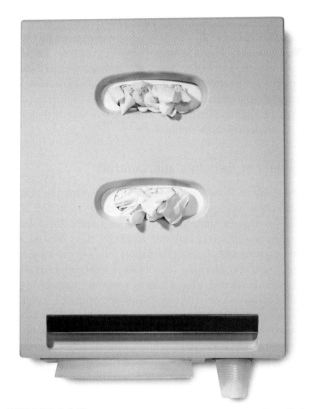

FIGURE 14-5 Wall-mounted dispensers organize supplies off of counters and protect supplies from spray or touch contamination. Dispenser material is more cleanable than cardboard dispensers. (Courtesy of Midmark Images.)

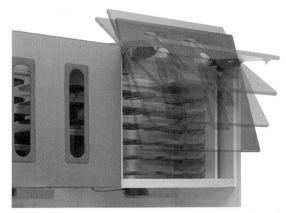

FIGURE 14-6 Cabinets protect stored items from touch and spray contamination. Foot-activated doors avoid contact contamination. (Courtesy of A-dec, Inc.)

and changed on schedule. Initially and periodically, it is helpful to observe and communicate with janitors and maintenance workers to insure that they are not undermining asepsis procedures performed by office workers, and that they are adequately trained.

ASEPTIC CONSIDERATIONS IN DENTAL EQUIPMENT SELECTION

Asepsis considerations have become a powerful driver of dental-equipment design and often enhance functional efficiency, along with the "clean" aesthetic that increasingly characterizes patient-care design. Cleanability and potential to resist contamination, both internally and externally, are key selling points for dental equipment, as are design elements that make infection control easier and quicker to achieve, and therefore more successful.

As environmental asepsis practices have evolved, various types of equipment, especially patient-care equipment in operatories, have been increasingly designed to be more cleanable (i.e., able to stand up to surface cleaning and disinfection, and have smoother surfaces). Impermeable barriers are used to prevent contamination

and reduce the need for chemical disinfection. Equipment with removable components that can be sterilized for reuse, or consists of single-use disposable items, further improves the ability to meet asepsis standards. Following are key equipment features that should be evaluated relative to asepsis:

1. External equipment design: shape and outer material have a direct impact on cleaning, disinfecting, and maintenance.
2. Equipment switches and controls: smooth or "hands-off" controls increase asepsis.
3. Internal potential for contamination, such as dental unit waterline contamination, is another key asepsis consideration when selecting and maintaining equipment.
4. Removable components of patient-care equipment that can be sterilized or are single-use disposable items are advantageous.
5. Equipment maintenance and manufacturers' directions are vital for asepsis, and must be realistic for the office to follow.
6. Electronic communications, records, and ancillary equipment can potentially bring asepsis advantages.

External Equipment Design

When selecting equipment, one should consider the contamination resistance and cleanability of an implement or device. These qualities often manifest themselves in a smooth, flowing, well-detailed appearance. While not a guarantee of asepsis, these characteristics can improve the success of infection-control efforts and communicate the practice's commitment to and concern for patient and professional protection and care.

Operatory equipment surface coverings protect high-technology systems from wear, moisture, and chemical and other damage. Seams, joints, connectors, and attachments should be as smooth and sealed as possible to limit contamination retention and seepage of surface liquids, such as disinfectants, into the underlying mechanisms. Materials should be selected that can withstand surface cleaners and disinfectants with minimal damage, and shapes should be simple, smooth, and easy to clean (Fig. 14-7).

Comfort and style motivate manufacturers to use cushioned chairs with colored and textured upholstery. Cloth-upholstered furnishings should be avoided in dental operatories, laboratories, and instrument-processing areas. Materials (e.g., vinyl) should be chosen to facilitate infection-control procedures. Since chairs can become contaminated during patient care, at least parts of them should be cleaned and disinfected between uses, or impermeable barriers should be used and changed between each patient to limit the use of liquid disinfectants on dental chair upholstery.

Equipment Switches and Controls

Equipment switches and controls have historically been a weak point in operatory asepsis. Toggle switches with complex shapes, undercuts, and open spaces are difficult to clean and disinfect, and unfortunately may allow liquids and other sources of contamination to enter inner mechanisms of the equipment (Fig. 14-8). Hand-operated touch controls on seamless flat surfaces are more easily cleaned, disinfected, and/or covered. Nontouch controls, such as foot pedals and electronic eye switches, are optimal. Alternative technologies, such as foot controls, avoid or reduce the need for hand contact with switches. Cordless (wireless technology) foot controls make interfacing with the devices more efficient and remove the inconvenience of having to clean and navigate around floor cords.

Internal Contamination and Equipment Cleanability

Water and compressed air delivered through internal tubing in dental equipment are two examples of how contamination may collect in the equipment and be difficult or impossible to detect, access, and remove. Equipment should be designed to avoid such build-up, or provide easy access to clean and maintain internal pathways, and

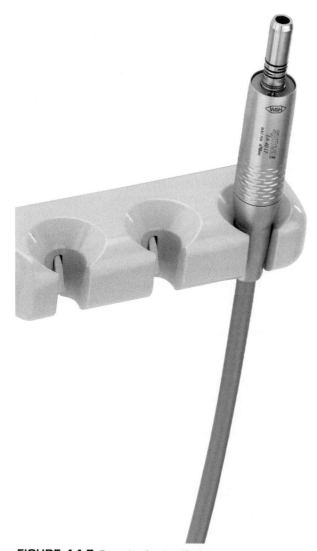

FIGURE 14-7 Example of a simplified equipment design that avoids undercuts, joints, and complex shapes that may make cleaning and disinfection difficult. Simple forms also facilitate easy placement and removal of barriers such as plastic sheets or sleeves. (Courtesy of A-dec, Inc.)

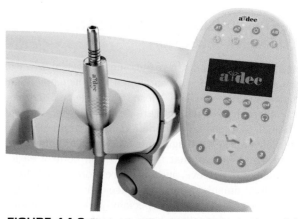

FIGURE 14-8 Flat touch-pad controls facilitate cleaning and disinfection, as well as placement of barrier sleeves or adhesive sheets. (Courtesy of A-dec, Inc.)

optimally make the internal maintenance of potentially contaminated areas, such as waterlines, an automatic feature rather than a time-consuming, labor-intensive procedure. Dental units with automatic waterline flush systems, installed filtration, or chemical treatment technology are examples of such systems. Periodic testing can confirm successful equipment control, and maintenance schedules should be managed carefully.

Alternative designs, such as external, removable, separate, sterilizable, and disposable water and air lines, make tubing more accessible and allow the delivery of sterile water and air for maximum asepsis. Peristaltic pumps, gravity drip bags, and bulb syringes, which are commonly seen in surgical settings, are examples of methods that can be used to bypass the dental unit waterlines and deliver clean or sterile water. Electrical dental handpieces, rather than compressed-air-driven handpieces, eliminate the air lines and therefore the potential for contamination in compressed air; however, they may still be water-cooled, so waterline contamination must still be controlled. Compressed-air units can become contaminated and should be fitted with filters or some other technology that can clean and dry the air before and after it is compressed.

Removable Components

For the highest level of asepsis, select patient treatment equipment with removable components to allow critical and semicritical devices to be sterilized, or single-use attachments that can be disposed of. Air-water syringe tips, high- and low-speed handpieces, and ultrasonic scalers are examples of attachments that should be removable and sterilizable for optimal asepsis.

Manufacturer Specifications and Maintenance

Equipment specification sheets indicating the building system (such as electrical or plumbing) requirements are necessary to properly integrate equipment into the office environment. This information must be supplied early in the process to ensure that provisions such as optimal numbers and locations of outlets, wiring, and fixtures are integrated into the office plan from the beginning. Not only will this make the design process more efficient, it will ensure that costly revisions are not required later in the process of design or (worse) construction. Equipment suppliers may be able to identify techniques of integrating equipment that have proved successful in other recent applications; this input often results in a much more sophisticated installation. Naturally, the manufacturer's requirements should be met to avoid invalidating any warrantees or levels of performance or effectiveness. Equipment must be accessible for maintenance, and maintenance procedures should be a managed and designated responsibility.

Digital Technology

Electronic information management impacts all aspects of the dental practice, such as record-keeping, data collection and management, diagnostics, and therapeutics. As paper charts are replaced with computerized records, the physical files that once were carried throughout the office (and perhaps outside the office), along with obvious cross-contamination potential, may bring other infection-control challenges. Electronic equipment can become contaminated from aerosols, splashes, or hand contact, and may be difficult to protect or clean and disinfect. Digital radiographs and other diagnostics replace older technology and offer improvements in asepsis, but may require special employee infection-control training and compliance. Keyboards and other devices that operators physically touch should be cleanable or covered to prevent contamination, or should use disposable components. Screens should be located where visibility is maximized for all who must see while being protected from contamination.

Ancillary Equipment: Asepsis Considerations

Ever-evolving equipment technologies may present infection-control challenges or trade-offs. For example, lasers may replace or decrease the use of scalpels, but they may also increase aerosolized contaminants unless specific suction and air filtration devices are installed. The first generations of digital radiography sensors are reusable semicritical components that cannot withstand heat sterilization, and thus require an alternative infection-control protocol. Later generations of new technologies typically improve asepsis options. Asepsis must be a key consideration when selecting new equipment. Examples of equipment that can pose infection-control challenges in operatories include the following:

a. microscopes

b. electrosurgery equipment

c. laser equipment

d. imaging equipment

e. intraoral cameras and computers

Equipment in Nonclinical Areas

In the employee zone, certain appliances, such as dishwashers, can make housekeeping more manageable. The refrigerator in the employee area should be large enough for, and restricted to, the storage of food and personal items. Separate refrigerators for patient or potentially contaminated items should be located in the clinical zone. Business office equipment can be a source of VOCs and particulate contamination, and should be kept clean to limit the spread of microorganisms by hand contact. Keyboards, telephones, electronic controls, and any frequently touched equipment or components should at least be cleaned and possibly disinfected daily, and more often as needed, such as during cold or influenza seasons.

SUMMARY

Input from the dental professional to the design team early in the process of office design, remodeling, or renovation is vital to office asepsis, and should include the overall layout, adequate space, mechanical systems, materials and finishes selection, and maintainability of the structures. Key aspects of dental equipment that affect asepsis include designs that avoid contamination and encourage safe practices, as well as surfaces, shapes, and materials that are cleanable and durable. Dental offices can be characterized by three different infection-control zones, or areas grouped together by similar functions, resulting in zone-specific infection-control standards. Clinical zones are areas dedicated to patient treatment or direct support of patient treatment, and require the highest degree of infection control in dental settings. Public zones are open to public access by patients and visitors or nondental workers, and employee zones include personal areas such as kitchens and lounges. These areas should be clean and sanitary, but are not subject to the strict infection-control standards of the clinical zone. Rooms or areas in each zone should be contiguous, or located directly next to other areas in the same infection-control zone to encourage a shared level of infection-control practices. The enduring impact of early office design decisions should facilitate asepsis and safety.

✔ Practical Dental Infection-Control Checklist

❏ When considering dental office design and equipment selection, do DHCP evaluate dental equipment features from an infection-control perspective?

❏ Are carpeting and cloth-upholstered furnishings avoided in dental operatories, laboratories, and instrument processing areas?

Review Questions

1. Which of the following statements is true?

   A. Information about asepsis is the single most important factor in dental office design that dental professionals should provide to architects.

   B. Asepsis should be a fundamental consideration in the initial design, renovation, periodic reevaluation, and ongoing maintenance of dental offices.

   C. Dental professionals should follow the lead of building designers in setting the asepsis standards for their office.

   D. The most important input from the dental professional to office designers relative to asepsis is the final approval of finishing details before occupancy.

2. The clinical zone:

   A. Should be located as near to the private bathroom as possible.

   B. Should not be near the front desk.

   C. Should be one contiguous aggregation of rooms and areas that share the highest infection-control standards and requirements.

   D. Should be maintained according to the highest standards of asepsis possible, and are most efficient if located throughout the office, alternating with private and public zones.

3. Dental offices are designed and engineered according to:

   A. Strict building regulations by OSHA, CDC, EPA, and FDA.

   B. Rules specific to dental buildings, created and enforced by ASHRAE.

   C. Local building codes and nonmandated standards written by professional organizations.

   D. Hospital building codes

4. When a dental office is located in an existing residential building, HVAC systems are likely to be inadequate to effectively manage air quality in dental offices or laboratories.

   A. True

   B. False

5. Physical barriers such as walls or panels may be necessary to prevent cross-contamination when space is limited.

   A. True

   B. False

6. Infection-control zones are

   A. Made up of rooms and areas grouped together by similar functions, resulting in zone-specific infection-control standards.

   B. Designed with different space allocations and layouts, plumbing, lighting, and air management and electrical systems, but share finishing materials and details.

   C. Different areas in the office that require different methods of asepsis maintenance because of the types of materials used for the floors, furniture, counters, and walls.

   D. All of the above.

7. Clinical rooms

A. Should be designed in an open, "universal design" way to accommodate free movement between shared work stations.

B. Should have three exits.

C. May be designed in any way as long as the surface materials are appropriate.

D. Should anticipate sequenced and/or shared work practices to avoid cross-contamination and inefficient flow patterns that might increase potential risks of occupational exposure.

8. HVAC systems control air quality, including

A. Comfort conditions such as temperature, humidity, and air flow.

B. Air contamination levels of chemicals, toxins, allergens, pathogens, and particulates.

C. Processes such as the filtration, trapping, detoxification, and irradiation of air contaminants.

D. All of the above.

9. Surface textures and relief details in clinical zones are less important today because barriers will be used.

A. True

B. False

10. Commissioning is

A. Not usually performed in small projects and is considered rarely necessary for new or renovated dental offices.

B. A process that allows the dental professional to ensure that the builders installed and connected all systems, and that the systems are operable and can be maintained.

C. Performed by architects, builders, and the OSHA inspector before occupancy.

D. A process that should include the dentist, office manager, and decorator.

11. Dental equipment surfaces should be selected to resist contamination retention and seepage of liquids into underlying mechanisms. This is best accomplished by

A. Tight joints

B. Smooth, seamless surfaces

C. Toggle switches

D. Completely covering all equipment with plastic barriers

12. Equipment switches and controls

A. Must be nontouch.

B. Are optimally nontouch, using alternatives to hand-operated switches, such as electronic-eye technology.

C. Must involve hand contact, but should be cleaned and disinfected after every patient.

D. Can be eliminated by computer-activated devices.

Critical Thinking

1. Does your office have an appropriate separate space for instrument cleaning and sterilization?

2. The dentist is planning to renovate the practice. Along with the planned renovation is the expectation that the dental chair and equipment in each operatory will be easier to clean and prepare between patient appointments. Go into one of the current operatories in your practice and develop a list of items and issues you need to address to accomplish that expectation.

SELECTED READINGS

CDC. Guidelines for infection control in dental health-care settings. MMWR 2003;51(RR-17):1–66.

Facility Guidelines Institute, American Institute of Architects (AIA) Academy of Architecture for Health, U.S. Dept. of Health and Human Services. 2006 Guidelines for Design and Construction of Healthcare Facilities. Washington, DC: AIA; 2006:1–34, 189–213.

Pollock R, Young JM. Infection-control considerations in dental office design. In: Cottone JA, Terezhalmy GT, Molinari JA, eds. Practical Infection Control in Dentistry. 2nd ed. Baltimore: Williams and Wilkins; 1996:281–293.

Sehulster LM, Chinn RYW, Arduino MJ, et al. Guidelines for environmental infection control in health-care facilities. Recommendations from CDC and the Healthcare Infection Control Practices Advisory Committee (HICPAC). Chicago, IL: American Society for Healthcare Engineering/American Hospital Association; 2004.

Tholen M. A Guide to Designing the Elegant Medical or Dental Office: The Largest Marketing Tool of Your Career. Madison, WI: Advanced Medical Publishing, Inc; 2006:2–22.

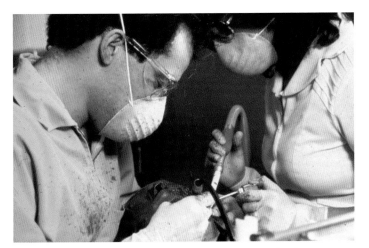

FIGURE I-1 A dentist and dental assistant using appropriate barrier techniques recommended in the mid-1980s, including a mask, gloves, protective eyewear, short-sleeve clinic attire, and a rubber dam on the patient. Red dye simulating saliva can be seen splashing on the face, hair, gloves, and chest of both the dentist and the dental assistant during a single, Class II operative procedure on a mandibular second molar.

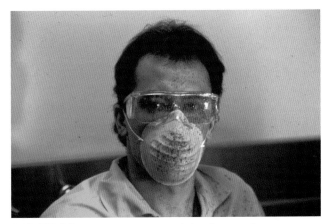

FIGURE I-2 The dentist after completing the operative procedure.

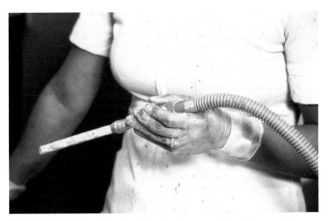

FIGURE I-3 The dental assistant after completing the operative procedure described in Figure I-1.

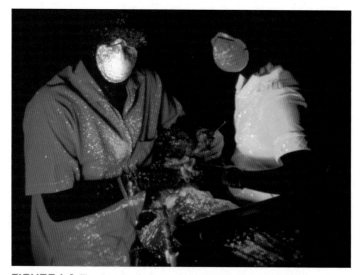

FIGURE I-4 The dental operatory after a single, Class II operative procedure on a mandibular second molar; fluorescent dye was used to trace saliva throughout the procedure.

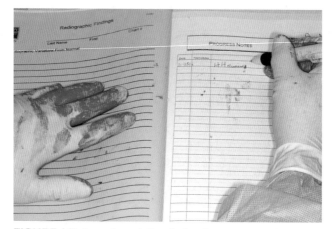

FIGURE I-5 Recording notations in the chart may transmit oral fluids to the papers if they are handled before gloves are removed and hands are washed.

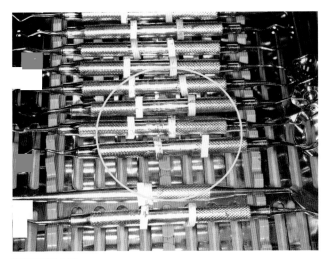

FIGURE I-6

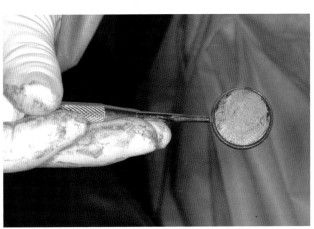

FIGURE I-7

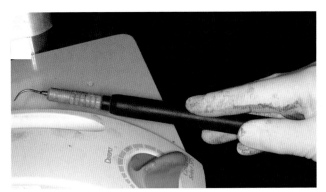

FIGURE I-8

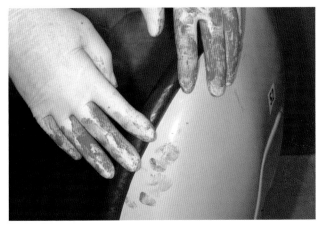

FIGURE I-9

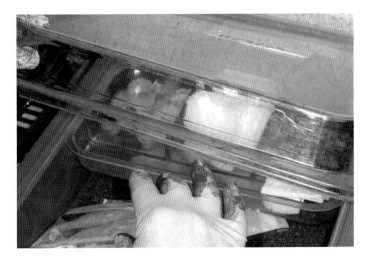

FIGURE I-10

FIGURES I-6 to I-10 The instrument tray, instruments, and equipment become contaminated with accumulated "saliva" as items are handled during treatment.

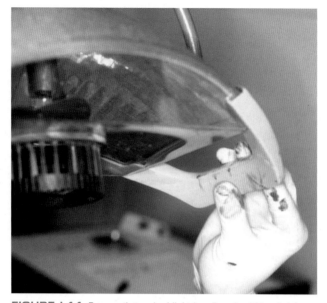

FIGURE I-11 Frequently-touched light handles should be disinfected or covered properly between patient appointments.

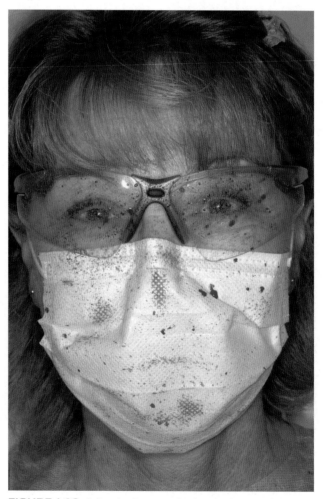

FIGURE I-12 Saliva may be transmitted to the face, mask, and glasses of the operator during the polishing procedure.

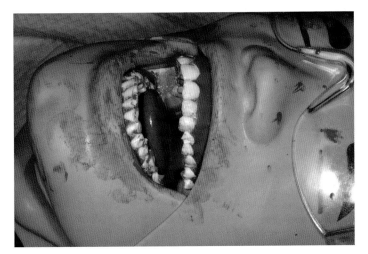

FIGURE I-13 Visualized saliva is also evident on the patient's face after prophylaxis.

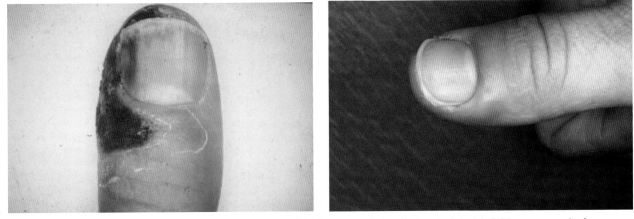

A

B

FIGURE I-14 Representative occupational microbial infections are noted on the hands of dental clinicians as a result of treating patients without wearing gloves. **(A)** Herpetic whitlow contracted from a patient who was asymptomatically shedding herpes simplex virus into the saliva. **(B)** An acute pyoderma from *Staphylococcus aureus* entering into an open cut in the finger.

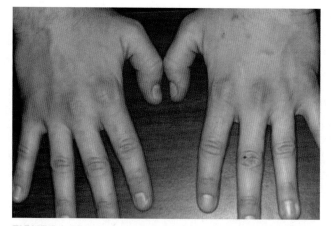

FIGURE I-15 Irritation contact dermatitis on the hands of a dental student caused by improper drying of hands after hand washing.

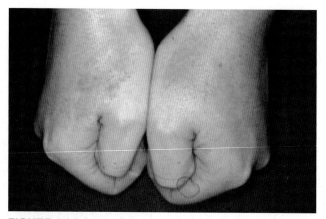

FIGURE I-16 Type I hypersensitivity reaction to NRL proteins in powdered latex gloves.

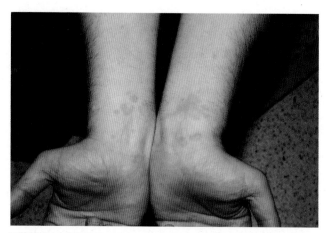

FIGURE I-17 Type IV allergic contact dermatitis 24 hours after wearing latex gloves. The reaction resolved within 96 hours with necrosis and sloughing of the affected tissue site.

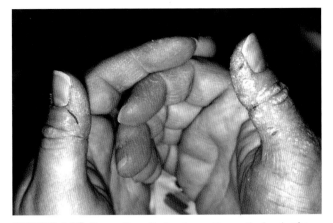

FIGURE I-18 Severe Type IV allergic reaction on the hands of a dental assistant following challenge with a glutaraldehyde chemical disinfectant/sterilant. The reaction had become increasingly more irritating and damaging to keratinized and deeper epithelial tissues over time with repeated direct contact of the chemical on the hands.

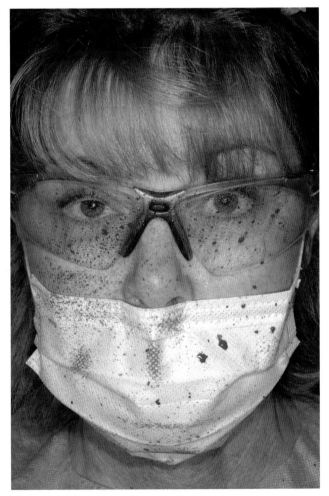

FIGURE I-19 Demonstration using the red saliva model described in Chapter 1, showing aerosolized "patient" spatter on the face of a dental hygienist after she used an ultrasonic scaler while improperly wearing her mask.

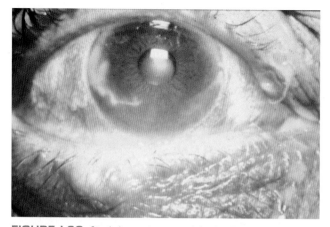

FIGURE I-20 *Staphylococcus aureus* infection in the eye of a dentist who was not wearing protective eyewear during an operative dentistry procedure on a patient. Note the acute inflammation and accumulation of a suppurative exudate around the eye. Aerosolized spatter generated during patient care can expose the eyes, the least protected parts of the body, to numerous microbial pathogens.

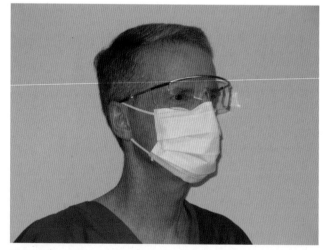

FIGURE I-21 A dental clinician wearing appropriate protective eyewear and a mask to protect the eyes and nose from both macroscopic (i.e., pieces of teeth, dental materials, or other visible particles) trauma and microscopic exposure from oral microorganisms in treatment aerosols and spatter.

IV

Infection Control Procedures and Protocols

15

Management of Occupational Exposures to Blood and Other Body Fluids

Jennifer A. Harte

John A. Molinari

LEARNING OBJECTIVES

After completion of this chapter individuals should be able to:

1 Describe the potential for transmission of bloodborne pathogens (BBPs) in dental settings.

2 Describe important factors that can influence the risk of infection following occupational exposures.

3 Describe the risks of infection after occupational exposure to HBV-, HCV-, or HIV-infected blood.

4 Describe the rationale for developing a postexposure management program.

5 Describe appropriate procedures that should be included in a postexposure management program for healthcare facilities.

6 Discuss the rationale for and use of specific recommended drugs for postexposure treatment involving possible exposures to HBV, HCV, and HIV.

KEY TERMS

Bloodborne pathogens: disease-producing microorganisms spread by contact with blood or other body fluids contaminated with blood from an infected person. Examples include HBV, HCV, and HIV.

Engineering controls: controls (e.g., sharps disposal containers, self-sheathing needles, and safer medical devices, such as sharps with engineered sharps injury protections and needleless systems) that isolate or remove the BBPs hazard from the workplace.

Hepatitis B immune globulin (HBIG): a product available for prophylaxis against HBV infection. HBIG is prepared from plasma containing high titers of anti-HBs and provides short-term protection (3–6 months).

Hepatitis B (HB) vaccine: HB immunization indicates that the person who received the HB vaccine has developed adequate HB surface antibody and is protected against HBV infection.

Occupational-exposure incident: an occupational-exposure incident can be defined as a percutaneous injury (e.g., needlestick or cut with a sharp object) or contact of mucous membrane or nonintact skin (e.g., exposed skin that is chapped, abraded, or afflicted with dermatitis) with potentially infectious blood, saliva, tissue, or other body fluids that may result from the performance of an employee's duties.

Other potentially infectious materials (OPIM): an OSHA term that refers to (a) the following human body fluids: semen, vaginal secretions, cerebrospinal fluid, synovial fluid, pleural fluid, pericardial fluid, peritoneal fluid, amniotic fluid, saliva in dental procedures, any body fluid that is visibly contaminated with blood, and all body fluids in situations where it is difficult or impossible to differentiate between body fluids; (b) any unfixed tissue or organ (other than intact skin) from a human (living or dead); and (c) HIV-containing cell or tissue cultures, organ cultures; HIV- or HBV-containing culture medium or other solutions; and blood, organs, or other tissues from experimental animals infected with HIV or HBV.

Percutaneous injury: an injury that penetrates the skin (e.g., needlestick, or cut with a sharp object).

Postexposure prophylaxis (PEP): the administration of medications following an occupational exposure in an attempt to prevent infection.

Qualified healthcare professional: any licensed healthcare provider who can provide counseling and perform all medical evaluations and procedures in accordance with the most current recommendations of the U.S. Department of Health and Human Services, including PEP when indicated.

Work practice controls: practices incorporated into the everyday work routine that reduce the likelihood of exposure by altering the manner in which a task is performed (e.g., prohibiting recapping of needles by a two-handed technique).

Preventing bloodborne virus transmission in healthcare facilities requires the implementation of a comprehensive, multifaceted program that includes compliance by those healthcare professionals who have occupational risks. Safeguards for avoiding exposure to blood and **other potentially infectious body materials (OPIM)** include the use of aseptic technique precautions, personal protective equipment (PPE), engineering and work practice controls, and immunization as primary strategies. Yet occupational exposures still occur despite the best efforts of healthcare providers to prevent them. An **occupational-exposure incident** may be defined as a needlestick or any puncture wound with a contaminated object, a splash of blood or body fluid onto mucous membranes, or a splash of blood or other body fluids onto nonintact skin. To help put this in proper perspective at the outset of this chapter, consider the fact that there are more than 8 million healthcare personnel (HCP) in the United States. Although precise numbers are not available, it

has been estimated that HCP may sustain as many as 600,000 percutaneous injuries annually. Multiple retrospective studies suggest that at least half of such accidents are not reported. When they occur, however, appropriate postexposure management is essential to reduce the risk of subsequent infection. While there are several respiratory, contact, and wound infections that could present dangerous sequelae for dental professionals, the following sections will focus on bloodborne occupational risks. The reader can find more information on the bloodborne viruses discussed by referring to Chapter 2 (HBV and HCV) and Chapter 3 (HIV).

When evaluating occupational exposures to fluids that might contain HBV, HCV, and HIV, blood and all body fluids containing visible blood are considered infectious. During dental procedures, saliva is predictably contaminated with blood. It can still be present in limited quantities even when blood is not visible. Therefore saliva is considered an OPIM by the Centers for Disease Control and Prevention (CDC) and the

Occupational Safety and Health Administration (OSHA). Current data and knowledge indicate that in dental treatment settings it is likely that only very small quantities of blood are present and the risks for transmission of HBV, HCV, and HIV are often small. However, despite this low risk of transmission, a **qualified healthcare professional** should evaluate any occupational exposure to saliva in dental settings, regardless of the presence of visible blood.

Dental practices and laboratories should establish written, step-by-step programs that include HB vaccination and postexposure management protocols. This program should also contain plans for reporting exposures in order to quickly evaluate the risk of infection, methods to inform employees about treatments available to help prevent infection, and ways to monitor side effects of treatments and determine whether infection occurs. Policies should be consistent with the practices and procedures for worker protection required by OSHA and with current United States Public Health Service (PHS) recommendations for managing occupational exposures to blood. The most recent CDC recommendations addressing the management of occupational blood exposures can be found in Table 15-1.

BLOODBORNE PATHOGENS AND OCCUPATIONAL-EXPOSURE RISKS FOR DENTISTRY

Bloodborne pathogens (BBPs) are disease-producing microorganisms spread by contact with blood or other body fluids that have been contaminated with blood from an infected person. Healthcare personnel are at risk for occupational exposure to BBPs, including HBV, HCV, and HIV. Exposures occur through needlesticks or cuts from other sharp instruments contaminated with an infected patient's blood or through contact of the eye, nose, mouth, or skin with a patient's blood. An occupational-exposure incident is defined as a percutaneous injury or contact of mucous membrane or nonintact skin with blood, saliva, tissue, or other body fluids that are potentially infectious. **Percutaneous injuries** are needlesticks or cuts with a sharp object. Nonintact skin is exposed skin that is chapped, abraded, or afflicted with dermatitis. Since occupational-exposure incidents might place dental personnel at risk for HBV, HCV, or HIV infection, these accidents should be evaluated immediately by a qualified healthcare professional following initial treatment of the exposure site. The CDC defines a qualified healthcare professional as any healthcare provider who can provide counseling and perform all medical evaluations and procedures in accordance with the most current recommendations of the PHS, including chemotherapeutic **postexposure prophylaxis (PEP)**

when indicated. In addition, this individual should be familiar with the unique nature of dental injuries so that he or she can provide appropriate guidance as needed for PEP. The importance of selecting a qualified healthcare professional *before* workers are placed at risk cannot be overemphasized, and this step is necessary to provide dental personnel with appropriate services. Dental schools and hospital dental practices can coordinate with departments that provide personnel health services. Since most dental practices are in ambulatory, private settings that do not have licensed medical staff and facilities to provide complete on-site health service programs, arrangements will have to be coordinated with external healthcare facilities. This might include an occupational health program of a hospital, a nearby educational institution, or healthcare facilities that offer personnel health services.

Important factors that influence the overall risk for occupational exposures to BBPs include the number of infected individuals in the patient population, and the type and number of blood contacts. It is important to note here that most exposures do not result in infection. Following a specific exposure, however, the risk of infection may vary with factors such as:

- the pathogen involved.
- the type of exposure.
- the amount of blood involved in the exposure.
- the amount of virus in the patient's blood at the time of exposure.

Hepatitis B Virus

As discussed in Chapter 2, healthcare occupational transmission of HBV occurs by direct exposure to blood and other infected body fluids. This hepadnavirus is relatively resistant compared to many other viruses, as it is capable of surviving in blood outside of the body and on inanimate environmental surfaces for approximately 1 week. HCP who have received the **hepatitis B (HB) vaccine** and have developed immunity to the virus are at virtually no risk for infection. The risk for a susceptible person from a single needlestick or a cut exposure to HBV-infected blood, however, ranges from 6% to 30%. The potential for viral infection in this instance depends on the HB e antigen (HBeAg) status of the source individual. Individuals who are both HB surface antigen (HBsAg)-positive and HBeAg-positive typically have much higher concentrations of virus in their blood and are more likely to transmit HBV than those who are HBeAg-negative. While there is a risk for HBV infection from exposures of mucous membranes or nonintact skin (i.e., chapped or abraded skin), there is no known risk for HBV infection from exposure to intact skin.

Table 15-1 Recommendations for Managing Occupational Blood Exposures

Establish written protocols for management of occupational exposures:
- Based on current PHS/CDC guidelines
- Review periodically
- Provide training to personnel
  - prevention and response to occupational exposures
- Identify a qualified healthcare professional who
  - is familiar with current PHS postexposure management recommendations, antiretroviral therapy, bloodborne disease transmission, and the OSHA BBP standard
  - will ensure prompt evaluation, treatment, management, and follow-up
  - will provide necessary counseling

Provide immediate care to the exposure site:
- Wash wounds and skin with soap and water
- Flush mucous membranes with water
- No evidence exists that using antiseptics for wound care or expressing fluid by squeezing the wound further reduces the risk of BBP transmission

Immediately report the exposure to the infection-control coordinator, who should:
- Initiate referral to a qualified healthcare professional
- Complete necessary reports

Include the following information in the postexposure report:
- date and time of exposure
- details of the procedure being performed
  - where and how the exposure occurred
  - type of device involved
    - how and when during its handling the exposure occurred
- Details of the exposure
  - type and amount of fluid or material
  - severity of the exposure
- Details about the exposure source (e.g., HBV, HCV, HIV status)
- Details about the exposed individual (e.g., HB vaccination and vaccine-response status)
- Details about counseling, postexposure management, and follow-up.

Evaluate the exposure
Determine risk associated with exposure
- **Exposures** posing risk of infection transmission
  - Percutaneous injury
  - Mucous membrane exposure
  - Nonintact skin exposure
  - Bites resulting in blood exposure to either person involved

- **Substances** posing risk of infection transmission
  - Blood
  - Fluids containing visible blood
  - Potentially infectious fluids (semen; vaginal secretions; saliva; and cerebrospinal, synovial, pleural, peritoneal, pericardial, and amniotic fluids) or tissue
  - Concentrated virus

- **Status**
  Determine infectious status of source (if not already known)
  - Presence of HBsAg
  - Presence of HCV antibody
  - Presence of HIV antibody*
  - For unknown sources, evaluate the likelihood of exposure to a source at high risk for HBV, HCV, or HIV infection
  - Do not test discarded needles

- **Susceptibility**
  Determine susceptibility of exposed person
  - HB vaccine status
  - HBV immune status if vaccine response status is unknown
  - Anti-HCV and ALT
  - HIV antibody

*Consider using rapid testing

Additional Resources
National Clinicians' Postexposure Prophylaxis Hotline (PEPline) http://www.ucsf.edu/hivcntr (888) 448-4911

Give PEP for exposures posing risk of infection transmission
- **HBV**
  - Give PEP as soon as possible, preferably within 24 hours
  - PEP can be given to pregnant women
- **HCV**-PEP not recommended
- **HIV**
  - Initiate PEP within hours of exposure
  - Offer pregnancy testing to all women of childbearing age not known to be pregnant
  - Seek expert consultation if viral resistance is suspected
  - Administer PEP for 4 weeks if tolerated

NOTE: In 2001 the CDC published guidelines for the management of occupational exposures to HBV, HCV, and HIV, and recommendations for PEP. The 2005 CDC guidelines only update the HIV recommendations and do not pertain to HBV and HCV. For HBV and HCV the 2001 guidelines should still be referenced.
Both the 2001 and 2005 CDC guidelines are available by visiting http://www.cdc.gov/ncidod/dhqp/gl_occupational.html.

Perform follow-up testing and provide counseling
- **HBV exposures**
  - Test for anti-HBs 1–2 months after last dose of vaccine if only vaccine is given
  - Follow-up not indicated if exposed person is immune to HBV or received HBIG PEP
- **HCV exposures**
  - Perform testing for anti-HCV and ALT 4–6 months after exposure
  - Perform HCV RNA testing at 4–6 weeks if earlier diagnosis of HCV infection is desired
  - Confirm repeatedly reactive anti-HCV EIAs with supplemental tests
- **HIV exposures**
  - Evaluate exposed persons taking PEP within 72 hours after exposure and monitor for drug toxicity for at least 2 weeks
  - Perform HIV-antibody testing for at least 6 months postexposure (e.g., at baseline, 6 weeks, 3 months, and 6 months)
  - Perform HIV antibody testing for illness compatible with an acute retroviral syndrome
  - Advise exposed persons to use precautions to prevent secondary transmission during the follow-up period

Courtesy of the USAF Dental Evaluation and Consultation Service Col Jennifer Harte. CDC. Updated U.S. Public Health Service guidelines for the management of occupational exposures to HBV, HCV, and HIV and recommendations for postexposure prophylaxis. MMWR 2001;50(RR-11); CDC. Updated U.S. Public Health Service guidelines for the management of occupational exposures to HIV and recommendations for postexposure prophylaxis. MMWR 2005;54(RR-9):1–17.

ALT, alanine aminotransferase; BBP, bloodborne pathogen; CDC, Centers for Disease Control and Prevention; EIA, enzyme immunoassay; HBV, hepatitis B virus; HBIG, hepatitis B immunoglobulin; HCV, hepatitis C virus; HIV, human immunodeficiency virus; PEP, postexposure prophylaxis; PHS, Public Health Service.

An exposure can be defined as a percutaneous injury (e.g., needlestick or cut with a sharp object) or contact of mucous membrane or nonintact skin (e.g., exposed skin that is chapped, abraded, or afflicted with dermatitis) with blood, saliva, tissue, or other body fluids that are potentially infectious. Exposure incidents might place dental healthcare personnel at risk for HBV, HCV, or HIV infection, and therefore should be evaluated immediately following treatment of the exposure site by a qualified healthcare professional.

Hepatitis C Virus

Based on limited studies, the risk for infection after a needlestick or cut exposure to HCV-infected blood is approximately 1.8% for health professionals. Recent data collected since the late 1980s suggest that, thanks to the implementation and routine use of standard (formerly universal) precautions, dental professionals have lowered their HCV occupational risks to the baseline level found within the general population. In addition, the risk following a blood exposure to the eye, nose or mouth is unknown, but is believed to be very small. However, HCV infection from a blood splash to the eye has been reported. There also has been a report of HCV transmission that may have resulted from exposure to nonintact skin, but there remains no known risk from exposure to intact skin.

Even with these accumulated data indicating a relatively low incidence among dental healthcare personnel (DHCP), HCV remains a major occupational concern. The most hazardous type of exposure that can increase the possibility of HCV infection is a needlestick injury. A second important feature of HCV healthcare risks is related to the virus replication cycle and the titers of infectious virions in the blood. HCV is present in concentrations ranging from only a few virions to 100,000 or more particles per milliliter of patient's blood. Although this reinforces its position as a greater infectious risk than HIV, the concentrations fall far below those routinely seen in HBV-infected persons.

Human Immunodeficiency Virus

The average risk of HIV infection after a needlestick or cut exposure to HIV-infected blood is 0.3%, or about one in 300. Stated another way, 99.7% of all healthcare provider-needlestick/cut exposures do not lead to HIV infection. As of this writing, there have not been any confirmed occupational HIV infections in DHCP since the first anti-HIV serologic assays were developed in 1984. Regarding mucous-membrane exposures, the risk after exposure of the eye, nose, or mouth to HIV-infected blood is estimated to be, on average, 0.1%, or one in 1,000. The risk after exposure of the skin to HIV-infected blood is estimated to be less than 0.1%. A small amount of blood on intact skin probably poses no risk at all. There have been no documented cases of HIV transmission because of an exposure involving a small amount of blood on intact skin, such as a few drops of blood on skin for a short period of time.

Bloodborne Pathogens and Aerosols

A visible spray is created during the use of air-water syringes and rotary dental and surgical instruments such as handpieces and ultrasonic scalers. This spray contains primarily a large-particle spatter of water, saliva, blood, microorganisms, and other debris. This spatter travels only a short distance and settles out quickly, landing on the floor, nearby operatory surfaces, dental personnel providing care, or the patient. This spatter can commonly be seen on face shields, protective eyewear, and other surfaces immediately after the dental procedure, but after a short time it may dry clear and not be easily detected. The spray may also contain some aerosol. Aerosols take considerable energy to generate, consist of particles less than 10 microns in diameter, and are not typically visible to the naked eye. Aerosols can remain airborne for extended periods of time and may be inhaled. Aerosols should not be confused with the large-particle spatter that makes up the bulk of the spray from handpieces and ultrasonic scalers. To prevent contact with splashes and spatter, dental personnel should position patients properly and make appropriate use of PPE (e.g., face shields, surgical masks, and gowns), rubber dams, and high-velocity air evacuation.

While it is known that BBPs can be transmitted through mucous-membrane exposure, there are no known instances of a BBP being transmitted by an aerosol in a clinical setting. In studies conducted in dental operatories and hemodialysis centers, HBsAg could not be detected in the air during the treatment of HB carriers, including during procedures known to generate aerosols. This suggests that detection of HIV in aerosols would also be uncommon, since the concentration of HIV in blood is generally lower that that of HBV. Finally, detection of HIV in an aerosol would not necessarily mean that HIV is readily transmissible by this route. In the healthcare setting, the major risks of HIV infection are blood contact because of percutaneous injuries and, to a lesser extent, mucous-membrane and skin contact. The possibility that HIV may be transmitted via aerosolized blood must be considered theoretical at this time.

POSTEXPOSURE MANAGEMENT AFTER AN INCIDENT

All occupational-exposure incidents should be treated as medical emergencies and tended to immediately. The importance of reporting and follow-up cannot be overstated. Support from all at-risk employees and their supervisors needs to be reinforced constantly in order for a program to have the best chance of successfully achieving its objectives. These objectives include the following:

1. Written policies and procedures to facilitate prompt reporting, evaluation, counseling, treatment, and medical follow-up of all occupational exposure should be available to all dental health professionals.

2. HCP should be educated about infection control and their responsibility in preventing cross-infection.

3. Prompt care should be provided to personnel who have experienced work-related exposures or occupational illnesses.
4. The confidentiality of exposed and source persons should be maintained.
5. Occupational risks in the dental facility or setting should be identified, and effective preventive measures instituted.
6. Follow-up testing should be available to all personnel who are concerned about possible infection through occupational exposure.
7. Employee misconceptions and fears concerning occupational infectious disease risks should be alleviated.

Although there may be variation in some of the specific details, a few fundamental components of a post-exposure management plan should be inherent in all programs:

1. Wounds and skin sites that have been in contact with blood or body fluids should be washed with soap and water; mucous membranes should be flushed with water. There is no evidence of benefit from applying antiseptics or disinfectants such as bleach or other caustic agents or squeezing ("milking") puncture sites.
2. The injury should be reported immediately to the employer or designated, responsible individual, and appropriate incident reporting forms completed.
3. It is very important to follow all instructions for immediate medical evaluation and follow-up care.

The example form shown in Figure 15-1 illustrates the inclusion of pertinent information about the exposure accident. When this is reviewed by the qualified healthcare professional during the initial evaluation of the incident, it can greatly assist in appropriately managing the occupational-exposure incident. This important information includes:

- The date and time of exposure.
- Details of the procedure being performed, including where and how the exposure occurred and whether the exposure involved a sharp device, the type and brand of device, and how and when during its handling the exposure occurred.
- Details of the exposure, including its severity and the type and amount of fluid or material. The severity of a percutaneous injury, for example, might be measured by the depth of the wound, gauge of the needle, and whether fluid was injected. For skin or mucous-membrane exposure, the estimated volume of material,

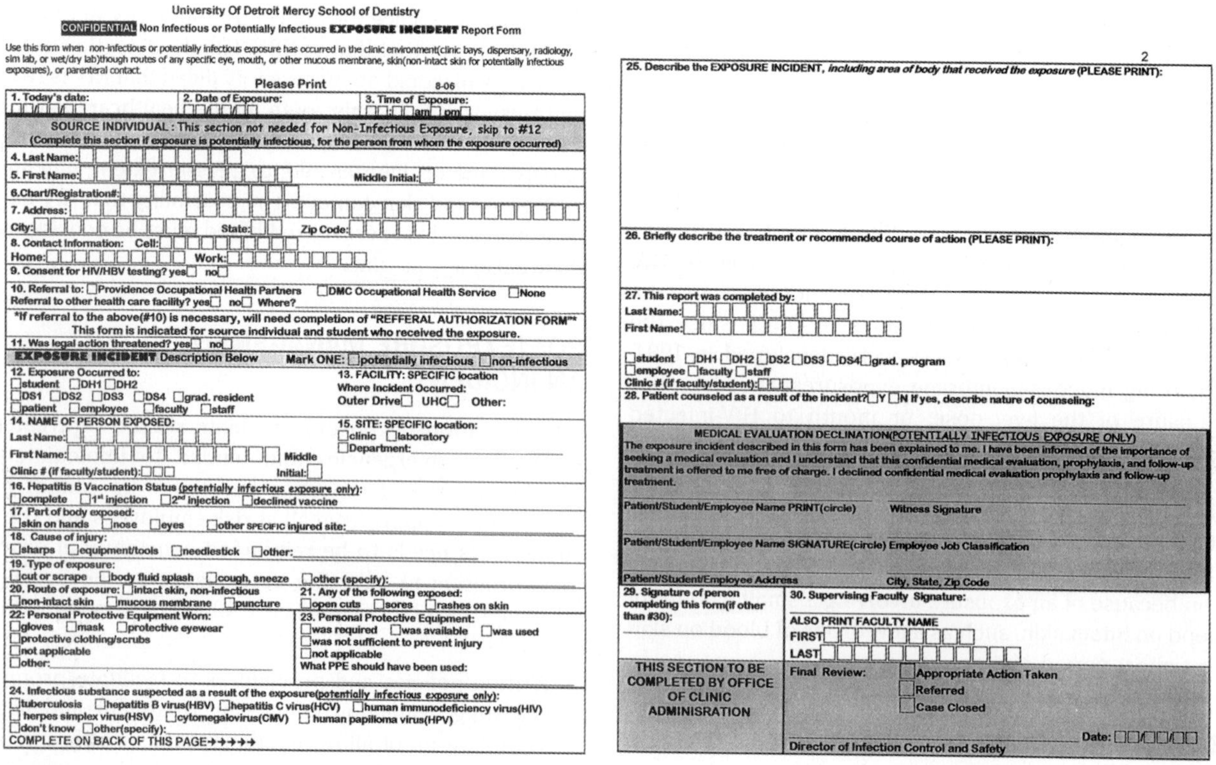

University Of Detroit Mercy School of Dentistry

CONFIDENTIAL Non Infectious or Potentially Infectious **EXPOSURE INCIDENT** Report Form

Use this form when non-infectious or potentially infectious exposure has occurred in the clinic environment(clinic bays, dispensary, radiology, sim lab, or wet/dry lab)though routes of any specific eye, mouth, or other mucous membrane, skin(non-intact skin for potentially infectious exposures), or parenteral contact.

Please Print 8-06

1. Today's date: ☐☐/☐☐/☐☐ 2. Date of Exposure: ☐☐/☐☐/☐☐ 3. Time of Exposure: ☐☐:☐☐am☐ pm☐

SOURCE INDIVIDUAL : This section not needed for Non-Infectious Exposure, skip to #12
(Complete this section if exposure is potentially infectious, for the person from whom the exposure occurred)

4. Last Name:
5. First Name: Middle Initial:
6.Chart/Registration#:
7. Address:
City: State: Zip Code:
8. Contact Information: Cell:
Home: Work:
9. Consent for HIV/HBV testing? yes☐ no☐
10. Referral to: ☐Providence Occupational Health Partners ☐DMC Occupational Health Service ☐None
Referral to other health care facility? yes☐ no☐ Where?
If referral to the above(#10) is necessary, will need completion of "REFFERAL AUTHORIZATION FORM"
This form is indicated for source individual and student who received the exposure.
11. Was legal action threatened? yes☐ no☐

EXPOSURE INCIDENT Description Below Mark ONE: ☐potentially infectious ☐non-infectious

12. Exposure Occurred to:
☐student ☐DH1 ☐DH2
☐DS1 ☐DS2 ☐DS3 ☐DS4 ☐grad. resident
☐patient ☐employee ☐faculty ☐staff

13. FACILITY: SPECIFIC location
Where Incident Occurred:
Outer Drive☐ UHC☐ Other:

14. NAME OF PERSON EXPOSED:
Last Name:
First Name: Middle Initial:
Clinic # (if faculty/student):

15. SITE: SPECIFIC location:
☐clinic ☐laboratory
☐Department:

16. Hepatitis B Vaccination Status (potentially infectious exposure only):
☐complete ☐1st injection ☐2nd injection ☐declined vaccine
17. Part of body exposed:
☐skin on hands ☐nose ☐eyes ☐other SPECIFIC injured site:
18. Cause of injury:
☐sharps ☐equipment/tools ☐needlestick ☐other:
19. Type of exposure:
☐cut or scrape ☐body fluid splash ☐cough, sneeze ☐other (specify):
20. Route of exposure: ☐intact skin, non-infectious
☐non-intact skin ☐mucous membrane ☐puncture
21. Any of the following exposed:
☐open cuts ☐sores ☐rashes on skin
22: Personal Protective Equipment Worn:
☐gloves ☐mask ☐protective eyewear
☐protective clothing/scrubs
☐not applicable
☐other:
23. Personal Protective Equipment:
☐was required ☐was available ☐was used
☐was not sufficient to prevent injury
☐not applicable
What PPE should have been used:
24. Infectious substance suspected as a result of the exposure(potentially infectious exposure only):
☐tuberculosis ☐hepatitis B virus(HBV) ☐hepatitis C virus(HCV) ☐human immunodeficiency virus(HIV)
☐ herpes simplex virus(HSV) ☐cytomegalovirus(CMV) ☐ human papilloma virus(HPV)
☐don't know ☐other(specify):
COMPLETE ON BACK OF THIS PAGE→→→→→

2

25. Describe the EXPOSURE INCIDENT, *including area of body that received the exposure* (PLEASE PRINT):

26. Briefly describe the treatment or recommended course of action (PLEASE PRINT):

27. This report was completed by:
Last Name:
First Name:
☐student ☐DH1 ☐DH2 ☐DS2 ☐DS3 ☐DS4☐grad. program
☐employee ☐faculty ☐staff
Clinic # (if faculty/student):
28. Patient counseled as a result of the incident?☐Y ☐N If yes, describe nature of counseling:

MEDICAL EVALUATION DECLINATION(POTENTIALLY INFECTIOUS EXPOSURE ONLY)
The exposure incident described in this form has been explained to me. I have been informed of the importance of seeking a medical evaluation and I understand that this confidential medical evaluation, prophylaxis, and follow-up treatment is offered to me free of charge. I declined confidential medical evaluation prophylaxis and follow-up treatment.

Patient/Student/Employee Name PRINT(circle) Witness Signature
Patient/Student/Employee Name SIGNATURE(circle) Employee Job Classification
Patient/Student/Employee Address City, State, Zip Code

29. Signature of person completing this form(if other than #30):
30. Supervising Faculty Signature:
ALSO PRINT FACULTY NAME
FIRST
LAST

THIS SECTION TO BE COMPLETED BY OFFICE OF CLINIC ADMINISRATION
Final Review: ☐Appropriate Action Taken ☐Referred ☐Case Closed
Director of Infection Control and Safety Date: ☐☐/☐☐/☐☐

FIGURE 15-1 Sample exposure-incident form.

duration of contact, and condition of skin should be noted. Other considerations involve noting whether the skin was chapped, abraded, or intact.

- Details regarding whether the source material was known to contain HIV or other BBPs, and, if the source was infected with HIV, the stage of disease, history of antiretroviral therapy, and viral load, if known.
- Details regarding the exposed person (e.g., HB vaccination and vaccine-response status).
- Details regarding counseling, postexposure management, and follow-up.

Each occupational exposure should be evaluated individually in terms of its potential to transmit HBV, HCV, and HIV, based on

- the type and amount of body substance involved,
- the type of exposure (e.g., percutaneous injury, mucous membrane or nonintact skin exposure, or bites resulting in blood exposure to either person involved),
- the infection status of the source,
- the susceptibility of the exposed person.

In the event the source individual cannot be identified because of certain types of accidents, such as an employee being injured while cleaning instruments from multiple patient appointments, or if the source cannot be tested, the circumstances of the exposure incident should be assessed by the qualified health professional to determine the likelihood of transmission of HBV, HCV, or HIV. Decisions regarding appropriate management should be handled on a case-by-case basis. Certain situations, as well as the type of exposure, may suggest an increased or decreased transmission risk. For example, it is helpful to know

- Where and under what circumstances did the accident occur? Exposure to a visibly bloody device would obviously suggest a higher-risk exposure than exposure to an instrument that has been processed through a washer-disinfector.
- What is the prevalence of HBV, HCV, or HIV in the population? An exposure that occurs in a geographic area where injectable-drug use is prevalent, or in an AIDS unit, would be considered epidemiologically to have a higher risk for transmission than one that occurs in a facility where no known HIV-infected patients are present.

Testing of needles and other sharp instruments implicated in an exposure, regardless of whether the source is known or unknown, is not recommended. The reliability and interpretation of findings in such circumstances are unknown, and testing might be hazardous to individuals handling the contaminated sharp instrument.

RECOMMENDATION OF DRUGS AS A COMPONENT OF A POSTEXPOSURE MANAGEMENT PLAN

In 2001 the CDC published guidelines for the management of occupational exposures to HBV, HCV, and HIV, and recommendations for PEP. In 2005 the CDC updated the HIV recommendations because the Food and Drug Administration (FDA) had approved new antiretroviral agents and additional information had become available regarding the use and safety of HIV PEP. The 2001 guidelines remain applicable for HBV and HCV postexposure recommendations.

HBV

Table 15-2 provides a summary of the recommendations for PEP following an exposure to HBV. **Hepatitis B immune globulin (HBIG)** and/or the HB vaccine may be recommended depending on the source person's infection status, the exposed person's vaccination status, and (if vaccinated) his/her response to the vaccine. Postexposure treatment should begin as soon as possible after exposure, preferably within 24 hours and no later than 7 days.

HCV

There is no postexposure treatment that will prevent HCV infection. However, the PHS recommends the following

- Perform testing for anti-HCV and certain liver enzymes 4–6 months after exposure.
- Perform HCV RNA testing at 4–6 weeks if an earlier diagnosis of HCV infection is desired.
- Confirm repeatedly reactive anti-HCV enzyme immunoassays with supplemental tests.

HIV

The PHS recommends antiretroviral agents from five classes of drugs currently available to treat HIV infection. The 2005 PHS guidelines provide guidance for two-or-more drug PEP regimens on the basis of the level of risk for HIV transmission represented by the exposure, such as those involving a larger volume of blood with a larger amount of HIV or a concern about drug-resistant HIV (Table 15-3). Treatment should be started as soon as possible, preferably within hours (as opposed to days) after the exposure. Although animal studies suggest that treatment is less effective when started more than 24–36 hours after exposure, the time frame after which no benefit is gained in humans is not known. Starting treatment after a longer period, such as 1 week, may be considered

Table 15-2 Recommended PEP for Exposure to HBV

Vaccination and antibody response status of exposed workers*	Treatment		
	Source HBsAg[†] positive	Source HBsAg[†] negative	Source unknown or not available for testing
Unvaccinated	HBIG[§] × + and initiate HB vaccine series[¶]	Initiate HB vaccine series	Initiate HB vaccine series
Previously vaccinated Known responder** Known nonresponder[††]	No treatment HBIG × 1 and initiate revaccination or HBIG × 2[§§]	No treatment No treatment	No treatment If known high-risk source, treat as if source were HBsAg-positive
Antibody response unknown	Test exposed person for anti-HBs[¶¶] 1. If adequate,** no treatment is necessary 2. If inadequate,[††] administer HBIG × 1 and vaccine booster	No treatment	Test exposed person for anti-HBs 1. If adequate,[¶] no treatment is necessary 2. If inadequate,[¶] administer vaccine booster and recheck titer in 1–2 months

Adapted from CDC. Updated U.S. Public Health Service guidelines for the management of occupational exposures to HBV, HCV, and HIV and recommendations for postexposure prophylaxis. MMWR 2001;50(RR-11):22.

*Persons who have previously been infected with HBV are immune to reinfection and do not require PEP.

[†]HBsAg.

[§]HB immune globulin; dose is 0.06 mL/kg intramuscularly.

[¶]HB vaccine.

**A responder is a person with adequate levels of serum antibody to HBsAg (i.e., anti-HBs ≥10 mIU/mL).

[††]A nonresponder is a person with inadequate response to vaccination (i.e., serum anti-HBs <10 mIU/mL).

[§§]The option of giving one dose of HBIG and reinitiating the vaccine series is preferred for nonresponders who have not completed a second three-dose vaccine series. For persons who previously completed a second vaccine series but failed to respond, two doses of HBIG are preferred.

[¶¶]Antibody to HBsAg.

for exposures that represent an increased risk of transmission. The exposed person should be reevaluated within 72 hours so that drug regimens can be altered as additional information becomes available. If a source patient is determined to be HIV-negative, PEP should be discontinued.

Differences in side effects associated with the use of these drugs may influence which drugs are selected in a specific situation. Recommendations are intended to provide guidance to clinicians and may be modified on a case-by-case basis. Determining which drugs and how many drugs to use, or when to change a treatment regimen, is largely a matter of judgment. Whenever possible, consulting an expert with experience in the use of antiviral drugs is advised, especially if a recommended drug is not available, the source patient's virus is likely to be resistant to one or more recommended drugs, or the drugs are poorly tolerated.

Unfortunately, individuals often fail to complete the recommended regiment because of the side effects they experience, such as nausea and diarrhea. These symptoms often can be managed with medications that target the specific symptoms without changing the treatment drugs. For the treatment to be most effective, it is important to complete the entire regimen of drugs. Additionally,

the drugs are very expensive and the employer is paying for the treatment. Therefore all individuals being treated should be strongly encouraged to seek counseling from a qualified healthcare provider before stopping treatment.

Rapid HIV-Antibody Testing

The use of FDA-approved rapid HIV-antibody tests for evaluating source patients has increased and is encouraged by the CDC. Rapid HIV-antibody tests can provide test results in as little as 20 minutes, so they can facilitate making timely decisions regarding the use of HIV PEP after occupational-exposure incidents and may prevent the unnecessary use of PEP and associated adverse symptoms. Additional information about rapid HIV-antibody tests is available by visiting the CDC Web site (http://www.cdc.gov/hiv/rapid_testing/).

PREVENTIVE MEASURES TO REDUCE OCCUPATIONAL RISKS

The majority of exposures in dentistry are preventable. Strategies to reduce the risk of blood contacts and prevent the transmission of HBV, HCV, and HIV include the use of the HB vaccine, standard precautions, devices with

Table 15-3 Recommended HIV PEP for Percutaneous Injuries

Exposure Type	Infection status of source				
	HIV-positive, class 1*	HIV-positive, class 2*	Source of unknown HIV status†	Unknown source§	HIV-negative
Less severe¶	Recommended basic 2-drug PEP	Recommend expanded ≥3-drug PEP	Generally, no PEP warranted; however, consider basic 2-drug PEP** for source with HIV risk factors††	Generally, no PEP warranted; however, consider basic 2-drug PEP** in settings in which exposure to HIV-infected persons is likely	No PEP warranted
More severe§§	Recommended expanded 3-drug PEP	Recommend expanded ≥3-drug PEP	Generally, no PEP warranted; however, consider basic 2-drug PEP** for source with HIV risk factors††	Generally, no PEP warranted; however, consider basic 2-drug PEP** in settings in which exposure to HIV-infected persons is likely	No PEP warranted

Adapted from CDC. Updated U.S. Public Health Service guidelines for the management of occupational exposures to HIV and recommendations for postexposure prophylaxis. MMWR 2005;54(RR-9):3.

*HIV-positive, class 1: asymptomatic HIV infection or know viral load (<1,500 ribonucleic acid copies/mL). HIV-positive, class 2: symptomatic HIV infection, acquired immunodeficiency syndrome, acute seroconversion, or known high viral load. If drug resistance is a concern, obtain expert consultation. Initiation of PEP should not be delayed pending expert consultation, and, because expert consultation alone cannot substitute for face-to-face counseling, resources should be available to provide immediate evaluation and follow-up care for all exposures.

†For example, deceased source person with no samples available for HIV testing.

§For example, a needle from a sharps disposal container.

¶For example, solid needle or superficial injury.

**The recommendation "consider PEP" indicates that PEP is optional; a decision to initiate PEP should be based on a discussion between the exposed person and the treating clinician regarding risks versus benefits of PEP.

††If PEP is offered and administered and the source is later determined to be HIV-negative, PEP should be discontinued.

§§For example, large-bore hollow needle, deep puncture, visible blood on device, or needle used in the patient's artery or vein.

features engineered to prevent sharp injuries, and modifications of work practices. Usually a combination of these practices is used. These approaches, along with training and education, have contributed to the decrease in percutaneous injuries among dentists during recent years.

Engineering controls isolate or remove the BBP hazard from the workplace and are considered to be the primary method to reduce exposures to blood and OPIM (e.g., saliva) from sharp instruments and needles. Whenever possible, engineering controls should be used as the primary method to reduce exposures to BBPs. Examples of engineering controls include sharps disposal containers, self-sheathing needles, safety scalpels with retractable blades or covers, and safer medical devices, such as sharps with engineered sharps injury protections and needleless systems (Fig. 15-2). Dental anesthetic syringes and needles that incorporate safety features have been developed for dental procedures, but the low injury rates in dentistry limit assessment of their effect on reducing injuries among dental workers. In most dental practices, none of the currently available dental anesthetic safety devices have been widely accepted as an alternative to the traditional dental anesthetic syringe. Therefore the importance of using work practice controls cannot be overlooked.

Work practice controls are behavior-based and intended to reduce the risk of blood exposure by changing the manner in which a task is performed. Examples include using a one-handed scoop technique (Fig. 15-3) or a needle recapping device (Fig. 15-4) to recap a needle; not bending or breaking needles before disposal; avoiding passing a syringe with an unsheathed needle;

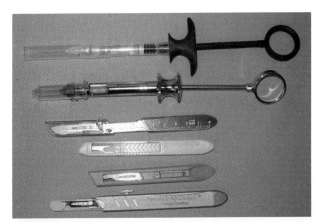

FIGURE 15-2 Examples of safety anesthetic devices and safety scalpels.

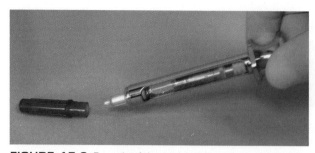

FIGURE 15-3 Example of the one-handed scoop technique for recapping a needle.

removing burs before disassembling the handpiece from the dental unit; using instruments, rather than fingers, to grasp needles, retract tissue, and load/unload needles and scalpels; placing used disposable syringes and needles, scalpel blades, and other sharp items in appropriate puncture-resistant containers located as close as feasible to where the items were used; and giving verbal announcements when passing sharps.

PPE consists of specialized clothing or equipment worn to protect against hazards. Examples include gloves, masks, protective eyewear with side shields, and gowns to prevent skin and mucous-membrane exposures.

SUMMARY

Current data indicate that the risk for transmitting HBV, HCV, and HIV in dental settings is low. However, a combination of pre-exposure HB vaccination, standard precautions, and engineering and work practice controls is the best means to minimize occupational exposures. Written policies and procedures to facilitate prompt reporting, evaluation, counseling, treatment, and medical follow-up of all occupational exposures should be available to all dental personnel. Additionally, rapid access to clinical

care, testing, counseling, and PEP for exposed personnel, and the testing of source patients are critical.

✓ Practical Dental Infection-Control Checklist

HBV Vaccination

❏ Is the HBV vaccination series offered to all DHCP with potential occupational exposure to blood or OPIM?

❏ Are U.S. Public Health Service/CDC recommendations always followed for HB vaccination, serologic testing, follow-up, and booster dosing?

❏ Are DHCP tested for anti-HBs 1–2 months after completion of the three-dose vaccination series?

  ❏ If no antibody response occurs to the primary vaccine series, do these DHCP complete a second three-dose vaccine series or are they evaluated to determine whether they are HBsAg-positive?

  ❏ At the completion of the second vaccine series, are DHCP retested for anti-HBs?

    ❏ If there is no response to the second three-dose series, are nonresponders tested for HBsAg?

❏ Are nonresponders to vaccination who are HBsAg-negative counseled regarding their susceptibility to HBV infection and precautions to take?

❏ Are employees provided with appropriate education regarding the risks of HBV transmission and the availability of the vaccine?

❏ Do employees who decline the vaccination sign a declination form to be kept on file with the employer?

Preventing Exposures to Blood and OPIM

❏ Are standard precautions (note: OSHA's Bloodborne Pathogen Standard retains the term *universal precautions*) used for all patient encounters?

❏ Are sharp items (e.g., needles, scalers, burs, lab knives, and wires) that are contaminated with patient blood and saliva treated as potentially infectious?

❏ Are engineering controls (e.g., sharps containers, automated instrument cleaners, safety needles, needle recapping devices) and work practice controls (e.g., one-handed scoop technique, placing sharps containers as close as possible to the point of use) used to prevent injuries?

❏ Does the dental office/clinic have a written, comprehensive program designed to minimize and manage DHCP exposures to blood and body fluids?

Engineering and Work Practice Controls

❏ Does the dental office/clinic identify, evaluate, and select devices with engineered safety features at least annually and as they become available on the market

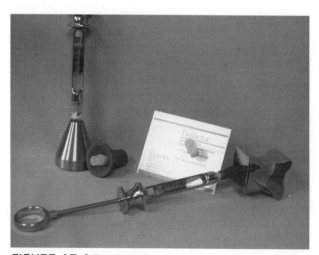

FIGURE 15-4 Examples of needle recapping devices.

(e.g., safer anesthetic syringes, retractable scalpel, or needleless IV systems)?

❑ Are employees directly responsible for patient care (e.g., dentists, hygienists, dental assistants) involved with the identification and selection of these devices?

❑ Are the results documented in the dental office/clinic's ECP?

❑ Are used disposable syringes and needles, scalpel blades, and other sharp items placed in appropriate puncture-resistant containers located as close as feasible to the area in which the items are used?

❑ Are sharps containers located in each dental operatory?

❑ Are sharps containers color-coded (e.g., red) or labeled appropriately (e.g., biohazard symbol)?

❑ When recapping needles, is a one-handed scoop technique or a mechanical device designed for holding the needle cap when recapping needles (e.g., between multiple injections and before removing from a nondisposable aspirating syringe)? Note: OSHA prohibits recapping used needles by using both hands or any other technique that involves directing the point of a needle toward any part of the body.

Postexposure Management and Prophylaxis

❑ Does the dental office/clinic follow CDC recommendations after percutaneous, mucous-membrane, or nonintact skin exposure to blood or OPIM?

❑ Does the dental office/clinic have a written comprehensive postexposure management and medical follow-up program?

❑ Do DHCP know the types of contact with blood or OPIM that can place them at risk for infection?

❑ Do DHCP know to report occupational injuries and exposures immediately?

❑ Does the dental office/clinic have a written plan establishing mechanisms for referral to a qualified healthcare professional for medical evaluation and follow-up?

❑ Does the program include policies and procedures for prompt reporting, evaluation, counseling, treatment, and medical follow-up of occupational exposures?

❑ When an occupational exposure occurs, does the exposure incident report contain the following information:

❑ Date and time of exposure?

❑ Details of the procedure being performed, including where and how the exposure occurred and whether the exposure involved a sharp device, the type and brand of device, and how and when during its handling the exposure occurred.

❑ Details of the exposure, including its severity and the type and amount of fluid or material? The severity of a percutaneous injury, for example, might be measured by the depth of the wound, gauge of the needle, and whether fluid was injected. For skin or mucous-membrane exposure, the estimated volume of material, duration of contact, and condition of skin should be noted. Other considerations involve noting whether the skin was chapped, abraded, or intact.

❑ Details regarding whether the source material was known to contain HIV or other BBPs, and, if the source was infected with HIV, the stage of disease, history of antiretroviral therapy, and viral load, if known.

❑ Details regarding the exposed person (e.g., HB vaccination and vaccine-response status)?

❑ Details regarding counseling, postexposure management, and follow-up?

Review Questions

1. An occupational-exposure incident is defined as a percutaneous injury or contact of mucous membrane or nonintact skin with

   A. blood, saliva, tissue, or other body fluids that are potentially infectious.

   B. blood, tissue, or other body fluids that are potentially infectious, but not saliva.

   C. blood only.

   D. none of the above.

2. Which of the following statements is false?

   A. Most occupational exposures do not result in infection.

   B. Following a specific exposure, the risk of infection will not vary with the amount of blood involved in the exposure.

   C. All occupational-exposure incidents should be treated as medical emergencies and tended to immediately.

   D. Wounds or skin sites that have been in contact with blood or body fluids should be washed with soap and water, and mucous membranes should be flushed with water.

3. Which of the following is true regarding PEP following a needlestick exposure to HIV-infected blood?

   A. The risk of developing HIV is 30% following a needlestick injury.

   B. PEP is not indicated.

   C. Initiate PEP within hours of the exposure.

4. Using a one-handed scoop technique to recap needles, avoiding passing unsheathed needles, and using instruments rather than fingers to retract tissues are examples of

   A. standard controls

   B. engineering controls

   C. work practice controls

5. _____ controls remove or isolate a hazard in the workplace and are frequently technology based.

   A. Sharps

   B. Engineering

   C. Work practice

   D. Standard

Critical Thinking

1. Does your dental office/clinic have a written program addressing the management of occupational exposure incidents?

2. Do you have an incident/injury report form? If yes, obtain a copy of the document and compare it with the sample form in this chapter.

3. During treatment you sustain a percutaneous injury with a bur.

   a. What is the first thing you should do, and why?

   b. To whom do you report the injury?

   c. What kind of information should be included in the injury report?

   d. If indicated, where will you go for your PEP treatment and follow-up?

4. What types of engineering and work practice controls are used in your dental office/clinic?

5. Go to one of the office's dental operatories. Demonstrate how you recap a needle on the anesthetic syringe.

SELECTED READINGS

CDC. Bloodborne pathogens and aerosols. Available at: http://www.cdc.gov/oralhealth/infectioncontrol/faq/aerosols.htm. Accessed January 15, 2008.

CDC. Exposure to blood: what health-care personnel need to know. Available at: http://www.cdc.gov/ncidod/dhqp/pdf/bbp/Exp_to_Blood.pdf. Accessed June 16, 2008.

CDC. Guidelines for infection control in dental health-care settings—2003. MMWR 2003;52(RR-17):1–66.

CDC. Guidelines for infection control in health-care personnel. Am J Infect Control 1998;26:289–354.

CDC. Guidelines for prevention of transmission of human immunodeficiency virus and hepatitis B virus to health-care and public-safety workers. MMWR 1989;38(S-6):1–36.

CDC. Sharps safety: be sharp, be safe. Available at http://www.cdc.gov/sharpssafety. Accessed June 16, 2008.

CDC. Update: universal precautions for prevention of transmission of human immunodeficiency virus, hepatitis B virus, and other bloodborne pathogens in health-care settings. MMWR 1988;37:377–382,387–388.

CDC. Updated U.S. Public Health Service guidelines for the management of occupational exposures to hepatitis B virus (HBV), hepatitis C virus (HCV), and human immunodeficiency virus (HIV) and recommendations for postexposure prophylaxis. MMWR 2001;50(RR-11).

CDC. Updated U.S. Public Health Service guidelines for the management of occupational exposures to HIV and recommendations for postexposure prophylaxis. MMWR 2005;54(RR-9):1–17.

Cleveland JL, Barker LK, Cuny EJ, et al. Preventing percutaneous injuries among dental healthcare personnel. J Am Dent Assoc 2007;138:169–178.

Cleveland JL, Barker L, Gooch BF, et al. Use of HIV postexposure prophylaxis (PEP) by dental healthcare personnel: an overview and updated recommendations. J Am Dent Assoc 2002;133:1619–1630.

Cleveland JL, Cardo DM. Occupational exposures to human immunodeficiency virus, hepatitis B virus, and hepatitis C virus: risk, prevention, and management. Dent Clinics North Am 2003;47:681–696.

Landrum ML, Wilson CH, Perri LP, et al. Usefulness of a rapid human immunodeficiency virus–1 antibody test for the management of occupational exposure to blood and body fluid. Infect Control Hosp Epidemiol 2005;26:768–774.

Osborn EHS, Papadakis MA, Gerberding JL. Occupational exposures to body fluids among medical students. A 7-year longitudinal study. Ann Intern Med 1999;130:45–51.

16

Instrument Processing and Recirculation

Jennifer A. Harte

John A. Molinari

LEARNING OBJECTIVES

After completion of this chapter individuals should be able to:

1   Discuss general instrument-processing and recirculation procedures.

2   Describe key design features of an instrument-processing area.

3   Describe the importance of cleaning instruments before sterilization procedures.

4   Describe the importance of packaging instruments before sterilization.

5   Discuss sterilizer loading procedures.

6   Discuss the importance of proper instrument storage and differentiate between time- and event-related storage practices.

KEY TERMS

Bioburden: the microbiological load (i.e., number of viable organisms in or on the object or surface) or organic material on a surface or object prior to decontamination or sterilization; also known as bioload or microbial load.

Chemical indicator: a device to monitor the sterilization process that changes color or form with exposure to one or more of the physical conditions within the sterilizing chamber (e.g., temperature and steam). Chemical indicators are intended to detect potential sterilization failures that could result from incorrect packaging, incorrect loading of the sterilizer, or malfunctions of the sterilizer. A "pass" response does not verify that the items are sterile.

Cleaning: the removal of visible soil and organic debris, either manually or mechanically, which results in a reduction in the number of microorganisms and the removal or organic matter, such as blood, tissue, and other biological material that may interfere with sterilization and disinfection. Cleaning is the first step in any sterilization or disinfection process.

Contaminated: state of having been in contact with microorganisms. As used in healthcare, it generally refers to microorganisms capable of producing disease or infection.

Event-related shelf life: a storage practice that recognizes that a package and its contents should remain sterile until some event causes the item(s) to become contaminated.

Food and Drug Administration (FDA): the FDA promotes and protects the public health by helping safe and effective products reach the market in a timely way; monitors products for continued safety after they are in use; and helps the public get the accurate, science-based information needed to improve health.

Instrument washer: an automated device designed to clean medical and dental instruments.

Ultrasonic cleaner: a device that uses waves of acoustic energy (a process known as "cavitation") to loosen and break up debris on instruments.

Washer-disinfector: an automated unit designed to clean and thermally disinfect instruments. Such units use a high-temperature cycle rather than a chemical bath.

Instrument processing and recirculation is a complex process that requires specialized equipment, adequate space, qualified dental healthcare personnel (DHCP), and multiple steps. Correct cleaning, packaging, sterilizer loading procedures, sterilization methods, and storage practices are essential to ensure that an instrument is adequately processed and safe for reuse on patients. This chapter covers cleaning, packaging, sterilizer loading procedures, and storage practices. Sterilization procedures, including equipment selection, and monitoring processes are discussed in Chapter 11.

INSTRUMENT-PROCESSING AREA DESIGN

Instrument processing should not take place in the operatory; a designated centralized area in the office should be used to control quality and ensure safety. Centralized processing may be more cost-effective because centralizing ultrasonic cleaners and sterilizers can result in cost savings for initial purchases, replacement, and repairs. The central processing area should be divided into sections for receiving, cleaning, and decontamination; preparation and packaging; sterilization; and storage. Ideally, walls or partitions should separate the sections to control traffic flow and contain contaminants generated during processing. When physical separation cannot be achieved, adequate spatial separation may be

satisfactory if the DHCP who process instruments are trained to use work practices that prevent contamination of clean areas. Space should be adequate for the volume of work anticipated and the items to be stored. Ventilation systems should control the heat generated by the sterilization equipment and provide easy access to the air filters for servicing. Comfortable working temperatures and humidity are necessary because DHCP will be wearing personal protective equipment (PPE). A hand-washing facility should be conveniently located. Automatically controlled pieces of equipment, such as faucets and soap dispensers, that use electronic sensors or foot controls are desirable. Table 16-1 lists other considerations for designing an instrument-processing area. The primary goal is to separate **contaminated** instruments from areas where clean items are packaged, sterilized, and stored.

HANDLING AND TRANSPORTING CONTAMINATED PATIENT-CARE ITEMS

Contaminated instruments should be handled as little as possible and carefully to prevent exposure to sharp instruments that can cause a percutaneous injury. Also of concern is exposure to microorganisms on contaminated instruments and devices through contact with nonintact skin on the hands or with mucous membranes

1. Space requirements may depend on
   • work flow patterns
   • clean and sterile storage space requirements
   • the need for separate areas for receiving, cleaning, and
     decontamination preparation and packaging; sterilization;
     and storage
   • types and amount of equipment and installation requirements
   • the workload and desired staffing

2. Mechanical/electrical requirements, in addition to routine electrical and
   plumbing, may include
   • pressurized gases and vacuum systems
   • adequate number of electrical outlets
   • a source for distilled or deionized water

3. Floors, walls, ceilings, and countertops:
   • Surfaces should be flush, smooth, nonporous, and uncarpeted.
   • Countertops should be chemical- and heat-resistant, and be able to
     hold tabletop sterilizers and other equipment.
   • Materials should be able to withstand frequent cleaning with
     chemical agents (e.g., environmental surface disinfectants).

of the eyes, nose, or mouth. All contaminated instruments and devices should be handled carefully by DHCP wearing heavy-duty utility gloves in addition to other appropriate PPE such as protective clothing, protective eyewear, masks, and head and shoe covers. Examination gloves do not provide adequate protection against sharps injuries. Instruments should be placed in an appropriate covered puncture-resistant container in the dental treatment area to limit cross-contamination and prevent percutaneous injuries during transport to the instrument-processing area. These carrying containers should be either red or labeled with the biohazard symbol.

RECEIVING, CLEANING, AND DECONTAMINATION

Reusable instruments, supplies, and equipment should be received, sorted, cleaned, and decontaminated in one section of the processing area. **Cleaning** (also called precleaning) is the most important step because if **bioburden** or debris, whether inorganic or organic matter, is not removed, it will interfere with microbial inactivation and can compromise the disinfection or sterilization process. Therefore cleaning should precede all disinfection and sterilization processes. Contaminated instruments should be handled carefully. DHCP should wear heavy-duty utility gloves, protective eyewear, a mask, and protective clothing. Head and shoe covers should be available to staff members if heavy contamination is expected.

If cleaning cannot be performed immediately, placing instruments in a puncture-resistant container or an ultrasonic cleaner and soaking them with detergent, a disinfectant/detergent, or an enzymatic cleaner will prevent drying of blood, saliva, and dental materials, and make cleaning easier and less time-consuming. This is often referred to as "presoaking." Using a liquid chemical sterilant/high-level disinfectant (e.g., glutaraldehyde) as a presoaking or holding solution is not recommended.

Considerations in selecting cleaning methods and equipment include the efficacy of the method, process, and equipment; compatibility with items to be cleaned; and occupational health and exposure risks. The use of automated cleaning equipment, such as **ultrasonic cleaners** or **instrument washers**, does not require presoaking or scrubbing of instruments and can increase productivity, improve cleaning effectiveness, and decrease worker exposure to blood and body fluids. Therefore, using automated equipment can be safer and more efficient than manually cleaning contaminated instruments.

In most dental offices, instruments are cleaned in an ultrasonic cleaner (Fig. 16-1) for a designated time period. The ultrasonic cleaner removes soil by a process that uses electrical energy to generate sound waves. When the sound waves travel through the liquid, millions of tiny bubbles are formed and burst continuously. This process is called cavitation and disrupts the bonds that hold debris on the surface of the instruments. For maximum decontamination, follow the manufacturer's instructions for operation of the equipment, including the operating time and amount and type of cleaning solutions. Do not use plain water or environmental surface disinfectants in the ultrasonic cleaner; use only solutions formulated specifically for use in an ultrasonic cleaner.

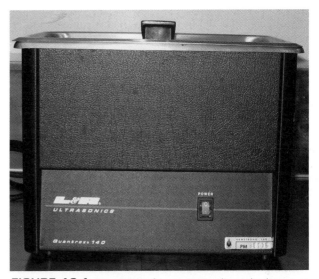

FIGURE 16-1 An example of a countertop ultrasonic cleaner.

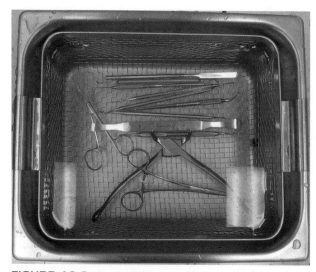

FIGURE 16-2 A perforated basket, tray, or rack should be used to keep instruments the proper distance from the bottom of the tank.

TABLE 16-2 Ultrasonic Cleaner Test Protocol

In the absence of the manufacturer's recommendations, the following procedure can be used:

1. Using standard lightweight or regular household aluminum foil, cut a piece of foil to fit the width of the cleaner chamber. For example, a tank 12 inches long × 6 inches wide × 5 inches deep would require a foil sample measuring 12 inches × 6 inches.

2. Prepare a fresh solution of ultrasonic cleaning solution and fill the tank according to the manufacturer's instructions. Do not turn the heater on for the test.

3. Insert the foil vertically into the cleaner chamber, with the length of the foil running the length of the chamber and the bottom of the foil about 1 inch above the bottom.

4. Holding the foil as steady as possible, turn on the ultrasonic cleaning unit for 20–60 seconds (if the unit is supplied with a high/low switch, it should be set in the high position).

5. Remove the foil sample and look for small indentations (pebbling) on the foil. Some holes may also be present.

6. With a properly functioning unit, the entire foil surface will be uniformly "peppered" (covered with a tiny pebbling effect). If areas greater than ½ inch square show no pebbling, the unit may require servicing.

The solution must completely cover the items for cleaning to occur. Cleaning solutions should be changed at least daily, or sooner if visibly contaminated. A perforated basket, tray, or rack should be used to keep instruments the proper distance from the bottom of the tank (Fig. 16-2). This allows the instruments to be easily rinsed under running water before they are placed into the ultrasonic cleaner filled with solution. Do not place items directly on the bottom of the tanks, because this reduces the amount of ultrasonic waves produced and may damage the unit. Always cover the unit when it is operating to decrease aerosols and avoid splashing and spattering of solution onto nearby surfaces. When the cleaning is complete, do not remove the instruments with your hands. Instead, remove the basket, drain, and thoroughly rinse the basket with the instruments under running water. Inspect the instruments for any residual blood or debris and dry thoroughly.

Ultrasonic cleaning equipment can be tested periodically for proper function. The aluminum foil test is a simple and fast method to check for an even distribution of the cleaning power in an ultrasonic cleaner. Manufacturers usually include test instructions in the operating manual and may even provide test kits. In the absence of manufacturer recommendations, the protocol in Table 16-2 may be used.

Instrument washers are becoming more popular in dental practices and can streamline the instrument-cleaning process (Fig. 16-3). Like ultrasonic cleaners they are available in a variety of sizes; however, they generally accommodate more instruments and use automated washing cycles compared to an ultrasonic cleaner. Instrument washers eliminate the need for manual presoaking or hand-scrubbing, rinsing, and drying. Some instrument washers, called **washer-disinfectors**, also have a high-temperature cycle to achieve high-level thermal disinfection along with cleaning. In hospitals or large clinics, a washer-sterilizer may be used. With this method, in addition to cleaning, the instruments are subjected to a short steam sterilization cycle. While instrument washers can increase productivity, improve cleaning effectiveness, and decrease workers' exposure to blood and body fluids, they are not a substitute for heat sterilization. The manufacturers' operating instructions and recommendations for cleaning solutions should always be followed. It is also important to remember that while these washers may appear to be similar to a home dishwasher, instrument-washing equipment is considered to be medical equipment and is regulated by the **Food and Drug Administration (FDA)**. Commercially available household dishwashers are not designed to process medical instruments and have not met the FDA requirements for safety and effectiveness. As such, the use of household dishwashers in dental settings is not a substitute for using a tested and approved instrument washer.

Because of the potential for injury from sharp instruments, hand-scrubbing should be avoided as much as possible. However, manual cleaning is sometimes unavoidable because the instruments are fragile or the automated equipment is being serviced or repaired. To avoid injury when manually scrubbing instruments, DHCP should wear heavy-duty utility gloves when handling or

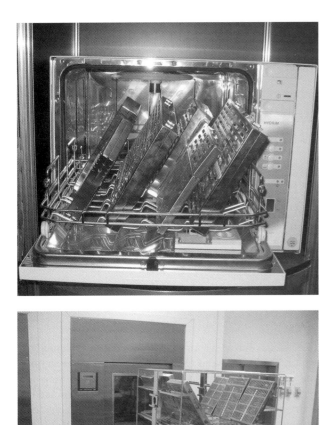

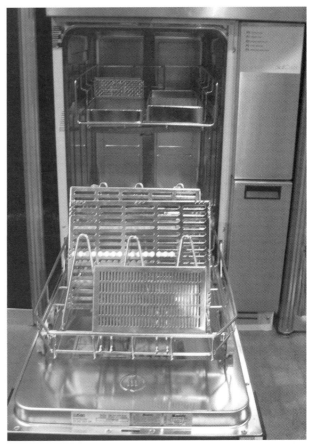

FIGURE 16-3 Instrument washers are available in a variety of sizes (left to right): countertop models, floor-standing, and large hospital-grade washer/sterilizers.

manually cleaning contaminated instruments and devices. Other recommendations include applying work practice controls, such as using a long-handled brush to keep the scrubbing hand away from sharp instruments, and cleaning instruments under water to decrease spatter. Individuals should never reach into trays or containers holding sharp instruments that cannot be seen, or sinks filled with soapy water in which sharp instruments have been placed.

PREPARATION AND PACKAGING

In another section of the processing area, cleaned instruments and other dental supplies should be inspected, assembled into sets or trays, and wrapped, packaged, or placed into container systems for sterilization. The purpose of packaging is to protect instruments from contamination after removal from the sterilizer and during storage. Therefore instruments must be packaged before being placed in the sterilizer, and quality packaging materials must be used to allow penetration of the sterilization agent and ensure that sterility is maintained.

A wide variety of packaging materials, such as bags, wraps, pouches, and wrapped perforated instrument cassettes are available to accommodate different practice considerations. See Table 16-3 for information to consider when selecting packaging materials. Self-sealing paper and plastic pouches that allow visual inspection of the sterile contents are very popular (Fig. 16-4). Instrument cassettes are another very useful and popular means of packing dental instruments. Cassettes are available in a variety of materials, sizes, and shapes (Fig. 16-5). Using instrument cassettes facilitates instrument processing and can significantly enhance organization of instruments. Cassettes can keep all of the instruments for a specific procedure together from the chairside procedure through cleaning,

TABLE 16-3 Factors to Consider When Selecting Packaging Materials

- Allows penetration of the sterilizing agent.

- Provides an adequate barrier to microorganisms.

- Is puncture- and tear-resistant.

- Can be sealed easily and completely.

- Contents can be easily removed while maintaining sterility.

- Is free of toxic elements and dyes.

- If fabric, is low-linting.

- Is cost-effective.

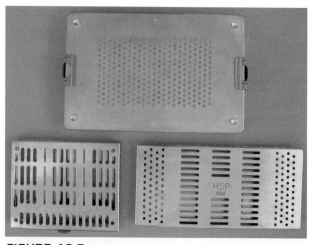

FIGURE 16-5 Instrument cassettes are available in a variety of materials, sizes, and shapes.

rinsing, drying, and sterilization. Following completion of dental treatment, instruments can be arranged in the cassette, transported to the instrument-processing area, and placed in the ultrasonic cleaner or instrument washer as a unit. The cassette can be rinsed and dried in this manner also. Therefore, with a cassette system, direct handling of potentially contaminated instruments is significantly reduced before sterilization. Furthermore, by having the instruments prearranged in the cassette, handling following sterilization is decreased. Different types and sizes of cassettes are available. It is important to follow the manufacturer's recommendations for cleaning, wrapping, and sterilizing the cassettes. Perforated cassettes are preferable, as completely solid containers may not allow steam or chemical vapor to reach the contents for sterilization to occur. It is also important to consider the size of the sterilizer and amount of storage space available, because cassettes can occupy more space than individual packages.

Packaging materials must be compatible and designed for the type of sterilization process being used

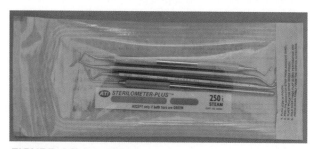

FIGURE 16-4 An example of a self-sealing paper/plastic pouch with instruments ready for sterilization.

(e.g., steam autoclave, dry heat, or unsaturated chemical vapor; Table 16-4) and cleared by the FDA. For example, the combination paper/plastic peel packages that are commonly used in the autoclave may burn when used in a dry-heat sterilizer. Inappropriate materials may compromise the sterilization process by not allowing the sterilizing agent to penetrate the packaging material. If there is any doubt about the packaging material, a spore test can be placed inside the package and processed through the sterilizer. Packaging materials must also be appropriate for the items being sterilized in terms of both the size of the instrument(s) and the number of instruments to be processed. For example, sharp instruments, such as explorers, may easily puncture paper packaging. Also, placing too many instruments in a pack may cause it to tear easily. The package should be sealed effectively to ensure that sterility is maintained. Some packages are self-sealing; others may require the use of sterilization indicator tape or heat sealing. Packages should never be sealed with metal closures such as staples or paper clips, as these could puncture the material and cause a break of sterility.

Hinged instruments, such as extraction forceps, scissors, and hemostats, should be processed open and unlocked to permit the sterilizing agent contact with all surfaces (Fig. 16-6). An internal **chemical indicator** should be placed in every package to ensure that the sterilizing agent has reached the inside of the packaging. In addition, an external chemical indicator, such as chemical indicator tape, should be used when the internal indicator cannot be seen from outside the package. A complete discussion of sterilization monitoring can be found in Chapter 11. After packaging is completed, the package should be labeled (Table 16-5). Automated labeling devices are available that can preprint the

TABLE 16-4 Sterilization Method and Packaging Material Compatibility

Sterilization Method	Packaging Material Requirements *		Comments
	Acceptable	*Unacceptable*	
Steam	• wrapped perforated metal trays/ cassettes • paper, plastic, cloth, paper/plastic peel pouches	• closed metal and glass containers	Must allow steam to penetrate
Dry Heat	• wrapped perforated metal trays/ cassettes • paper bags • aluminum foil • polyfilm plastic tubing	• plastic and paper bags that cannot withstand dry heat temperatures	Must not insulate items from heat and must not be destroyed by the temperature used
Unsaturated Chemical Vapor	• wrapped perforated metal trays/ cassettes • paper or paper plastic peel pouches	• closed metal trays and sealed glass jars	Vapors must be allowed to precipitate on contents and must not react with packaging material; plastics should not contact sides of the sterilizer

*Use only materials approved by the sterilizer manufacturer.

information on self-adhesive labels. This provides an efficient method for creating legible and standardized labels. If a handwritten label is used, the marking pen should be indelible, nonbleeding, and nontoxic. Felt-tip ink pens or a very soft lead pencil may be used. Do not write on paper or cloth wrapping materials. Peel packages should be labeled on the plastic portion or on the self-sealing tab.

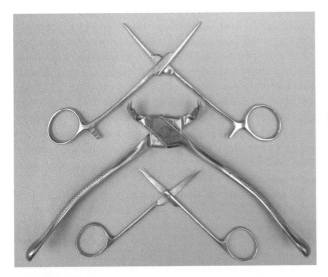

FIGURE 16-6 Hinged instruments, such as hemostats, extraction forceps, and scissors, should be processed open and unlocked to permit the sterilizing agent to contact all surfaces.

STERILIZATION

The sterilization section of the processing area should include the sterilization equipment and related supplies, with adequate space for loading, unloading, and cooldown. Manufacturer and local building code specifications will determine placement and room ventilation requirements.

Heat-tolerant dental instruments usually are sterilized by steam under pressure (autoclaving), dry heat, or unsaturated chemical vapor. All sterilizations should be performed with the use of medical sterilization equipment cleared by FDA and according to the manufacturer's instructions. A complete discussion of sterilization equipment can be found in Chapter 11.

TABLE 16-5 Information to Include on the Package Label

• Sterilizer identification number
• Load number
• Operator's initials
• An indefinite shelf-life label (if using event-related shelf life) with the date of sterilization, or, if using time-related shelf-life policies, an expiration date
• Package contents

Courtesy of the USAF Dental Evaluation and Consultation Service.

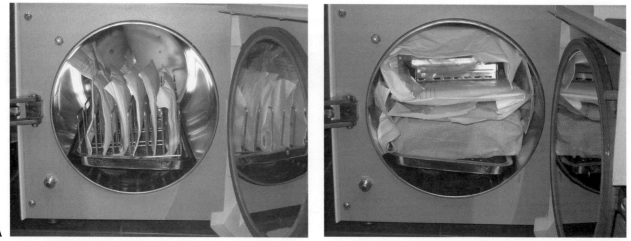

A   B

FIGURE 16-7 Correct loading of a tabletop sterilizer **(A)** and an example of an overloaded sterilizer **(B)**.

The manufacturer's instructions for loading the sterilizer should be followed. Correct loading of the sterilizer chamber is essential. Items to be sterilized should be arranged to permit free circulation of the sterilizing agent (e.g., steam, chemical vapor, or dry heat). Overloading the sterilizer chamber can increase sterilizer warm-up times and may prevent thorough contact of the sterilizing agent with all items in the sterilizer. Accessories, such as racks or trays, are usually provided with the sterilizer, or can be purchased separately, to help users with proper loading procedures. Underloading the chamber may cause damage to the instruments from overheating. Generally, packages should be placed in the chamber on their edges so that the sterilizing agent can contact every surface of every article to be sterilized (Fig. 16-7). Instrument packs should be allowed to dry inside the sterilizer chamber before they are removed and handled. Packs should not be touched until they are cool and dry, because hot packs act as wicks, absorbing moisture and hence bacteria from hands and the environment. Also, wet packs can tear easily.

STORAGE OF STERILIZED ITEMS AND CLEAN DENTAL SUPPLIES

The storage area should be clean and dry, and should contain enclosed storage units for sterile items and clean patient-care supplies. Closed cabinets limit dust accumulation and inadvertent contact with the sterile items. The shelves or drawers should be cleaned and disinfected on a regular basis (e.g., once a week). Sterile instruments or patient-care items should not be stored where they may become wet, such as under a sink, because even a small leak could compromise the integrity of the packaging material. Also, storage of supplies on the floor should be avoided. Shipping boxes and other cardboard cartons should not be used in sterile storage areas because they have potentially been exposed to high microbial contami-

nation and they serve as a reservoir for dust. Packages should be handled only when absolutely necessary to avoid unnecessary contamination. By developing a stock rotation policy in the dental office, DHCP can ensure that older packages are used first and prevent waste because of expiration. This principle is sometimes referred to as "first in, first out." Proper care and storage of packaged, sterilized instruments will help ensure that they will remain sterile until the package is opened at the time of use.

The shelf life of sterilized instruments is the period during which an item is considered safe for use. It depends on the quality of the packaging material, storage conditions, conditions during transport, and the amount of handling an item has received. Instruments should never be stored unpackaged because an unwrapped item has no shelf life. Storage practices for wrapped sterilized instruments can be either time- or event-related. Although the issue of shelf life has been addressed by several organizations, including the Centers for Disease Control and Prevention (CDC), Association of Operating Room Nurses (AORN), Association for the Advancement of Medical Instrumentation (AAMI), and The Joint Commission, these organizations no longer make specific recommendations regarding expiration policies of sterilized items. Most facilities have adopted event-related shelf-life practices, as opposed to placing expiration dates on packages.

The **event-related shelf life** approach recognizes that the product should remain sterile indefinitely, unless an event (e.g., torn or wet packaging) causes it to become contaminated. Instead of placing an expiration (i.e., time-related) date on the package, an indefinite shelf-life label with the date of sterilization is placed on the package. Placing the date of sterilization facilitates the retrieval of processed items in the event of a sterilization failure. In addition to other labeling information, the package label should contain the following statement (or similar wording): "indefinite shelf life unless integrity of the package is compromised." With either time- or event-related shelf-life storage, inspect all packages at the time of use, and if the packaging is compromised (e.g., torn, wet, or punctured), do not use the item(s). The item(s) must be recleaned, repackaged, and resterilized before use.

SUMMARY

Instrument processing and recirculation involve multiple steps. Correct cleaning, packaging, sterilizer loading procedures, sterilization methods, and storage practices are essential to ensure that an instrument is adequately processed and safe for reuse on patients. It is important for the office staff to be familiar with each procedure. Office infection-control plans and training programs should include comprehensive information about this process.

✔ Practical Dental Infection-Control Checklist

Instrument-Processing Area

❏ Does the dental office/clinic have a central instrument-processing area?

❏ Do personnel working in the instrument-processing area receive initial and recurring training?

❏ Is the instrument-processing area divided—physically or, at a minimum, spatially—into distinct areas for receiving, cleaning, and decontamination; preparation and packaging; sterilization; and storage?

❏ Are DHCP trained to use work practices that prevent contamination of clean areas?

❏ Are instruments stored in an area away from where contaminated instruments are held or cleaned?

Receiving, Cleaning, and Decontamination Work Area

❏ Is the handling of loose contaminated instruments minimized during transport to the instrument-processing area to minimize exposure potential (e.g., by using work-practice controls, such as carrying instruments in a covered container)?

❏ Is all visible blood and other contamination from dental instruments and devices removed by cleaning before sterilization or disinfection procedures?

❏ Is automated cleaning equipment (e.g., an ultrasonic cleaner or washer-disinfector) used to remove debris to improve cleaning effectiveness and decrease worker exposure to blood?

❏ Are work-practice controls used that minimize contact with sharp instruments if manual cleaning is necessary (e.g., using a long-handled brush)?

❏ Do DHCP wear puncture- and chemical-resistant/heavy-duty utility gloves for instrument cleaning and decontamination procedures?

❏ Do DHCP wear appropriate PPE (e.g., mask, protective eyewear, and gown) when splashing or spraying is anticipated during cleaning?

❏ Is the tabletop ultrasonic cleaner periodically tested (e.g., with a foil test) for proper function?

Preparation and Packaging

❏ Are dental instruments/items inspected for cleanliness and dried before they are wrapped or placed in containers designed to maintain sterility during storage (e.g., cassettes and organizing trays)?

❏ Is an internal chemical indicator placed in each package?

❏ Is an external indicator also used if the internal indicator cannot be seen from outside the package?

❏ Is either the FDA-cleared container system (e.g., instrument cassette) or wrapping compatible with the type of sterilization process used?

❏ Are packages labeled with the following information:

  ❏ sterilization identification number (if there is more than one sterilizer in the office/clinic)?

  ❏ load number?

  ❏ operator's initials?

  ❏ either an expiration date or the date sterilized (i.e., event-related)?

Storage Area for Sterilized Items and Clean Dental Supplies

❏ Does the dental office/clinic use date- or event-related shelf-life storage practices for wrapped, sterilized instruments and devices?

  ❏ If event-related packaging is used, is the date of sterilization placed on the package label to facilitate the retrieval of processed items in the event of a sterilization failure?

  ❏ If multiple sterilizers are used in the facility, is a sterilizer number or identification placed on the package label to facilitate the retrieval of processed items in the event of a sterilization failure?

❏ Are all wrapped packages of sterilized instruments inspected before they are opened, to ensure that the barrier wrap has not been compromised during storage?

❏ Are instruments/items recleaned, repackaged, and resterilized if the instrument package material has been compromised (e.g., wet, torn, or damaged)?

❏ Are sterile items and dental supplies stored in covered or closed cabinets if possible?

❏ Is a "first in, first out" storage policy used?

Review Questions

1. Cleaning, disinfecting, and sterilizing instruments in a designated central processing area controls both quality and personnel safety.

    A. True

    B. False

2. What types of PPE should be available when instruments are being cleaned?

    A. puncture- and chemical-resistant, heavy-duty utility gloves; masks; eye protection; protective clothing; head and shoe covers

    B. puncture- and chemical-resistant, heavy-duty utility gloves; masks; protective clothing; head and shoe covers

    C. puncture- and chemical-resistant, heavy-duty utility gloves; masks; eye protection

3. Which of the following is true regarding instrument cleaning?

    A. Using a washer-disinfector eliminates the need for heat sterilization.

    B. Using automated cleaning equipment is less time-efficient than hand-scrubbing instruments.

    C. Using automated equipment is more time-efficient, improves cleaning effectiveness, and is safer than hand-scrubbing instruments.

    D. A and C

4. Packaging instruments before sterilization is necessary to

    A. protect instruments from corrosion during cleaning.

    B. protect instruments from contamination after sterilization.

    C. protect instruments from the sterilizing agent.

    D. all of the above.

5. Using instrument cassettes can

    A. make instrument processing more efficient

    B. increase organization of instruments

    C. decrease handling of contaminated instruments

    D. eliminate corrosion

    E. A, B, C

    F. all of the above

6. With event-related shelf-life policies, which of the following would be an indication to not use the package?

    A. The package is torn.

    B. The package is wet.

    C. The expiration date has passed.

    D. A and B

    E. All of the above.

Critical Thinking

1. Go to the instrument-processing area in your dental office/clinic.

    a. How many functional areas do you have?

    b. How are instruments cleaned? If automated cleaning equipment is not used, what measures are taken to prevent injury when instruments are hand-scrubbed?

    c. Does the office use instrument cassettes? What are some advantages to using instrument cassettes?

2. How do you load your sterilizer? Why is it important to follow the manufacturer's instructions when loading the sterilizer?

3. Why is it important to allow packages to dry inside the sterilizer?

4. Obtain a package of instruments that has been sterilized.

    a. Does your office/clinic use time- or event-related expiration dating? What is the difference between the two methods?

    b. Is there an external indicator on the package? Does it indicate the package has been through the sterilizer? How do you know?

    c. After opening the package, do you observe an internal chemical indicator? Does it indicate the package has been through the sterilizer? How do you know?

SELECTED READINGS

AAMI, American National Standards Institute. Comprehensive guide to steam sterilization and sterility assurance in healthcare facilities. ANSI/AAMI ST79:2006. Arlington, VA: Association for the Advancement of Medical Instrumentation; 2006.

AAMI, American National Standards Institute. Steam sterilization and sterility assurance in healthcare facilities. ANSI/AAMI ST46:2002. Arlington, VA: Association for the Advancement of Medical Instrumentation; 2002.

AAMI, American National Standards Institute. Steam sterilization and sterility assurance using table-top sterilizers in office-based, ambulatory-care medical, surgical, and dental facilities. ANSI/AAMI ST40-1998. Arlington, VA: Association for the Advancement of Medical Instrumentation; 1998.

Cardo DM, Sehulster LM. Central sterile supply. In: Mayhall CG, ed. Hospital Epidemiology and Infection Control. 2nd ed. Philadelphia, PA: Lippincott Williams & Wilkins; 1999:1023–1030.

CDC. Guidelines for infection control in dental health-care settings–2003. MMWR 2003;52(RR-17):1–66.

Mayworm D. Sterile shelf life and expiration dating. J Hosp Supply Process Distrib 1984;2:32–35.

Miller CH, Palenik CJ. Instrument processing. In: Miller CH, Palenik DJ, eds. Infection Control and Management of Hazardous Materials for the Dental Team. 3rd ed. St. Louis: Mosby; 2005:191–241.

Miller CH, Palenik CJ. Sterilization, disinfection, and asepsis in dentistry. In: Block SS, ed. Disinfection, Sterilization, and Preservation. 5th ed. Philadelphia, PA: Lippincott Williams & Wilkins; 2001:1049–1068.

Miller CH, Tan CM, Beiswanger MA, et al. Cleaning dental instruments: measuring the effectiveness of an instrument washer/disinfector. Am J Dent 2000;13:39–43.

Molinari JA, Harte JA. Dental services. In: APIC Text of Infection Control and Epidemiology. 2nd ed. Washington, DC: APIC; 2005:51-1–51-23.

U.S. Department of Labor, Occupational Safety, and Health Administration. 29 CFR Part 1910.1030. Occupational exposure to bloodborne pathogens; needlesticks and other sharps injuries; final rule. Fed Regist 2001;66:5317–5325. [As amended from and includes 29 CFR Part 1910.1030. Occupational exposure to bloodborne pathogens; final rule. Fed Regist 1991;56:64174–64182.]

U.S. Department of Labor, Occupational Safety, and Health Administration. OSHA instruction: enforcement procedures for the occupational exposure to bloodborne pathogens. Directive CPL 2-2.69. Washington, DC: U.S. Department of Labor, Occupational Safety and Health Administration; 2001.

17

Role for Single-Use Disposable Items

Jennifer A. Harte

John A. Molinari

LEARNING OBJECTIVES

After completion of this chapter individuals should be able to:

1 Describe the role for single-use disposable items in dentistry.

2 Give examples of commonly used single-use disposable items in dentistry.

3 Describe advantages and disadvantages of using single-use disposable items.

Disposable item: see "single-use disposable item."

Regulated waste: liquid or semiliquid blood or other potentially infectious materials (OPIM); contaminated items that would release blood or OPIM in a liquid or semiliquid state if compressed; items that are caked with dried blood or OPIM and are capable of releasing the material during handling; contaminated sharps; and pathological and micro-biological wastes containing blood or OPIM.

Single-use disposable item: a device intended to be used on one patient and then discarded appropriately;

these items are not intended to be reprocessed (cleaned, disinfected, or sterilized) and used on another patient.

Surface barrier: material that prevents the penetration of microorganisms, particulates, and fluids. Barrier choices range from inexpensive plastic food wrap to commercially available custom-made covers.

Unit dose: the amount of material that is sufficient to accomplish a particular procedure to prevent cross-contam-ination. The material is dispensed before patient contact, and any excess is discarded at completion.

A disposable, or single-use, device is designed to be used on one patient and then discarded. **Disposable items** are not intended to be cleaned and sterilized for reuse on another patient, because they are usually not heat-tolerant and cannot be reliably cleaned. The labeling on the single-use item may or may not identify the device as single-use or disposable, and does not include instructions for reprocessing. In other words, if an item is not labeled single-use or disposable and does not include instructions for reprocessing, it should be used once and disposed of appropriately. Single-use devices were introduced into healthcare set-tings in the 1960s and promoted as being convenient and easy to use. Today numerous single-use or disposable items are commonly used in the dental office (Fig. 17-1).

EXAMPLES OF SINGLE-USE DISPOSABLE ITEMS

Examples of **single-use disposable items** include anes-thetic carpules, syringe needles, scalpel blades, pro-phylaxis cups and brushes, matrix bands, wooden and plastic wedges, dental dams, saliva ejectors, and plastic orthodontic brackets. Sometimes disposable items have reusable, heat-tolerant alternatives; these include high-volume evacuator tips, impression trays, prophy-laxis angles, dental burs, and air/water syringe tips. In many instances the reusable version of these items is difficult to clean adequately, and it may be safer, easier, and more cost-effective to use the disposable version. Any single-use device or item (e.g., cotton rolls, gauze, and irrigating syringes) used during oral surgical pro-cedures should be sterile at the time of use. It is com-mon for manufacturers to provide these items in sterile unit-dose packages.

Disposable safety devices are becoming more popu-lar. Several disposable safety scalpels and safety anes-thetic syringes/needles are available that do not require

the blade or needle to be removed before disposal, which helps protect users from accidental sharps injuries (Fig. 17-2).

Surface barriers used to protect equipment and other environmental surfaces in dental treatment areas include clear plastic wrap, bags, sheets, tubing, and plastic-backed paper or other materials that are impervious to moisture. These barriers are disposable and should be removed and discarded between patients. The primary

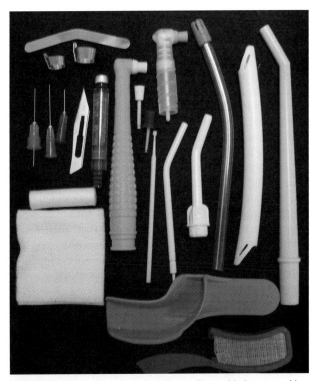

FIGURE 17-1 Examples of single-use disposable items used in dentistry.

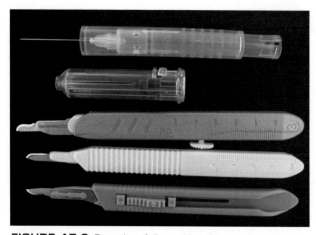

FIGURE 17-2 Examples of disposable safety needles and scalpels.

personal protective equipment (PPE) used in dental settings consists of gloves, masks, protective eyewear, and protective clothing such as gowns or jackets. Gloves and masks are to be changed between patients and not reused. Disposable or reusable versions of protective gowns, some face shields, and protective eyewear are available; however, reusable versions may be more cost-effective.

ADVANTAGES AND DISADVANTAGES OF USING SINGLE-USE DISPOSABLE ITEMS

Using disposable items enhances infection control by eliminating the risk of patient-to-patient transmission of infectious microorganisms because the item is discarded and not used on another patient. Another advantage is that time-consuming cleaning and sterilization procedures are eliminated. The disadvantages of disposables include the addition of nonbiodegradable plastic materials to the environment upon disposal. Also, some disposables may not function as well as their reusable counterparts, and disposable items may be more expensive. It is important to remember that when determining the cost-effectiveness of the disposable vs. the reusable item, one should consider the cost, time, and materials involved in decontaminating and reprocessing the reusable item, and not just the cost of the disposable item.

DISPOSAL OF SINGLE-USE ITEMS

The majority of single-use disposable items can be discarded in the regular trash. However, some items meet the Occupational Safety and Health Administration's definition of **regulated waste** and need to be discarded in special containers. For example, needles, scalpel blades, and any other sharp items must be disposed of in sharps containers. Any disposable item, such as gauze, that would release blood or saliva if squeezed or compressed, or that is caked with dried blood or saliva must be disposed of in a biohazard bag. In addition to the federal regulations regarding regulated waste, dental personnel should be familiar with their local and state regulations.

COMPLIANCE OF USE

Inspection of healthcare facilities can identify a wide variety of single-use, disposable patient-care items. The question remains, however: Are they being used as mandated and directed by the manufacturer? Two points must be considered to address this question:

1. Health professionals today are not too far removed from a time when reuse was much more common than disposal.

2. Compliance with recommended procedures and precautions continues to present challenges to accepted infection-control goals.

To illustrate the first point, many dental clinicians remember using the same pair of latex gloves during treatment of multiple patients. This primarily occurred prior to dentistry's acceptance and implementation of CDC and ADA infection-control recommendations. Gloves often were changed when they became sticky from washing with a liquid antiseptic or when they developed visible defects. Reuse of plastic saliva ejectors and prophylaxis cups after washing and immersion in chemical disinfectants/sterilants was also observed in some practices, and the list could be expanded further. Unfortunately, regulatory agencies historically have had to deal with the issue of compliance to ascertain which practices constitute a dangerous misuse of disposable devices. As recently as 1999, a survey conducted by the National Center for Policy Analysis (NCPA) to investigate hospital recycling of medical items found that nearly half of the 132 hospitals surveyed reused medical devices designed for single use. Items inappropriately reused on different patients included plastic catheters.

While long-term, accumulated scientific and clinical evidence is not available for the cross-infection potential presented by reuse of most disposable devices, accumulated data show that reuse of disposable needles and other sharps devices presents substantial risks for exposed patients. This was most recently demonstrated in a CDC report of four hepatitis outbreaks that occurred among patients between 2000 and 2002. One of these outbreaks involved the routine reuse of syringes and needles by a nurse anesthetist during clinic sessions. By the time the investigation of cases was concluded, a total of 69 hepatitis C virus (HCV) and

31 hepatitis B virus (HBV) infections were identified as probably being traceable to this person's practices. The nurse anesthetist ceased to reuse needles after a complaint was filed by staff nurses, and since that time no evidence of HCV or HBV transmission associated with treatment has been detected.

Although the lack of compliance with basic infection-control principles and practices for single-use disposable needles and syringes was apparent and serious in this instance, misuse of other disposable devices may not present with the same indirect infection risks. The most common outcome may be a lessening of the overlap and effectiveness of one's total chain of infection control. The ripple effect caused by what seems to be a minor infraction can reduce the margin of reinforcement and overlap each component of a prevention program. As evidence of this, the FDA has repeatedly taken the position that it is not aware of any data that would establish conditions for the safe, effective cleaning and subsequent resterilization and/or reuse of any disposable medical devices, and it has urged those who reprocess devices to submit additional data to show that their procedures are safe.

SUMMARY

Disposable items are not intended to be cleaned and sterilized for reuse on another patient, because they are usually not heat-tolerant and cannot be reliably cleaned. A variety of single-use disposable items are available for use in dentistry, and when used appropriately may enhance an infection-control program (Table 17-1).

TABLE 17-1 Key Points to Remember When Using Single-Use Disposable Items

1. Disposable items are not intended to be cleaned and sterilized for reuse on another patient, because they are usually not heat-tolerant and cannot be reliably cleaned.

2. Handle disposable items aseptically.
   - If an item is stored in a bulk container or package, use an aseptic technique when retrieving it (e.g., use sterile cotton pliers to retrieve an item for use).
   - Dispense disposable items in small amounts (i.e., **unit dose**) sufficient for care of one patient before treatment begins and discard whatever is not used.

3. Any single-use device or item (e.g., cotton rolls, gauze, and irrigating syringes) used during oral surgical procedures should be sterile at the time of use.

4. Follow federal, state, and local regulations when disposing of single-use disposable items.

✔ Practical Dental Infection-Control Checklist

Single-Use (Disposable) Devices

❑ Are single-use devices used for one patient only and disposed of appropriately?

Aseptic Technique for Parenteral Medications

❑ Are aseptic techniques followed when using single- or multiple-dose medication vials and IV fluids?

❑ Are single-dose vials used for parenteral medications when possible?

❑ Are single-dose medication vials used for one patient only and disposed of appropriately?

❑ Are IV fluid bags and equipment used for one patient and disposed of appropriately?

❑ Are sterile devices (i.e., needle, syringe) used to enter single- or multiple-dose medication vials?

❑ Are manufacturer and/or local policies followed in terms of storage, use, and expiration?

❑ If multidose vials are used, is the access diaphragm cleaned with 70% alcohol before a sterile device (i.e., needle or syringe) is inserted into the vial?

❑ Are multidose vials kept away from the immediate patient treatment area to prevent inadvertent contamination by spray or spatter?

❑ Is the multidose vial discarded if sterility is compromised?

Review Questions

1. A disposable, or single-use, device is designed to be used on one patient and then discarded.
   A. True
   B. False

2. If a disposable device is used during an oral surgical procedure, it must be sterile at the time of use.
   A. True
   B. False

3. Using disposable items enhances infection control by eliminating the risk of patient-to-patient transmission of infectious microorganisms because
   A. the item is cleaned and disinfected before use on another patient.
   B. the item is discarded and not used on another patient.
   C. extra steps are necessary during the cleaning process.
   D. A and C

4. All disposable items can be discarded with the regular trash.
   A. True
   B. False

Critical Thinking

1. Make a list of the single-use disposable items you use in your dental office/clinic? Can you list several advantages and disadvantages of using single-use disposable items?

2. Can you think of any items you are currently using that have a disposable alternative that may be easier and more cost-effective to use?

3. A new employee says he has an idea that will save money. He states that at another office where he worked, they cleaned and "soaked" the prophy cups and were able to use them several times. How do you explain to him that it is not acceptable to reuse a disposable item?

SELECTED READINGS

CDC. Guidelines for infection control in dental health-care settings—2003. MMWR 2003;52(RR-17):1–66.

CDC. Transmission of hepatitis B and C viruses in outpatient settings–New York, Oklahoma, and Nebraska, 2000–2002. MMWR 2003;52:901–906.

Food and Drug Administration. Labeling recommendations for single-use devices reprocessed by third parties and hospitals; final guidance for industry and FDA. Rockville, MD: U.S. Department of Health and Human Services, Food and Drug Administration; 2001.

National Center for Policy Analysis. Health issues; hospitals "recycling" single-use medical items. http://www.ncpa.org/pi/health/pd091599c.html. Accessed July 10, 2008.

U.S. Department of Labor, Occupational Safety, and Health Administration. 29 CFR Part 1910.1030. Occupational exposure to bloodborne pathogens; needlesticks and other sharps injuries; final rule. Fed Regist 2001;66:5317–5325. [As amended from and includes 29 CFR Part 1910.1030. Occupational exposure to bloodborne pathogens; final rule. Fed Regist 1991;56:64174–64182.]

18

Infection Control in Dental Radiography

Jennifer A. Harte

John A. Molinari

LEARNING OBJECTIVES

After completion of this chapter individuals should be able to:

1 Describe general infection-control practices before, during, and after radiographic procedures.

2 Describe techniques to minimize contamination of equipment and environmental surfaces during intraoral and extraoral radiographic procedures.

3 Describe techniques to minimize contamination of radiographic processing equipment and the darkroom.

4 Discuss special infection-control considerations for digital radiography sensors and associated computer equipment.

The same infection-control practices used to eliminate or minimize disease transmission during patient treatment also apply to dental radiographic procedures. However, in addition to the potential to cross-contaminate equipment and environmental surfaces in the treatment area, dental healthcare personnel (DHCP) are faced with several unique infection-control challenges. Transporting contaminated films from the treatment area to the darkroom increases the potential for cross-contamination outside of the treatment area. Also, with the increasing popularity of digital radiography, DHCP are faced with new challenges of preventing cross-contamination of the digital sensor and computer equipment in the treatment room. Of concern is the digital sensor that is used instead of radiographic film, because currently it cannot be heat sterilized. Additionally, disinfection or barrier protection of associated computer equipment in the treatment room must not be overlooked.

GENERAL INFECTION-CONTROL PRACTICES BEFORE, DURING, AND AFTER RADIOGRAPHIC PROCEDURES

The potential for cross-contamination exists during the exposure and processing of dental radiographs. Standard precautions apply and measures must be taken to reduce or eliminate the cross-contamination, even though disease transmission has not been documented. Just as with operative, surgical, periodontal, prosthodontic, or endodontic procedures, infection-control measures to protect both patients and staff are necessary during radiographic procedures. These procedures are briefly reviewed in this chapter and discussed in detail in previous chapters.

Personal Protective Equipment (PPE) and Hand Hygiene

When dental radiography procedures are performed, the possibility exists that DHCP will contact blood, blood-contaminated saliva, or mucous membranes. Gloves must be worn when taking radiographs and handling contaminated film packets. As a reminder, gloves are not a substitute for hand hygiene. DHCP must wash their hands before gloving and after removing gloves. Powder-free gloves are recommended because powder can affect the film's emulsion layer and cause image artifacts. A surgical mask, protective eyewear, and gown also should be considered if spattering of blood or other body fluids is likely. For example, it would be recommended to wear additional PPE when treating patients with gagging problems or respiratory infections such as the common cold.

Environmental Infection Control

The potential to cross-contaminate equipment and environmental surfaces is high if **aseptic technique** is not practiced. Table 18-1 presents surfaces that are likely to become contaminated during radiography procedures. As a general rule, the best way to minimize contamination of environmental surfaces is to touch as few surfaces as possible. Since radiographic equipment, such as the x-ray tube head and control panels, is often difficult to clean, surface barriers are effective in preventing contamination of these clinical contact surfaces (Fig. 18-1). Barriers should not interfere with access to the controls either visually or mechanically. Clear disposable plastic wrap, plastic sheets or tubing, plastic-backed paper, or other material impervious to moisture are effective barriers. Once gloves have been donned and exposure of film begins, DHCP should touch only barrier-protected surfaces.

TABLE 18-1 Examples of Clinical Contact Surfaces Likely to Become Contaminated During Radiography Procedures

• The entire tube head (including the swivel arms used to turn the tube head)

• The entire extension device

• Arm rest, chair controls, and head rest

• Exposure panel (including all adjustment knobs and exposure buttons)

• Work areas/countertops onto which exposed film packets or film-holding devices are laid

• Any other surface likely to be contacted that is not operated via a foot control (e.g., light switch, faucet handles)

If surface barriers are used, the barriers must be changed between patients. If barriers are not used, equipment that is contaminated must be cleaned and disinfected with an Environmental Protection Agency (EPA)-registered hospital disinfectant of low- (i.e., HIV and HBV claim) to intermediate-level (i.e., tuberculocidal claim) activity. An **intermediate-level disinfectant** should be used when the surface is visibly contaminated with blood or saliva. PPE (e.g., gloves, surgical mask, protective eyewear, and gowns) should be worn until cleaning and disinfection are complete. If lead aprons and thyroid collars become contaminated, they should be cleaned and disinfected before the next patient is seated.

Radiographic Supplies

All necessary supplies, equipment, and instruments should be prepared before the patient is seated. Dispensing only the amount necessary for each procedure, commonly known as unit dosing, minimizes cross contamination. In addition, unit dosing reduces both chairside time and DHCP contact with environmental surfaces. Table 18-2 provides examples of items to unit dose for dental radiography procedures.

Cleaning, Disinfecting, and Sterilizing Radiographic Instruments

Many radiographic supplies, such as bitewing tabs, cotton rolls, and some film-stabilizing devices, are disposable (i.e., used once and disposed of appropriately). Using disposable items eliminates the need for sterilization between patients. Because most of the reusable radiographic instruments, such as film-stabilizing devices, are heat tolerant, they should be cleaned and heat-sterilized before patient use.

INTRAORAL AND EXTRAORAL RADIOGRAPHIC PROCEDURES

For intraoral radiographic procedures, infection-control procedures can be simplified by using films with protective barriers (Fig. 18-2). DHCP can purchase films with plastic barrier covers that protect the film from contamination and reduce processing time. After the radiograph is exposed, if the barrier is carefully opened, the underlying uncontaminated film packet can be dropped onto a

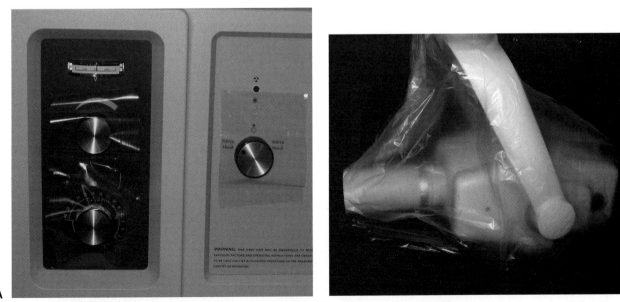

A   B

FIGURE 18-1 An example of a barrier-protected control panel **(A)** and a tube head **(B)**.

TABLE 18-2 Examples of Items to Prepare Before Seating the Patient

- Surface barriers
- Powder-free gloves
- Radiographic film(s)
- Sterile or disposable film holders
- Cotton rolls/gauze
- Paper towels
- Lead apron and thyroid collar

TABLE 18-3 Infection-Control Hints for Intraoral Radiographic Procedures

1. Use films protected with plastic barrier packets whenever possible.

2. To minimize contamination of environmental surfaces:
   - touch as few surfaces as possible;
   - use foot controls for chair adjustment and film exposure;
   - remove the lead apron with clean, ungloved hands to avoid contamination.

3. Keep unused and exposed films separate:
   - place unused films on a tray or paper towel;
   - wipe off excess saliva and place exposed films in a plastic cup labeled with the patient's name, being careful not to contaminate the outside of the cup since it will be used to transport films to the darkroom.

4. Do not place contaminated film-holding devices on non–barrier-protected surfaces.

clean surface or into a plastic cup for transport to the processing area (Fig. 18-2). DHCP can then open the film packet with clean, ungloved hands in the processing area. A study has shown that correctly placed film barriers can prevent contamination by preventing fluid penetration. If film barriers are not used, additional precautions are necessary when opening the film packets during processing. This will be addressed in the Processing Procedures section. Review Table 18-3 for several ways to reduce the potential for cross-contamination during intraoral radiographic procedures.

Because contamination from blood or saliva is highly unlikely during extraoral radiographic procedures, such as taking a panoramic radiograph, the infection-control practices that should be followed are more straightforward. With panoramic machines, the main infection-control concern is the bite guide, which can be disposable, reusable, and heat-sterilized between each patient, or barrier-protected. For hygienic purposes, the patient chin rest, head-positioning guides, and handgrips can be barrier-protected or cleaned after film exposure. If barriers are used, they should be placed before positioning the patient. The patient can be asked to remove the contaminated barrier on the bite guide or the disposable bite guide and place it in the regular waste container, or DHCP can remove the contaminated item while wearing gloves. Since oral secretions normally do not contaminate extraoral cassettes, they can be handled with ungloved hands and no other infection-control measures will be necessary for processing.

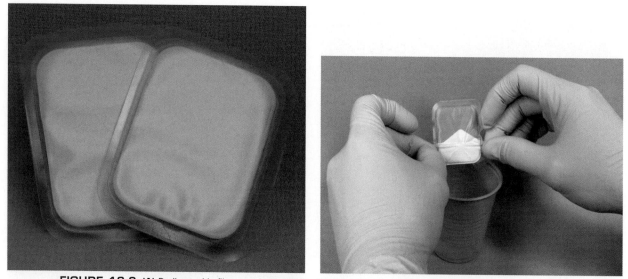

FIGURE 18-2 (A) Radiographic film protected with plastic barrier covers. **(B)** Opening the barrier-protected film wearing gloves.

TRANSITION FROM THE TREATMENT AREA TO THE DARKROOM

Any reusable instruments should be left in the treatment room and cleaned up according to standard office procedures. After film exposure, all film packets should be wiped dry. When using films with protective plastic barriers, carefully remove the barrier covers (Fig. 18-2) and dispose of them appropriately before leaving the treatment room. If protective barriers are not used on the films, the contaminated film packets should be placed on a tray or in a plastic cup to allow the film to be transported to the processing area without being touched. Be careful not to contaminate the outside of the carrying container. Do not transport films in clinic jacket pockets. Regardless of which technique is used, gloves and other PPE can then be removed and hands washed. The films are now ready for transport to the processing area.

PROCESSING PROCEDURES

Care should be taken when unwrapping films to avoid contamination of the developing equipment and surrounding environmental surfaces. Using films with protective barriers helps to minimize contamination in the darkroom. If barriers are not used and/or the film is contaminated, it is necessary to take precautions when using a **daylight loader** or portable darkroom. In particular, care must be taken to avoid contaminating the protective sleeves or flaps that allow access to the chamber while minimizing light exposure (Fig. 18-3). The sleeves are commonly made of cloth or rubber and, if contaminated, cannot be adequately cleaned and disinfected. As a result, the use of day-

light loaders is discouraged. Table 18-4 compares infection-control procedures that are necessary when developing films in a darkroom and when using a daylight loader.

DIGITAL RADIOGRAPHY INFECTION-CONTROL CONSIDERATIONS

Digital Sensors

Because of its clinical advantages, **digital radiography** is becoming more popular in dentistry; however, it presents new infection-control challenges. Because a darkroom is not necessary for digital radiography, concerns about cross-contamination during darkroom activities are eliminated. Intraoral **digital sensors** come into contact with mucous membranes, and therefore ideally should be cleaned and heat-sterilized or high-level-disinfected between patients. At this time, however, sensors cannot withstand heat sterilization or complete immersion in a high-level disinfectant. Until technology permits this, the Centers for Disease Control and Prevention (CDC) recommends at a minimum that the sensor be barrier-protected by using a **Food and Drug Administration (FDA)-cleared barrier** to reduce gross contamination during use. Although wireless technology is becoming available, many sensors still have a connecting cord. It is also necessary to ensure that the barrier extends onto any section of the cord that may contact mucous membranes. Because the use of a barrier does not always protect against contamination, after the barrier is removed the device should be cleaned and disinfected with an EPA-registered, intermediate-level disinfectant after each

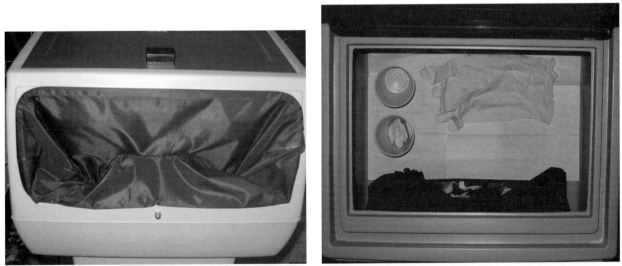

FIGURE 18-3 When using a daylight loader **(A)**, place a pair of gloves, contaminated film in a plastic cup, barriers, and an extra plastic cup for waste materials on the loader floor **(B)**.

TABLE 18-4 Infection-Control Procedures in a Darkroom vs. Using a Daylight Loader

	In a Darkroom	Using a Daylight Loader
Films with protective plastic covers	1. Open the film packets carefully to avoid touching the film; place the films in the developer. Note: It is recommended to remove the barrier in the area where the radiograph was exposed, and to transport the uncontaminated film packets in a cup to the processing area (Fig. 18-2).	
Films without protective plastic covers	1. Prepare a work area near the processor with the plastic cup of contaminated films, a clean paper towel, and a second plastic cup. 2. Don a new pair of gloves (preferably powder free). 3. With gloved hands, open the film packets carefully to avoid touching the film. Drop the exposed film onto the clean paper towel. 4. Place the contaminated film packaging materials into the second plastic cup. 5. Discard the plastic cups, remove and discard gloves, perform hand hygiene. 6. With clean, ungloved hands, place the films in the developer.	1. With clean hands, prepare the inside of the daylight loader by placing a barrier on the bottom of the chamber. 2. Place a clean pair of gloves (preferably powder free), the cup of contaminated films, and a second plastic cup on the barrier inside the daylight loader. 3. Close the top of the daylight loader. 4. Place clean hands through the sleeves and don the clean gloves. 5. With gloved hands, open the film packets carefully to avoid touching the film. Drop the exposed film onto the clean paper towel. 6. Place the contaminated film packaging materials in the second plastic cup. 7. Remove gloves, place films in the developing slots and pull ungloved hands through the sleeves. 8. Open the top of the daylight loader, wrap all the trash in the barrier, remove, and discard. Do not remove contaminated items through the protective sleeves. 9. Perform hand hygiene.

patient (Fig. 18-4). This will also minimize the potential for device-associated infections. One study determined that a brand of commercially available plastic barriers used to protect dental digital radiography sensors failed at a substantial rate (44%). This rate dropped to 6% when latex finger cots were used in conjunction with the plastic barrier. Because digital radiography sensors vary by manufacturer or type of device in their ability to be sterilized or high level disinfected, manufacturers should be consulted regarding appropriate barrier and disinfection/sterilization procedures.

Computer Equipment

Computer equipment in patient treatment areas that are used for digital radiography or other procedures is an-

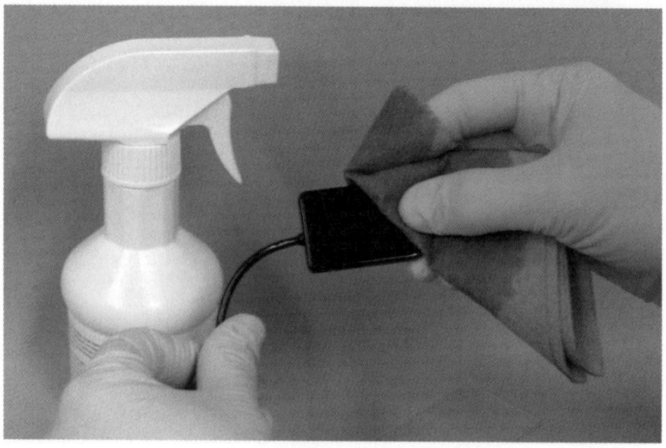

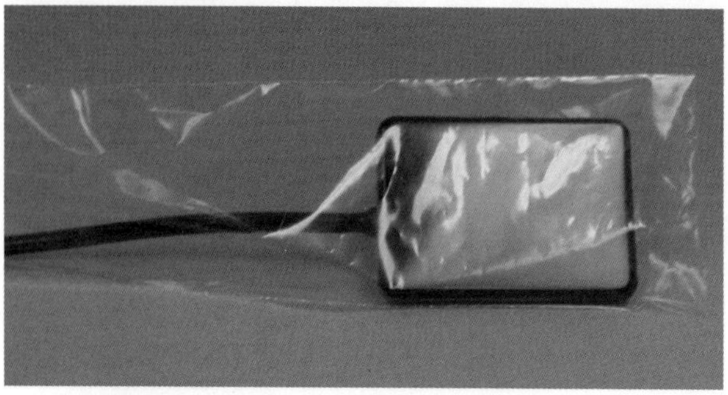

FIGURE 18-4 A digital radiographic sensor with barrier protection **(A)**, and recommended cleaning and disinfection procedures following barrier removal **(B)**.

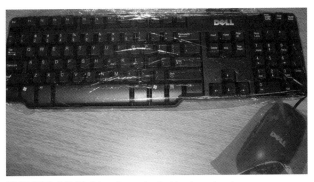

FIGURE 18-5 A barrier-protected keyboard and mouse.

other infection-control concern. The basic principles of cleaning and disinfecting clinical contact surfaces used routinely in the dental operatory also apply to computer equipment. Avoiding contamination is important because many computer-related items cannot be properly cleaned and disinfected or sterilized. A computer keyboard and mouse are excellent examples of difficult items to clean. Studies have shown that computer equipment can serve as a potential reservoir for infectious agents. The best results with the least damage to the equipment are obtained by following the manufacturer's directions; however, most computer companies provide only basic cleaning instructions for their computer hardware, and rarely do they offer instructions for disinfection in healthcare settings. One study demonstrated that keyboards could be successfully decontaminated using disinfectant wipes without causing functional or cosmetic damage after 300 disinfection cycles. Also, computer equipment is being designed that can tolerate the use of liquid disinfectant products. Examples include liquid-proof mice and keyboards. Computer equipment that can tolerate the use of liquid disinfectant products may be preferable and easier to maintain. If the cleaning and disinfecting products used in the dental practice are not compatible with the computer equipment, the computer equipment should be covered with a plastic barrier when contamination is likely. Reusable form-fitted barriers that can be cleaned and disinfected between patients are available for keyboards. If the barrier is disposable, it should be changed between patients (Fig. 18-5).

SUMMARY

Radiographic procedures involve multiple steps, and the potential for cross-contamination within and outside the treatment area is high if aseptic technique is not followed. To protect both patients and staff members, office infection-control plans and training programs should include dental radiographic infection-control practices.

✓ Practical Dental Infection-Control Checklist

General Considerations

❑ Do DHCP wear gloves and use when exposing radiographs and handling contaminated film packets?

❑ Is other PPE (e.g., protective eyewear, mask, and gown) used, as appropriate, if spattering of blood or other body fluids is likely?

❑ Are heat-tolerant or disposable intraoral devices (e.g., film-holding and positioning devices) used whenever possible?

❑ Are heat-tolerant devices cleaned and heat-sterilized between patients?

❑ Are exposed radiographs handled and transported in an aseptic manner to prevent contamination of developing equipment?

Digital Radiography

❑ When using digital radiography sensors, are FDA-cleared barriers employed to protect the sensor from contamination?

❑ After the barrier is removed, is the digital radiography sensor cleaned and disinfected with an EPA-registered hospital disinfectant with intermediate-level activity (i.e., tuberculocidal claim) between patients?

❑ Does the dental office/clinic consult with the manufacturer regarding methods of disinfection and sterilization of digital radiography sensors, and protection of associated computer hardware?

Review Questions

1. Infection-control practices in dental radiography

   A. are the same as those used during other dental procedures.

   B. are not necessary since dental handpieces are not used.

   C. require the application of special precautions.

   D. are not necessary since there is minimal contact with blood or other potentially infectious materials (OPIM).

2. Standard precautions do not apply when taking dental radiographs.

   A. True

   B. False

3. Which of the following are potential sources of cross-contamination when taking dental radiographs?

   A. film packets

   B. control panels on radiography equipment

   C. environmental surfaces (e.g., countertops)

   D. A and B only

   E. all of the above

4. Hand-washing is not necessary when taking intraoral dental radiographs because gloves are always worn.

   A. True

   B. False

5. Gloves must always be worn when taking intraoral radiographs and handling contaminated film packets. Other types of PPE (e.g., mask, protective eyewear, long-sleeved gown) are required if contamination with blood or OPIM is anticipated.

   A. The first statement is true. The second statement is false.

   B. The first statement is false. The second statement is true.

   C. Both statements are true.

   D. Both statements are false.

6. Which of the following statements about environmental surface barriers is false?

   A. Surface barriers are simple to use and can shorten patient turnaround time.

   B. Surface barriers should not interfere with access to control panels.

   C. Surface barriers should not be used on items that are difficult to clean and disinfect.

   D. If surface barriers are used, the barriers must be changed between patients.

7. Unit dosing for intraoral radiographs

   A. minimizes cross-contamination.

   B. is recommended before beginning the radiographic procedure.

   C. refers to dispensing supplies in amounts appropriate for each patient procedure.

   D. all of the above

8. Which of the following statements is false?

   A. Ideally, during film exposure, surfaces should be barrier protected.

   B. Film(s) should be dried (following film exposure and before glove removal) to remove excess saliva or blood.

   C. Films should be transported to the darkroom for processing in your clinic jacket pocket.

   D. Reusable heat-tolerant film holders or positioning devices should be heat-sterilized between patients.

9. The use of radiographic film barriers is a simple way to maintain infection-control measures by protecting film packets from contamination, and can reduce preparation and processing time.

   A. True

   B. False

10. What infection-control measures are recommended for digital radiography sensors?

    A. Heat-sterilize the sensor between patients.

    B. Immerse in a high-level disinfectant for 10 hours between patients.

    C. Barrier-protect, clean, and disinfect with an intermediate-level disinfectant.

    D. No special procedures are necessary because the sensor is not placed intraorally.

Critical Thinking

1. Obtain a radiographic film packet. Demonstrate how you would handle it after exposing the radiograph on the patient.

2. You just started using digital radiography in the dental office/clinic. You notice that the digital sensor cannot be heat-sterilized or immersed in a high-level disinfectant. What infection-control measures will you apply to minimize cross-contamination between patients? What type of infection-control measures do you take to protect the associated computer equipment?

3. Why are different infection-control practices used for intraoral and extraoral radiographic procedures?

SELECTED READINGS

American Academy of Oral and Maxillofacial Radiology. American Academy of Oral and Maxillofacial Radiology infection control guidelines for dental radiographic procedures. Oral Surg Oral Med Oral Pathol 1983;55:421–426.

American Dental Association Council on Scientific Affairs. An update on radiographic practices: information and recommendations. J Am Dent Assoc 2001;132:234–238.

Bachman CE, White JM, Goodis HE, et al. Bacterial adherence and contamination during radiographic processing. Oral Surg Oral Med Oral Pathol 1990;70:669–673.

Bajuscak RE, Hall EH, Giambarresi LI, et al. Bacterial contamination of dental radiographic film. Oral Surg Oral Med Oral Pathol 1993;76:661–663.

Bartoloni JA, Charlton DG, Flint DJ. Infection control practices in dental radiology. Gen Dent 2003;51:264–271.

CDC. Guidelines for infection control in dental healthcare settings–2003. MMWR 2003;52(RR-17):1–66.

Crawford JJ. Clinical Asepsis in Dentistry. Mesquite, TX: Oral Medicine Press; 1987:27–35.

Haring JI, Jansen L. Infection control and the dental radiographer. In: Dental Radiography: Principles and Techniques. 2nd ed. Philadelphia: WB Saunders; 2000:194–204

Hartmann B, Benson M, Junger A, et al. Computer keyboard and mouse as reservoir of pathogens in an intensive care unit. J Clin Monit Comput 2004;18:7–12.

Hokett SD, Honey JR, Ruiz F, et al. Assessing the effectiveness of direct digital radiography barrier sheaths and finger cots. J Am Dent Assoc 2000;131:463–467.

Langland OE, Langlais RP. Radiology infection control procedures. In: Principles of Dental Imaging. Baltimore: Lippincott, Wilkins & Wilkins; 1997:69–84.

Neely AN, Weber JM, Daviau P, et al. Computer equipment used in patient care within a multihospital system: recommendations for cleaning and disinfection. Am J Infect Control 2005;33:233–237.

Rutala WA, White MS; Gergen MF, et al. Bacterial contamination of keyboards: efficacy and functional impact of disinfectants. Infect Control Hosp Epidemiol 2006;27:372–377.

Schultz M, Gill J, Zubairi S, et al. Bacterial contamination of computer keyboards in a teaching hospital. Infect Control Hosp Epidemiol 2003;24:302–303.

Stanczyk DA, Paunovich ED, Broome JC, et al. Microbiologic contamination during dental radiographic film processing. Oral Surg Oral Med Oral Pathol 1993;76:112–119.

White SC, Glaze S. Interpatient microbiological cross-contamination after dental radiographic examination. J Am Dent Assoc 1978;96:801–804.

Wolfgang L. Analysis of a new barrier infection control system for dental radiographic film. Compend Contin Educ Dent 1992;1:68–71.

19

Infection Control in the Dental Laboratory

Virginia A. Merchant

LEARNING OBJECTIVES

After completion of this chapter individuals should be able to:

1 Explain the need for infection control in the dental laboratory.

2 Explain the requirements for infection control in both in-office and commercial dental laboratories.

3 Explain the methods for disinfection of dental impressions and the limitations posed by certain impression materials.

4 Choose an appropriate disinfectant based on the type of impression material used.

5 Appropriately disinfect other items transported to and from the dental laboratory.

6 Choose an appropriate disinfectant for prostheses and other laboratory-produced items.

7 Appropriately sterilize or disinfect items used chairside in prosthodontic and orthodontic procedures.

8 Explain the unit-dose concept.

KEY TERMS

Intermediate-level disinfectant: a liquid chemical germicide registered by the Environmental Protection Agency (EPA) as a hospital disinfectant and with a label claim of potency as a tuberculocidal. Intermediate-level disinfection is a process that inactivates most vegetative bacteria, most fungi, and some viruses, but cannot be relied on to inactivate resistant microorganisms, such as mycobacteria or bacterial spores.

Rinse-spray-rinse-spray: a disinfection method whereby an item that has been or potentially can be contaminated

with oral secretions is rinsed under running water and then sprayed with disinfectant. This method is most appropriate for items that are not easily wiped (as in the spray-wipe-spray method).

Unit dosing: the amount of material that is sufficient to accomplish a particular procedure to prevent cross-contamination. The material is dispensed before patient contact, and any excess is discarded at completion.

Before we understood the need for universal precautions (now called standard precautions) in all areas of dentistry, the need for infection control in the dental laboratory was rarely considered, and primarily focused on the handling of items from "high-risk" patients. In 1978, the American Dental Association (ADA) first published specific recommendations for infection control in the dental laboratory. Subsequent ADA recommendations and the guidelines from the Centers for Disease Control and Prevention (CDC) have included infection-control recommendations for the dental laboratory.

Aside from certain pieces of equipment, few items are unique to the dental laboratory environment. Most items that require infection control in the dental laboratory originate in the dental operatory or are returned there from the laboratory. Several of these are composed of heat-sensitive materials and are subject to distortion.

Dental impressions are contaminated with saliva and sometimes blood. Prostheses and appliances are often "tried in" in the process of their construction, and thus go from laboratory to operatory and back again. Patient prostheses and appliances that require laboratory repair are often grossly contaminated. All of these items are potentially infectious and must be either disinfected or sterilized before being handled in the laboratory. Alternatively, such items and any items fabricated from them can be handled as contaminated; however, they then pose an additional risk of cross-contaminating other devices and materials in the laboratory. Figure 19-1 provides a flowchart of infection-control procedures for common items shipped between the dental office and the dental laboratory.

Prostheses, appliances, and related items constructed in the laboratory that are to be inserted into the patient's

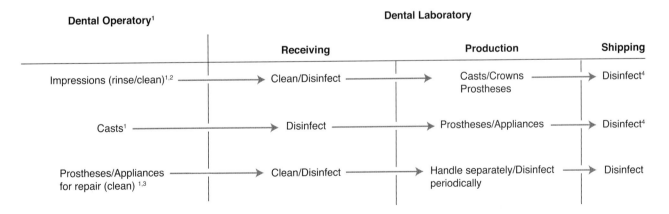

¹ Ideally, contaminated items to be transported to the dental laboratory should be disinfected before shipping. If not, they must be labeled BIOHAZARD.
² All impressions should be rinsed under running water immediately after removal from the patient's mouth. If still visibly contaminated, clean.
³ Any item work by a patient is grossly contaminated and must be cleaned and disinfected prior to further handling.
⁴ If the laboratory practices routine infection control, new prostheses and appliances are considered "clean" but must be disinfected prior to delivery of the patient. This disinfection step may be accomplished in either the dental laboratory or the dental office.

FIGURE 19-1 Flowchart of selected laboratory infection-control procedures.

mouth must also be rendered "noninfectious" prior to delivery. These prosthodontic and orthodontic items, along with their associated handling or construction in the dental laboratory, offer some relatively unique challenges to infection control. Several reviews that have addressed infection control in the dental laboratory and as related to prosthodontics are listed at the end of this chapter.

STERILIZATION VS. DISINFECTION

In most cases, **intermediate-level disinfection** is sufficient for decontaminating items handled in the dental laboratory. The primary concern is preventing exposure of employees to infectious microorganisms, and the cross-contamination of cases being processed. Only items that ultimately will come in contact with mucous membranes require sterilization; however, routine sterilization of items that can withstand heat enhances the overall laboratory infection-control program and further reduces the potential for cross-contamination. If a laboratory item that will come into contact with mucous membranes cannot be heat-sterilized (e.g., acrylic appliances), disinfection using an Environmental Protection Agency (EPA)-registered hospital disinfectant with at least intermediate-level (i.e., tuberculocidal) activity is acceptable if laboratory infection-control protocols are adequate to prevent cross-contamination. Some dental laboratories are now equipped with heat sterilizers (usually autoclaves) that can be used to sterilize heat-stable items.

The routine cleaning and disinfection of environmental surfaces and equipment in the dental laboratory should be comparable to that practiced in the dental office. Laboratory staff should use EPA-registered hospital disinfectants with low- (HIV, HBV effectiveness claim) to intermediate-level (tuberculocidal claim) activity depending on the degree of contamination.

THE DENTAL LABORATORY

Dental laboratories range from small in-office laboratories containing a single lathe and sink to large commercial laboratories. In either circumstance, regulations as defined by the Occupational Safety and Health Administration (OSHA) apply for occupational exposure to bloodborne pathogens. Infection-control protocols for in-office laboratories must be included in the dental office's overall exposure-control plan. Commercial laboratories are subject to the same OSHA regulations as dental offices and are required to have their own exposure-control plans.

Refer to the appropriate text chapters for information related to OSHA regulations, disease transmission, personal protection (including hand-washing and immunizations), surface disinfection, and sterilization methods.

Personal Protective Equipment (PPE)

PPE must be used when handling contaminated items in the laboratory. Depending on the amount of contamination or the task being performed, PPE (e.g., gloves, masks, protective eyewear, and gowns) is indicated. In the dental laboratory following disinfection or sterilization to decontaminate an item, most items can then be handled as noninfectious if separate "clean" work areas are available.

Following decontamination of laboratory items, some type of gown or laboratory coat is still recommended in the work area to protect the employee's clothes, and other barriers are often required as a safety precaution. A National Institute of Occupational Safety and Health (NIOSH)-approved dust/mist face mask and eye protection (e.g., protective eyewear with side shields or a face shield) must be worn when operating lathes, model trimmers, or other rotary equipment. Safety shields and ventilation systems are also required when using mounted rotary equipment, such as lathes, to reduce the risk of aerosols, spatter, and projectiles.

If gloves are worn during operation of a lathe, extreme caution must be taken to avoid injury resulting from the glove being caught in the lathe. The risk of infection when handling contaminated items is considered greater than the physical hazard; therefore, gloves should be worn when necessary and appropriate caution exercised.

Communication with the Dental Laboratory

The dental practitioner should communicate with the dental laboratory regarding infection-control procedures used in the dental office. Ideally, contaminated items should be disinfected prior to transport from the dental office to the laboratory and vice versa. Both parties should be aware of the disinfection methods used by the other. Items that have been disinfected should be labeled to so indicate; otherwise, the laboratory or dental office should assume that they are contaminated and disinfect them as appropriate. When returning items to the dental office, National Association of Dental Laboratories (NADL)-member laboratories label bags containing disinfected appliances with a sticker indicating that the contents have been disinfected by the laboratory for the protection of the dentist, staff, and patient (Fig. 19-2).

Communication and understanding can avoid duplication of effort and possible adverse effects on the materials. Some clinicians have recommended that disinfection should be left to the laboratory to avoid duplication, and in certain geographic locations this is the accepted policy. If so, OSHA regulations require that contaminated

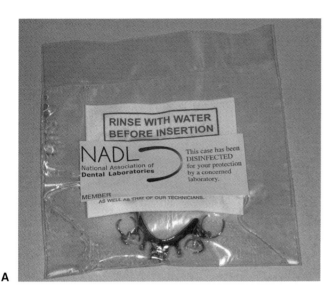

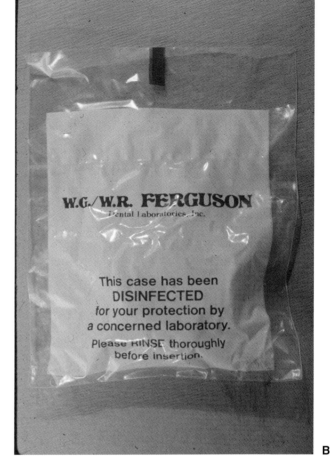

FIGURE 19-2 (A,B) Many commercial laboratories label disinfected items shipped from the laboratory to the dental office.

items be shipped or otherwise transported in closed containers that do not leak and are either colored red or identified with a biohazard label (Fig. 19-3). The CDC guidelines state that laboratory materials should be cleaned and disinfected before being manipulated in the laboratory, but do not specify at what point this should

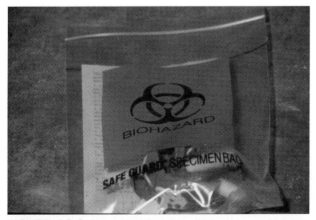

FIGURE 19-3 Impression shipped in a biohazard bag with a separate compartment for the work authorization.

occur. If either the laboratory or the dental office is uncertain of the status of disinfection, the process should be repeated.

The In-Office Laboratory

In its simplest form, the in-office laboratory consists of an area designated for laboratory adjustments of dental prostheses and/or pouring stone models of dental impressions. Dental impressions and prostheses that have been inserted into the mouth are contaminated and must be handled as such or decontaminated before laboratory manipulations are performed.

Potential cross-contamination problems arise in the dental office primarily because of the need to make quick adjustments on dental prostheses that have been either tried-in in the patient's mouth or worn by the patient. Items should be disinfected before adjustment to prevent contamination of the lathe and transmission of microorganisms via aerosols. The use of sterilized (e.g., rag wheels and burs) or **unit dosing** materials (e.g., pumice and polishing compounds) decreases the potential for cross-contamination. The prosthesis must also be disinfected before it is returned to the patient.

The Commercial Dental Laboratory

The NADL, which has been instrumental in developing infection-control protocols for dental laboratories, recommends the disinfection of all items received from the dental office, and all appliances before shipping. A manual and video training program, available to NADL member laboratories, details infection-control protocols for receiving, production, and shipping areas. Because they are subject to OSHA regulations, commercial laboratories must have exposure control plans similar to those developed for the dental office.

Procedures for the Dental Laboratory

Several organizations and individuals have proposed designating specific areas for various purposes in laboratories. A strict adherence to these designated purposes acts as a barrier system, reducing the potential for cross-contamination.

Receiving Area

The receiving area should be separate from the production area. Incoming cases should be unpacked carefully by an individual wearing PPE (Fig. 19-4). Unless the employee knows that the case was adequately disinfected in the dental office, it should be immediately disinfected upon receipt with an EPA-registered tuberculocidal disinfectant. As a precaution, most commercial laboratories disinfect all incoming items. Items that are visibly contaminated should be cleaned prior to disinfection.

Items should be disinfected before being transferred to case pans to avoid contamination of the pan (Fig. 19-5). Case pans must be cleaned and disinfected prior to reuse

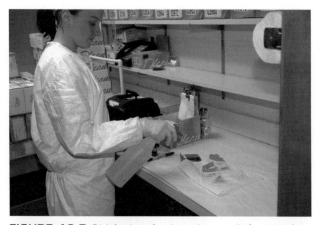

FIGURE 19-5 Disinfection of an incoming case before transfer to a case pan. (Photograph courtesy of Olson Dental Company, Inc.)

to avoid cross-contamination. Work authorizations shipped in direct contact with a contaminated item are also contaminated and should be placed in a plastic bag before transfer to the production area.

Packing materials should be discarded, and not reused, to prevent cross-contamination. Most laboratory waste, with the exception of sharps, can be disposed of in the regular trash. Sharps must be disposed of in accordance with OSHA, state, and local regulations.

Employees working in the receiving area must remove PPE before moving to another area that is considered to be uncontaminated. All environmental surfaces in the receiving area should be cleaned and disinfected at least daily with an EPA-registered hospital disinfectant with low- to intermediate-level activity.

Production Area

Separate areas should be designated for new work and repairs. If these areas are adequately separated and all incoming cases are known to be disinfected, employees can handle new cases as noninfectious once they have been decontaminated. Given the uncertainty of decontamination of acrylic devices that have been worn by a patient, full PPE is advisable when handling these items, and every effort should be made to avoid cross-contamination from such items. Because of the porous nature of acrylics, periodic disinfection of repair work following grinding procedures is recommended.

All work surfaces should be cleaned and disinfected with an EPA-registered hospital low- to intermediate-level disinfectant on a regular basis, but at least daily. Pumice should be mixed with green soap and a disinfectant, such as an iodophor or chlorine compound, and should be changed when contaminated or at least daily. Ragwheels and brushes should be changed at least daily and after each case for repairs or when contaminated. These should be heat-sterilized if possible, but at a minimum

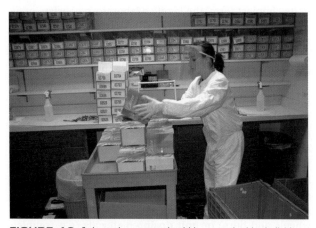

FIGURE 19-4 Incoming cases should be unpacked by individuals wearing full protective equipment. (Photograph courtesy of Olson Dental Company, Inc., Clinton Township, MI.)

cleaned and disinfected. When disposable items are available, the need for cleaning and disinfection of reusable items is eliminated. Unit doses of pumice and polishing compound prevent cross-contamination during polishing of repairs. Plastic wrap or other barriers can be used to cover pumice pans and work surfaces, simplifying cleanup.

Equipment should be cleaned and sterilized or disinfected as appropriate, usually on at least a daily basis. Avoiding contamination of sensitive equipment by properly disinfecting items received from the dental office and using barriers whenever possible is preferable to repeated exposures to chemical disinfectants or sterilization cycles.

Shipping Area

If prostheses or appliances are disinfected prior to shipping to the dental office, they should be labeled accordingly and shipped in a sealed plastic bag (Fig. 19-2). Disinfected acrylic items should be stored and shipped in a sealed bag containing a small amount of diluted mouthwash. Only new packing materials should be used to avoid cross-contamination.

Consultation Room

If patients are seen in the dental laboratory for purposes of shade verification, infection-control procedures must be the same as those used in the dental office, with proper cleaning and disinfection after each patient appointment. In states where denturism is legal, the denturist must follow the same infection-control precautions as a dentist.

Clean Dental Laboratories

Some dental laboratories operate as clean laboratories and only accept items that have been appropriately decontaminated prior to transport as evidenced on the work authorization. This system works most effectively in a closed environment where the dentists and the laboratory are all a part of some larger organization (e.g., military facilities and dental schools). In such a system, no special precautions are required in the receiving area. The production and shipping areas are handled in the same manner as described above for the standard dental laboratory.

DENTAL IMPRESSIONS

Although dental impressions were one of the first laboratory items to be considered contaminated and a potential infection-control problem, the first extensive study on disinfection of impressions was not published until 1981 (Storer and McCabe, 1981). Traditionally, impressions were rinsed under running water after being removed from the mouth to visibly eliminate saliva and blood.

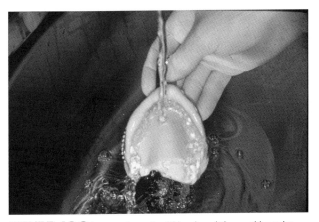

FIGURE 19-6 Impressions should be rinsed thoroughly under running tap water both before and after disinfection.

Although rinsing significantly reduces the numbers of microorganisms in most cases, it does not decontaminate the impression. Chairside rinsing of impressions remains the first step in successful infection control in the laboratory (Fig. 19-6).

Several investigations have evaluated the effects of various disinfectant products on different types of impression materials. Although most of these studies evaluated the dimensional stability of impression materials, other investigations have addressed the wettability of impressions following disinfection or effects on surface detail reproduction and hardness of resultant casts. A few studies have evaluated the effectiveness of disinfecting impressions, but they extrapolated results from the efficacy of the disinfectants on other surfaces. The majority of studies that actually evaluated effectiveness looked at elimination of vegetative bacteria or fungi; only a few studies have considered viruses.

Based on their research findings, some authors have recommended preparations for disinfecting impressions that are not approved as hospital-level disinfectants or have been shown in other studies to have adverse effects on the particular impression material. Other investigations have evaluated the effects of disinfectants on impression materials using inadequate exposure times for the disinfectant tested. Given the porosity of impression materials, the recommended exposure times probably should be longer than those for hard surfaces, rather than shorter.

As a result of the multiple experimental protocols used, and the variety of impression materials and disinfectant solutions available, research findings have sometimes been contradictory. Researchers have occasionally reported statistically significant effects that are not necessarily significant clinically. A small dimensional change or effect on the physical properties of die stone may be within the acceptable range for the particular impression

TABLE 19-1 **Guide for Selecting Appropriate Disinfection Methods for Items Transported to or from the Dental Laboratory**

Item	Method*	Recommended Disinfectants	Comments
Appliances Metal/acrylic All metal	Immersion is preferred; alternatively, spray all surfaces until thoroughly wet.	Chlorine compounds or iodophors Glutaraldehydes[†]	Rinse thoroughly following disinfection
Articulators/facebows	Spray-wipe-spray	Iodophors or phenolics	Facebow forks should be heat-sterilized before reuse.
Casts	Spray until wet or immerse.	Chlorine compounds or iodophors	Disinfectant may be prepared using slurry water (saturated calcium sulfate). Should not be disinfected until fully set (24 hours). Do not ship until fully dried.
Custom Impression Trays (acrylic)	Immerse or spray until wet	Chlorine compounds, iodophors, or phenolics	Do not reuse! Discard.
Impressions	Immersion disinfection preferred.		Heat-sterilize reusable impression trays. Discard plastic trays after use.
Irreversible hydrocolloid (alginate)	Use only disinfectants with short-term exposure times (no more than 10 minutes for alginates).	Chlorine compounds or iodophors. Phenolic sprays may be used on alginates.	Short-term immersion in glutaraldehydes[†] has been shown to be acceptable, but time is inadequate for disinfection.
Reversible hydrocolloid	Use caution with immersion disinfection.		Do not immerse in alkaline glutaraldehyde[†]
Polysulfide rubber Silicone rubber	Disinfect by immersion	Glutaraldehydes,[†] chlorine compounds, iodophors, phenolics	Disinfectants that require more than 30-minute exposures are not recommended.
Polyether	Disinfect by immersion with caution! Use only disinfectants with short-term exposure times (no more than 10 minutes).	Chlorine compounds, iodophors, or phenolics	ADA also recommends glutaraldehydes[†]; however, short-term exposures are essential to avoid distortion.
ZOE impression paste	Disinfection by immersion preferred.	Glutaraldehydes[†] or iodophors	Not compatible with chlorine compounds! Phenolic sprays may be used.
Impression compound	Spraying may be used for bite registrations.	Iodophors or chlorine compounds	Phenolic sprays may be used.
Prostheses	Immerse in disinfectant. Use caution to avoid corrosion of metal! NEVER expose unglazed porcelain to any disinfectant (must handle as contaminated).		Clean "old" prostheses by scrubbing with hand-wash antiseptic or sonication prior to disinfection.
Removable (acrylic/porcelain) Removable (metal/acrylic) Fixed (metal/porcelain)		Chlorine compounds or iodophors Chlorine compounds or iodophors Glutaraldehydes,[†] chlorine compounds, or iodophors	Rinse thoroughly following disinfection; store in diluted mouthwash.
Shade Guides	Immerse or spray-wipe-spray	Iodophors or phenolics	Final wipe with water or alcohol to avoid discoloration.
Wax Rims/Wax Bites	Rinse-spray-rinse-spray	Iodophors or phenolics	Rinse again following disinfection.

*Exposure time to disinfectant should be that recommended by the disinfectant manufacturer. All items must be thoroughly rinsed (15 seconds minimum) under running tap water following disinfection.

[†]Glutaraldehyde-based products should be used only if another disinfectant is not readily available. When used, appropriate precautions, including closed containers to limit vapor release, chemically-resistant gloves and aprons, face shields, and adequate ventilation, are essential. All items must be thoroughly and carefully rinsed.

Modification of table originally published in Merchant VA. Dental laboratory infection control. Operatory Infection Control Update 1995;3:3.

ZOE, zinc oxide eugenol.

material or stone and thus have no clinically discernible effect on the final product. Some significant differences, such as increased hardness of stone, are actually positive effects that result in an improved final product. Because of the variety of materials used, it is recommended that dental healthcare personnel (DHCP) consult with manufacturers regarding the stability of specific materials during disinfection.

Disinfection Method

Immersion, spraying, and short-term submersion have been recommended for disinfection of impressions. Immersion is the preferred method for disinfection. Spraying is an alternative method, but it poses the risk of not covering all surfaces of the impression, especially undercuts. Additionally, because the disinfectant runs off and pools, much of the impression is exposed to disinfectant for only a brief time, rather than the exposure time recommended for disinfection. Despite this, DHCP often choose to spray impressions because the same disinfectant product can be used that is used to disinfect environmental surfaces in the dental operatory, and less disinfectant is used. Short-term submersion or "dunking," an alternative to spraying, presents some of the same problems as spraying and requires excess disinfectant. The primary argument against immersion has been the concern that hydrophilic materials will become distorted from imbibing the water or disinfectant solution. Research has repeatedly shown this to be clinically unfounded if short disinfection times (less than 30 minutes) and the appropriate disinfectant are used (refer to Table 19-1).

Rinsing is the first step in the cleaning process. Impressions should be rinsed thoroughly under running tap water immediately after removal from the mouth to eliminate as much bioburden as possible, and again after disinfection to remove residual disinfectant from the impression surface. Impressions that contain residual bioburden should be further cleaned prior to disinfection. A camel-hair brush (artist's brush) with half-inch bristles dipped in a liquid detergent is an effective means of removing excess bioburden, but increases the risk of cross-contamination. An alternative would be to use disposable brushes. The addition of dental stone powder can further enhance cleaning. The impression should be rinsed again with water to remove residual detergent and debris before disinfection.

Impressions can be immersed in disinfectant in a variety of containers. Reusable plastic or glass containers that can be disinfected, or inexpensive, disposable, zipper-closure plastic bags are convenient for this purpose (Fig. 19-7). If an impression is sprayed with disinfectant, it must be sprayed on all sides until it is thoroughly wet and then covered (i.e., wrapped with plastic or otherwise enclosed) to prevent drying and allow exposure for the recommended disinfection time. Impressions should

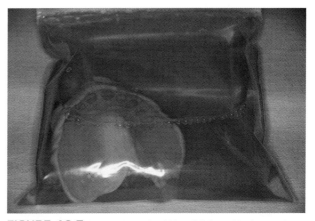

FIGURE 19-7 Impressions should be disinfected by immersion in an appropriate disinfectant for the time recommended for tuberculocidal disinfection. Zipper-closure plastic bags are convenient for this purpose.

always be rinsed under running water to remove residual disinfectant following disinfection. Some large commercial laboratories have designed efficient methods for disinfecting multiple cases simultaneously (Fig. 19-8).

No single disinfectant is compatible with all impression materials. Some of the newer or more recently approved disinfectants have not been evaluated for any or all impression materials. The recommendations in this chapter are based on available research data and generally do not address untested disinfectants or disinfectants that have not been approved as hospital-level disinfectants. Only disinfectants that are EPA-registered as a hospital disinfectant with tuberculocidal activity should be used for disinfection of impressions. Glutaraldehyde-based preparations are discussed in this chapter and can be used to disinfect laboratory items; however, their use is discouraged because they are highly toxic and require special precautions when being used, as discussed in Chapter 11. Alternative disinfectant products are available to successfully and safely disinfect laboratory items, and should be used whenever possible.

When selecting a disinfectant, one should consider the type of impression material, the disinfectants available in the dental office or laboratory, and the number of impressions to be disinfected per day. Disinfectant solutions should not be used repeatedly for disinfection of impressions.

The exposure or immersion time for a particular disinfectant should be at least that recommended by the disinfectant manufacturer, and in general no longer than recommended to avoid adverse effects on the impression or cast. Impression materials that are hydrophilic should be disinfected with a product that requires a minimum time for disinfection, preferably no more than 10 minutes. Caution should be exercised when following recommendations for disinfecting a particular

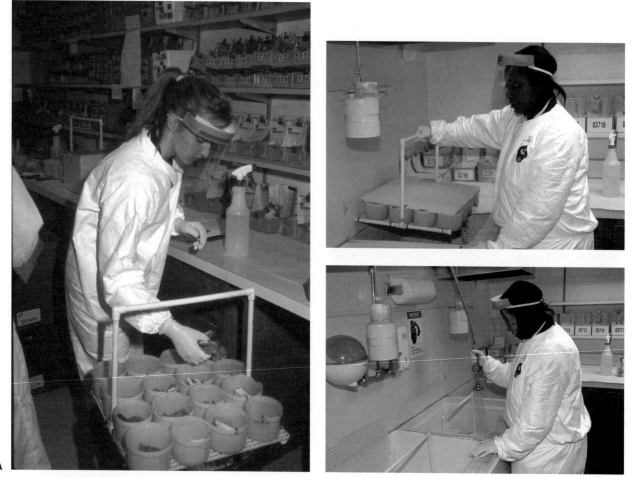

FIGURE 19-8 (A) Incoming impressions are loaded into labeled compartments (a companion label is attached to the work authorization) on a large tray. **(B)** The tray is covered and lowered into a vat of disinfectant for 10 minutes. **(C)** The disinfected impressions are rinsed thoroughly with tap water. (Photographs courtesy of Olson Dental Company, Inc.)

impression material, because some manufacturers have recommended disinfectant exposure times that are inconsistent with the recommendations of the disinfectant manufacturers. To avoid adverse effects, impressions should not be immersed in a disinfectant for any longer than recommended for disinfection and must never be shipped in disinfectant.

When using a newer disinfectant that has not been tested by research studies, the dental laboratory or dental office should perform its own testing to ascertain compatibility with impression materials. Caution is especially recommended when disinfecting hydrophilic impressions or using a disinfectant with a high alcohol content. Studies in Europe and Australia have evaluated disinfectants that are not registered in the United States as hospital disinfectants. Several studies have determined that a sodium dichloroisocyanurate solution (10,000 ppm available chlorine) used as an immersion disinfectant is effective and does not compromise the accuracy of alginate impressions; however, this preparation is not currently recommended for use as a hospital disinfectant in the United States.

Elastomeric Impressions

Several investigations have shown that polysulfides and silicones are relatively stable and can be disinfected without adverse effects by immersion in most disinfectants recommended for use in dentistry. Although they are hydrophilic, polyether impressions can also be disinfected by immersion, but exposure times should be kept to a minimum (10 minutes). Disinfectants that require exposure times longer than 10 minutes for tuberculocidal disinfection should be avoided with polyethers. Table 19-1 summarizes the commercially available disinfectant categories that have been tested and recommended for disinfection of elastomeric impression materials, plus suggested methods.

Immersion in acid glutaraldehyde actually improves the surface detail reproduction of elastomeric impressions (Johnson et al, 1988). Immersion in disinfectants increases the wettability of polysulfide (all disinfectants tested) and polyether (only chlorine dioxide), has no effect on the wettability of hydrophobic addition silicones, and decreases the wettability of hydrophilic addition silicones (Pratten et al, 1990).

Hydrocolloid Impressions

Several investigators have evaluated disinfection of irreversible hydrocolloid or alginate, sometimes with contradictory results. Based on these findings, the ADA recommended disinfecting alginates by immersion in diluted hypochlorite, iodophor, or glutaraldehyde with phenolic buffer (a product that is no longer available). Several investigators have reported significant adverse effects on specific materials with disinfectants that are nonreactive with other alginates, suggesting that caution should be exercised. Given the hydrophilic nature of the material, a minimal disinfection time is recommended; however, studies have shown no adverse effect on the dimensional stability of alginates when the appropriate disinfectant is used.

Several studies have confirmed that alginates harbor significantly higher levels of bacteria than silicone rubber impressions. It is postulated that the porosity of alginate might account for this difference. At least two studies (Gerhardt and Sydiskis, 1991; McNeill et al, 1992) have shown that virus absorbs to alginates; therefore, conscientious disinfection is paramount.

Limited data are available regarding disinfection of reversible hydrocolloid; however, research data suggest that there is no effect on the dimensional accuracy of impressions immersed in an iodophor diluted 1:213, 5.25% sodium hypochlorite diluted 1:10, or 2% acid glutaraldehyde diluted 1:4. Immersion in 2% alkaline glutaraldehyde has significant adverse effects on the impressions and resultant dies. Table 19-1 summarizes the recommendations for hydrocolloid impressions.

Zinc Oxide Eugenol (ZOE) and Compound Impressions

Limited data are available regarding disinfection of ZOE and compound impressions. Adverse effects have been reported for ZOE immersed for 16 hours in diluted hypochlorite and on compound with all of the disinfectants tested (hypochlorite, formaldehyde, and 2% alkaline glutaraldehyde). Follow-up studies using times recommended for tuberculocidal disinfection confirm these adverse effects and suggest appropriate product categories for immersion disinfection, as presented in Table 19-1.

DENTAL PROSTHESES AND APPLIANCES

Iodophors and chlorine-based compounds are generally recommended for disinfection of removable prostheses. Although both of these disinfectants are somewhat corrosive, studies have shown little effect on a chrome-cobalt alloy with short-term exposures (10 minutes) to either iodophors or 1:10 hypochlorite. Pitting of heat-cured denture base resin has been shown to occur after only 10 minutes of immersion in a glutaraldehyde with phenolic buffer (no longer available), although immersion in 2% alkaline glutaraldehyde did not damage the acrylic surface. Given the tissue toxicity of glutaraldehydes and phenolics, however, iodophors or chlorine compounds are preferred for disinfection of acrylic appliances (refer to Table 19-1).

New prostheses and appliances constructed in a laboratory where all incoming items are properly disinfected and standard disinfection techniques are practiced routinely are considered industrially clean following production. These items must be disinfected, however, before they are placed in the patient's mouth. This disinfection step may be done in the dental laboratory or the dental office. Items must never be shipped or stored in disinfectant. Acrylic items that should remain moist may be stored in water or diluted mouthwash following disinfection and rinsing.

Fixed metal/porcelain prostheses are actually sterile following porcelain firing/glazing, but if they are not handled aseptically after this step, they must be disinfected before delivery to the patient. They may be disinfected by immersion in glutaraldehydes for the time recommended for tuberculocidal inactivation by the disinfectant manufacturer, but extreme caution must be used to avoid patient exposure to the disinfectant. In addition, several clinical sources have confirmed that fixed prostheses can be disinfected by short-term immersion in diluted hypochlorite without apparent harm to the device. The higher the content of noble metal, the less the likelihood of adverse effects on the metal. Care should be taken to minimize the exposure times of metals to potentially corrosive chemicals. Iodophors, phenolics, or quat alcohols might be used as well, but no data are available to substantiate this. Any device that has been immersed in a disinfectant must be rinsed thoroughly before insertion into the patient's mouth.

Unglazed porcelain should not be exposed to any disinfectant, and porcelain firing/glazing will sterilize. Fixed metal prostheses can be sterilized with ethylene oxide or even by autoclaving if desired. Orthodontic appliances can be handled in a similar manner.

Prostheses or appliances that have been worn by patients should be thoroughly cleaned prior to disinfection by scrubbing with a brush and an antiseptic hand wash chairside or by cleaning in an ultrasonic unit.

Calculus and other deposits must be removed prior to disinfection. Stone and plaster removal solution may be useful for devices with extensive deposits. This method should be followed by cleaning with a detergent or cleanser. Note that denture cleansers, including those made for ultrasonic cleaning in the dental office, are cleaners and cannot substitute for appropriate disinfection. Some of these products have limited antimicrobial activity; however, they cannot be assumed to eliminate all classes of microorganisms.

Dentures or other acrylic appliances that have been worn by patients and require repair should be cleaned and disinfected before handling, but should probably be handled as contaminated (i.e., with gloves) even after disinfection. The porous nature of acrylic makes such devices difficult to adequately disinfect. It is recommended that such devices be redisinfected following grinding.

DISINFECTION OF WAX BITES, WAX RIMS, CASTS, CUSTOM IMPRESSION TRAYS, AND BITE REGISTRATIONS

Wax rims and wax bites should be disinfected by the spray-wipe-spray method using an intermediate-level (i.e., tuberculocidal activity) spray disinfectant. **Rinse-spray-rinse-spray** may be more appropriate for wax bites (Fig. 19-9). For adequate disinfection, these items should remain wet with disinfectant for the time recommended by the manufacturer. After the second spray, they can be enclosed in a sealed plastic bag or wrapped in plastic wrap for the recommended disinfection time. These items should be rinsed again following disinfection to remove any residual disinfectant.

Bite registrations made of materials such as ZOE or compound can be handled in the same manner as impressions of the same materials. These registrations can also

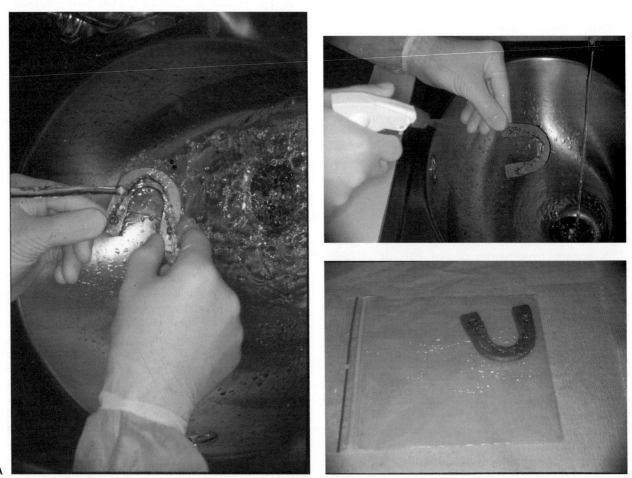

FIGURE 19-9 **(A)** Wax bites should be rinsed. **(B)** They should then be sprayed, rinsed again, and sprayed a second time. **(C)** Following the second spray, the wax bite should be enclosed in plastic for the time recommended for tuberculocidal disinfection.

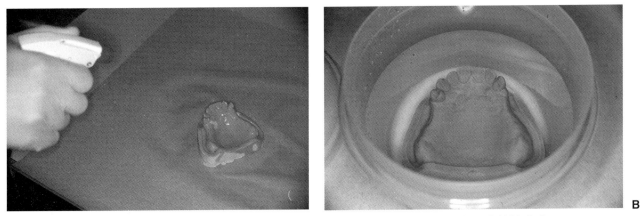

A   B

FIGURE 19-10 (A,B) Stone casts can be sprayed until wet or immersed in 1:10 hypochlorite or 1:213 iodophor.

be disinfected, using the rinse-spray-rinse-spray technique, with most EPA-registered hospital-level tuberculocidal disinfectants employed as sprays. (Chlorine compounds should not be applied to ZOE.) After disinfection, the registration should be rinsed again to remove residual disinfectant.

Dental casts are difficult to disinfect; therefore, it is preferable to disinfect the impression. If necessary, one can disinfect stone casts either by spraying them until wet or immersing them in a 1:10 dilution of sodium hypochlorite or an iodophor (Fig. 19-10). Placing casts on their ends may facilitate drainage after they are sprayed with the disinfectant. Casts should be fully set (i.e., stored for at least 24 hours) before any disinfection process is conducted. Sarma and Neiman (1990) submerged die stone models in a variety of disinfectants and found that 1:10 sodium hypochlorite and 1:213 iodophor produced no to minimal undesirable physical effects on set die stone. Several authors have recommended using a solution of saturated calcium sulfate ($CaSO_4$, slurry water) as the diluent for disinfectants to be used on stone casts to avoid damage to the cast surface. Disinfected casts that are to be shipped should be thoroughly dried before they are wrapped for shipment.

Several investigators have recommended adding disinfectants to gypsum during mixing, as all or part of the liquid, when pouring casts. Although such applications have a potential role in infection control, they do not solve the problem of the contaminated impression or tray as a source of infectious microorganisms, nor are they likely to eliminate all microbes that potentially can contaminate the surface of the cast.

Custom acrylic resin impression trays should be disinfected before use with a surface-disinfectant spray or immersion in either 1:213 iodophor or 1:10 sodium hypochlorite. They should be rinsed thoroughly to remove any residual disinfectant and allowed to dry fully prior to

use. After they are used in the mouth, custom trays should be discarded.

OTHER PROSTHODONTIC AND ORTHODONTIC ITEMS

Heat-stable items, such as facebow forks, orthodontic pliers, and metal impression trays, that come in contact with oral tissues must be heat-sterilized. Other sterilizable items used chairside, such as all-metal spatulas and stainless-steel bowls used for ice or water baths, should also be heat-sterilized. Polishing strips, points, wheels, disks, brushes, and burs used chairside should be discarded after use (if disposable) or heat-sterilized.

Articulators and facebows should be cleaned and disinfected following manipulations chairside. Wood-handled spatulas should be cleaned and disinfected (Fig. 19-11). Other items, such as Hanau torches, should be disinfected

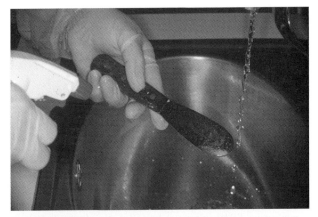

FIGURE 19-11 Wood-handled spatulas can be cleaned and disinfected using the rinse-spray-rinse-spray method.

after use or the area to be touched should be covered with a barrier, such as plastic wrap, to prevent contamination. Rubber mixing bowls can be autoclaved but will become distorted if they are overheated or undergo repeated exposures. Therefore, they should be cleaned and disinfected following use chairside.

Items such as shade guides should be cleaned and disinfected to avoid cross-contamination. If iodophors are used on shade guides, they should be wiped with water or alcohol following the exposure time to remove any residual disinfectant. If phenolics are used on any item that may come in contact with skin or mucous membranes, extreme caution must be used and careful rinsing must follow.

The unit-dosing concept minimizes cross-contamination during prosthodontic procedures. This refers to the dispensing of an amount of material that is sufficient to accomplish a particular procedure, prior to patient contact, with any excess being discarded at completion. Some waste is involved, but the use of unit-dose materials prevents cross-contamination of impression materials, waxes, compound, petroleum jelly, indelible pencils, and other items.

SUMMARY

Protection of dental laboratory as well as dental office employees from bloodborne pathogens is mandated by OSHA regulations. Infection-control protocols must be applied in the dental laboratory in the same manner as in the dental office. Many of the items transported between the dental office and the dental laboratory are potential sources of infectious microorganisms. Dental impressions, prostheses, appliances, and related materials can be rendered noninfectious without adverse effects to the material if the proper protocols are followed. New prostheses and appliances must also be disinfected before they are delivered to the patient. Communication of infection-control procedures between the dental practice and the dental laboratory is an important part of a successful infection-control program.

✔ Practical Dental Infection-Control Checklist

❏ Do DHCP use PPE when handling items received in the laboratory until they have been decontaminated?

❏ Before they are handled in the laboratory, are all dental prostheses and prosthodontic materials (e.g., impressions, bite registrations, occlusal rims, and extracted teeth) cleaned, disinfected, and rinsed by using an EPA-registered hospital disinfectant with at least intermediate-level (i.e., tuberculocidal claim) activity?

❏ Does the dental office/clinic consult with manufacturers regarding the stability of specific materials (e.g., impression materials) relative to disinfection procedures?

❏ Is specific information regarding the disinfection techniques (e.g., solution used and duration) used included when laboratory cases are sent off-site or returned?

❏ Are heat-tolerant items used in the mouth (e.g., metal impression trays and face-bow forks) cleaned and heat-sterilized?

❏ Are manufacturers' instructions followed regarding cleaning and sterilizing or disinfecting items that become contaminated but do not normally contact the patient (e.g., burs, polishing points, rag wheels, articulators, case pans, and lathes)?

❏ If the manufacturers' instructions are unavailable, are heat-tolerant items cleaned and heat-sterilized or cleaned and disinfected with an EPA-registered hospital disinfectant with low- (HIV, HBV effectiveness claim) to intermediate-level (tuberculocidal claim) activity, depending on the degree of contamination?

Review Questions

1. Dental laboratory personnel are required to wear PPE

   A. when handling contaminated items.

   B. when operating a lathe, model trimmer, or other rotary equipment.

   C. in all areas of the laboratory.

   D. only to protect their clothes.

   E. A and B only.

2. OSHA regulations require contaminated items that are shipped or transported to be in closed containers that

   A. do not leak.

   B. are colored red or identified with a biohazard label.

   C. Both A and B.

   D. Neither A nor B.

3. The first step in successful cleaning and disinfection of dental impressions is

   A. chairside rinsing under running tap water.

   B. cleaning with soap and water prior to shipping.

   C. spraying with disinfectant upon arrival in the laboratory.

   D. dunking of impressions in disinfectant prior to pouring with stone.

   E. overnight immersion in disinfectant.

4. If not handled properly, which of the following items has the greatest risk of transmitting infectious microorganisms to dental laboratory personnel?

   A. alginate impressions

   B. casts formed from silicone impressions

   C. dentures submitted for repair

   D. RPD frameworks that have been "tried in"

5. Which of the following statements is correct?

   A. Laboratory cases from patients with infectious diseases must be labeled as "high risk."

   B. New prostheses and appliances constructed in a laboratory that routinely disinfects all incoming cases do not require disinfection before they are delivered to the patient.

   C. Stone casts that are fully set may be disinfected by immersion in 1:10 sodium hypochlorite or by spraying until wet.

   D. The preferred method for disinfection of impressions is spraying.

6. Wax rims and wax bites are best disinfected by

   A. immersion in disinfectant.

   B. spray-wipe-spray-wipe.

   C. rinse-spray-rinse-spray.

   D. none of the above.

Critical Thinking

1. Obtain a laboratory prescription used in your dental office/clinic. How do you communicate infection-control procedures (e.g., disinfection) performed before shipping the item to the laboratory? Why is communication between the dental lab and office important?

2. Explain how you would disinfect an impression before shipping it to the dental laboratory.

3. A patient comes in with a broken denture. What infection-control measures would you take to disinfect the denture before it is sent to the dental laboratory for repair?

SELECTED READINGS

Al-Omari WM, Glyn Jones JC, Hart P. A microbiological investigation following the disinfection of alginate and addition cured silicone rubber impression materials. Eur J Prosthodont Restor Dent 1998;6:97–101.

Al-Omari WM, Glyn Jones JC, Wood DJ. The effect of disinfecting alginate and addition cured silicone rubber impression materials on the physical properties of impressions and resultant casts. Eur J Prosthodont Restor Dent 1998;6:103–109.

American Dental Association Council on Dental Materials and Equipment. Disinfection of impressions. J Am Dent Assoc 1991;122:110.

American Dental Association Council on Scientific Affairs and ADA Council on Dental Practice. Infection-control recommendations for the dental office and the dental laboratory. J Am Dent Assoc 1996;127:672–680.

Boden J, Likeman P, Clark R. Some effects of disinfecting solutions on the properties of alginate impression material and dental stone. Eur J Prosthodont Restor Dent 2001;9:131–135.

CDC. Guidelines for infection control in dental health-care settings–2003. MMWR 2003;52(RR-17):1–66.

Gerhardt DE, Sydiskis RJ. Impression materials and virus. J Am Dent Assoc 1991;122:51–54.

Hussain SMA, Tredwin CJ, Nesbit M, et al. The effect of disinfection on irreversible hydrocolloid and type III gypsum casts. Eur J Prosthodont Restor Dent 2006;14:50–54.

Ivanovski S, Savage NW, Brockhurst PJ, et al. Disinfection of dental stone casts: antimicrobial effects and physical property alterations. Dent Mater 1995;11:19–23.

Jagger DC, Al Jabra O, Harrison A, et al. The effect of a range of disinfectants on the dimensional accuracy of some impression materials. Eur J Prosthodont Restor Dent 2004;12:154–160.

Johnson GH, Chellis KD, Gordon GE, et al. Dimensional stability and detail reproduction of irreversible hydrocolloid and elastomeric impressions disinfected by immersion. J Prosthet Dent 1998;79:446–453.

King AH, Matis B. Infection control of in-office dental laboratories. Dent Clinics North Am 1991;35:415–426.

Kugel G, Perry RD, Ferrari M, et al. Disinfection and communication practices: a survey of U. S. dental laboratories. J Am Dent Assoc 2000;131:786–792.

McNeill MRJ, Coulter WA, Hussey DL. Disinfection of irreversible hydrocolloid impressions: a comparative study. Int J Prosthodont 1992;5:563–567.

Merchant VA. Dental laboratory infection control. Operatory Infect Control Update 1995;3:1–8.

Merchant VA. An update on infection control in the dental laboratory. Quintessence Dent Technol 1997;20:157–169.

National Association of Dental Laboratories (NADL) Health and Safety Committee: Infection Control Compliance Manual for Dental Laboratories. Alexandria, Virginia, National Association of Dental Laboratories, 1992.

Naylor WP. Infection control in prosthodontics. Dent Clin North Am 1992;36:809–831.

Organization for Safety and Asepsis Procedures Foundation: position paper on laboratory asepsis, November 1998. Available at http://www.osap.org/displaycommon.cfm?an=1&subarticlenbr=38. Accessed July 2008.

Owen CP, Goolam R. Disinfection of impression materials to prevent viral cross contamination: a review and a protocol. Int J Prosthodont 1993;6:480–494.

Plummer KD, Wakefield CW. Practical infection control in dental laboratories. Gen Dent 1994;42:545–548.

Pratten DH, Covey DA, Sheats RD. Effect of disinfectant solutions on the wettability of elastomeric materials. J Prosthet Dent 1990;63:223–227.

Sarma AC, Neiman R. A study of the effect of disinfectant chemicals on physical properties of die stone. Quintessence Int 1990;21:53–59.

Storer R, McCabe JF. An investigation of methods available for sterilising impressions. Br Dent J 1981;151:217–219.

Tullner JB, Commette JA, Moon PC. Linear dimensional changes in dental impressions after immersion in disinfectant solutions. J Prosthet Dent 1988;64:25–31.

20

Medical Waste Management

Kathy Neveu

Jennifer A. Harte

John A. Molinari

LEARNING OBJECTIVES

After completion of this chapter individuals should be able to:

1 Describe regulation of medical waste.

2 Define and give examples of nonregulated and regulated medical waste.

3 List appropriate protocols for disposal of medical waste.

4 List components of a dental office medical waste management plan.

KEY TERMS

Environmental Protection Agency (EPA): the mission of the EPA is to protect human health and the environment; the EPA works to develop and enforce regulations that implement environmental laws enacted by Congress.

Infectious waste: hazardous waste capable of causing infections in humans, including contaminated animal waste, human blood and blood products, isolation waste, pathological waste, and discarded sharps (needles, scalpels, or broken medical instruments).

Medical waste: any solid waste generated in the diagnosis, treatment, or immunization of human beings.

Occupational Safety and Health Administration (OSHA): established in 1971, OSHA aims to ensure worker safety and health in the United States by working with employers and employees to create better working environments; sets and enforcing standards; provides training, outreach, and education; establishes partnerships; and encourages continual improvement in workplace safety and health.

Other Potentially Infectious Materials (OPIM): an OSHA term That refers to (a) the following human body fluids: semen, vaginal secretions, cerebrospinal fluid, synovial fluid, pleural fluid, pericardial fluid, peritoneal fluid, amniotic fluid, saliva in dental procedures, any body fluid that is visibly contaminated with blood, and all body fluids in situations where it is difficult or impossible to differentiate between body fluids; (b) any unfixed tissue or organ (other than intact skin) from a human (living or dead); and (c) HIV-containing cell or tissue cultures, organ cultures, and HIV- or HBV-containing culture medium or other solutions; and blood, organs, or other tissues from experimental animals infected with HIV or HBV.

Regulated waste: liquid or semiliquid blood or OPIM; contaminated items that would release blood or OPIM in a liquid or semiliquid state if compressed; items that are caked with dried blood or OPIM and are capable of releasing these materials during handling; contaminated sharps; and pathological and microbiological wastes containing blood or OPIM.

In the late 1980s, public concern began to rise because of local and national media reports of medical wastes being indiscriminately discarded in common trash bins or washing ashore, and concerns regarding dwindling landfill space (Fig. 20-1). Additionally, media reports that were not based on scientific evidence increased fears of the potential for transmission of infectious diseases, specifically human immunodeficiency virus (HIV). Studies have compared the microbial load and diversity of microorganisms in residential waste with waste from multiple healthcare settings, general waste from hospitals, and other healthcare facilities such as dental practices and clinical laboratories. Accumulated data suggest that such waste is no more infective than residential waste.

Medical wastes require careful disposal and containment before they are collected and consolidated for treatment. Individuals need to be aware of regulations established by the **Environmental Protection Agency (EPA)**, **Occupational Safety and Health Administration (OSHA)**, and Department of Transportation (DOT). Readers need to be aware that many of these waste streams are also regulated at the state and local level. It is beyond the scope of this chapter to cover specific state and local requirements. In addition to guidance from regulatory agencies, the Centers for Disease Control and Prevention (CDC) has made recommendations to healthcare facilities, including dental practices, pertaining to medical waste management. All of these measures are designed to protect the workers who generate medical wastes and who manage the wastes from the point of generation to disposal. This chapter provides information on managing medical waste in the dental healthcare setting.

REGULATIONS AND GUIDANCE FOR MEDICAL WASTE

Medical waste can be defined as any solid waste generated in a healthcare facility—or, in other words, waste generated during the diagnosis, treatment, or immunization of human beings. Most medical waste generated in

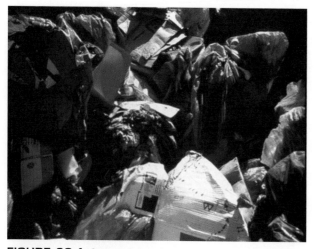

FIGURE 20-1 Open and closed bags of medical waste found in trash bins outside of a hospital.

the United States is regulated at the state and local level. Regulations can vary from state to state, so it is important to be familiar with the laws that apply to your state. State medical waste regulations identify categories of medical waste and the treatment or decontamination of such waste. Additional information on state medical waste programs and regulations can be found by visiting the EPA Web site at http://www.epa.gov/epaoswer/other/medical/programs.htm. Also, local regulations may apply concerning the disposal and handling of medical waste. Several categories of medical waste are governed by federal regulations. In the dental setting, medical waste containing mercury or other toxic metals may be governed by the Resource Conservation and Recovery Act (RCRA) hazardous waste regulation. The Food and Drug Administration (FDA) regulates medical devices, such as sharps containers designed to safely contain used needles and other sharp objects. OSHA regulates medical waste in the workplace, and the U.S. Postal Service regulates medical waste in the postal system.

TYPES OF WASTE IN THE DENTAL SETTING

There are two basic types of waste found in the dental setting: nonregulated and regulated medical waste. The majority of contaminated or soiled items in the dental setting are considered to be general medical waste and therefore can be disposed of with the general office trash. Examples of medical waste that usually do not require special disposal include used gloves, masks, gowns, lightly soiled gauze and other cotton products, and environmental surface barriers, such as plastic wrap, used to cover equipment during treatment. Also included in the general waste category are single-use disposable items used during patient treatment, such as plastic saliva ejectors, high-volume evacuator tips, prophylaxis angles, mouth mirrors, and air water syringe tips.

Regulated waste, as defined in the OSHA Bloodborne Pathogens Standard, is liquid or semiliquid blood or **other potentially infectious materials (OPIM)**; contaminated items that would release blood or OPIM in a liquid or semiliquid state if compressed; items that are caked with dried blood or OPIM and are capable of releasing these materials during handling; contaminated sharps; and pathological and microbiological wastes containing blood or OPIM. Regulated medical waste is only a limited subset of waste, comprising 9% to 15% of total waste in hospitals and 1% to 2% of total waste in dental settings. Regulated medical waste requires special storage, handling, neutralization, and disposal, and in addition to federal regulations, state and local rules and regulations may also apply. Examples of regulated waste found in dental healthcare settings are solid waste soaked or saturated with blood or saliva (e.g., gauze saturated with blood after surgery), extracted teeth, surgically removed hard and soft tissues, and contaminated sharp items (e.g., needles,

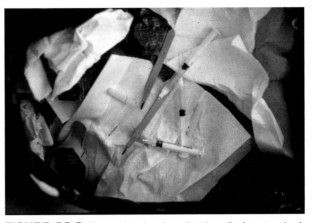

FIGURE 20-2 Nonregulated and regulated medical waste mixed in the same general disposal container. This represents inappropriate waste management and presents an increased potential for accidental exposures by healthcare providers.

scalpel blades, and wires). In addition to wearing personal protection equipment (PPE) when handling medical waste, it is important to remember a basic axiom of waste disposal: Do not mix waste categories (Fig. 20-2).

MANAGING REGULATED WASTE IN A DENTAL HEATHCARE SETTING

OSHA has dictated initial measures for discarding regulated waste. These procedures are designed to protect the workers who generate medical wastes and who manage the wastes from point of generation to disposal. For nonsharp regulated waste, a single leak-resistant, color-coded or biohazard-labeled container (e.g., a biohazard bag) is usually adequate (Table 20-1). The bag must be sturdy and the waste must be able to be discarded without contaminating the bag's exterior. Exterior con-

TABLE 20-1 Regulated Waste Container Requirements

According to the OSHA Bloodborne Pathogens Standard, regulated waste should be placed in containers that are
- closable;

- constructed to contain all contents and prevent leakage of fluids during handling, storage, transport or shipping;

- puncture-resistant if discarding contaminated sharps;

- marked with fluorescent orange or orange-red labels with lettering and symbols in a contrasting color (red bags or red containers may be substituted for labels);

- closed prior to removal to prevent spillage or protrusion of contents during handling, storage, transport, or shipping.

tamination or puncturing of the bag requires placement in a second biohazard bag. All bags should be securely closed for disposal. Puncture-resistant color-coded or biohazard-labeled containers (i.e., sharps containers) located at the point of use are used as containment for scalpel blades, needles, syringes, and unused sterile sharps. Additional OSHA requirements for labeling and containers are described in Table 20-1.

Dental facilities should dispose of medical waste regularly to avoid accumulation. Any facility that generates regulated medical waste should have a written plan for its management that complies with federal, state, and local regulations to ensure health and environmental safety. Recommended objectives of the plan should include, but are not limited to: rendering **infectious waste** safe for disposal; ensuring there is minimal risk to patients, staff, visitors, and the community; meeting all applicable federal, state, and local regulations; educating dental health-care personnel (DHCP) regarding the office waste management plan; and establishing a record-keeping system. Although multiple steps are involved in handling medical waste, the process can be broken down into several components as described below and in Table 20-2.

Managing Contaminated Sharps

Contaminated sharps are considered capable of transmitting disease, and therefore are considered to be regulated waste. Examples in the dental setting include needles, scalpel blades, suture needles, dental burs, endodontic files, reamers, broaches, instruments, and broken glass. These devices pose a significant occupational hazard to individuals who handle and dispose of them. OSHA requires that sharp items must be placed in appropriate puncture-resistant containers (Table 20-1) located as close as feasible to where the items were used (Fig. 20-3). It would be best to have a sharps container in each dental operatory. Also, used needles should never be recapped or otherwise manipulated by using both hands, or any other technique that involves directing the point of a needle toward any part of the body. Never bend or break needles before disposal, because this practice requires unnecessary manipulation. It is also important to wear appropriate PPE when handling sharp objects. This recommendation includes the use of heavy-duty utility gloves, since routine exam gloves do not protect against needlestick injuries.

A medical waste hauler and disposal service can remove contaminated sharps containers; however, this can be expensive because the cost is usually based on weight. As a result, if it is legally permissible, some offices may choose to treat their sharps containers by steam sterilization (i.e., autoclaving) before disposal. A written step-by-step operating protocol for rendering waste noninfectious should be included in your office waste

---

TABLE 20-2 Recommended Components of a Dental Office Waste Management Program*

Designate
- Assign program oversight responsibility to an individual who is knowledgeable about applicable federal, state, and local regulations (e.g., the office infection-control coordinator).
- Define and identify regulated and nonregulated waste items in the dental office.

Educate
- Ensure that DHCP who handle and dispose of regulated medical waste are trained in appropriate handling and disposal methods, and informed of the possible health and safety hazards.

Handle
- To prevent exposure to contaminated materials, always wear appropriate PPE when handling regulated waste. For example:
  - Wear heavy-duty utility gloves when handling sharp items.
  - Wear heavy-duty utility gloves, protective eyewear, mask, and protective clothing when handling blood products or blood or body-fluid soaked or caked materials.

Segregate
- To minimize handling and simplify disposal, separate waste at the point of creation.
- Place waste in appropriate containers. For example:
  - Discard sharps immediately into a sharps disposal container.
  - Place nonsharp regulated waste into a single leak-resistant color-coded or biohazard-labeled container (e.g., biohazard bag).

Label/Package
- To protect patients, staff, visitors, and the public from potential exposure to infectious materials, package waste appropriately. For example:
  - Regulated waste must be placed in a container that has a biohazard label or is color-coded red to identify the contents.
  - Sharp items must be placed in a rigid puncture-proof biohazard-labeled container or one that is color-coded red and disposed of when the indicated capacity has been reached.

Storage/Disposal
- Store medical waste in sealed containers until it is picked up by a contracted medical waste hauler or processed in the dental office.
- Label the storage area with a biohazard symbol and limit access.
- Dispose of medical waste as soon as possible following federal, state, and local regulations.

Record Keeping
- The generating facility is responsible for ensuring that the waste hauler is using acceptable and correct methods when removing and disposing of medical waste (often referred to as the cradle-to-grave concept).
- Check your waste hauler's credentials—the EPA usually approves waste haulers.
- Obtain paperwork describing shipment, the manner in which the waste was treated, and its final site of disposal.

*State and local regulations may apply.

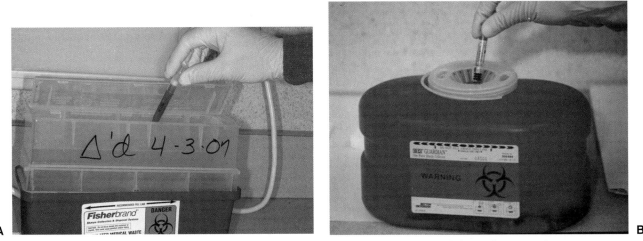

FIGURE 20-3 Disposal of **(A)** a contaminated needle and **(B)** a used anesthetic carpule into a sharps container. It is important to replace containers as soon as the contents reach the fill line, or sooner, as required by state and local regulations.

management plan. When sterilizing sharps containers before disposal,

1. Ensure that the sharps container can be autoclaved.
2. Monitor the sterilization process (e.g., use mechanical, chemical, and biological indicators).
3. Do not completely fill the sharps container.
4. If vents are present, leave them open.
5. Place the container in an upright position in the autoclave.
6. Process the containers for 40–60 minutes.
7. Allow the containers to cool before closing the vents.
8. Label and dispose of the sterilized sharps container according to state and local regulations.

Managing Blood and Other Body Fluid Waste

According to OSHA, contaminated items that would release blood or OPIM (i.e., saliva) in a liquid or semiliquid state if compressed, or items that are caked with dried blood or OPIM and are capable of releasing these materials during handling, are considered to be regulated waste. In the dental setting, this commonly applies to gauze and other cotton products used during an oral surgical procedure such as a tooth extraction or periodontal surgery. If the gauze product is saturated with blood or saliva and would release blood or saliva when squeezed, it must be disposed of in a container that meets the special criteria for regulated waste (Table 20-1).

Containers with blood or saliva, such as that suctioned during an oral surgical procedure, can be inactivated according to state-approved treatment technologies or

carefully poured down a utility sink drain or toilet. Because of the potential for splash and aerosolization, appropriate PPE, such as gloves, protective eyewear, mask, and protective clothing, should be worn when performing these tasks. There is no evidence that bloodborne diseases have been transmitted from contact with raw or treated sewage. Multiple bloodborne pathogens, particularly viruses, are not stable in the environment for long periods of time, and the disposal of limited quantities of blood and other body fluids into the sanitary sewer is considered a safe method for disposing of these waste materials. Some areas may have limits to the amount of blood or body fluid products that may be disposed of by this method or not allow disposal by this method. There may also be requirements regarding pretreatment procedures before disposal. Readers should always be aware of applicable state and local regulations.

Managing Extracted Teeth and Other Tissues

Extracted teeth and surgically removed hard and soft tissues are considered to be potentially infectious by OSHA and must be disposed of in medical waste containers as outlined by OSHA's Bloodborne Pathogens Standard (Table 20-1). Always use a leak-proof, color-coded, and labeled container such as a biohazard bag to contain nonsharp waste. Extracted teeth can be returned to patients on request, at which time provisions of the federal OSHA standard no longer apply. Again, some state and local regulations may be more stringent, so it is best to be knowledgeable about applicable regulations in your local area.

Extracted teeth containing dental amalgam should not be placed in a medical waste container (e.g., a red bag, biohazard bag, or sharps container) or regular trash intended for incineration for final disposal. This is because mercury can be released into the environment as a result of the extremely high temperatures used in the incineration process. Some commercial metal-recycling companies accept extracted teeth with metal restorations, including amalgam. State and local regulations should be consulted regarding disposal of the amalgam. The American Dental Association (ADA) has published "Best Management Practices for Amalgam Waste," which discusses disposal of teeth with amalgam restorations as well as other amalgam waste generated in the dental setting. Additional information can be found by visiting the ADA Web site at http://www.ada.org.

If it is legally permissible in your state or local area, human tissues may be neutralized and disposed of with the regular office trash. Neutralization is most commonly done by steam sterilization (i.e., autoclaving). While steam sterilization is the easiest and most economical method, using an unsaturated chemical vapor sterilizer (i.e., chemiclave) is also acceptable. Dry-heat sterilization is not acceptable for neutralizing this type of waste in healthcare settings. States often require that the treatment methods selected be monitored. For example, a biological indicator or spore test would be required. Chemical and mechanical monitoring may also be required. Place the waste in an autoclavable plastic or paper-plastic bag or pouch and run a standard cycle. After sterilizing the waste, it may be best to place the waste in a sealed box or bag for disposal because some waste haulers refuse to pick up blood-covered items. Extracted teeth containing amalgam restorations must not be heat-sterilized because of the potential health hazards associated with mercury vaporization and exposure. Disposal options for extracted teeth containing amalgam restorations have been addressed by the ADA (http://www.ada.org).

Extracted Teeth in Educational Settings

Extracted teeth are occasionally collected and used for preclinical or postgraduate educational training. The teeth should be cleansed of visible blood and gross debris, and maintained in a hydrated state in a well-constructed container with a secure lid to prevent leakage during transport. The container should also be labeled with the biohazard symbol. Because the recommendation is to autoclave these teeth before clinical exercises, use of the most economical storage solution (e.g., water or saline) might be practical.

Before they are used in an educational setting, the teeth should be heat-sterilized to allow for safe handling (Table 20-3). Pantera and Shuster demonstrated elimination of microbial growth using an autoclave cycle for 40 minutes. Autoclaving teeth for preclinical laboratory exercises does not alter their physical properties suffi-

TABLE 20-3 Recommended Steps for Sterilizing Amalgam-Free Teeth for Use in an Educational Setting

1. Wear PPE (e.g., gloves, mask, protective eyewear) when handling extracted teeth.

2. Do not heat-sterilize any teeth containing amalgam. If it is necessary to use extracted teeth containing amalgam, immerse in 10% formalin for 2 weeks before use in an educational setting.

3. Clean and thoroughly rinse any amalgam-free teeth to be sterilized.

4. Place amalgam-free teeth in a heat-resistant glass container.

5. Fill the heat-resistant container no more than halfway with deionized or distilled water or saline, and cover loosely (e.g., place foil over the top of the beaker, use a cork to close a flask).

6. Process through a steam sterilizer at 121°C for 40 minutes using a fluid or liquid cycle.

7. At the end of the cycle, remove the container slowly without shaking to prevent the water from boiling over.

(Oral communication courtesy of Chris H. Miller, PhD, Indiana University School of Dentistry.)

ciently to compromise the learning experience. It is unknown, however, whether autoclave sterilization of extracted teeth affects the dentinal structure such that the chemistry and microchemical relationship between dental materials and the dentin is affected for purposes of dental materials research.

Using teeth that do not contain amalgam is preferable because they can be safely autoclaved. Extracted teeth containing amalgam restorations must not be heat-sterilized because of the potential health hazards associated with mercury vaporization and exposure. If extracted teeth containing amalgam restorations are to be used, immersion in 10% formalin solution for 2 weeks has been found to be an effective method for disinfecting both the internal and external structures of the teeth. When using formalin, the manufacturer's Material Safety Data Sheet (MSDS) should be reviewed for occupational safety and health concerns, and to ensure compliance with OSHA recommendations.

SUMMARY

There are two basic types of waste found in the dental setting: nonregulated and regulated medical waste. Medical wastes require careful disposal and containment before collection and consolidation for treatment. In addition to being aware of federal regulations, it is important to be familiar with state and local regulations also. Any facility that generates regulated medical waste should have a written plan for its management that complies with federal, state, and local regulations, and dental facilities should ensure that DHCP who handle and dispose of regulated medical waste are educated in appropriate handling and disposal methods, and informed of the possible health and safety hazards.

✓ Practical Dental Infection-Control Checklist

Management of Regulated Medical Waste in Dental Healthcare Facilities

❏ Does the dental office/clinic have a written medical waste management program?

❏ Does disposal of regulated medical waste follow federal, state, and local regulations?

❏ Are DHCP who handle and dispose of regulated medical waste trained in appropriate handling and disposal methods, and informed of the possible health and safety hazards?

❏ Is a color-coded or labeled container that prevents leakage (e.g., biohazard bag) used to contain non-sharp regulated medical waste?

❏ Are sharp items (e.g., needles, scalpel blades, broken metal instruments, and burs) placed in an appropriate sharps container (e.g., puncture resistant, color-coded, and leakproof)?

❏ Is the container closed immediately before removal or replacement to prevent spillage or protrusion of contents during handling, storage, transport, or shipping?

❏ While wearing appropriate PPE, do DHCP pour blood, suctioned fluid, or other liquid waste carefully into a drain connected to a sanitary sewer system, if local sewage discharge requirements are met and the state has declared this an acceptable method of disposal?

Spills of Blood and Body Substances

❏ Are spills of blood or OPIM cleaned and decontaminated with an EPA-registered hospital disinfectant with low- (i.e., HBV and HIV label claims) to intermediate-level (i.e., tuberculocidal claim) activity, depending on the size of the spill and the surface porosity?

Handling of Extracted Teeth

❏ Are extracted teeth disposed of as regulated medical waste unless returned to the patient?

❏ Are extracted teeth containing amalgam disposed of appropriately (i.e., not placed in regulated medical waste intended for incineration)?

   ❏ Does the dental office/clinic follow the ADA Best Management Practices for Amalgam Waste (http://www.ada.org)?

❏ Are extracted teeth cleaned and placed in a leakproof container, labeled with a biohazard symbol, and kept hydrated during transport to educational institutions or a dental laboratory?

❏ Are teeth that do not contain amalgam heat-sterilized before they are used for educational purposes?

Review Questions

1. Which of the following is an example of regulated waste?

   A. blood-spattered mask

   B. light-handle barrier

   C. blood-stained gauze

   D. contaminated needle

   E. all of the above

2. According to the OSHA Bloodborne Pathogens Standard, a sharps disposal container must be

   A. closed before removal to prevent spillage during handling, storage, transport, or shipping.

   B. red or marked with fluorescent orange or orange-red labels.

   C. puncture resistant.

   D. A and B only

   E. all of the above

3. Which of the following statements is false?

   A. Containers with blood or saliva can be carefully poured down a utility sink drain or toilet if legally permissible by state and local regulations.

   B. Extracted teeth and surgically removed hard and soft tissues are considered to be potentially infectious by OSHA and must be disposed of as regulated medical waste.

   C. Extracted teeth containing amalgam restorations can be disposed of in medical waste containers that will be incinerated.

   D. Sharps disposal containers should be located as close as possible to the point of use.

   E. To prevent exposure to contaminated materials, always wear appropriate PPE when handling regulated waste.

4. The majority of contaminated or soiled items in the dental setting are considered to be general medical waste and therefore can be disposed of with the general office trash.

   A. True

   B. False

5. You have properly handled regulated waste, and a waste hauler has removed it from the dental office. If the hauler disposes it improperly, you will not be held responsible. It is out of your hands.

A. True

B. False

> ## Critical Thinking
>
> 1. Make a list of all the types of waste that are considered to be regulated waste in your dental office/clinic.
> 2. How do you dispose of extracted teeth in your office/clinic? What do you do if the extracted tooth contains amalgam?

SELECTED READINGS

American Dental Association. Best management practices for amalgam waste. Available at http://www.ada.org/prof/resources/topics/topics_amalgamwaste.pdf. Accessed July 2008.

CDC. Guidelines for environmental infection control in health-care facilities: recommendations of CDC and the Healthcare Infection Control Practices Advisory Committee (HICPAC). MMWR 2003;52(RR-10):1–42.

CDC. Guidelines for infection control in dental health-care settings–2003. MMWR 2003;52(RR-17):1–66.

CDC. National Institute for Occupational Safety and Health. Selecting, evaluating, and using sharps disposal containers. DHHS publication no. (NIOSH) 97–111. Cincinnati, OH: U.S. Department of Health and Human Services, Public Health Service, CDC, National Institute for Occupational Safety and Health; 1998.

CDC. Perspectives in disease prevention and health promotion. Summary of the Agency for Toxic Substances and Disease Registry report to Congress: the public health implications of medical waste. MMWR 1990;39:822–824.

Greene R. State and territorial association on alternate treatment technologies. Technical Assistance Manual: State Regulatory Oversight of Medical Waste Treatment Technologies. 2nd ed. Washington, DC: U.S. Environmental Protection Agency; 1994.

Hedrick E, Wideman JM. Waste management. In: APIC Text of Infection Control and Epidemiology. Washington, DC: APIC; 2005:104-1–104-12.

Miller CH, Palenik CJ. Waste management. In: Miller CH, Palenik DJ, eds. Infection Control and Management of Hazardous Materials for the Dental Team. 3rd ed. St. Louis: Mosby; 2005:321–331.

Palenik CJ. Managing regulated waste in dental environments. J Contemp Dent Pract 2003;4:76.

Pantera Jr EA, Schuster GS. Sterilization of extracted human teeth. J Dent Educ 1990;54:283–285.

Parsell DE, Stewart BM, Barker JR, et al. The effect of steam sterilization on the physical properties and perceived cutting characteristics of extracted teeth. J Dent Educ 1998;62:260–263.

Rutala WA, Mayhall CG. Medical waste. Infect Control Hosp Edidemiol 1992;13:38–48.

Schulein TM. Infection control for extracted teeth in the teaching laboratory. J Dent Educ 1994;58:411–413.

Tate WH, White RR. Disinfection of human teeth for educational purposes. J Dent Educ 1991;55:583–585.

U.S. Department of Labor, Occupational Safety and Health Administration. 29 CFR 1910.1200. Hazard communication. Fed Regist 1994;59:17479.

U.S. Department of Labor, Occupational Safety and Health Administration. 29 CFR Part 1910.1030. Occupational exposure to bloodborne pathogens; needlesticks and other sharps injuries; final rule. Fed Regist 2001;66:5317–5325. [As amended from and includes 29 CFR Part 1910.1030. Occupational exposure to bloodborne pathogens; final rule. Fed Regist 1991;56:64174–64182.]

U.S. Department of Labor, Occupational Safety and Health Administration. OSHA instruction: enforcement procedures for the occupational exposure to bloodborne pathogens. Directive no. CPL 2-2.69. Washington, DC: U.S. Department of Labor, Occupational Safety and Health Administration; 2001.

U.S. Environmental Protection Agency. 40 CFR Part 60. Standards of performance for new stationary sources and emission guidelines for existing sources: hospital/medical/infectious waste incinerators; final rule. Fed Regist 1997;62:48347–48391.

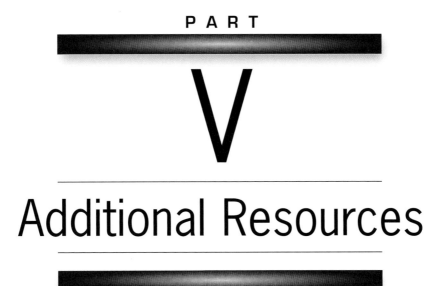

PART

V

Additional Resources

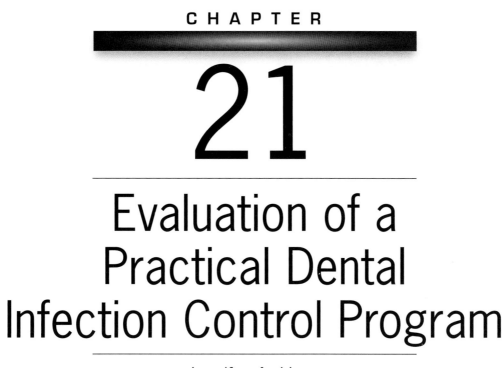

Evaluation of a Practical Dental Infection Control Program

Jennifer A. Harte

✓ Dental Infection-Control Program Administration/Personnel Health Elements

Program Administration

❏ Does the dental office/clinic have a written infection-control program for dental healthcare personnel (DHCP) to prevent or reduce the risk of disease transmission that includes

❏ establishment and implementation of policies, procedures, and practices (in conjunction with selection and use of technologies and products) to prevent work-related injuries and illnesses among DHCP, and

❏ healthcare-associated infections among patients?

❏ Does the infection-control program

❏ embody the principles of infection control and occupational health,

❏ reflect current science, and

❏ adhere to relevant federal, state, and local regulations and statutes?

❏ Does the dental office/clinic have access to the most current copies of the following:

❏ Centers for Disease Control and Prevention (CDC) dental infection-control guidelines? (available by visiting http://www.cdc.gov/oralhealth)

❏ Occupational Safety and Health Administration (OSHA) regulations? (both federal OSHA [available by visiting http://www.osha.gov] and, if applicable, state OSHA)?

❏ Appropriate state and local requirements (e.g., state dental board requirements)?

❏ Are standard precautions used for all patient encounters?

❏ Are transmission-based precautions applied when patients who require additional precautions receive treatment in the dental office/clinic?

❏ Does the dental office/clinic have a written exposure control plan (ECP)?

❏ Does the dental office/clinic have an assigned infection-control coordinator (e.g., dentist or other DHCP) who is knowledgeable, or willing to be trained, managing the program?

Personnel Health Elements of an Infection-Control Program

❏ Does the dental office/clinic have a written health program for DHCP, including policies, procedures, and guidelines for

❏ education and training;

❏ immunizations;

❏ exposure prevention;

❏ postexposure management;

❏ medical conditions, work-related illness, and associated work restrictions;

❏ contact dermatitis and latex hypersensitivity; and

❏ maintenance of records, data management, and confidentiality?

Education and Training

❏ Have all personnel received training regarding occupational exposure to potentially infectious agents and infection-control procedures/protocols appropriate for and specific to their assigned duties:

❏ upon initial employment/assignment,

❏ when new tasks or procedures affect the employee's occupational exposure, and

❏ at a minimum, annually?

❏ Is the educational information appropriate in content and vocabulary to the educational level, literacy, and language of DHCP?

Immunizations

❏ Does the dental office/clinic have a written comprehensive policy regarding immunizing DHCP, including a list of all required and recommended immunizations?

❏ Are DHCP referred to a prearranged qualified healthcare professional or to their own healthcare professional to receive all appropriate immunizations based on the latest recommendations as well as their medical history and risk for occupational exposure?

Exposure Prevention/Postexposure Management

❏ Does the dental office/clinic have a comprehensive postexposure management and medical follow-up program, not only for bloodborne pathogens, but other diseases as well (e.g., tuberculosis)?

❏ Does the program include policies and procedures for prompt reporting, evaluation, counseling, treatment, and medical follow-up of occupational exposures?

❏ Does the dental office/clinic have a written plan establishing mechanisms for referral to a qualified healthcare professional to ensure prompt and appropriate delivery of preventive services, occupationally related medical services, and postexposure management with any necessary medical evaluation and follow-up?

Medical Conditions, Work-Related Illness, and Work Restrictions

❑ Does the dental office/clinic have comprehensive written policies regarding work restriction and exclusion (including a statement of authority defining who can implement such policies) readily available to all DHCP?

  ❑ Do the policies for work restriction and exclusion encourage DHCP to seek appropriate preventive and curative care and report their illnesses, medical conditions, or treatments that can render them more susceptible to opportunistic infection or exposures?

  ❑ Are DHCP protected against lost wages, benefits, and job status in the event of such an illness or medical condition?

❑ Does the dental office/clinic have policies and procedures for evaluation, diagnosis, and management of DHCP with suspected or known occupational contact dermatitis?

  ❑ Does the dental office/clinic seek a definitive diagnosis by a qualified healthcare professional for any DHCP with suspected latex allergy to carefully determine its specific etiology and appropriate treatment, as well as work restrictions and accommodations?

Records Maintenance, Data Management, and Confidentiality

❑ Does the dental office/clinic establish and maintain confidential medical records (e.g., immunization records and documentation of tests received as a result of occupational exposure) for all DHCP?

❑ Is this in compliance with all applicable federal, state, and local laws regarding medical record-keeping and confidentiality?

✔ Preventing Transmission of Bloodborne Pathogens

Hepatitis B Virus (HBV) Vaccination

❑ Is the HBV vaccination series offered to all DHCP with potential occupational exposure to blood or other potentially infectious materials (OPIM)?

❑ Are U.S. Public Health Service/CDC recommendations always followed for hepatitis B vaccination, serologic testing, follow-up, and booster dosing?

❑ Are DHCP tested for anti-HBs 1–2 months after completion of the three-dose vaccination series?

  ❑ If no antibody response to the primary vaccine series occurs, do these DHCP complete a second three-dose vaccine series, or are they evaluated to determine whether they are HBsAg-positive?

❑ At the completion of the second vaccine series, are DHCP retested for anti-HBs?

  ❑ If there is no response to the second three-dose series, are nonresponders tested for HBsAg?

❑ Are nonresponders to vaccination who are HBsAg-negative counseled regarding their susceptibility to HBV infection and precautions to take?

❑ Are employees provided with appropriate education regarding the risks of HBV transmission and the availability of the vaccine?

❑ Do employees who decline the vaccination sign a declination form to be kept on file with the employer?

Preventing Exposures to Blood and OPIM

❑ Are standard precautions (note: OSHA's Bloodborne Pathogen Standard retains the term "universal precautions") used for all patient encounters?

❑ Does the dental office/clinic have a written, comprehensive program designed to minimize and manage DHCP exposures to blood and body fluids?

❑ Are sharp items (e.g., needles, scalers, burs, lab knives, and wires) that are contaminated with patient blood and saliva treated as potentially infectious?

❑ Are engineering controls (e.g., sharps containers, automated instrument cleaners, safety needles, and needle recapping devices) and work practice controls (e.g., the one-handed scoop technique, and placing sharps containers as close as possible to the point of use) used to prevent injuries?

Engineering and Work Practice Controls

❑ Does the dental office/clinic identify, evaluate, and select devices with engineered safety features at least annually and as they become available on the market (e.g., safer anesthetic syringes, retractable scalpel, or needleless IV systems)?

  ❑ Are employees who are directly responsible for patient care (e.g., dentists, hygienists, and dental assistants) involved with the identification and selection of these devices?

  ❑ Are the results documented in the dental office/clinic's ECP?

❑ Are used disposable syringes and needles, scalpel blades, and other sharp items placed in appropriate puncture-resistant containers located as close as feasible to the area in which the items are used?

  ❑ Are sharps containers located in each dental operatory?

  ❑ Are sharps containers color-coded (e.g., red) or labeled appropriately (e.g., with a biohazard symbol)?

❏ When recapping needles, is a one-handed scoop technique or a mechanical device designed for holding the needle cap when recapping needles (e.g., between multiple injections and before removing from a nondisposable aspirating syringe)? Note: OSHA prohibits recapping used needles by using both hands or any other technique that involves directing the point of a needle toward any part of the body.

Postexposure Management and Prophylaxis

❏ Does the dental office/clinic follow CDC recommendations after percutaneous, mucous-membrane, or non-intact skin exposure to blood or OPIM?

❏ Does the dental office/clinic have a written comprehensive postexposure management and medical follow-up program?

  ❏ Do DHCP know the types of contact with blood or OPIM that can place them at risk for infection?

  ❏ Do DHCP know to report occupational injuries and exposures immediately?

  ❏ Does the dental office/clinic have a written plan establishing mechanisms for referral to a qualified healthcare professional for medical evaluation and follow-up?

  ❏ Does the program include policies and procedures for prompt reporting, evaluation, counseling, treatment, and medical follow-up of occupational exposures?

  ❏ When an occupational exposure occurs, does the exposure incident report contain the following information:

    ❏ Date and time of exposure?

    ❏ Details of the procedure being performed, including where and how the exposure occurred and whether the exposure involved a sharp device, the type and brand of device, and how and when during its handling the exposure occurred?

    ❏ Details of the exposure, including its severity and the type and amount of fluid or material involved? The severity of a percutaneous injury, for example, might be measured by the depth of the wound, gauge of the needle, and whether fluid was injected. For skin or mucous-membrane exposure, the estimated volume of material, duration of contact, and condition of skin should be noted. Other considerations involve noting whether the skin was chapped, abraded, or intact.

    ❏ Details regarding whether the source material was known to contain HIV or other bloodborne pathogens, and, if the source was infected with HIV, the stage of disease, history of antiretroviral therapy, and viral load, if known?

    ❏ Details regarding the exposed person (e.g., hepatitis B vaccination and vaccine-response status)?

    ❏ Details regarding counseling, postexposure management, and follow-up?

✔ Hand Hygiene

General Considerations

❏ Do DHCP perform hand hygiene

  ❏ when hands are visibly contaminated with blood or OPIM?

  ❏ after barehanded touching of inanimate objects likely to be contaminated by blood, saliva, or respiratory secretions?

  ❏ before and after treating each patient?

  ❏ before donning gloves?

  ❏ immediately after removing gloves?

❏ Do DHCP perform hand hygiene with either nonantimicrobial or antimicrobial soap and water when hands are visibly dirty or contaminated with blood or OPIM?

❏ If hands are not visibly soiled, do DHCP use an alcohol-based hand rub according to the manufacturer's instructions?

❏ Before performing oral surgical procedures, do DHCP perform surgical hand antisepsis before donning sterile surgeon's gloves following the manufacturer's instructions by using an antimicrobial soap and water?

  ❏ If an alcohol-based surgical hand-scrub product with persistent activity is used, are hands cleaned with soap and water and dried before the waterless product is applied?

❏ Are liquid hand-care products stored in either disposable closed containers or closed containers that can be washed and dried before refilling?

  ❏ Are reusable dispensers or containers for soap or lotion washed and dried before refilling?

Special Considerations for Hand Hygiene and Glove Use

❏ Are hand lotions used to prevent skin dryness associated with hand washing?

❏ Is the compatibility of lotion and antiseptic products considered?

❏ Is the effect of petroleum or other oil emollients on the integrity of gloves considered during product selection and glove use?

❑ Do DHCP keep fingernails short with smooth, filed edges to allow thorough cleaning and prevent glove tears?

❑ Are DCHP discouraged from using artificial fingernails?

❑ If hand or nail jewelry is worn, is it removed if it makes donning gloves more difficult or compromises the fit and integrity of the glove?

✔ Personal Protective Equipment (PPE)

General Considerations

❑ Is PPE available in a variety of types and sizes?

❑ Is PPE donned and removed in a manner that minimizes further spread of contamination?

❑ Is contaminated laundry (e.g., reusable PPE) placed in an appropriately marked container according to local policy?

❑ Is PPE removed before leaving the work area?

Masks, Protective Eyewear, and Face Shields

❑ Do DHCP wear eye protection with solid side shields and a surgical mask, or a face shield and a surgical mask, to protect mucous membranes of the eyes, nose, and mouth during procedures likely to generate splashing or spattering of blood or other body fluids?

> ❑ Is a National Institute for Occupational Safety and Health (NIOSH)-approved disposable particulate respirator mask (PRM) worn when airborne isolation precautions are required (e.g., for protection against diseases spread through the air, such as tuberculosis)?

❑ Do DHCP always wear a mask when wearing a face shield?

❑ Do DHCP change masks between patients or during patient treatment if the mask becomes wet?

❑ Is reusable facial protective equipment (e.g., clinician and patient protective eyewear or face shields) cleaned with soap and water, or, if visibly soiled, cleaned and disinfected between patients?

Protective Clothing

❑ Do DHCP wear protective clothing (e.g., a long-sleeved reusable or disposable gown, laboratory coat, or uniform) that covers personal clothing and skin (e.g., forearms) likely to be soiled with blood, saliva, or OPIM?

❑ Do DHCP change protective clothing if it is visibly soiled?

❑ Do DHCP change protective clothing immediately or as soon as feasible if it is penetrated by blood or other potentially infectious fluids?

❑ Do DHCP remove barrier protection, including gloves, masks, eyewear, and gowns, before departing the work area (e.g., dental patient care, instrument processing, or laboratory area)?

Gloves

❑ Does the dental office/clinic ensure that appropriate gloves in the correct size are readily accessible?

❑ Do DHCP wear medical gloves when a potential exists for contacting blood, saliva, OPIM, or mucous membranes?

❑ Do DHCP wear a new pair of medical gloves for each patient, remove them promptly after use, and wash hands immediately to avoid transferring microorganisms to other patients or environments?

❑ Do DHCP remove gloves that are torn, cut, or punctured as soon as feasible and wash their hands before regloving?

❑ Are appropriate gloves (e.g., puncture- and chemical-resistant utility gloves) used when cleaning instruments and performing housekeeping tasks involving contact with blood or OPIM?

❑ Does the dental office/clinic consult with glove manufacturers regarding the chemical compatibility of the glove material and dental materials used?

Sterile Surgeon's Gloves and Double Gloving during Oral Surgical Procedures

❑ Are sterile surgeon's gloves worn when performing oral surgical procedures?

Head and Shoe Covers

❑ Are head and shoe covers available if personnel request them?

❑ Are head and shoe covers worn if contamination is likely?

✔ Contact Dermatitis and Latex Hypersensitivity

❑ Are DHCP educated regarding the signs, symptoms, and diagnoses of skin reactions associated with frequent hand hygiene and glove use?

❑ Are all patients screened for latex allergy (e.g., take health history and refer for medical consultation when latex allergy is suspected)?

❑ Is a latex-safe environment available for patients and DHCP with latex allergy?

❑ Are emergency treatment kits with latex-free products available at all times?

☑️ Sterilization and Disinfection of Patient-Care Items

General Considerations

❏ Are FDA-cleared medical devices used for sterilization and are the manufacturer's instructions followed for correct use and maintenance?

❏ Are reusable critical and semicritical dental instruments cleaned and heat-sterilized before each use?

❏ Are packages allowed to dry in the sterilizer before they are handled to avoid contamination?

❏ If available, are heat-stable semicritical alternatives used?

❏ Have heat-sensitive semicritical instruments been replaced with heat-tolerant or disposable versions?

  ❏ If heat-stable alternatives are not available, are heat-sensitive critical and semicritical instruments reprocessed by using FDA-cleared sterilant/high-level disinfectants or an FDA-cleared low-temperature sterilization method (e.g., ethylene oxide)?

   ❏ Are the manufacturer's instructions followed for use of chemical sterilants/high-level disinfectants?

   ❏ If single-use disposable instruments are used, are they used only once and disposed of correctly?

❏ Are noncritical patient-care items barrier-protected or cleaned, or, if visibly soiled, cleaned and disinfected after each use with an EPA-registered hospital disinfectant?

  ❏ If an item is visibly contaminated with blood, is an EPA-registered hospital disinfectant with a tuberculocidal claim (i.e., intermediate level) used?

❏ Are DHCP aware of all OSHA guidelines for exposure to chemical agents used for disinfection and sterilization?

Instrument-Processing Area

❏ Does the dental office/clinic have a central instrument-processing area?

❏ Do personnel working in the instrument-processing area receive initial and recurring training?

❏ Is the instrument-processing area divided physically or, at a minimum, spatially into distinct areas for receiving, cleaning, and decontamination; preparation and packaging; sterilization; and storage?

❏ Are DHCP trained to use work practices that prevent contamination of clean areas?

❏ Are instruments stored in an area away from where contaminated instruments are held or cleaned?

Receiving, Cleaning, and Decontamination Work Area

❏ Is the handling of loose contaminated instruments minimized during transport to the instrument processing area (e.g., by using work-practice controls, such as carrying instruments in a covered container, to minimize exposure potential)?

❏ Is all visible blood and other contamination from dental instruments and devices removed by cleaning before sterilization or disinfection procedures are performed?

❏ Is automated cleaning equipment (e.g., ultrasonic cleaner or washer-disinfector) used to remove debris to improve cleaning effectiveness and decrease worker exposure to blood?

❏ Are work-practice controls used that minimize contact with sharp instruments if manual cleaning is necessary (e.g., a long-handled brush)?

❏ Do DHCP wear puncture- and chemical-resistant/heavy-duty utility gloves for instrument cleaning and decontamination procedures?

❏ Do DHCP wear appropriate PPE (e.g., mask, protective eyewear, and gown) when splashing or spraying is anticipated during cleaning?

❏ Is the tabletop ultrasonic cleaner periodically tested (e.g., foil test) for proper function?

Preparation and Packaging

❏ Are dental instruments/items inspected for cleanliness and dried before they are wrapped or placed in containers designed to maintain sterility during storage (e.g., cassettes and organizing trays)?

❏ Is an internal chemical indicator placed in each package?

❏ Is an external indicator also used if the internal indicator cannot be seen from outside the package?

❏ Is either the FDA-cleared container system (e.g., instrument cassette) or wrapping compatible with the type of sterilization process used?

❏ Are packages labeled with the following information:

  ❏ sterilization identification number (if there is more than one sterilizer in the office/clinic)?

  ❏ load number?

  ❏ operator's initials?

  ❏ either an expiration date or the date sterilized (i.e., event-related)?

Sterilization of Unwrapped Instruments

❏ Although it is not recommended as a routine practice, if instruments are sterilized unwrapped, is there a written policy for how these instruments will be labeled and stored?

❑ Are instruments cleaned and dried before the unwrapped sterilization cycle?

❑ Are mechanical and chemical indicators used for each unwrapped sterilization cycle (i.e., is an internal chemical indicator placed among the instruments or items to be sterilized)?

❑ Are unwrapped instruments allowed to dry and cool in the sterilizer before they are handled to avoid contamination and thermal injury?

❑ Are semicritical instruments that are sterilized unwrapped and will be used immediately or within a short time handled aseptically during removal from the sterilizer and transport to the point of use?

❑ Are critical instruments that are sterilized unwrapped and intended for immediate reuse removed from the sterilizer and transported to the point of use in a manner that maintains sterility (e.g., transported in a sterile covered container)?

❑ When storing critical items, are they always wrapped before sterilization?

Implantable Devices

❑ Are implantable devices always wrapped before sterilization?

❑ Is a biological indicator used for every sterilizer load that contains an implantable device?

   ❑ When sterilizing an implantable device, are results verified before the implantable device is used, whenever possible?

Sterilization Monitoring

❑ Are mechanical, chemical, and biological monitors used according to the manufacturer's instructions to ensure the effectiveness of the sterilization process?

❑ Is each load monitored with mechanical (e.g., time, temperature, and pressure) and chemical indicators?

   ❑ Are the chemical indicators designed for the sterilization process being used (i.e., steam, dry heat, chemical vapor)?

   ❑ Is a chemical indicator placed on the inside of each package?

   ❑ Is an external indicator also used if the internal indicator cannot be seen from outside the package?

❑ Are items/packages placed correctly and loosely into the sterilizer so as not to impede penetration of the sterilant?

❑ Are instrument packages only used if mechanical or chemical indicators indicate adequate processing?

❑ Are sterilizers monitored at least weekly by using a biological indicator (i.e., spore test) with a matching control (i.e., the biological indicator and control are from same lot number)?

   ❑ Is the spore test designed for the type of sterilizer being used (i.e., steam, dry heat, chemical vapor)?

   ❑ In addition to at least weekly spore testing, is the sterilizer tested

      ❑ whenever a new type of packaging material or tray is used?

      ❑ after new sterilization personnel are trained?

      ❑ during initial uses of a new sterilizer?

      ❑ during the first run after repair of a sterilizer?

      ❑ with every implantable device, and are devices withheld from use until results of the test are known?

      ❑ after any other change in sterilizing procedures?

❑ If a prevacuum steam autoclave is used, is air removal testing performed daily or according to the manufacturer's instructions?

❑ Does the dental office/clinic have a written protocol to manage a sterilizer failure (i.e., a positive spore test)?

   ❑ After a positive spore test:

      ❑ Is the sterilizer removed from service and are sterilization procedures reviewed (e.g., work practices and use of mechanical and chemical indicators) to determine whether operator error could be responsible?

      ❑ Is the sterilizer retested by using biological, mechanical, and chemical indicators after any identified procedural problems are corrected?

      ❑ If the repeat spore test is negative, and mechanical and chemical indicators are within normal limits, is the sterilizer returned to service?

   ❑ If the repeat spore test is positive:

      ❑ Is the sterilizer removed from service until it has been inspected or repaired, or the exact reason for the positive test has been determined?

      ❑ To the extent possible, are all items that have been processed since the last negative spore test recalled and reprocessed?

      ❑ Before the sterilizer is placed back in service, is the sterilizer rechallenged with biological indicator tests in three consecutive empty-chamber sterilization cycles (or three fully loaded chamber sterilization cycles if using a tabletop sterilizer) after the cause of the sterilizer failure has been determined and corrected?

❑ Are sterilization records (i.e., mechanical, chemical, and biological) maintained in compliance with state and local regulations?

Storage Area for Sterilized Items and Clean Dental Supplies

❑ Does the dental office/clinic use date- or event-related shelf-life storage practices for wrapped, sterilized instruments and devices?

   ❑ If event-related packaging is used, is the date of sterilization placed on the package label to facilitate the retrieval of processed items in the event of a sterilization failure?

   ❑ If multiple sterilizers are used in the facility, is a sterilizer number or identification placed on the package label to facilitate the retrieval of processed items in the event of a sterilization failure?

❑ Are all wrapped packages of sterilized instruments inspected before they are opened to ensure the barrier wrap has not been compromised during storage?

❑ Are instruments/items recleaned, repackaged, and resterilized if the instrument package material has been compromised (e.g., wet, torn, or damaged)?

❑ Are sterile items and dental supplies stored in covered or closed cabinets, if possible?

❑ Is a "first in, first out" storage policy used?

✔ Environmental Infection Control

General Considerations

❑ Are manufacturers' instructions followed for the correct use of cleaning and EPA-registered hospital disinfecting products?

   ❑ Are products used that are intended only for environmental surfaces (i.e., low- to intermediate-level disinfectant products)? Note: liquid chemical sterilants and high-level disinfectants are not to be used for disinfection of environmental surfaces.

   ❑ Before disinfection, are surfaces cleaned according to manufacturers' instructions?

   ❑ After cleaning, is the disinfectant allowed to remain on the treated surface for the longest recommended contact time on the product label?

❑ Do DHCP use PPE, as appropriate, when cleaning and disinfecting environmental surfaces?

❑ When considering dental office design and equipment selection, do DHCP evaluate dental equipment features from an infection-control perspective?

Clinical Contact Surfaces

❑ Are surface barriers used to protect clinical contact surfaces, particularly those that are difficult to clean (e.g., switches on dental equipment), and are the surface barriers changed between patients?

❑ Are clinical contact surfaces that are not barrier-protected cleaned and disinfected using an EPA-registered hospital disinfectant with a low- (i.e., HIV and HBV label claims) to intermediate-level (i.e., tuberculocidal claim) activity after each patient?

   ❑ Is an intermediate-level disinfectant used if the surface is visibly contaminated with blood?

Housekeeping Surfaces

❑ Are housekeeping surfaces (e.g., floors, walls, and sinks) cleaned with a detergent and water or an EPA-registered hospital disinfectant/detergent on a routine basis (depending on the nature of the surface and type and degree of contamination) and as appropriate, based on the location in the facility, and when visibly soiled?

❑ Are mops and cloths cleaned after use and allowed to dry before reuse, or are single-use, disposable mop heads or cloths used?

❑ Are fresh cleaning or EPA-registered disinfecting solutions prepared daily and as instructed by the manufacturer?

❑ Are walls, blinds, and window curtains cleaned in patient-care areas when they are visibly dusty or soiled?

Spills of Blood and Body Substances

❑ Are spills of blood or OPIM cleaned and decontaminated with an EPA-registered hospital disinfectant with low- (i.e., HBV and HIV label claims) to intermediate-level (i.e., tuberculocidal claim) activity, depending on the size of the spill and the surface porosity?

Carpet and Cloth Furnishings

❑ Are carpeting and cloth-upholstered furnishings avoided in dental operatories, laboratories, and instrument-processing areas?

Dental Operatory Asepsis

At the beginning of the day before the first patient, do DHCP:

❑ perform initial hand washing of the day?

❑ don appropriate PPE and clean and disinfect operatory surfaces?

❑ turn on the dental unit and other equipment in the operatory?

❑ keep countertops uncluttered by removing unnecessary items?

❑ place disposable surface barriers on clinical contact surfaces?

During patient treatment do DHCP perform all treatment to minimize cross-contamination by:

❑ keeping their hands away from their face?

❏ limiting the surfaces touched?

❏ changing gloves when torn or heavily contaminated?

❏ using a dental (rubber) dam?

❏ using high-volume evacuation?

❏ using engineering and work practice controls to minimize injury with contaminated sharps?

❏ not touching or writing in the dental record while wearing gloves?

❏ not touching radiographs while wearing gloves?

❏ not picking up the telephone while wearing gloves?

❏ not touching non–barrier-protected computer equipment while wearing gloves?

❏ not using items dropped on the floor?

❏ not entering drawers/cabinets with contaminated gloves?

  ❏ If it is necessary to retrieve an item during treatment that is in a cabinet or drawer, is aseptic technique used (e.g., using a sterile cotton forceps to retrieve the item, using an overglove, or removing gloves and washing hands)?

Between patients (operatory turnover), do DHCP:

❏ don appropriate PPE?

❏ flush any device connected to the air/waterlines for a minimum of 20–30 seconds after each patient—including dental handpiece(s), air/water syringes, ultrasonic scalers, and Cavitron units?

❏ remove burs from dental handpieces and disconnect all devices from the dental unit?

❏ remove all surface barriers without touching the underlying surface and discard appropriately?

❏ clean and disinfect contaminated surfaces that were not barrier-protected, including patient safety glasses?

❏ remove PPE (clean and disinfect reusable PPE) and wash hands?

At the end of the day, do DHCP:

❏ don appropriate PPE?

❏ clean and disinfect clinical contact surfaces, dental unit surfaces, and countertops?

❏ clean high-volume evacuator, low-volume suction lines, and suction/amalgam traps using an approved evacuation system cleaner according to the manufacturer's instructions?

❏ leave the dental operatory "clean and clear"?

Once a week, do DHCP:

❏ clean and disinfect the main evacuation system trap?

❏ clean and disinfect the outside of drawers and cabinets?

❏ clean and disinfect operatory and laboratory floors?

Management of Regulated Medical Waste in Dental Healthcare Facilities

❏ Does the dental office/clinic have a written medical waste management program?

❏ Does disposal of regulated medical waste follow federal, state, and local regulations?

❏ Are DHCP who handle and dispose of regulated medical waste trained in appropriate handling and disposal methods, and informed of the possible health and safety hazards?

❏ Is a color-coded or labeled container that prevents leakage (e.g., biohazard bag) used to contain non-sharp regulated medical waste?

❏ Are sharp items (e.g., needles, scalpel blades, broken metal instruments, and burs) placed in an appropriate sharps container (e.g., puncture resistant, color-coded, and leakproof)?

❏ Is the container closed immediately before removal or replacement to prevent spillage or protrusion of contents during handling, storage, transport, or shipping?

❏ While wearing appropriate PPE, do DHCP pour blood, suctioned fluids, or other liquid waste carefully into a drain connected to a sanitary sewer system, if local sewage discharge requirements are met and the state has declared this an acceptable method of disposal?

✓ Dental Unit Waterlines, Biofilm, and Water Quality

General Considerations

❏ Is water that meets EPA regulatory standards for drinking water (i.e., ≤500 CFU/mL of heterotrophic water bacteria) used for routine dental treatment output water?

❏ Does the dental office/clinic consult with the dental unit manufacturer for appropriate methods and equipment to maintain the recommended quality of dental water?

❏ Are recommendations for monitoring water quality provided by the manufacturer of the unit or waterline treatment product followed?

❏ Is water and air discharged for a minimum of 20–30 seconds after each patient, from any device connected to the dental water system that enters the patient's mouth (e.g., handpieces, ultrasonic scalers, and air/water syringes)?

❏ Does the dental office/clinic consult with the dental unit manufacturer on the need for periodic maintenance of antiretraction mechanisms?

Boil-Water Advisories

❏ If a boil-water advisory is in effect, does the dental office/clinic have a written protocol to follow? If yes, does it include:

  ❏ not delivering water from the public water system to the patient through the dental operative unit, ultrasonic scaler, or other dental equipment that uses the public water system?

  ❏ not using water from the public water system for dental treatment, patient rinsing, or hand washing?

  ❏ using antimicrobial-containing products that do not require water for use (e.g., alcohol-based hand rubs) for hand washing? Note: If hands are visibly contaminated, use bottled water, if available, and soap for hand washing or an antiseptic towelette.

❏ When the boil-water advisory is canceled, does the dental clinic/office have a written protocol to follow? If yes, does it include:

  ❏ following guidance given by the local water utility regarding adequate flushing of waterlines? Note: If no guidance is provided, are dental waterlines and faucets flushed for 1–5 minutes before using for patient care?

  ❏ disinfecting/cleaning dental waterlines as recommended by the dental unit manufacturer?

✔ Dental Handpieces and Other Devices Attached to Air and Waterlines

❏ Are handpieces and other intraoral instruments that can be removed from the air and waterlines of dental units cleaned and heat-sterilized between patients?

❏ Are the manufacturer's instructions followed for cleaning, lubrication, and sterilization of handpieces and other intraoral instruments that can be removed from the air and waterlines of dental units?

❏ Are patients advised not to close their lips tightly around the tip of the saliva ejector to evacuate oral fluids?

✔ Dental Radiography

General Considerations

❏ Do DHCP wear gloves when exposing radiographs and handling contaminated film packets?

❏ Is other PPE (e.g., protective eyewear, mask, and gown) used, as appropriate, if spattering of blood or other body fluids is likely?

❏ Are heat-tolerant or disposable intraoral devices (e.g., film-holding and positioning devices) used whenever possible?

❏ Are heat-tolerant devices cleaned and heat-sterilized between patients?

❏ Are exposed radiographs handled and transported in an aseptic manner to prevent contamination of developing equipment?

Digital Radiography

❏ When using digital radiography sensors, are FDA-cleared barriers used to protect the sensor from contamination?

❏ After the barrier is removed, is the digital radiography sensor cleaned and disinfected with an EPA-registered hospital disinfectant with intermediate-level (i.e., tuberculocidal claim) activity, between patients?

❏ Does the dental office/clinic consult with the manufacturer for methods of disinfection and sterilization of digital radiography sensors and for protection of associated computer hardware?

✔ Aseptic Technique for Parenteral Medications

❏ Are aseptic techniques followed when using single- or multiple-dose medication vials and IV fluids?

❏ Are single-dose vials for parenteral medications used when possible?

  ❏ Are single-dose medication vials used for one patient only and disposed of appropriately?

❏ Are IV fluid bags and equipment used for one patient and disposed of appropriately?

❏ Are sterile devices (i.e., needle, syringe) used to enter single- or multiple-dose medication vials?

❏ Are manufacturer and/or local policies followed for storage, use, and expiration policies?

❏ If multidose vials are used, is the access diaphragm cleaned with 70% alcohol before a sterile device (i.e., needle and syringe) is inserted into the vial?

  ❏ Are multidose vials kept away from the immediate patient treatment area to prevent inadvertent contamination by spray or spatter?

  ❏ Is the multidose vial discarded if sterility is compromised?

✔ Single-Use (Disposable) Devices

❏ Are single-use devices used for one patient only and disposed of appropriately?

✔ Preprocedural Mouth Rinses

❏ Are preprocedural mouth rinses considered as a means to reduce the level of oral microorganisms in aerosols and spatter generated during routine dental procedures?

✔ Oral Surgical Procedures

❑ Before performing oral surgical procedures, do DHCP perform surgical hand antisepsis before donning sterile surgeon's gloves following the manufacturer's instructions by using an antimicrobial soap and water?

  ❑ If an alcohol-based surgical hand-scrub product with persistent activity is used, are hands cleaned with soap and water and dried before the waterless product is applied?

❑ Do DHCP wear sterile surgeon's gloves when performing oral surgical procedures?

❑ Do DHCP use sterile saline or sterile water as a coolant/irrigant when performing oral surgical procedures?

✔ Handling of Biopsy Specimens

❑ During transport, are biopsy specimens placed in a sturdy, leakproof container labeled with the biohazard symbol?

❑ If a biopsy specimen container is visibly contaminated, is the outside of the container cleaned and disinfected, or is it placed in an impervious bag labeled with the biohazard symbol?

✔ Handling of Extracted Teeth

❑ Are extracted teeth disposed of as regulated medical waste unless returned to the patient?

❑ Are extracted teeth containing amalgam disposed of appropriately (i.e., not placed in regulated medical waste intended for incineration)?

  ❑ Does the dental office/clinic follow the American Dental Association (ADA) Best Management Practices for Amalgam Waste (http://www.ada.org)?

❑ Are extracted teeth cleaned and placed in a leakproof container, labeled with a biohazard symbol, and kept hydrated during transport to educational institutions or a dental laboratory?

❑ Are teeth that do not contain amalgam heat-sterilized before they are used for educational purposes?

✔ Dental Laboratory

❑ Do DHCP use PPE when handling items received in the laboratory until they have been decontaminated?

❑ Before they are handled in the laboratory, are all dental prostheses and prosthodontic materials (e.g., impressions, bite registrations, occlusal rims, and extracted teeth) cleaned, disinfected, and rinsed by using an EPA-registered hospital disinfectant with at least intermediate-level (i.e., tuberculocidal claim) activity?

❑ Does the dental office/clinic consult with manufacturers regarding the stability of specific materials (e.g., impression materials) relative to disinfection procedures?

❑ Is specific information regarding disinfection techniques (e.g., solution used and duration) included when laboratory cases are sent off-site and on their return?

❑ Are heat-tolerant items used in the mouth (e.g., metal impression trays and face-bow forks) cleaned and heat-sterilized?

❑ Are manufacturers' instructions followed for cleaning and sterilizing or disinfecting items that become contaminated but do not normally contact the patient (e.g., burs, polishing points, rag wheels, articulators, case pans, and lathes)?

❑ If the manufacturer's instructions are unavailable, are heat-tolerant items cleaned and heat-sterilized or cleaned and disinfected with an EPA-registered hospital disinfectant with low- (HIV, HBV effectiveness claim) to intermediate-level (tuberculocidal claim) activity, depending on the degree of contamination?

✔ *Mycobacterium tuberculosis*

❑ Are all DHCP educated regarding the recognition of signs, symptoms, and transmission of tuberculosis (TB)?

❑ Is a baseline tuberculin skin test (TST; preferably a two-step test) conducted for all DHCP who might have contact with persons with suspected or confirmed active TB, regardless of the risk classification of the setting?

❑ Is each patient assessed for a history of TB as well as symptoms indicative of TB and documented on the medical history form?

❑ Are CDC recommendations followed for

  ❑ developing, maintaining, and implementing a written TB infection-control plan?

  ❑ managing a patient with suspected or active TB?

  ❑ completing a community risk-assessment to guide employee TSTs and follow-up?

  ❑ managing DHCP with TB disease?

❑ If a patient is known or suspected to have active TB, is he evaluated away from other patients and DHCP?

❑ When not being evaluated, does the patient wear a surgical mask or is he instructed to cover his mouth and nose when coughing or sneezing?

❑ Is elective dental treatment deferred until the patient is noninfectious?

❑ Are patients who require urgent dental treatment referred to a previously identified facility with TB engineering controls and a respiratory protection program?

✓ Program Evaluation

❏ Does the dental office/clinic routinely evaluate the office infection-control program, including evaluation of performance indicators?

Critical Thinking

1. Using this checklist examine your written operating instructions, training programs, records, and daily practices to ensure compliance with infection control procedures. If deficiencies or problems are identified, discuss what your plans are for improving your infection control program.

SELECTED READINGS

CDC. Guidelines for infection control in dental health-care settings–2003. MMWR 2003;52(RR-17):1–66.

Organization for Safety and Asepsis Procedures. Infection control in practice: OSAP chart and checklist. 2004;3:1–9. Available online at http://www.osap.org/displaycommon.cfm?an=1&subarticlenbr=370. Accessed July 2008.

USAF Dental Evaluation and Consultation Service. In Control Fact Sheet Number 10, USAF Dental Infection Control Program Check-Up, 2004. Available online at https://decs.nhgl.med.navy.mil/4QTR04/incontrolfactsheet10.htm. Accessed July 2008.

U.S. Department of Labor, Occupational Safety and Health Administration. 29 CFR Part 1910.1030. Occupational exposure to bloodborne pathogens; needlesticks and other sharps injuries; final rule. Fed Regist 2001;66:5317–5325. [As amended from and includes 29 CFR Part 1910.1030. Occupational exposure to bloodborne pathogens; final rule. Fed Regist 1991;56:64174–64182.]

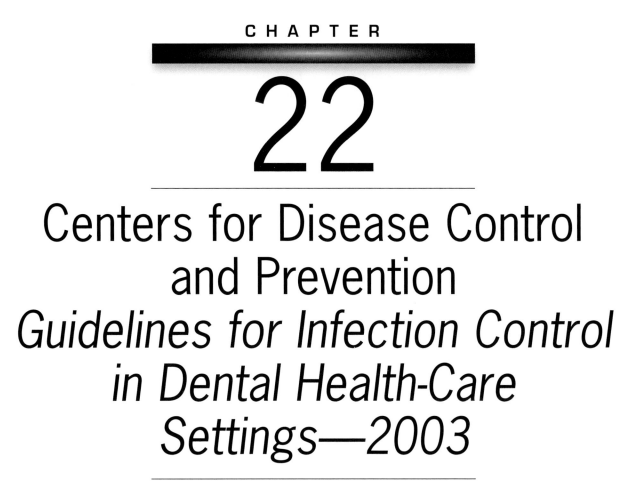

22

Centers for Disease Control and Prevention
Guidelines for Infection Control in Dental Health-Care Settings—2003

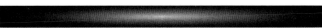

The Centers for Disease Control and Prevention (CDC)'s most recent *Guidelines for Infection Control in Dental Health-Care Settings—2003* was published in a supplement to the *Morbidity and Mortality Weekly Report* on December 19, 2003. The guidelines have two parts. The first part provides the background and scientific evidence on which the recommendations are based. The second part contains the recommendations (reprinted below). These recommendations were developed in collaboration with and after review by authorities on infection control from the CDC and other public agencies, academia, and private and professional organizations.

In addition to providing dental practitioners with the scientific rationale for the recommendations, the CDC guidelines present dental practitioners with the information needed to make educated choices when selecting infection control processes, methods and products. Regulatory and legal issues preclude the CDC from commenting on the efficacy or effectiveness of specific products. Also, because there are usually several ways to achieve the desired end result, the CDC refrains from making specific recommendations on protocols or techniques. This textbook should help users with "how-to" techniques and methods to develop safe and efficient work practices to achieve the recommendations.

The complete set of recommendations and rankings from the 2003 CDC publication follow. Reference numbers appearing in parentheses refer to the first part of the full set of guidelines, which can be accessed by visiting the CDC Web site at http://www.cdc.gov/oralhealth/infectioncontrol/index.htm. If desired, readers can match the references later with the full document.

GUIDELINES FOR INFECTION CONTROL IN DENTAL HEALTH-CARE SETTINGS—2003

Prepared by
William G. Kohn, DDS,[1] Amy S. Collins, MPH,[1] Jennifer L. Cleveland, DDS,[1] Jennifer A. Harte, DDS,[2] Kathy J. Eklund, MHP,[3] Dolores M. Malvitz, DrPH[1]

[1]*Division of Oral Health, National Center for Chronic Disease Prevention and Health Promotion, CDC, Atlanta, Georgia*
[2]*United States Air Force Dental Investigation Service, Great Lakes, Illinois*
[3]*Forsyth Institute, Boston, Massachusetts*

RECOMMENDATIONS

Each recommendation is categorized on the basis of existing scientific data, theoretical rationale, and applicability. Rankings are based on the system used by CDC and the Healthcare Infection Control Practices Advisory Committee (HICPAC) to categorize recommendations:

Category IA. Strongly recommended for implementation and strongly supported by well-designed experimental, clinical, or epidemiologic studies.

Category IB. Strongly recommended for implementation and supported by experimental, clinical, or epidemiologic studies and a strong theoretical rationale.

Category IC. Required for implementation as mandated by federal or state regulation or standard. When IC is used, a second rating can be included to provide the basis of existing scientific data, theoretical rationale, and applicability. Because of state differences, the reader should not assume that the absence of an IC implies the absence of state regulations.

Category II. Suggested for implementation and supported by suggestive clinical or epidemiologic studies or a theoretical rationale.

Unresolved issue. No recommendation. Insufficient evidence or no consensus regarding efficacy exists.

I. PERSONNEL HEALTH ELEMENTS OF AN INFECTION-CONTROL PROGRAM

A. General Recommendations

1. Develop a written health program for DHCP that includes policies, procedures, and guidelines for education and training; immunizations; exposure prevention and postexposure management; medical conditions, work-related illness, and associated work restrictions; contact dermatitis and latex hypersensitivity; and maintenance of records, data management, and confidentiality (IB) (*5,16–18,22*).
2. Establish referral arrangements with qualified healthcare professionals to ensure prompt and appropriate provision of preventive services, occupationally related medical services, and postexposure management with medical follow-up (IB, IC) (*5,13,19,22*).

B. Education and Training

1. Provide DHCP 1) on initial employment, 2) when new tasks or procedures affect the employee's occupational exposure, and 3) at a minimum, annually, with education and training regarding occupational exposure to potentially infectious agents and infection-control procedures/protocols appropriate for and specific to their assigned duties (IB, IC) (*5,11,13,14,16,19,22*).
2. Provide educational information appropriate in content and vocabulary to the educational level, literacy, and language of DHCP (IB, IC) (*5,13*).

C. Immunization Programs

1. Develop a written comprehensive policy regarding immunizing DHCP, including a list of all required and recommended immunizations (IB) (*5,17,18*).
2. Refer DHCP to a prearranged qualified healthcare professional or to their own healthcare

professional to receive all appropriate immunizations based on the latest recommendations as well as their medical history and risk for occupational exposure (IB) (*5,17*).

D. Exposure Prevention and Postexposure Management

1. Develop a comprehensive postexposure management and medical follow-up program (IB, IC) (*5,13,14,19*).
   a. Include policies and procedures for prompt reporting, evaluation, counseling, treatment, and medical follow-up of occupational exposures.
   b. Establish mechanisms for referral to a qualified healthcare professional for medical evaluation and follow-up.
   c. Conduct a baseline TST, preferably by using a two-step test, for all DHCP who might have contact with persons with suspected or confirmed infectious TB, regardless of the risk classification of the setting (IB) (*20*).

E. Medical Conditions, Work-Related Illness, and Work Restrictions

1. Develop and have readily available to all DHCP comprehensive written policies regarding work restriction and exclusion that include a statement of authority defining who can implement such policies (IB) (*5,22*).
2. Develop policies for work restriction and exclusion that encourage DHCP to seek appropriate preventive and curative care and report their illnesses, medical conditions, or treatments that can render them more susceptible to opportunistic infection or exposures; do not penalize DHCP with loss of wages, benefits, or job status (IB) (*5,22*).
3. Develop policies and procedures for evaluation, diagnosis, and management of DHCP with suspected or known occupational contact dermatitis (IB) (*32*).
4. Seek definitive diagnosis by a qualified healthcare professional for any DHCP with suspected latex allergy to carefully determine its specific etiology and appropriate treatment as well as work restrictions and accommodations (IB) (*32*).

F. Records Maintenance, Data Management, and Confidentiality

1. Establish and maintain confidential medical records (e.g., immunization records and documentation of tests received as a result of occupational exposure) for all DHCP (IB, IC) (*5,13*).
2. Ensure that the practice complies with all applicable federal, state, and local laws regarding medical recordkeeping and confidentiality (IC) (*13,34*).

II. PREVENTING TRANSMISSION OF BLOODBORNE PATHOGENS

A. HBV Vaccination

1. Offer the HBV vaccination series to all DHCP with potential occupational exposure to blood or other potentially infectious material (IA, IC) (*2,13,14,19*).
2. Always follow U.S. Public Health Service/CDC recommendations for hepatitis B vaccination, serologic testing, follow-up, and booster dosing (IA, IC) (*13,14,19*).
3. Test DHCP for anti-HBs 1–2 months after completion of the 3-dose vaccination series (IA, IC) (*14,19*).
4. DHCP should complete a second 3-dose vaccine series or be evaluated to determine if they are HBsAg-positive if no antibody response occurs to the primary vaccine series (IA, IC) (*14,19*).
5. Retest for anti-HBs at the completion of the second vaccine series. If no response to the second 3-dose series occurs, nonresponders should be tested for HBsAg (IC) (*14,19*).
6. Counsel nonresponders to vaccination who are HBsAg-negative regarding their susceptibility to HBV infection and precautions to take (IA, IC) (*14,19*).
7. Provide employees appropriate education regarding the risks of HBV transmission and the availability of the vaccine. Employees who decline the vaccination should sign a declination form to be kept on file with the employer (IC) (*13*).

B. Preventing Exposures to Blood and OPIM

1. General recommendations
   a. Use standard precautions (OSHA's bloodborne pathogen standard retains the term universal precautions) for all patient encounters (IA, IC) (*11,13,19,53*).
   b. Consider sharp items (e.g., needles, scalers, burs, lab knives, and wires) that are contaminated with patient blood and saliva as potentially infective and establish engineering controls and work practices to prevent injuries (IB, IC) (*6,13,113*).
   c. Implement a written, comprehensive program designed to minimize and manage DHCP exposures to blood and body fluids (IB, IC) (*13,14,19,97*).
2. Engineering and work-practice controls
   a. Identify, evaluate, and select devices with engineered safety features at least annually

and as they become available on the market (e.g., safer anesthetic syringes, blunt suture needle, retractable scalpel, or needleless IV systems) (IC) (*13,97,110–112*).

   b. Place used disposable syringes and needles, scalpel blades, and other sharp items in appropriate puncture-resistant containers located as close as feasible to the area in which the items are used (IA, IC) (*2,7,13,19, 113,115*).

   c. Do not recap used needles by using both hands or any other technique that involves directing the point of a needle toward any part of the body. Do not bend, break, or remove needles before disposal (IA, IC) (*2,7, 8,13,97,113*).

   d. Use either a one-handed scoop technique or a mechanical device designed for holding the needle cap when recapping needles (e.g., between multiple injections and before removing from a nondisposable aspi- rating syringe) (IA, IC) (*2,7,8,13,14,113*).

3. Postexposure management and prophylaxis

   a. Follow CDC recommendations after percuta- neous, mucous membrane, or nonintact skin exposure to blood or other potentially infectious material (IA, IC) (*13,14,19*).

III. HAND HYGIENE

A. General Considerations

1. Perform hand hygiene with either a nonantimi- crobial or antimicrobial soap and water when hands are visibly dirty or contaminated with blood or other potentially infectious material. If hands are not visibly soiled, an alcohol-based hand rub can also be used. Follow the manu- facturer's instructions (IA) (*123*).

2. Indications for hand hygiene include

   a. when hands are visibly soiled (IA, IC);

   b. after barehanded touching of inanimate objects likely to be contaminated by blood, saliva, or respiratory secretions (IA, IC);

   c. before and after treating each patient (IB);

   d. before donning gloves (IB); and

   e. immediately after removing gloves (IB, IC) (*7–9,11,13,113,120–123,125,126,138*).

3. For oral surgical procedures, perform surgical hand antisepsis before donning sterile sur- geon's gloves. Follow the manufacturer's instructions by using either an antimicrobial soap and water, or soap and water followed by drying hands and application of an alcohol- based surgical hand-scrub product with persistent activity (IB) (*121–123,127–133, 144,145*).

4. Store liquid hand-care products in either dis- posable closed containers or closed contain- ers that can be washed and dried before refill- ing. Do not add soap or lotion to (i.e., top off) a partially empty dispenser (IA) (*9,120,122, 149,150*).

B. Special Considerations for Hand Hygiene and Glove Use

1. Use hand lotions to prevent skin dryness asso- ciated with handwashing (IA) (*153,154*).

2. Consider the compatibility of lotion and anti- septic products and the effect of petroleum or other oil emollients on the integrity of gloves during product selection and glove use (IB) (*2,14,122,155*).

3. Keep fingernails short with smooth, filed edges to allow thorough cleaning and prevent glove tears (II) (*122,123,156*).

4. Do not wear artificial fingernails or extenders when having direct contact with patients at high risk (e.g., those in intensive care units or operating rooms) (IA) (*123,157–160*).

5. Use of artificial fingernails is usually not rec- ommended (II) (*157–160*).

6. Do not wear hand or nail jewelry if it makes donning gloves more difficult or compromises the fit and integrity of the glove (II) (*123,142,143*).

IV. PPE

A. Masks, Protective Eyewear, and Face Shields

1. Wear a surgical mask and eye protection with solid side shields or a face shield to protect mucous membranes of the eyes, nose, and mouth during procedures likely to generate splashing or spattering of blood or other body fluids (IB, IC) (*1,2,7,8,11,13,137*).

2. Change masks between patients or during patient treatment if the mask becomes wet (IB) (*2*).

3. Clean with soap and water, or if visibly soiled, clean and disinfect reusable facial protective equipment (e.g., clinician and patient protec- tive eyewear or face shields) between patients (II) (*2*).

B. Protective Clothing

1. Wear protective clothing (e.g., reusable or dis- posable gown, laboratory coat, or uniform) that covers personal clothing and skin (e.g., fore- arms) likely to be soiled with blood, saliva, or OPIM (IB, IC) (*7,8,11,13,137*).

2. Change protective clothing if visibly soiled (*134*); change immediately or as soon as feasi- ble if penetrated by blood or other potentially infectious fluids (IB, IC) (*13*).

3. Remove barrier protection, including gloves, mask, eyewear, and gown before departing work area (e.g., dental patient care, instrument processing, or laboratory areas) (IC) (*13*).

C. Gloves

1. Wear medical gloves when a potential exists for contacting blood, saliva, OPIM, or mucous membranes (IB, IC) (*1,2,7,8,13*).
2. Wear a new pair of medical gloves for each patient, remove them promptly after use, and wash hands immediately to avoid transfer of microorganisms to other patients or environments (IB) (*1,7,8,123*).
3. Remove gloves that are torn, cut, or punctured as soon as feasible and wash hands before regloving (IB, IC) (*13,210,211*).
4. Do not wash surgeon's or patient examination gloves before use or wash, disinfect, or sterilize gloves for reuse (IB, IC) (*13,138,177,212,213*).
5. Ensure that appropriate gloves in the correct size are readily accessible (IC) (*13*).
6. Use appropriate gloves (e.g., puncture- and chemical-resistant utility gloves) when cleaning instruments and performing housekeeping tasks involving contact with blood or OPIM (IB, IC) (*7,13,15*).
7. Consult with glove manufacturers regarding the chemical compatibility of glove material and dental materials used (II).

D. Sterile Surgeon's Gloves and Double Gloving During Oral Surgical Procedures

1. Wear sterile surgeon's gloves when performing oral surgical procedures (IB) (*2,8,137*).
2. No recommendation is offered regarding the effectiveness of wearing two pairs of gloves to prevent disease transmission during oral surgical procedures. The majority of studies among HCP and DHCP have demonstrated a lower frequency of inner glove perforation and visible blood on the surgeon's hands when double gloves are worn; however, the effectiveness of wearing two pairs of gloves in preventing disease transmission has not been demonstrated (Unresolved issue).

V. CONTACT DERMATITIS AND LATEX HYPERSENSITIVITY

A. General Recommendations

1. Educate DHCP regarding the signs, symptoms, and diagnoses of skin reactions associated with frequent hand hygiene and glove use (IB) (*5,31,32*).
2. Screen all patients for latex allergy (e.g., take health history and refer for medical consultation when latex allergy is suspected) (IB) (*32*).

3. Ensure a latex-safe environment for patients and DHCP with latex allergy (IB) (*32*).
4. Have emergency treatment kits with latex-free products available at all times (II) (*32*).

VI. STERILIZATION AND DISINFECTION OF PATIENT-CARE ITEMS

A. General Recommendations

1. Use only FDA-cleared medical devices for sterilization and follow the manufacturer's instructions for correct use (IB) (*248*).
2. Clean and heat-sterilize critical dental instruments before each use (IA) (*2,137,243,244,246, 249,407*).
3. Clean and heat-sterilize semicritical items before each use (IB) (*2,249,260,407*).
4. Allow packages to dry in the sterilizer before they are handled to avoid contamination (IB) (*247*).
5. Use of heat-stable semicritical alternatives is encouraged (IB) (*2*).
6. Reprocess heat-sensitive critical and semicritical instruments by using FDA-cleared sterilant/high-level disinfectants or an FDA-cleared low-temperature sterilization method (e.g., ethylene oxide). Follow manufacturer's instructions for use of chemical sterilants/high-level disinfectants (IB) (*243*).
7. Single-use disposable instruments are acceptable alternatives if they are used only once and disposed of correctly (IB, IC) (*243,383*).
8. Do not use liquid chemical sterilants/high-level disinfectants for environmental surface disinfection or as holding solutions (IB, IC) (*243,245*).
9. Ensure that noncritical patient-care items are barrier-protected or cleaned, or if visibly soiled, cleaned and disinfected after each use with an EPA-registered hospital disinfectant. If visibly contaminated with blood, use an EPA-registered hospital disinfectant with a tuberculocidal claim (i.e., intermediate level) (IB) (*2,243,244*).
10. Inform DHCP of all OSHA guidelines for exposure to chemical agents used for disinfection and sterilization. Using this report, identify areas and tasks that have potential for exposure (IC) (*15*).

B. Instrument Processing Area

1. Designate a central processing area. Divide the instrument processing area, physically or, at a minimum, spatially, into distinct areas for 1) receiving, cleaning, and decontamination; 2) preparation and packaging; 3) sterilization; and 4) storage. Do not store instruments in an

area where contaminated instruments are held or cleaned (II) (*173,247,248*).

2. Train DHCP to employ work practices that prevent contamination of clean areas (II).

C. Receiving, Cleaning, and Decontamination Work Area

1. Minimize handling of loose contaminated instruments during transport to the instrument processing area. Use work-practice controls (e.g., carry instruments in a covered container) to minimize exposure potential (II). Clean all visible blood and other contamination from dental instruments and devices before sterilization or disinfection procedures (IA) (*243,249–252*).

2. Use automated cleaning equipment (e.g., ultrasonic cleaner or washer-disinfector) to remove debris to improve cleaning effectiveness and decrease worker exposure to blood (IB) (*2,253*).

3. Use work-practice controls that minimize contact with sharp instruments if manual cleaning is necessary (e.g., long-handled brush) (IC) (*14*).

4. Wear puncture- and chemical-resistant/heavy-duty utility gloves for instrument cleaning and decontamination procedures (IB) (*7*).

5. Wear appropriate PPE (e.g., mask, protective eyewear, and gown) when splashing or spraying is anticipated during cleaning (IC) (*13*).

D. Preparation and Packaging

1. Use an internal chemical indicator in each package. If the internal indicator cannot be seen from outside the package, also use an external indicator (II) (*243,254,257*).

2. Use a container system or wrapping compatible with the type of sterilization process used and that has received FDA clearance (IB) (*243,247,256*).

3. Before sterilization of critical and semicritical instruments, inspect instruments for cleanliness, then wrap or place them in containers designed to maintain sterility during storage (e.g., cassettes and organizing trays) (IA) (*2,247,255,256*).

E. Sterilization of Unwrapped Instruments

1. Clean and dry instruments before the unwrapped sterilization cycle (IB) (*248*).

2. Use mechanical and chemical indicators for each unwrapped sterilization cycle (i.e., place an internal chemical indicator among the instruments or items to be sterilized) (IB) (*243,258*).

3. Allow unwrapped instruments to dry and cool in the sterilizer before they are handled to avoid contamination and thermal injury (II) (*260*).

4. Semicritical instruments that will be used immediately or within a short time can be sterilized unwrapped on a tray or in a container

system, provided that the instruments are handled aseptically during removal from the sterilizer and transport to the point of use (II).

5. Critical instruments intended for immediate reuse can be sterilized unwrapped if the instruments are maintained sterile during removal from the sterilizer and transport to the point of use (e.g., transported in a sterile covered container) (IB) (*258*).

6. Do not sterilize implantable devices unwrapped (IB) (*243,247*).

7. Do not store critical instruments unwrapped (IB) (*248*).

F. Sterilization Monitoring

1. Use mechanical, chemical, and biological monitors according to the manufacturer's instructions to ensure the effectiveness of the sterilization process (IB) (*248,278,279*).

2. Monitor each load with mechanical (e.g., time, temperature, and pressure) and chemical indicators (II) (*243,248*).

3. Place a chemical indicator on the inside of each package. If the internal indicator is not visible from the outside, also place an exterior chemical indicator on the package (II) (*243, 254,257*).

4. Place items/packages correctly and loosely into the sterilizer so as not to impede penetration of the sterilant (IB) (*243*).

5. Do not use instrument packs if mechanical or chemical indicators indicate inadequate processing (IB) (*243,247,248*).

6. Monitor sterilizers at least weekly by using a biological indicator with a matching control (i.e., biological indicator and control from same lot number) (IB) (*2,9,243,247,278,279*).

7. Use a biological indicator for every sterilizer load that contains an implantable device. Verify results before using the implantable device, whenever possible (IB) (*243,248*).

8. The following are recommended in the case of a positive spore test:
   a. Remove the sterilizer from service and review sterilization procedures (e.g., work practices and use of mechanical and chemical indicators) to determine whether operator error could be responsible (II) (*8*).
   b. Retest the sterilizer by using biological, mechanical, and chemical indicators after correcting any identified procedural problems (II).
   c. If the repeat spore test is negative, and mechanical and chemical indicators are within normal limits, put the sterilizer back in service (II) (*9,243*).

9. The following are recommended if the repeat spore test is positive:
   a. Do not use the sterilizer until it has been inspected or repaired or the exact reason for the positive test has been determined (II) (*9,243*).
   b. Recall, to the extent possible, and reprocess all items processed since the last negative spore test (II) (*9,243,283*).
   c. Before placing the sterilizer back in service, rechallenge the sterilizer with biological indicator tests in three consecutive empty chamber sterilization cycles after the cause of the sterilizer failure has been determined and corrected (II) (*9,243,283*).
10. Maintain sterilization records (i.e., mechanical, chemical, and biological) in compliance with state and local regulations (IB) (*243*).

G. Storage Area for Sterilized Items and Clean Dental Supplies

1. Implement practices on the basis of date- or event-related shelf-life for storage of wrapped, sterilized instruments and devices (IB) (*243,284*).
2. Even for event-related packaging, at a minimum, place the date of sterilization, and if multiple sterilizers are used in the facility, the sterilizer used, on the outside of the packaging material to facilitate the retrieval of processed items in the event of a sterilization failure (IB) (*243,247*).
3. Examine wrapped packages of sterilized instruments before opening them to ensure the barrier wrap has not been compromised during storage (II) (*243,284*).
4. Reclean, repack, and resterilize any instrument package that has been compromised (II).
5. Store sterile items and dental supplies in covered or closed cabinets, if possible (II) (*285*).

VII. ENVIRONMENTAL INFECTION CONTROL

A. General Recommendations

1. Follow the manufacturers' instructions for correct use of cleaning and EPA-registered hospital disinfecting products (IB, IC) (*243–245*).
2. Do not use liquid chemical sterilants/high-level disinfectants for disinfection of environmental surfaces (clinical contact or housekeeping) (IB, IC) (*243–245*).
3. Use PPE, as appropriate, when cleaning and disinfecting environmental surfaces. Such equipment might include gloves (e.g., puncture- and chemical-resistant utility), protective clothing (e.g., gown, jacket, or lab coat), and protective eyewear/face shield, and mask (IC) (*13,15*).

B. Clinical Contact Surfaces

1. Use surface barriers to protect clinical contact surfaces, particularly those that are difficult to clean (e.g., switches on dental chairs) and change surface barriers between patients (II) (*1,2,260,288*).
2. Clean and disinfect clinical contact surfaces that are not barrier-protected, by using an EPA-registered hospital disinfectant with a low- (i.e., HIV and HBV label claims) to intermediate-level (i.e., tuberculocidal claim) activity after each patient. Use an intermediate-level disinfectant if visibly contaminated with blood (IB) (*2,243,244*).

C. Housekeeping Surfaces

1. Clean housekeeping surfaces (e.g., floors, walls, and sinks) with a detergent and water or an EPA-registered hospital disinfectant/detergent on a routine basis, depending on the nature of the surface and type and degree of contamination, and as appropriate, based on the location in the facility, and when visibly soiled (IB) (*243,244*).
2. Clean mops and cloths after use and allow to dry before reuse; or use single-use, disposable mop heads or cloths (II) (*243,244*).
3. Prepare fresh cleaning or EPA-registered disinfecting solutions daily and as instructed by the manufacturer. (II) (*243,244*).
4. Clean walls, blinds, and window curtains in patient-care areas when they are visibly dusty or soiled (II) (*9,244*).

D. Spills of Blood and Body Substances

1. Clean spills of blood or OPIM and decontaminate surface with an EPA-registered hospital disinfectant with low- (i.e., HBV and HIV label claims) to intermediate-level (i.e., tuberculocidal claim) activity, depending on size of spill and surface porosity (IB, IC) (*13,113*).

E. Carpet and Cloth Furnishings

1. Avoid using carpeting and cloth-upholstered furnishings in dental operatories, laboratories, and instrument processing areas (II) (*9,293–295*).

F. Regulated Medical Waste

1. General Recommendations
   a. Develop a medical waste management program. Disposal of regulated medical waste must follow federal, state, and local regulations (IC) (*13,301*).
   b. Ensure that DHCP who handle and dispose of regulated medical waste are trained in appropriate handling and disposal methods and informed of the possible health and safety hazards (IC) (*13*).

2. Management of Regulated Medical Waste in Dental Healthcare Facilities

   a. Use a color-coded or labeled container that prevents leakage (e.g., biohazard bag) to contain nonsharp regulated medical waste (IC) (*13*).

   b. Place sharp items (e.g., needles, scalpel blades, orthodontic bands, broken metal instruments, and burs) in an appropriate sharps container (e.g., puncture resistant, color-coded, and leakproof). Close container immediately before removal or replacement to prevent spillage or protrusion of contents during handling, storage, transport, or shipping (IC) (*2,8,13,113,115*).

   c. Pour blood, suctioned fluids, or other liquid waste carefully into a drain connected to a sanitary sewer system, if local sewage discharge requirements are met and the state has declared this an acceptable method of disposal. Wear appropriate PPE while performing this task (IC) (*7,9,13*).

VIII. DENTAL UNIT WATERLINES, BIOFILM, AND WATER QUALITY

A. General Recommendations

1. Use water that meets EPA regulatory standards for drinking water (i.e., ≤500 CFU/mL of heterotrophic water bacteria) for routine dental treatment output water (IB, IC) (*341,342*).

2. Consult with the dental unit manufacturer for appropriate methods and equipment to maintain the recommended quality of dental water (II) (*339*).

3. Follow recommendations for monitoring water quality provided by the manufacturer of the unit or waterline treatment product (II).

4. Discharge water and air for a minimum of 20–30 seconds after each patient, from any device connected to the dental water system that enters the patient's mouth (e.g., handpieces, ultrasonic scalers, and air/water syringes) (II) (*2,311,344*).

5. Consult with the dental unit manufacturer on the need for periodic maintenance of antiretraction mechanisms (IB) (*2,311*).

B. Boil-Water Advisories

1. The following apply while a boil-water advisory is in effect:

   a. Do not deliver water from the public water system to the patient through the dental operative unit, ultrasonic scaler, or other dental equipment that uses the public water system (IB, IC) (*341,342,346,349,350*).

   b. Do not use water from the public water system for dental treatment, patient rinsing, or handwashing (IB, IC) (*341,342,346,349,350*).

   c. For handwashing, use antimicrobial-containing products that do not require water for use (e.g., alcohol-based hand rubs). If hands are visibly contaminated, use bottled water, if available, and soap for handwashing or an antiseptic towelette (IB, IC) (*13,122*).

2. The following apply when the boil-water advisory is canceled:

   a. Follow guidance given by the local water utility regarding adequate flushing of waterlines. If no guidance is provided, flush dental waterlines and faucets for 1–5 minutes before using for patient care (IC) (*244,346, 351,352*).

   b. Disinfect dental waterlines as recommended by the dental unit manufacturer (II).

IX. SPECIAL CONSIDERATIONS

A. Dental Handpieces and Other Devices Attached to Air and Waterlines

1. Clean and heat-sterilize handpieces and other intraoral instruments that can be removed from the air and waterlines of dental units between patients (IB, IC) (*2,246,275,356,357,360,407*).

2. Follow the manufacturer's instructions for cleaning, lubrication, and sterilization of handpieces and other intraoral instruments that can be removed from the air and waterlines of dental units (IB) (*361–363*).

3. Do not surface-disinfect, use liquid chemical sterilants, or ethylene oxide on handpieces and other intraoral instruments that can be removed from the air and waterlines of dental units (IC) (*2,246,250,275*).

4. Do not advise patients to close their lips tightly around the tip of the saliva ejector to evacuate oral fluids (II) (*364–366*).

B. Dental Radiology

1. Wear gloves when exposing radiographs and handling contaminated film packets. Use other PPE (e.g., protective eyewear, mask, and gown) as appropriate if spattering of blood or other body fluids is likely (IA, IC) (*11,13*).

2. Use heat-tolerant or disposable intraoral devices whenever possible (e.g., film-holding and positioning devices). Clean and heat-sterilize heat-tolerant devices between patients. At a minimum, high-level disinfect semicritical heat-sensitive devices, according to manufacturer's instructions (IB) (*243*).

3. Transport and handle exposed radiographs in an aseptic manner to prevent contamination of developing equipment (II).
4. The following apply for digital radiography sensors:
   a. Use FDA-cleared barriers (IB) (*243*).
   b. Clean and heat-sterilize, or high-level disinfect, between patients, barrier-protected semicritical items. If the item cannot tolerate these procedures then, at a minimum, protect with an FDA-cleared barrier and clean and disinfect with an EPA-registered hospital disinfectant with intermediate-level (i.e., tuberculocidal claim) activity, between patients. Consult with the manufacturer for methods of disinfection and sterilization of digital radiology sensors and for protection of associated computer hardware (IB) (*243*).

C. Aseptic Technique for Parenteral Medications
1. Do not administer medication from a syringe to multiple patients, even if the needle on the syringe is changed (IA) (*378*).
2. Use single-dose vials for parenteral medications when possible (II) (*376,377*).
3. Do not combine the leftover contents of single-use vials for later use (IA) (*376,377*).
4. The following apply if multidose vials are used:
   a. Cleanse the access diaphragm with 70% alcohol before inserting a device into the vial (IA) (*380,381*).
   b. Use a sterile device to access a multiple-dose vial and avoid touching the access diaphragm. Both the needle and syringe used to access the multidose vial should be sterile. Do not reuse a syringe even if the needle is changed (IA) (*380,381*).
   c. Keep multidose vials away from the immediate patient treatment area to prevent inadvertent contamination by spray or spatter (II).
   d. Discard the multidose vial if sterility is compromised (IA) (*380,381*).
5. Use fluid infusion and administration sets (i.e., IV bags, tubings and connections) for one patient only and dispose of appropriately (IB) (*378*).

D. Single-Use (Disposable) Devices
1. Use single-use devices for one patient only and dispose of them appropriately (IC) (*383*).

E. Preprocedural Mouth Rinses
1. No recommendation is offered regarding use of preprocedural antimicrobial mouth rinses to prevent clinical infections among DHCP or patients. Although studies have demonstrated that a preprocedural antimicrobial rinse (e.g., chlorhexidine gluconate, essential oils, or povidone-iodine) can reduce the level of oral microorganisms in aerosols and spatter generated during routine dental procedures and can decrease the number of microorganisms introduced in the patient's bloodstream during invasive dental procedures (*391–399*), the scientific evidence is inconclusive that using these rinses prevents clinical infections among DHCP or patients (see discussion, Preprocedural Mouth Rinses) (Unresolved issue).

F. Oral Surgical Procedures
1. The following apply when performing oral surgical procedures:
   a. Perform surgical hand antisepsis by using an antimicrobial product (e.g., antimicrobial soap and water, or soap and water followed by alcohol-based hand scrub with persistent activity) before donning sterile surgeon's gloves (IB) (*127–132,137*).
   b. Use sterile surgeon's gloves (IB) (*2,7,121, 123,137*).
   c. Use sterile saline or sterile water as a coolant/irrigatant when performing oral surgical procedures. Use devices specifically designed for delivering sterile irrigating fluids (e.g., bulb syringe, single-use disposable products, and sterilizable tubing) (IB) (*2,121*).

G. Handling of Biopsy Specimens
1. During transport, place biopsy specimens in a sturdy, leakproof container labeled with the biohazard symbol (IC) (*2,13,14*).
2. If a biopsy specimen container is visibly contaminated, clean and disinfect the outside of a container or place it in an impervious bag labeled with the biohazard symbol, (IC) (*2,13*).

H. Handling of Extracted Teeth
1. Dispose of extracted teeth as regulated medical waste unless returned to the patient (IC) (*13,14*).
2. Do not dispose of extracted teeth containing amalgam in regulated medical waste intended for incineration (II).
3. Clean and place extracted teeth in a leakproof container, labeled with a biohazard symbol, and maintain hydration for transport to educational institutions or a dental laboratory (IC) (*13,14*).
4. Heat-sterilize teeth that do not contain amalgam before they are used for educational purposes (IB) (*403,405,406*).

I. Dental Laboratory

1. Use PPE when handling items received in the laboratory until they have been decontaminated (IA, IC) (2,7,11,13,113).

2. Before they are handled in the laboratory, clean, disinfect, and rinse all dental prostheses and prosthodontic materials (e.g., impressions, bite registrations, occlusal rims, and extracted teeth) by using an EPA-registered hospital disinfectant having at least an intermediate-level (i.e., tuberculocidal claim) activity (IB) (2,249,252,407).

3. Consult with manufacturers regarding the stability of specific materials (e.g., impression materials) relative to disinfection procedures (II).

4. Include specific information regarding disinfection techniques used (e.g., solution used and duration), when laboratory cases are sent off-site and on their return (II) (2,407,409).

5. Clean and heat-sterilize heat-tolerant items used in the mouth (e.g., metal impression trays and face-bow forks) (IB) (2,407).

6. Follow manufacturers' instructions for cleaning and sterilizing or disinfecting items that become contaminated but do not normally contact the patient (e.g., burs, polishing points, rag wheels, articulators, case pans, and lathes). If manufacturer instructions are unavailable, clean and heat-sterilize heat-tolerant items or clean and disinfect with an EPA-registered hospital disinfectant with low- (HIV, HBV effectiveness claim) to intermediate-level (tuberculocidal claim) activity, depending on the degree of contamination (II).

J. Laser/Electrosurgery Plumes/Surgical Smoke

1. No recommendation is offered regarding practices to reduce DHCP exposure to laser plumes/surgical smoke when using lasers in dental practice. Practices to reduce HCP exposure to laser plumes/surgical smoke have been suggested, including use of a) standard precautions (e.g., high-filtration surgical masks and possibly full face shields) (437); b) central room suction units with in-line filters to collect particulate matter from minimal plumes; and c) dedicated mechanical smoke exhaust systems with a high-efficiency filter to remove substantial amounts of laser-plume particles. The effect of the exposure (e.g., disease transmission or adverse respiratory effects) on DHCP from dental applications of lasers has not been adequately evaluated (see previous discussion, Laser/ Electrosurgery Plumes or Surgical Smoke) (Unresolved issue).

K. *Mycobacterium tuberculosis*

1. General Recommendations
   a. Educate all DHCP regarding the recognition of signs, symptoms, and transmission of TB (IB) (20,21).
   b. Conduct a baseline TST, preferably by using a two-step test, for all DHCP who might have contact with persons with suspected or confirmed active TB, regardless of the risk classification of the setting (IB) (20).
   c. Assess each patient for a history of TB as well as symptoms indicative of TB and document on the medical history form (IB) (20,21).
   d. Follow CDC recommendations for 1) developing, maintaining, and implementing a written TB infection-control plan; 2) managing a patient with suspected or active TB; 3) completing a community risk-assessment to guide employee TSTs and follow-up; and 4) managing DHCP with TB disease (IB) (2,21).

2. The following apply for patients known or suspected to have active TB:
   a. Evaluate the patient away from other patients and DHCP. When not being evaluated, the patient should wear a surgical mask or be instructed to cover mouth and nose when coughing or sneezing (IB) (20,21).
   b. Defer elective dental treatment until the patient is noninfectious (IB) (20,21).
   c. Refer patients requiring urgent dental treatment to a previously identified facility with TB engineering controls and a respiratory protection program (IB) (20,21).

L. Creutzfeldt-Jakob Disease (CJD) and Other Prion Diseases

1. No recommendation is offered regarding use of special precautions in addition to standard precautions when treating known CJD or vCJD patients. Potential infectivity of oral tissues in CJD or vCJD patients is an unresolved issue. Scientific data indicate the risk, if any, of sporadic CJD transmission during dental and oral surgical procedures is low to nil. Until additional information exists regarding the transmissibility of CJD or vCJD during dental procedures, special precautions in addition to standard precautions might be indicated when treating known CJD or vCJD patients; a list of such precautions is provided for consideration without recommendation (see Creutzfeldt-

Jakob Disease and Other Prion Diseases) (Unresolved issue).

M. Program Evaluation

1. Establish routine evaluation of the infection-control program, including evaluation of performance indicators, at an established frequency (II) (*470–471*).

NOTE: The complete CDC *Guidelines for Infection Control in Dental Health-Care Settings—2003*, including the background, tables, appendices, and references, are available by visiting http://www.cdc.gov/oralhealth/infectioncontrol/index.htm.

Critical Thinking

1. Do you have a copy of the CDC Guidelines for Infection Control in Dental Health-Care Settings—2003? If not, do you know how to obtain a copy of the guidelines?

2. Some state dental licensing boards adopt CDC recommendations as the standard of care in their state. Do you know if your state follows CDC recommendations?

CHAPTER

23

Occupational Safety and Health Administration (OSHA) Bloodborne Pathogens Standard*

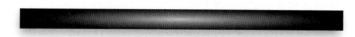

*Reprinted from: U.S. Department of Labor, Occupational Safety and Health Administration. 29 CFR Part 1910.1030. Occupational exposure to bloodborne pathogens; needlesticks and other sharps injuries; final rule. Federal Register 2001;66:5317–5325. [As amended from and includes 29 CFR Part 1910.1030. Occupational exposure to bloodborne pathogens; final rule. Federal Register 1991;56:64174–64182.]

294

XI. THE STANDARD

General Industry

Part 1910 of title 29 of the Code of Federal Regulations is amended as follows:

PART 1910-[AMENDED]

Subpart Z—[Amended]. 1. The general authority citation for subpart Z of 29 CFR part 1910 continues to read as follows and a new citation for § 1910.1030 is added:

Authority: Secs 6 and 8, Occupational Safety and Health Act. 29 U.S.C. 655, 657, Secretary of Labor's Orders Nos. 12—71 (36 FR 8754), 8—76 (41 FR 25059), or 9—83 (48 FR 35736) as applicable; and 29 CFR part 1911.

Section 1910.10130 also issued under 29 U.S.C. 653.

2. Section 1910.1030 is added to read as follows (includes 2001 update; new or updated items annotated by "•"):

§1910.30 Bloodborne Pathogens

(a) Scope and Application. This section applies to all occupational exposure to blood or other potentially infectious materials as defined by paragraph (b) of this section.

(b) Definitions. For purposes of this section, the following shall apply:

Assistant Secretary means the Assistant Secretary of Labor for Occupational Safety and Health, or designated representative.

Blood means human blood, human blood components, and products made from human blood.

Bloodborne Pathogens means pathogenic microorganisms that are present in human blood and can cause disease in humans. These pathogens include, but are not limited to, hepatitis B virus (HBV) and human immunodeficiency virus (HIV).

Clinical Laboratory means a workplace where diagnostic or other screening procedures are performed on blood or other potentially infectious materials.

Contaminated means the presence or the reasonably anticipated presence of blood or other potentially infectious materials on an item or surface.

Contaminated Laundry means laundry which has been soiled with blood or other potentially infectious materials or may contain sharps.

Contaminated Sharps means any contaminated object that can penetrate the skin including, but not limited to, needles, scalpels, broken glass, broken capillary tubes, and exposed ends of dental wires.

Decontamination means the use of physical or chemical means to remove, inactivate, or destroy bloodborne pathogens on a surface or item to the point where they are no longer capable of transmitting infectious particles and the surface or item is rendered safe for handling, use, or disposal.

Director means the Director of the National Institute for Occupational Safety and Health, U.S. Department of Health and Human Services, or designated representative.

•Engineering Controls means controls (e.g., sharps disposal containers, self-sheathing needles, safer medical devices, such as sharps with engineered sharps injury protections and needleless systems) that isolate or remove the bloodborne pathogens hazard from the workplace.

Exposure Incident means a specific eye, mouth, other mucous membrane, non-intact skin, or parenteral contact with blood or other potentially infectious materials that results from the performance of an employee's duties.

Handwashing facilities means a facility providing an adequate supply of running potable water, soap and single use towels or hot air drying machines.

Licensed Healthcare Professional is a person whose legally permitted scope of practice allows him or her to independently perform the activities required by paragraph (f) Hepatitis B Vaccination and Post-exposure Evaluation and Follow-up.

HBV means hepatitis B virus.

HIV means human immunodeficiency virus.

Needleless systems means a device that does not use needles for: (1) The collection of bodily fluids or withdrawal of body fluids after initial venous or arterial access is established; (2) The administration of medication or fluids; or (3) Any other procedure involving the potential for occupational exposure to bloodborne pathogens due to percutaneous injuries from contaminated sharps.

Occupational Exposure means reasonably anticipated skin, eye, mucous membrane, or parenteral contact with blood or other potentially infectious materials that may result from the performance of an employee's duties.

Other Potentially Infectious Materials means (1) The following human body fluids: semen, vaginal secretions, cerebrospinal fluid, synovial fluid, pleural fluid, pericardial fluid, peritoneal fluid, amniotic fluid, saliva in dental procedures, any body fluid that is visibly contaminated with blood, and all body fluids in situations where it is difficult or impossible to differentiate between body fluids; (2) Any unfixed tissue or organ (other than intact skin) from a human (living or dead); and (3) HIV-containing cell or tissue cultures, organ cultures, and HIV- or HBV-containing culture medium or other solutions; and blood, organs, or other tissues from experimental animals infected with HIV or HBV.

Parenteral means piercing mucous membranes or the skin barrier through such events as needlesticks, human bites, cuts, and abrasions.

Personal Protective Equipment is specialized clothing or equipment worn by an employee for protection against a hazard. General work clothes (e.g., uniforms, pants, shirts or blouses) not intended to function as protection against a hazard are not considered to be personal protective equipment.

Production Facility means a facility engaged in industrial-scale, large-volume or high concentration production of HIV or HBV.

Regulated Waste means liquid or semi-liquid blood or other potentially infectious materials; contaminated items that would release blood or other potentially infectious materials in a liquid or semi-liquid state if compressed; items that are caked with dried blood or other potentially infectious materials and are capable of releasing these materials during handling; contaminated sharps; and pathological and microbiological wastes containing blood or other potentially infectious materials.

Research Laboratory means a laboratory producing or using research-laboratory-scale amounts of HIV or HBV. Research laboratories may produce high concentrations of HIV or HBV but not in the volume found in production facilities.

•**Sharps with Engineered Sharps Injury Protections** means a nonneedle sharp or a needle device used for withdrawing body fluids, accessing a vein or artery, or administering medications or other fluids, with a built-in safety feature or mechanism that effectively reduces the risk of an exposure incident.

Source Individual means any individual, living or dead, whose blood or other potentially infectious materials may be a source of occupational exposure to the employee. Examples include, but are not limited to, hospital and clinic patients; clients in institutions for the developmentally disabled; trauma victims; clients of drug and alcohol treatment facilities; residents of hospices and nursing homes; human remains; and individuals who donate or sell blood or blood components.

Sterilize means the use of a physical or chemical procedure to destroy all microbial life including highly resistant bacterial endospores.

Universal Precautions is an approach to infection control. According to the concept of Universal Precautions, all human blood and certain human body fluids are treated as if known to be infectious for HIV, HBV, and other bloodborne pathogens.

Work Practice Controls means controls that reduce the likelihood of exposure by altering the manner in which a task is performed (e.g., prohibiting recapping of needles by a two-handed technique).

(c) Exposure Control —

(1) Exposure Control Plan.

  (i) Each employer having an employee(s) with occupational exposure as defined by paragraph (b) of this section shall establish a written Exposure Control Plan designed to eliminate or minimize employee exposure.

  (ii) The Exposure Control Plan shall contain at least the following elements:

    (A) The exposure determination required by paragraph (c)(2),

    (B) The schedule and method of implementation for paragraphs (d) Methods of Compliance, (e) HIV and HBV Research Laboratories and Production Facilities, (f) Hepatitis B Vaccination and Post-Exposure Evaluation and Follow-up, (g) Communication of Hazards to Employees, and (h) Recordkeeping, of this standard, and

    (C) The procedure for the evaluation of circumstances surrounding exposure incidents as required by paragraph (f)(3)(i) of this standard.

  (iii) Each employer shall ensure that a copy of the Exposure Control Plan is accessible to employees in accordance with 29 CFR 1910.1020(e).

  (iv) The Exposure Control Plan shall be reviewed and updated at least annually and whenever necessary to reflect new or modified tasks and procedures which affect occupational exposure and to reflect new or revised employee positions with occupational exposure. The review and update of such plans shall also:

    •(A) Reflect changes in technology that eliminate or reduce exposure to bloodborne pathogens; and

    •(B) Document annually consideration and implementation of appropriate commercially available and effective safer medical devices designed to eliminate or minimize occupational exposure.

  •(v) An employer who is required to establish an Exposure Control Plan shall solicit input from non-managerial employees responsible for direct patient care who are potentially exposed to injuries from contaminated sharps in the identification, evaluation, and selection of effective engineering and work practice controls and shall document the solicitation in the Exposure Control Plan.

  (vi) The Exposure Control Plan shall be made available to the Assistant Secretary and the

Director upon request for examination and copying.

(2) Exposure Determination.

(i) Each employer who has an employee(s) with occupational exposure as defined by paragraph (b) of this section shall prepare an exposure determination. This exposure determination shall contain the following:

(A) A list of all job classifications in which all employees in those job classifications have occupational exposure;

(B) A list of job classifications in which some employees have occupational exposure, and

(C) A list of all tasks and procedures or groups of closely related task and procedures in which occupational exposure occurs and that are performed by employees in job classifications listed in accordance with the provisions of paragraph (c)(2)(i)(B) of this standard.

(ii) This exposure determination shall be made without regard to the use of personal protective equipment.

(d) Methods of Compliance —

(1) General. Universal precautions shall be observed to prevent contact with blood or other potentially infectious materials. Under circumstances in which differentiation between body fluid types is difficult or impossible, all body fluids shall be considered potentially infectious materials.

(2) Engineering and Work Practice Controls.

(i) Engineering and work practice controls shall be used to eliminate or minimize employee exposure. Where occupational exposure remains after institution of these controls, personal protective equipment shall also be used.

(ii) Engineering controls shall be examined and maintained or replaced on a regular schedule to ensure their effectiveness.

(iii) Employers shall provide handwashing facilities which are readily accessible to employees.

(iv) When provision of handwashing facilities is not feasible, the employer shall provide either an appropriate antiseptic hand cleanser in conjunction with clean cloth/paper towels or antiseptic towelettes. When antiseptic hand cleansers or towelettes are used, hands shall be washed with soap and running water as soon as feasible.

(v) Employers shall ensure that employees wash their hands immediately or as soon as feasible after removal of gloves or other personal protective equipment.

(vi) Employers shall ensure that employees wash hands and any other skin with soap and water, or flush mucous membranes with water immediately or as soon as feasible following contact of such body areas with blood or other potentially infectious materials.

(vii) Contaminated needles and other contaminated sharps shall not be bent, recapped, or removed except as noted in paragraphs (d)(2)(vii)(A) and (d)(2)(vii)(B) below. Shearing or breaking of contaminated needles is prohibited.

(A) Contaminated needles and other contaminated sharps shall not be bent, recapped or removed unless the employer can demonstrate that no alternative is feasible or that such action is required by a specific medical or dental procedure.

(B) Such bending, recapping or needle removal must be accomplished through the use of a mechanical device or a one-handed technique.

(viii) Immediately or as soon as possible after use, contaminated reusable sharps shall be placed in appropriate containers until properly reprocessed. These containers shall be:

(A) Puncture resistant;

(B) Labeled or color-coded in accordance with this standard;

(C) Leakproof on the sides and bottom; and

(D) In accordance with the requirements set forth in paragraph (d)(4)(ii)(E) for reusable sharps.

(ix) Eating, drinking, smoking, applying cosmetics or lip balm, and handling contact lenses are prohibited in work areas where there is a reasonable likelihood of occupational exposure.

(x) Food and drink shall not be kept in refrigerators, freezers, shelves, cabinets or on countertops or benchtops where blood or other potentially infectious materials are present.

(xi) All procedures involving blood or other potentially infectious materials shall be performed in such a manner as to minimize splashing, spraying, spattering, and generation of droplets of these substances.

(xii) Mouth pipetting/suctioning of blood or other potentially infectious materials is prohibited.

(xiii) Specimens of blood or other potentially infectious materials shall be placed in a container which prevents leakage during collection, handling, processing, storage, transport, or shipping.

(A) The container for storage, transport, or shipping shall be labeled or color-coded according to paragraph (g)(1)(i) and closed prior to being stored, transported, or shipped. When a facility utilizes Universal Precautions in the handling of all specimens, the labeling/color-coding of specimens is not necessary provided containers are recognizable as containing specimens. This exemption only applies while such specimens/containers remain within the facility. Labeling or color-coding in accordance with paragraph (g)(1)(i) is required when such specimens/containers leave the facility.

(B) If outside contamination of the primary container occurs, the primary container shall be placed within a second container which prevents leakage during handling, processing, storage, transport, or shipping and is labeled or color-coded according to the requirements of this standard.

(C) If the specimen could puncture the primary container, the primary container shall be placed within a secondary container which is puncture-resistant in addition to the above characteristics.

(xiv) Equipment which may become contaminated with blood or other potentially infectious materials shall be examined prior to servicing or shipping and shall be decontaminated as necessary, unless the employer can demonstrate that decontamination of such equipment or portions of such equipment is not feasible.

(A) A readily observable label in accordance with paragraph (g)(1)(i)(H) shall be attached to the equipment stating which portions remain contaminated.

(B) The employer shall ensure that this information is conveyed to all affected employees, the servicing representative, and/or the manufacturer, as appropriate, prior to handling, servicing, or shipping so that appropriate precautions will be taken.

(3) Personal Protective Equipment —

(i) **Provision.** When there is occupational exposure, the employer shall provide, at no cost to the employee, appropriate personal protective equipment such as, but not limited to, gloves, gowns, laboratory coats, face shields or masks and eye protection, and mouthpieces, resuscitation bags, pocket masks, or other ventilation devices. Personal protective equipment will be considered "appropriate" only if it does not permit blood or other potentially infectious materials to pass through to or reach the employee's work clothes, street clothes, undergarments, skin, eyes, mouth, or other mucous membranes under normal conditions of use and for the duration of time which the protective equipment will be used.

(ii) **Use.** The employer shall ensure that the employee uses appropriate personal protective equipment unless the employer shows that the employee temporarily and briefly declined to use personal protective equipment when, under rare and extraordinary circumstances, it was the employee's professional judgment that in the specific instance its use would have prevented the delivery of healthcare or public safety services or would have posed an increased hazard to the safety of the worker or co-worker. When the employee makes this judgement, the circumstances shall be investigated and documented in order to determine whether changes can be instituted to prevent such occurrences in the future.

(iii) **Accessibility.** The employer shall ensure that appropriate personal protective equipment in the appropriate sizes is readily accessible at the worksite or is issued to employees. Hypoallergenic gloves, glove liners, powderless gloves, or other similar alternatives shall be readily accessible to those employees who are allergic to the gloves normally provided.

(iv) **Cleaning, Laundering, and Disposal.** The employer shall clean, launder, and dispose of personal protective equipment required by paragraphs (d) and (e) of this standard, at no cost to the employee.

(v) **Repair and Replacement.** The employer shall repair or replace personal protective equipment as needed to maintain its effectiveness, at no cost to the employee.

(vi) If a garment(s) is penetrated by blood or other potentially infectious materials, the garment(s) shall be removed immediately or as soon as feasible.

(vii) All personal protective equipment shall be removed prior to leaving the work area.

(viii) When personal protective equipment is removed it shall be placed in an appropriately designated area or container for storage, washing, decontamination or disposal.

(ix) **Gloves.** Gloves shall be worn when it can be reasonably anticipated that the employee may have hand contact with blood, other potentially infectious materials, mucous membranes, and non-intact skin; when performing vascular access procedures except as specified in paragraph (d)(3)(ix)(D); and when handling or touching contaminated items or surfaces.

(A) Disposable (single use) gloves, such as surgical or examination gloves, shall be replaced as soon as practical when contaminated or as soon as feasible if they are torn, punctured, or when their ability to function as a barrier is compromised.

(B) Disposable (single use) gloves shall not be washed or decontaminated for re-use.

(C) Utility gloves may be decontaminated for re-use if the integrity of the glove is not compromised. However, they must be discarded if they are cracked, peeling, torn, punctured, or exhibit other signs of deterioration or when their ability to function as a barrier is compromised.

(D) If an employer in a volunteer blood donation center judges that routine gloving for all phlebotomies is not necessary then the employer shall:

(1) Periodically reevaluate this policy;

(2) Make gloves available to all employees who wish to use them for phlebotomy;

(3) Not discourage the use of gloves for phlebotomy; and

(4) Require that gloves be used for phlebotomy in the following circumstances:

(i) When the employee has cuts, scratches, or other breaks in his or her skin;

(ii) When the employee judges that hand contamination with blood may occur, for example, when performing phlebotomy on an uncooperative source individual; and

(iii) When the employee is receiving training in phlebotomy.

(x) **Masks, Eye Protection, and Face Shields.** Masks in combination with eye protection devices, such as goggles or glasses with solid side shields, or chin-length face shields, shall be worn whenever splashes, spray, spatter, or droplets of blood or other potentially infectious materials may be generated and eye, nose, or mouth contamination can be reasonably anticipated.

(xi) **Gowns, Aprons, and Other Protective Body Clothing.** Appropriate protective clothing such as, but not limited to, gowns, aprons, lab coats, clinic jackets, or similar outer garments shall be worn in occupational exposure situations. The type and characteristics will depend upon the task and degree of exposure anticipated.

(xii) Surgical caps or hoods and/or shoe covers or boots shall be worn in instances when gross contamination can reasonably be anticipated (e.g., autopsies, orthopaedic surgery).

(4) Housekeeping —

(i) **General.** Employers shall ensure that the worksite is maintained in a clean and sanitary condition. The employer shall determine and implement an appropriate written schedule for cleaning and method of decontamination based upon the location within the facility, type of surface to be cleaned, type of soil present, and tasks or procedures being performed in the area.

(ii) All equipment and environmental and working surfaces shall be cleaned and decontaminated after contact with blood or other potentially infectious materials.

(A) Contaminated work surfaces shall be decontaminated with an appropriate disinfectant after completion of procedures; immediately or as soon as feasible when surfaces are overtly contaminated or after any spill of blood or other potentially infectious materials; and at the end of the work shift if the surface may have become contaminated since the last cleaning.

(B) Protective coverings, such as plastic wrap, aluminum foil, or imperviously-backed absorbent paper used to cover equipment and environmental surfaces, shall be removed and replaced as soon as feasible when they become overtly contaminated or at the end of the work-shift if they may have become contaminated during the shift.

(C) All bins, pails, cans, and similar receptacles intended for reuse which have a reasonable likelihood for becoming contaminated with blood or other potentially infectious materials shall be inspected and decontaminated on a regularly scheduled basis and cleaned and decontaminated immediately or as soon as feasible upon visible contamination.

(D) Broken glassware which may be contaminated shall not be picked up directly with the hands. It shall be cleaned up using mechanical means, such as a brush and dust pan, tongs, or forceps.

(E) Reusable sharps that are contaminated with blood or other potentially infectious materials shall not be stored or processed in a manner that requires employees to reach by hand into the containers where these sharps have been placed.

(iii) **Regulated Waste —**

(A) **Contaminated Sharps Discarding and Containment.**

(1) Contaminated sharps shall be discarded immediately or as soon as feasible in containers that are:

  (i) Closable;

  (ii) Puncture resistant;

  (iii) Leakproof on sides and bottom; and

  (iv) Labeled or color-coded in accordance with paragraph (g)(1)(i) of this standard.

(2) During use, containers for contaminated sharps shall be:

  (i) Easily accessible to personnel and located as close as is feasible to the immediate area where sharps are used or can be reasonably anticipated to be found (e.g., laundries);

  (ii) Maintained upright throughout use; and

  (iii) Replaced routinely and not be allowed to overfill.

(3) When moving containers of contaminated sharps from the area of use, the containers shall be:

  (i) Closed immediately prior to removal or replacement to prevent spillage or protrusion of contents during handling, storage, transport, or shipping;

  (ii) Placed in a secondary container if leakage is possible. The second container shall be:

    (A) Closable;

    (B) Constructed to contain all contents and prevent leakage during handling, storage, transport, or shipping; and

    (C) Labeled or color-coded according to paragraph (g)(1)(i) of this standard.

(4) Reusable containers shall not be opened, emptied, or cleaned manually or in any other manner which would expose employees to the risk of percutaneous injury.

(B) **Other Regulated Waste Containment—**

(1) Regulated waste shall be placed in containers which are:

  (i) Closable;

  (ii) Constructed to contain all contents and prevent leakage of fluids during handling, storage, transport or shipping;

  (iii) Labeled or color-coded in accordance with paragraph (g)(1)(i) this standard; and

  (iv) Closed prior to removal to prevent spillage or protrusion of contents during handling, storage, transport, or shipping.

(2) If outside contamination of the regulated waste container occurs, it shall be placed in a second container. The second container shall be:

  (i) Closable;

  (ii) Constructed to contain all contents and prevent leakage of fluids during handling, storage, transport or shipping;

  (iii) Labeled or color-coded in accordance with paragraph (g)(1)(i) of this standard; and

  (iv) Closed prior to removal to prevent spillage or protrusion of contents during handling, storage, transport, or shipping.

(C) Disposal of all regulated waste shall be in accordance with applicable regulations of the United States, States and Territories, and political subdivisions of States and Territories.

(iv) **Laundry.**

(A) Contaminated laundry shall be handled as little as possible with a minimum of agitation.

(1) Contaminated laundry shall be bagged or containerized at the location where it was used and shall not be sorted or rinsed in the location of use.

(2) Contaminated laundry shall be placed and transported in bags or containers labeled or color-coded in accordance with paragraph (g)(1)(i) of this standard. When a facility utilizes Universal Precautions in the handling of all soiled laundry, alternative labeling or color-coding is sufficient if it permits all employees to recognize the containers as requiring compliance with Universal Precautions.

(3) Whenever contaminated laundry is wet and presents a reasonable likelihood of soak-through of or leakage from the bag or container, the laundry shall be placed and transported in bags or containers which prevent soak-through and/or leakage of fluids to the exterior.

(B) The employer shall ensure that employees who have contact with contaminated laundry wear protective gloves and other appropriate personal protective equipment.

(C) When a facility ships contaminated laundry off-site to a second facility which does not utilize Universal Precautions in the handling of all laundry, the facility generating the contaminated laundry must place such laundry in bags or containers which are labeled or color-coded in accordance with paragraph (g)(1)(i).

(e) HIV and HBV Research Laboratories and Production Facilities.

(1) This paragraph applies to research laboratories and production facilities engaged in the culture, production, concentration, experimentation, and manipulation of HIV and HBV. It does not apply to clinical or diagnostic laboratories engaged solely in the analysis of blood, tissues, or organs. These requirements apply in addition to the other requirements of the standard.

(2) Research laboratories and production facilities shall meet the following criteria:

(i) **Standard Microbiological Practices.** All regulated waste shall either be incinerated or decontaminated by a method such as

autoclaving known to effectively destroy bloodborne pathogens.

(ii) **Special Practices.**

(A) Laboratory doors shall be kept closed when work involving HIV or HBV is in progress.

(B) Contaminated materials that are to be decontaminated at a site away from the work area shall be placed in a durable, leakproof, labeled or color-coded container that is closed before being removed from the work area.

(C) Access to the work area shall be limited to authorized persons. Written policies and procedures shall be established whereby only persons who have been advised of the potential biohazard, who meet any specific entry requirements, and who comply with all entry and exit procedures shall be allowed to enter the work areas and animal rooms.

(D) When other potentially infectious materials or infected animals are present in the work area or containment module, a hazard warning sign incorporating the universal biohazard symbol shall be posted on all access doors. The hazard warning sign shall comply with paragraph (g)(1)(ii) of this standard.

(E) All activities involving other potentially infectious materials shall be conducted in biological safety cabinets or other physical-containment devices within the containment module. No work with these other potentially infectious materials shall be conducted on the open bench.

(F) Laboratory coats, gowns, smocks, uniforms, or other appropriate protective clothing shall be used in the work area and animal rooms. Protective clothing shall not be worn outside of the work area and shall be decontaminated before being laundered.

(G) Special care shall be taken to avoid skin contact with other potentially infectious materials. Gloves shall be worn when handling infected animals and when making hand contact with other potentially infectious materials is unavoidable.

(H) Before disposal all waste from work areas and from animal rooms shall either be incinerated or decontaminated by a method such as autoclaving known to effectively destroy blood-borne pathogens.

(I) Vacuum lines shall be protected with liquid disinfectant traps and high-efficiency particulate air (HEPA) filters or filters of equivalent or superior efficiency and which are checked routinely and maintained or replaced as necessary.

(J) Hypodermic needles and syringes shall be used only for parenteral injection and aspiration of fluids from laboratory animals and diaphragm bottles. Only needle-locking syringes or disposable syringe-needle units (i.e., the needle is integral to the syringe) shall be used for the injection or aspiration of other potentially infectious materials. Extreme caution shall be used when handling needles and syringes. A needle shall not be bent, sheared, replaced in the sheath or guard, or removed from the syringe following use. The needle and syringe shall be promptly placed in a puncture-resistant container and autoclaved or decontaminated before reuse or disposal.

(K) All spills shall be immediately contained and cleaned up by appropriate professional staff or others properly trained and equipped to work with potentially concentrated infectious materials.

(L) A spill or accident that results in an exposure incident shall be immediately reported to the laboratory director or other responsible person.

(M) A biosafety manual shall be prepared or adopted and periodically reviewed and updated at least annually or more often if necessary. Personnel shall be advised of potential hazards, shall be required to read instructions on practices and procedures, and shall be required to follow them.

(iii) **Containment Equipment.**

(A) Certified biological safety cabinets (Class I, II, or III) or other appropriate combinations of personal protection or physical containment devices, such as special protective clothing, respirators, centrifuge safety cups, sealed centrifuge rotors, and containment caging for animals, shall be used for all activities with other potentially infectious materials that pose a threat of exposure to droplets, splashes, spills, or aerosols.

(B) Biological safety cabinets shall be certified when installed, whenever they are moved and at least annually.

(3) HIV and HBV research laboratories shall meet the following criteria:

(i) Each laboratory shall contain a facility for hand washing and an eye wash facility which is readily available within the work area.

(ii) An autoclave for decontamination of regulated waste shall be available.

(4) HIV and HBV production facilities shall meet the following criteria:

(i) The work areas shall be separated from areas that are open to unrestricted traffic flow within the building. Passage through two sets of doors shall be the basic requirement for entry into the work area from access corridors or other contiguous areas. Physical separation of the high-containment work area from access corridors or other areas or activities may also be provided by a double-doored clothes-change room (showers may be included), airlock, or other access facility that requires passing through two sets of doors before entering the work area.

(ii) The surfaces of doors, walls, floors and ceilings in the work area shall be water resistant so that they can be easily cleaned. Penetrations in these surfaces shall be sealed or capable of being sealed to facilitate decontamination.

(iii) Each work area shall contain a sink for washing hands and a readily available eye wash facility. The sink shall be foot, elbow, or automatically operated and shall be located near the exit door of the work area.

(iv) Access doors to the work area or containment module shall be self-closing.

(v) An autoclave for decontamination of regulated waste shall be available within or as near as possible to the work area.

(vi) A ducted exhaust-air ventilation system shall be provided. This system shall create directional airflow that draws air into the work area through the entry area. The exhaust air shall not be recirculated to any other area of the building, shall be discharged to the outside, and shall be dispersed away from occupied areas and air intakes. The proper direction of the airflow shall be verified (i.e., into the work area).

(5) Training Requirements. Additional training requirements for employees in HIV and HBV research laboratories and HIV and HBV production facilities are specified in paragraph (g)(2)(ix).

(f) Hepatitis B Vaccination and Post-exposure Evaluation and Follow-up —

(1) General.

(i) The employer shall make available the hepatitis B vaccine and vaccination series to all employees who have occupational exposure, and post-exposure evaluation and follow-up to all employees who have had an exposure incident.

(ii) The employer shall ensure that all medical evaluations and procedures including the hepatitis B vaccine and vaccination series and post-exposure evaluation and follow-up, including prophylaxis, are:

(A) Made available at no cost to the employee;

(B) Made available to the employee at a reasonable time and place;

(C) Performed by or under the supervision of a licensed physician or by or under the supervision of another licensed healthcare professional; and

(D) Provided according to recommendations of the U.S. Public Health Service current at the time these evaluations and procedures take place, except as specified by this paragraph (f).

(iii) The employer shall ensure that all laboratory tests are conducted by an accredited laboratory at no cost to the employee.

(2) Hepatitis B Vaccination.

(i) Hepatitis B vaccination shall be made available after the employee has received the training required in paragraph (g)(2)(vii)(I) and within 10 working days of initial assignment to all employees who have occupational exposure unless the employee has previously received the complete hepatitis B vaccination series, antibody testing has revealed that the employee is immune, or the vaccine is contraindicated for medical reasons.

(ii) The employer shall not make participation in a prescreening program a prerequisite for receiving hepatitis B vaccination.

(iii) If the employee initially declines hepatitis B vaccination but at a later date while still covered under the standard decides to accept the vaccination, the employer shall make available hepatitis B vaccination at that time.

(iv) The employer shall assure that employees who decline to accept hepatitis B vaccination offered by the employer sign the statement in Appendix A.

(v) If a routine booster dose(s) of hepatitis B vaccine is recommended by the U.S. Public Health Service at a future date, such booster dose(s) shall be made available in accordance with section (f)(1)(ii).

(3) Post-exposure Evaluation and Follow-up. Following a report of an exposure incident, the employer shall make immediately available to the exposed employee a confidential medical evaluation and follow-up, including at least the following elements:

(i) Documentation of the route(s) of exposure, and the circumstances under which the exposure incident occurred;

(ii) Identification and documentation of the source individual, unless the employer can establish that identification is infeasible or prohibited by state or local law;

(A) The source individual's blood shall be tested as soon as feasible and after consent is obtained in order to determine HBV and HIV infectivity. If consent is not obtained, the employer shall establish that legally required consent cannot be obtained. When the source individual's consent is not required by law, the source individual's blood, if available, shall be tested and the results documented.

(B) When the source individual is already known to be infected with HBV or HIV, testing for the source individual's known HBV or HIV status need not be repeated.

(C) Results of the source individual's testing shall be made available to the exposed employee, and the employee shall be informed of applicable laws and regulations concerning disclosure of the identity and infectious status of the source individual.

(iii) Collection and testing of blood for HBV and HIV serological status;

(A) The exposed employee's blood shall be collected as soon as feasible and tested after consent is obtained.

(B) If the employee consents to baseline blood collection, but does not give consent at that time for HIV serologic testing, the sample shall be preserved for at least 90 days. If, within 90 days of the exposure incident, the employee elects to have the baseline sample tested, such testing shall be done as soon as feasible.

(iv) Post-exposure prophylaxis, when medically indicated, as recommended by the U.S. Public Health Service;

(v) Counseling; and

(vi) Evaluation of reported illnesses.

(4) Information Provided to the Healthcare Professional.

(i) The employer shall ensure that the healthcare professional responsible for the employee's Hepatitis B vaccination is provided a copy of this regulation.

(ii) The employer shall ensure that the healthcare professional evaluating an employee after an exposure incident is provided the following information:

(A) A copy of this regulation;

(B) A description of the exposed employee's duties as they relate to the exposure incident;

(C) Documentation of the route(s) of exposure and circumstances under which exposure occurred;

(D) Results of the source individual's blood testing, if available; and

(E) All medical records relevant to the appropriate treatment of the employee including vaccination status which are the employer's responsibility to maintain.

(5) Healthcare Professional's Written Opinion. The employer shall obtain and provide the employee with a copy of the evaluating healthcare professional's written opinion within 15 days of the completion of the evaluation.

(i) The healthcare professional's written opinion for Hepatitis B vaccination shall be limited to whether Hepatitis B vaccination is indicated for an employee, and if the employee has received such vaccination.

(ii) The healthcare professional's written opinion for post-exposure evaluation and follow-up shall be limited to the following information:

(A) That the employee has been informed of the results of the evaluation; and

(B) That the employee has been told about any medical conditions resulting from exposure to blood or other potentially infectious materials which require further evaluation or treatment.

(iii) All other findings or diagnoses shall remain confidential and shall not be included in the written report.

(6) Medical Recordkeeping. Medical records required by this standard shall be maintained in accordance with paragraph (h)(1) of this section.

(g) Communication of Hazards to Employees —

(1) Labels and Signs —

(i) **Labels.**

(A) Warning labels shall be affixed to containers of regulated waste, refrigerators and freezers containing blood or other potentially infectious material; and other containers used to store, transport or ship blood or other potentially infectious materials, except as provided in paragraph (g)(1)(i)(E), (F) and (G).

(B) Labels required by this section shall include the following legend:

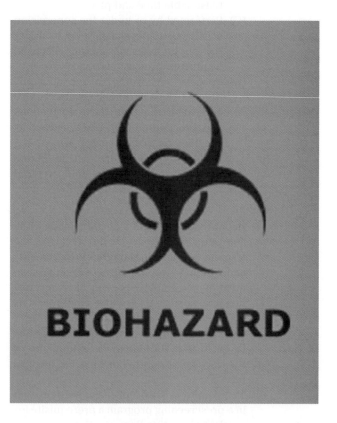

(C) These labels shall be fluorescent orange or orange-red or predominantly so, with lettering and symbols in a contrasting color.

(D) Labels shall be affixed as close as feasible to the container by string, wire, adhesive, or other method that prevents their loss or unintentional removal.

(E) Red bags or red containers may be substituted for labels.

(F) Containers of blood, blood components, or blood products that are labeled as to their contents and have been released for transfusion or other clinical use are exempted from the labeling requirements of paragraph (g).

(G) Individual containers of blood or other potentially infectious materials that are placed in a labeled container during storage, transport, shipment or disposal are exempted from the labeling requirement.

(H) Labels required for contaminated equipment shall be in accordance with this paragraph and shall also state which portions of the equipment remain contaminated.

(I) Regulated waste that has been decontaminated need not be labeled or color-coded.

(ii) **Signs.**

(A) The employer shall post signs at the entrance to work areas specified in paragraph (e), HIV and HBV Research Laboratory and Production Facilities, which shall bear the following legend:
(Name of the Infectious Agent)
(Special requirements for entering the area)
(Name, telephone number of the laboratory director or other responsible person.)

(B) These signs shall be fluorescent orange-red or predominantly so, with lettering and symbols in a contrasting color.

(2) Information and Training.

(i) Employers shall ensure that all employees with occupational exposure participate in a training program which must be provided at no cost to the employee and during working hours.

(ii) Training shall be provided as follows:

(A) At the time of initial assignment to tasks where occupational exposure may take place;

(B) At least annually thereafter.

(iii) [Reserved]

(iv) Annual training for all employees shall be provided within one year of their previous training.

(v) Employers shall provide additional training when changes such as modification of tasks or procedures or institution of new tasks or procedures affect the employee's occupational exposure. The additional training may be limited to addressing the new exposures created.

(vi) Material appropriate in content and vocabulary to educational level, literacy, and language of employees shall be used.

(vii) The training program shall contain at a minimum the following elements:

(A) An accessible copy of the regulatory text of this standard and an explanation of its contents;

(B) A general explanation of the epidemiology and symptoms of bloodborne diseases;

(C) An explanation of the modes of transmission of bloodborne pathogens;

(D) An explanation of the employer's exposure control plan and the means by which the employee can obtain a copy of the written plan;

(E) An explanation of the appropriate methods for recognizing tasks and other activities that may involve exposure to blood and other potentially infectious materials;

(F) An explanation of the use and limitations of methods that will prevent or reduce exposure including appropriate engineering controls, work practices, and personal protective equipment;

(G) Information on the types, proper use, location, removal, handling, decontamination and disposal of personal protective equipment;

(H) An explanation of the basis for selection of personal protective equipment;

(I) Information on the hepatitis B vaccine, including information on its efficacy, safety, method of administration, the benefits of being vaccinated, and that the vaccine and vaccination will be offered free of charge;

(J) Information on the appropriate actions to take and persons to contact in an emergency involving blood or other potentially infectious materials;

(K) An explanation of the procedure to follow if an exposure incident occurs, including the method of reporting the incident and the medical follow-up that will be made available;

(L) Information on the post-exposure evaluation and follow-up that the employer is required to provide for the employee following an exposure incident;

(M) An explanation of the signs and labels and/or color coding required by paragraph (g)(1); and

(N) An opportunity for interactive questions and answers with the person conducting the training session.

(viii) The person conducting the training shall be knowledgeable in the subject matter covered by the elements contained in the training program as it relates to the workplace that the training will address.

(ix) Additional Initial Training for Employees in HIV and HBV Laboratories and Production Facilities. Employees in HIV or HBV research laboratories and HIV or HBV production facilities shall receive the following initial training in addition to the above training requirements.

(A) The employer shall assure that employees demonstrate proficiency in standard microbiological practices and techniques and in the practices and operations specific to the facility before being allowed to work with HIV or HBV.

(B) The employer shall assure that employees have prior experience in the handling of human pathogens or tissue cultures before working with HIV or HBV.

(C) The employer shall provide a training program to employees who have no prior experience in handling human pathogens. Initial work activities shall not include the handling of infectious agents. A progression of work activities shall be assigned as techniques are learned and proficiency is developed. The employer shall assure that employees participate in work activities involving infectious agents only after proficiency has been demonstrated.

(h) Recordkeeping —

(1) Medical Records.

(i) The employer shall establish and maintain an accurate record for each employee with occupational exposure, in accordance with 29 CFR 1910.1020.

(ii) This record shall include:

(A) The name and social security number of the employee;

(B) A copy of the employee's hepatitis B vaccination status including the dates of all the hepatitis B vaccinations and any medical records relative to the employee's ability to receive vaccination as required by paragraph (f)(2);

(C) A copy of all results of examinations, medical testing, and follow-up procedures as required by paragraph (f)(3);

(D) The employer's copy of the healthcare professional's written opinion as required by paragraph (f)(5); and

(E) A copy of the information provided to the healthcare professional as required by paragraphs (f)(4)(ii)(B)(C) and (D).

(iii) Confidentiality. The employer shall ensure that employee medical records required by paragraph (h)(1) are:

(A) Kept confidential; and

(B) Not disclosed or reported without the employee's express written consent to any person within or outside the workplace except as required by this section or as may be required by law.

(iv) The employer shall maintain the records required by paragraph (h) for at least the duration of employment plus 30 years in accordance with 29 CFR 1910.1020.

(2) Training Records.

(i) Training records shall include the following information:

(A) The dates of the training sessions;

(B) The contents or a summary of the training sessions;

(C) The names and qualifications of persons conducting the training; and

(D) The names and job titles of all persons attending the training sessions.

(ii) Training records shall be maintained for 3 years from the date on which the training occurred.

(3) Availability.

(i) The employer shall ensure that all records required to be maintained by this section shall be made available upon request to the Assistant Secretary and the Director for examination and copying.

(ii) Employee training records required by this paragraph shall be provided upon request for examination and copying to employees, to employee representatives, to the Director, and to the Assistant Secretary.

(iii) Employee medical records required by this paragraph shall be provided upon request for examination and copying to the subject employee, to anyone having written consent of the subject employee, to the Director, and to the Assistant Secretary in accordance with 29 CFR 1910.1020.

(4) Transfer of Records.

(i) The employer shall comply with the requirements involving transfer of records set forth in 29 CFR 1910.1020(h).

(ii) If the employer ceases to do business and there is no successor employer to receive and retain the records for the prescribed period, the employer shall notify the Director, at least three months prior to their disposal and transmit them to the Director, if required by the Director to do so, within that three month period.

(5) Sharps Injury Log.

(i) The employer shall establish and maintain a sharps injury log for the recording of percutaneous injuries from contaminated sharps. The information in the sharps injury log shall be recorded and maintained in such manner as to protect the confidentiality of the injured employee. The sharps injury log shall contain, at a minimum

(A) The type and brand of device involved in the incident,

(B) The department or work area where the exposure incident occurred, and

(C) An explanation of how the incident occurred.

(ii) The requirement to establish and maintain a sharps injury log shall apply to any employer who is required to maintain a log of occupational injuries and illnesses under 29 CFR 1904.

(iii) The sharps injury log shall be maintained for the period required by 29 CFR 1904.6.

(i) Dates—

(1) Effective Date. The standard shall become effective on March 6, 1992.

(2) The Exposure Control Plan required by paragraph (c) of this section shall be completed on or before May 5, 1992.

(3) Paragraph (g)(2) Information and Training and (h) Recordkeeping shall take effect on or before June 4, 1992.

(4) Paragraphs (d)(2) Engineering and Work Practice Controls, (d)(3) Personal Protective Equipment, (d)(4) Housekeeping, (e) HIV and HBV Research Laboratories and Production Facilities, (f) Hepatitis B Vaccination and Post-Exposure Evaluation and Follow-Up, and (g)(1) Labels and Signs, shall take effect July 6, 1992.

[56 FR 64004, Dec. 06, 1991, as amended at 57 FR 12717, April 13, 1992; 57 FR 29206, July 1, 1992; 61 FR 5507, Feb. 13, 1996; 66 FR 5325 Jan., 18, 2001; 71 FR 16672 and 16673, April 3, 2006]

APPENDIX A TO SECTION 1910.1030: HEPATITIS B VACCINE DECLINATION (MANDATORY)

I understand that due to my occupational exposure to blood or other potentially infectious materials I may be at risk of acquiring hepatitis B virus (HBV) infection. I have been given the opportunity to be vaccinated with hepatitis B vaccine, at no charge to myself. However, I decline hepatitis B vaccination at this time. I understand that by declining this vaccine, I continue to be at risk of acquiring hepatitis B, a serious disease. If in the future I continue to have occupational exposure to blood or other potentially infectious materials and I want to be vaccinated with hepatitis B vaccine, I can receive the vaccination series at no charge to me.

Critical Thinking

At one of your upcoming practice meetings where all dentists, hygienists, assistants, office staff, and lab technicians are present, set aside a specified amount of time to discuss one aspect of the practice's adherence to OSHA and infection-control protocols. Each person should be able to contribute his or her opinions regarding compliance and areas for possible improvement, if needed. Over time, where different areas are discussed at meetings, it would be interesting to re-evaluate personnel compliance with stated recommendations and regulations.

Appendix

ANSWERS TO THE REVIEW QUESTIONS

Chapter 1

No review questions

Chapter 2

1. A
2. B
3. A
4. A
5. B
6. C
7. C
8. D
9. D
10. E

Chapter 3

1. B
2. D
3. E
4. C
5. C
6. B

Chapter 4

1. D
2. D
3. A
4. B
5. C
6. C
7. A
8. B
9. A
10. A

Chapter 5

1. C
2. D
3. E
4. E
5. C
6. F
7. A
8. A

Chapter 6

1. C
2. F
3. E
4. F

Chapter 7

1. B
2. E
3. A
4. B
5. C
6. A
7. D
8. D
9. C
10. E

Chapter 8

1. A
2. D
3. A
4. E
5. B
6. B
7. B
8. A
9. C
10. F
11. C
12. A

Chapter 9

1. D
2. F
3. C
4. B
5. E
6. C
7. B
8. A
9. D
10. D

Chapter 10

1. A
2. B
3. A
4. D

Chapter 11

1. C
2. B
3. D
4. C
5. B
6. C
7. B
8. B
9. A
10. B

Chapter 12

1. B
2. C
3. A
4. B
5. A
6. E
7. D
8. A

Chapter 13

1. B
2. E
3. B
4. F

Chapter 14

1. B
2. C
3. C
4. A
5. A
6. A
7. D
8. D
9. B
10. B
11. B
12. B

Chapter 15

1. A
2. B
3. C
4. C
5. B

Chapter 16

1. A
2. A
3. C
4. B
5. E
6. D

Chapter 17

1. A
2. A
3. B
4. B

Chapter 18

1. A
2. B
3. E
4. B
5. C
6. C
7. D
8. C
9. A
10. C

Chapter 19

1. E
2. C
3. A
4. C
5. C
6. C

Chapter 20

1. D
2. E
3. C
4. A
5. B

Chapter 21

No review questions

Chapter 22

No review questions

Chapter 23

No review questions

Glossary

Acquired immunodeficiency syndrome (AIDS): a disease of the body's immune system caused by the human immunodeficiency virus (HIV). AIDS is characterized by the death of CD4 cells (an important part of the body's immune system), which leaves the body vulnerable to life-threatening conditions such as infections and cancers.

Active immunization: see "vaccination."

Acute retroviral syndrome (ARS): also known as primary HIV infection or acute HIV infection, it refers to the period of rapid HIV replication that occurs 2 to 4 weeks after infection by HIV. Acute HIV infection is characterized by a drop in CD4 cell counts and an increase in HIV levels in the blood. Some, but not all, individuals experience flu-like symptoms during this period of infection. These symptoms can include fever, inflamed lymph nodes, sore throat, and rash. These symptoms may last from a few days to 4 weeks and then go away.

Aerosol: particles of respirable size generated by both humans and environmental sources that can remain viable and airborne for extended periods in the indoor environment; commonly generated in dentistry during use of handpieces, ultrasonic scalers, and air/water syringes.

Air removal test: a diagnostic test for prevacuum steam sterilizers that checks for the sterilizer's ability to remove air from the chamber.

Airborne transmission: a means of spreading infection in which airborne droplet nuclei are inhaled by the susceptible host.

Alcohol-based hand rub: an alcohol-containing preparation designed for application to the hands to reduce the number of viable microorganisms on the hands. In the United States, such preparations usually contain 60% to 95% ethanol or isopropanol. These waterless antiseptic agents do not require the use of exogenous water. After such an agent is applied, the hands are rubbed together until the agent has dried.

Allergic contact dermatitis: a type IV or delayed-hypersensitivity reaction resulting from contact with a chemical allergen (e.g., poison ivy and certain components of patient care gloves), generally localized to the contact area. Reactions occur slowly over 12 to 48 hours.

American Society of Heating, Refrigerating, and Air-Conditioning Engineers (ASHRAE): international technical society organized to advance the arts and sciences of heating, ventilation, air conditioning, and refrigeration. ASHRAE develops standards for refrigeration processes and the design and maintenance of indoor environments. ASHRAE publishes voluntary consensus standards designed to define minimum values or acceptable performance. ASHRAE is accredited by the American National Standards Institute (ANSI) and follows ANSI's requirements for due process and standards development.

Anaphylaxis (immediate anaphylactic hypersensitivity): a severe and sometimes fatal Type 1 reaction in a susceptible person after a second exposure to a specific antigen (e.g., food, pollen, proteins in latex gloves, or penicillin) after previous sensitization. Anaphylaxis is characterized commonly by respiratory symptoms, itching, hives, and rarely by shock and death (anaphylactic shock).

Anicteric: not associated with jaundice.

Antibiotic: a substance that fights bacteria.

Antibody: a protein found in the blood that is produced in response to foreign substances (e.g., bacteria or viruses) invading the body. Antibodies protect the body from disease by binding to these organisms and destroying them.

Antigen: a foreign substance, usually protein or carbohydrate substance (as a toxin or enzyme) capable of stimulating an immune response, usually the production of antibodies.

Antigenic drift: a minor change in surface antigens that results from point mutations in a gene segment; may result in an epidemic since the protection that remains from past exposure to similar viruses is incomplete.hem

Antigenic shift: a major change in one or both surface antigens (hemaggluton and neuraminidase) that occurs at varying intervals; may result in a worldwide pandemic if the virus is efficiently transmitted from person to person.

Antimicrobial soap: a soap (i.e., detergent) containing an antiseptic agent.

Antiretroviral therapy: treatment with drugs that inhibit the ability of retroviruses (such as HIV) to multiply in the body. The antiretroviral therapy recommended for HIV infection is referred to as highly active antiretroviral therapy (HAART), which uses a combination of medications to attack HIV at different points in its life cycle.

Antiseptic: a germicide that is used on skin or living tissue for the purpose of inhibiting or destroying microorganisms. Examples include alcohols, chlorhexidine, chlorine, hexachlorophene, iodine, chloroxylenol (PCMX), quaternary ammonium compounds, and triclosan.

Antiseptic hand rub: the process of applying an antiseptic hand-rub product to all surfaces of the hands to reduce the number of microorganisms present.

Antiseptic hand wash: washing hands with water and soap or detergents containing an antiseptic agent.

Artificial fingernails: substances or devices applied or added to the natural nails to augment or enhance the wearer's own nails. They include, but are not limited to, bondings, tips, wrappings, and tapes.

Asepsis: prevention from contamination with microorganisms; includes sterile conditions on tissues, on materials, and in rooms, as obtained by excluding, removing, or killing organisms.

Aseptic technique: a procedure that breaks the cycle of cross-infection and ideally eliminate cross-contamination.

Attenuated (live) vaccines: preparations derived from live, wild-type, disease-causing microorganisms. They are modified in vitro by repeated culturing with resultant weakening of their virulence prior to their use in immunization. After vaccination into immune competent hosts, they are able to replicate in the body for a period of time, but do not cause disease.

Autoclave: an instrument for sterilization that uses moist heat under pressure.

Bacteria: tiny one-celled organisms present throughout the environment that require a microscope to be seen. While not all bacteria are harmful, some cause disease. Examples of bacterial disease include diphtheria, pertussis, tetanus, *Haemophilus influenza*, and pneumococcus (pneumonia).

Bacterial count: a method of estimating the number of bacteria per unit sample. The term also refers to the estimated number of bacteria per unit sample, usually expressed as colony-forming units (CFUs) per square centimeter (cm^2) per milliliter (mL).

Bead sterilizer (endodontic dry-heat sterilizer): a device that uses small glass beads (1.2–1.5 mm diameter) and high temperatures (217–232°C/423–450°F) for brief exposures (e.g., 45 seconds) to inactivate microorganisms. The term is a misnomer because it is not cleared by the FDA as a sterilizer.

Bioburden: the microbiological load (i.e., number of viable organisms in or on the object or surface) or organic material on a surface or object prior to decontamination, or sterilization, also known as "bioload" or "microbial load."

Biofilm: a microbially-derived sessile community characterized by cells that are irreversibly attached to a substratum or interface to each other, are embedded in a matrix of extracellular polymeric substances that they have produced, and exhibit an altered phenotype with respect to growth rate and gene transcription.

Biological indicator: a device to monitor the sterilization process that consists of a standardized population of bacterial spores known to be resistant to the mode of sterilization being monitored. Biological indicators indicate whether all the parameters necessary for sterilization were present.

Bloodborne pathogens: disease-producing microorganisms spread by contact with blood or other body fluids contaminated with blood from an infected person. Examples include hepatitis B virus (HBV), hepatitis C virus (HCV), and human immunodeficiency virus (HIV).

Bloodborne Pathogens Standard: a standard developed, promulgated, and enforced by the Occupational Safety and Health Administration (OSHA) directing employers to protect employees from occupational exposure to blood and other potentially infectious material.

Boil-water advisory: a public health announcement that the public should boil tap water before drinking it; when issued, the public should assume the water is unsafe to drink.

Building code: regulations established by a recognized agency describing design loads, procedures, and construction details for structures, usually applying to a designated political jurisdiction (e.g., city, county, or state).

Building systems: mechanical, electrical, plumbing, air-handling, and communication equipment and structures in buildings.

Carrier: an individual who harbors a disease agent and may transmit the infection without demonstrating apparent symptoms.

Caseation necrosis: necrosis that transforms tissue into a dry, cheese-like mass.

Cellular immunity (cell-mediated immunity): immune responses and effects caused by sensitized lymphocytes or activated macrophages.

Centers for Disease Control and Prevention (CDC): one of the 13 major operating components of the Department of Health and Human Services (HHS), which is the principal agency in the United States government for protecting the health and safety of all Americans and providing essential human services, especially for those people who are least able to help themselves.

Chemical indicator: a device used to monitor a sterilization process that changes color or form with exposure to one or more physical conditions within a sterilizing chamber (e.g., temperature or steam). Chemical indicators are intended to detect potential sterilization failures that could result from incorrect packaging, incorrect loading of the sterilizer, or malfunctions of the sterilizer. A "pass" response does not verify that the items are sterile.

Chemical sterilant: chemicals used for the purpose of destroying all forms of microbial life, including bacterial spores.

Chemical vapor sterilizer (chemiclave): an instrument for sterilization that uses hot formaldehyde vapors under pressure.

Chronic: of long duration.

Circulation space: space allocated for movement of people and equipment through an office and/or building.

Cirrhosis: chronic liver disease characterized by progressive destruction and regeneration of liver cells and increased connective tissue formation.

Cleaning: the removal of visible soil and organic debris, either manually or mechanically, which results in a reduction in the number of microorganisms and the removal or organic matter, such as blood, tissue, and other biological material that may interfere with sterilization and disinfection. Cleaning is the first step in any sterilization or disinfection process.

Clinical contact surface: a surface contaminated from patient materials either from direct spray or spatter generated during dental procedures or by contact with dental healthcare personnel (DHCP)'s gloved hands. These surfaces can subsequently contaminate other instruments, devices, hands, or gloves. Examples of such surfaces include light handles, switches, dental radiograph equipment, dental chairside computers, reusable containers of dental materials, drawer handles, faucet handles, countertops, pens, telephones, and doorknobs.

Clinical zone: office areas dedicated to patient treatment or direct support of patient treatment, including patient treatment rooms (operatories), dental laboratories, instrument-processing rooms/areas, radiography procedure and processing areas, and patient recovery areas. Clinical zones require the highest degree of infection control in dental settings. Aseptic technique and correct office and equipment design should contain and control contaminants within the clinical zone.

Colony-forming unit (CFU): the minimum number of separable cells on the surface of or in semisolid agar medium that gives rise to a visible colony of progeny is on the order of tens of millions. CFUs may consist of pairs, chains, and clusters, as well as single cells, and are often expressed as CFU per milliliter (CFU/mL).

Commissioning: an inspection and evaluation process to verify and document that the facility and all of its systems and assemblies are planned, designed, installed, tested, operated, and maintained to meet the owner's project requirements. Commissioning is performed after construction and before occupation of a building.

Contaminated: state of having been in contact with microorganisms. As used in health care, it generally refers to microorganisms capable of producing disease or infection.

Contiguous zones: rooms or areas located directly next to other areas in the same infection-control zones, allowing uninterrupted flow and use while applying a shared level of infection-control practices.

Control biological indicator: a biological indicator from the same lot as a test indicator that is left unexposed to the sterilization cycle and then incubated to verify the viability of the test indicator. The control indicator should yield positive results for bacterial growth.

Critical: the category of medical devices or instruments that are introduced directly into the human body, either into or in contact with the bloodstream or normally sterile areas of the body (e.g., surgical instruments and scalpels). These items are so called because of the substantial risk of acquiring infection if the item is contaminated with microorganisms at the time of use.

Cross-contamination: passage of microorganisms from one person or inanimate object to another.

Cross-infection: passage of microorganisms from one person to another.

Daylight loader: equipment attached to an automatic film processor that shields an area from light, allowing films to be unwrapped in regular lighting.

Decontamination: a process or treatment that renders a medical device, instrument, or environmental surface safe to handle. According to OSHA, "the use of physical or chemical means to remove, inactivate, or destroy bloodborne pathogens on a surface or item to the point where they are no longer capable of transmitting infectious particles and the surface or item is rendered safe for handling, use, or disposal" [29 CFR 1910.1030].

Dental healthcare personnel (DHCP): refers to all paid and unpaid personnel in the dental healthcare setting who might be occupationally exposed to infectious materials, including body substances and contaminated supplies, equipment, environmental surfaces, water, or air. DHCP include dentists, dental hygienists, dental assistants, dental laboratory technicians (in-office and commercial), students and trainees, contractual personnel, and other persons not directly involved in patient care but potentially exposed to infectious agents (e.g., administrative, clerical, housekeeping, maintenance, or volunteer personnel).

Dental treatment water: nonsterile water used for dental therapeutic purposes, including irrigation of nonsurgical operative sites and cooling of high-speed rotary and ultrasonic instruments.

Detergents: compounds that possess a cleaning action and have hydrophilic and lipophilic parts. Although products used for hand washing or antiseptic hand wash in a healthcare setting represent various types of detergents, the term "soap" is used to refer to such detergents in this book. Detergents make no antimicrobial claims on the label.

Digital radiography: a technique for capturing a radiographic image using an appropriate radiation source and a sensor instead of radiographic film; the image is sent to a computer monitor for viewing.

Digital sensor: a detector used intraorally instead of x-ray film when taking radiographs; the image is sent to a computer monitor for viewing.

Direct contact transmission: physical transfer of microorganisms between a susceptible host and an infected or colonized person.

Disinfectant: a chemical agent used on inanimate (i.e., nonliving) objects (e.g., floors, walls, and sinks) to destroy virtually all recognized pathogenic microorganisms, but not necessarily all microbial forms (e.g., bacterial endospores). The EPA groups disinfectants according to whether the product label claims it to be a "limited," "general," or "hospital" disinfectant.

Disinfection: the destruction of pathogenic and other kinds of microorganisms by physical or chemical means. Disinfection is less lethal than sterilization because it destroys most recognized pathogenic microorganisms, but not necessarily all microbial forms, such as bacterial spores. Disinfection does not ensure the margin of safety associated with sterilization processes.

Disposable item: see "single-use disposable item."

Droplet nuclei: particles 5 μm or less in diameter that are formed by dehydration of airborne droplets containing microorganisms that can remain suspended in the air for long periods of time.

Droplets: small particles of moisture (e.g., spatter) that may be generated when a person coughs or sneezes, or when water is converted to a fine mist by an aerator or shower head. These particles are intermediate in size between drops and droplet nuclei. Although they may still contain infectious microorganisms, they tend to quickly settle out from the air, so any risk of disease transmission is generally limited to persons in close proximity to the droplet source.

Dry heat: used to sterilize materials that might be damaged in the presence of water vapor.

Dry-heat sterilizer: an instrument for sterilization that uses heated air; dry-heat sterilizers used in dentistry include static-air and forced-air types.

Emollients (humectants): ingredients in hand-hygiene and hand-care products that add moisture to skin and reduce skin dryness.

Employee zone: areas used primarily by dental workers for non–patient-treatment activities, including kitchens, lounges, closets and storage, private restrooms, and private offices. Correct office design and aseptic practices should protect the employee zone from contamination generated in other areas, and should not allow transfer of potentially infectious or contaminated materials out of the area to other parts of the office.

Endotoxin: the lipopolysaccharide of Gram-negative bacteria, the toxic character of which resides in the lipid protein. Endotoxins can produce pyrogenic reactions in persons exposed to their bacterial component.

Engineering controls: controls (e.g., sharps disposal containers, self-sheathing needles, and safer medical devices, such as sharps with engineered sharps injury protections and needleless systems) that isolate or remove the bloodborne pathogens hazard from the workplace.

Environmental Protection Agency (EPA): the mission of the EPA is to protect human health and the environment; the EPA works to develop and enforce regulations that implement environmental laws enacted by Congress.

Event-related shelf life: a storage practice that recognizes that a package and its contents should remain sterile until some event causes the item(s) to become contaminated.

Exposure time: the period of time during a sterilization or disinfection process in which items are exposed to the sterilant or disinfectant at the parameters specified by the manufacturer (e.g., time, concentration, temperature, and pressure).

Flash sterilization: process designed for the steam sterilization of unwrapped patient-care items for immediate use. Currently, the time required for flash sterilization depends on the type of sterilizer and the type of item (i.e., porous vs. nonporous) involved. This process is usually only used in emergency situations (e.g., when a short turnaround time is needed).

Food and Drug Administration (FDA): the FDA promotes and protects the public health by helping safe and effective products reach the market in a timely way, monitors products for continued safety after they are in use, and helps the public get the accurate, science-based information needed to improve health.

Food and Drug Administration (FDA)-cleared barrier: a product recognized by the FDA as being safe and effective for use on patients.

Fulminant: occurring suddenly, rapidly, and with great intensity.

Gamma globulin: generally any serum protein that exhibits antibody activity.

Glycocalyx: a gelatinous polysaccharide and/or polypeptide outer covering. The glycocalyx can be identified by negative staining techniques. The glycocalyx is referred to as a capsule if it is firmly attached to the cell wall, or as a slime layer if it is loosely attached. This material, which is produced by bacteria, forms the structural matrix of biofilm.

Gravity displacement sterilizer: a type of steam sterilizer in which incoming steam displaces residual air through a port or drain in or near the bottom (usually) of the sterilizer chamber.

Guidelines for the Design and Construction of Health Care Facilities: a joint publication of the American Institute of Architects (AIA), the Facility Guidelines Institute, and the U.S. Department of Health and Human Services. This publication attempts to address the specific requirements for best building practices of specialized clinical environments, and is often directly referenced by local and state building codes.

Hand hygiene: a general term that applies to hand washing, antiseptic hand wash, antiseptic hand rub, and surgical hand antisepsis.

Hand washing: washing hands with plain (i.e., nonantimicrobial) soap and water.

Healthcare-associated infection: any infection associated with a medical or surgical intervention. The term "healthcare-associated" replaces "nosocomial," which is limited to adverse infectious outcomes occurring in hospitals.

Heating, ventilation, and air conditioning (HVAC): a system that provides heating, ventilating, and/or cooling within or associated with a building.

Hepatitis: an inflammation of the liver. The most common cause is infection with one of the five hepatitis viruses; hepatitis can also be caused by other viruses, bacteria, parasites, and toxic reactions to drugs, alcohol, and chemicals.

Hepatitis B immune globulin (HBIG): a product available for prophylaxis against HBV infection. HBIG is prepared from plasma containing high titers of anti-HBs and provides short-term protection (3–6 months).

Hepatitis B vaccination: having received hepatitis B vaccine; hepatitis B immunization indicates that the person who received hepatitis B vaccine has developed adequate hepatitis B surface antibody and is protected against HBV infection.

Heterotrophic bacteria: those bacteria that require an organic carbon source for growth (i.e., they derive energy and carbon from organic compounds). The modifier "mesophilic" describes bacteria that grow best within the middle ranges of environmental temperature.

High-level disinfectant: a liquid chemical germicide registered by the FDA used in the disinfection process for critical and semicritical patient-care devices that inactivates vegetative bacteria, mycobacteria, fungi, and viruses, but not necessarily high numbers of bacterial spores. The FDA further defines a high-level disinfectant as a sterilant used under the same contact conditions except for a shorter contact time.

Highly active antiretroviral therapy (HAART): the name given to treatment regimens that aggressively suppress HIV replication and progression of HIV disease. The usual HAART regimen combines three or more anti-HIV drugs.

Hospital disinfectant: a germicide that is registered by EPA for use on inanimate objects in hospitals, clinics, dental offices, or any other medical-related facility. Efficacy is demonstrated against *Salmonella enterica* (formerly *Salmonella choleraesuis*), *Staphylococcus aureus*, and *Pseudomonas aeruginosa*.

Housekeeping surface: environmental surfaces (e.g., floors, walls, ceilings, and tabletops) that are not involved in direct delivery of patient care in healthcare facilities.

Human immunodeficiency virus (HIV): the virus that causes acquired immunodeficiency syndrome (AIDS). HIV is in the retrovirus family, and two types have been identified: HIV-1 and HIV-2. HIV-1 is responsible for most HIV infections throughout the world, while HIV-2 is found primarily in West Africa.

Humoral immunity: immunity because of specific immunoglobulins (i.e., antibodies) in blood or other tissues.

Iatrogenic: induced inadvertently by healthcare personnel (HCP) or by medical treatment or diagnostic procedures. Used especially in reference to an infectious disease or other complication of medical treatment.

Icteric: related to or marked by jaundice.

Illumination Engineering Society of North America (IESNA): an organization that establishes and issues standards for building illumination.

Immunization: the act of artificially inducing immunity or providing protection against a disease.

Implantable device: according to the FDA, a "device that is placed into a surgically or naturally formed cavity of the human body if it is intended to remain there for a period of 30 days or more" [21 CFR 812.3(d)].

Inactivated (killed) vaccines: produced by growing bacteria or viruses in vitro and then inactivating the whole organisms with chemicals or heat. They cannot replicate in the body after administration as an immunizing agent.

Independent water reservoir: a container used to hold water or other solutions and supply it to handpieces and air/water syringes attached to a dental unit. The independent reservoir, which isolates the unit from the public water system, may be provided as original equipment or as a retrofit device on all modern dental units.

Indirect contact transmission: contact of a susceptible host with a contaminated, intermediate object, usually inanimate.

Indoor air quality (IAQ): the quality of the facility's indoor air, including sensory comforts such as temperature, humidity, and air flow, or levels of contamination by chemicals, toxins, allergens, pathogens, and particulates.

Infection control: policies and procedures used to prevent or reduce the potential for disease transmission.

Infection control office zones: office areas grouped together by similar functions, resulting in zone-specific infection-control standards.

Infectious waste: hazardous waste capable of causing infections in humans, including contaminated animal waste, human blood and blood products, isolation waste, pathological waste, and discarded sharps (needles, scalpels, or broken medical instruments).

Inflammation: a fundamental immunological and pathological process that occurs following any injury to tissue, such as that following the establishment and multiplication of microorganisms.

Instrument washer: an automated device designed to clean medical and dental instruments.

Intermediate-level disinfectant: a liquid chemical germicide registered by the EPA as a hospital disinfectant and with a label claim of potency as a tuberculocidal. Intermediate-level disinfection is a process that inactivates most vegetative bacteria, most fungi, and some viruses, but cannot be relied on to inactivate resistant microorganisms such as mycobacteria or bacterial spores.

Irritation contact dermatitis: the development of dry, itchy, irritated areas on the skin, which can result from frequent hand washing and gloving as well as exposure to chemicals. This condition is not an allergic reaction.

Jaundice: a yellowish staining of the skin, mucous membranes, and sclera with bilirubin and other bile pigments.

Latex: a milky white fluid extracted from the rubber tree *Hevea brasiliensis* that contains the rubber material cis-1,4 polyisoprene.

Latex allergy: a type I or immediate anaphylactic hypersensitivity reaction to the proteins found in natural rubber latex.

Low-level disinfectant: a liquid chemical germicide registered by the EPA as a hospital disinfectant. OSHA requires low-level disinfectants to also have a label claim for potency against HIV and HBV if used for disinfecting clinical contact surfaces. Low-level disinfection is a process that will inactivate most vegetative bacteria, some fungi, and some viruses, but cannot be relied on to inactivate resistant microorganisms (e.g., mycobacteria or bacterial spores).

Lymphocytes: a type of infection-fighting white blood cell found in blood, lymph, and lymphoid tissue.

Mechanical indicator: devices (e.g., gauges, meter, display, and printout) that display an element of the sterilization process (e.g., time, temperature, and pressure).

Medical waste: any solid waste generated in the diagnosis, treatment, or immunization of human beings.

Multiresistant organisms: microorganisms that demonstrate resistance to multiple antibiotic medications.

Mycobacterium tuberculosis (M. tuberculosis): the namesake member organism of the *M. tuberculosis* complex, and the most common causative infectious agent of tuberculosis (TB) disease in humans. At times, the species name refers to the entire *M. tuberculosis* complex, which includes *M. bovis* and five other related species.

N-95 respirator: one of nine types of disposable particulate respirators; "95" refers to the percentage of particles filtered (see "particulate respirator").

National Institute for Occupational Safety and Health (NIOSH): the federal agency responsible for conducting research and making recommendations for the prevention of work-related disease and injury. The institute is part of the CDC.

Noncritical: the category of medical items or surfaces that carry the least risk of disease transmission. This category has been expanded to include not only noncritical medical devices but also environmental surfaces. Noncritical medical devices (e.g., a blood pressure cuff) touch only unbroken (nonintact) skin. Noncritical environmental surfaces can be further divided into clinical contact surfaces (e.g., a light handle) and housekeeping surfaces (e.g., floors and countertops).

Nosocomial infection: an infection acquired in a hospital as a result of medical care; now referred to as a healthcare-associated infection (see "healthcare-associated infection").

Occupational exposure incident: an occupational exposure incident can be defined as a percutaneous injury (e.g., needlestick or cut with a sharp object) or contact of mucous membrane or nonintact skin (e.g., exposed skin that is chapped, abraded, or afflicted with dermatitis) with blood, saliva, tissue, or other body fluids that are potentially infectious that may result from the performance of an employee's duties.

Occupational Safety and Health Administration (OSHA): established in 1971, OSHA aims to ensure worker safety and health in the United States by working with employers and employees to create better working environments; sets and enforcing standards; provides training, outreach, and education; establishes partnerships; and encourages continual improvements in workplace safety and health.

Opportunistic infection: infection caused by normally nonpathogenic microorganisms in a host whose resistance has been decreased or compromised.

Oral surgical procedure: involves an incision, excision, or reflection of tissue that exposes normally sterile areas of the oral cavity. Examples include biopsy, periodontal surgery, apical surgery, implant surgery, and surgical extractions of teeth (e.g., removal of erupted or nonerupted teeth requiring elevation of the mucoperiosteal flap, removal of bone or sectioning of teeth, and suturing if needed).

Other potentially infectious materials (OPIM): an OSHA term that refers to (a) the following human body fluids: semen, vaginal secretions, cerebrospinal fluid, synovial fluid, pleural fluid, pericardial fluid, peritoneal fluid, amniotic fluid, saliva in dental procedures, any body fluid that is visibly contaminated with blood, and all body fluids in situations where it is difficult or impossible to differentiate between body fluids; (b) any unfixed tissue or organ (other than intact skin) from a human (living or dead); and (c) HIV-containing cell or tissue cultures, organ cultures, and HIV- or HBV-containing culture medium or other solutions; and blood, organs, or other tissues from experimental animals infected with HIV or HBV.

Particulate respirator: also known as "air-purifying respirators" because they protect by filtering particles out of the air you breathe. Workers can wear any one of the particulate respirators for protection against diseases spread through the air, if they are NIOSH-approved and have been properly fit-tested and maintained. NIOSH-approved disposable respirators are marked with the manufacturer's name, the part number (P/N), the protection provided by the filter (e.g., N-95), and "NIOSH"; the number 95 refers to the percentage of particles filtered.

Percutaneous injury: an injury that penetrates the skin (e.g., needlestick, or cut with a sharp object).

Persistent activity: prolonged or extended activity that prevents or inhibits the proliferation or survival of microorganisms after application of the product. This activity may be demonstrated by sampling a site several minutes or hours after application and observing bacterial antimicrobial effectiveness when compared with a baseline level. In the past, this property was also called "residual activity." Both substantive and nonsubstantive active ingredients can show a persistent antimicrobial effect if they lower the number of bacteria significantly during the hand-washing period. Substantivity is an attribute of certain active ingredients that adhere to the stratum corneum (i.e., remain on the skin after rinsing or drying) to provide an inhibitory effect on the growth of bacteria remaining on the skin.

Personal protective equipment (PPE): specialized clothing or equipment (e.g., gloves, masks, protective eyewear, and gowns) worn by an employee for protection against a hazard. General work clothes (e.g., uniforms, pants, shirts, and blouses) that are not intended to function as protection against a hazard are not considered to be PPE.

Plain soap: soaps or detergents that do not contain antimicrobial agents or contain very low concentrations of such agents that are effective solely as preservatives; also referred to as nonantimicrobial soap.

Planktonic: collective name for free-floating microbiological organisms dispersed in solution, as in the case of free-swimming plankton.

Postexposure prophylaxis: the administration of medications following an occupational exposure in an attempt to prevent infection.

Potable (drinking) water: water suitable for drinking per applicable public health standards.

Preprocedural mouth rinse: a mouth rinse used by patients before a dental procedure, intended to produce a transient reduction in the overall numbers of microorganisms in the oral cavity.

Prevaccum steam sterilizer: a type of steam sterilizer in which air is removed from the chamber and the load by means of pressure and vacuum excursions at the beginning of the cycle.

Product vaccine: detoxified antigenic products that are produced by bacteria and used in certain vaccine regimens. Detoxification of microbial exotoxins with formalin yields a toxoid that is used for immunization.

Public zone: areas of the office open to public access by patients and visitors or nondental workers, including the reception room, hallways, public restrooms, business office, conference rooms, and utility rooms/areas. These areas should be clean and sanitary, but are not subject to the strict infection-control standards of the clinical zone.

Qualified healthcare professional: any licensed healthcare provider who can provide counseling and perform all medical evaluations and procedures in accordance with the most current recommendations of the U.S. Department of Health and Human Services, including postexposure prophylaxis when indicated.

Regulated waste: liquid or semiliquid blood or other potentially infectious material (OPIM); contaminated items that would release blood or OPIM in a liquid or semiliquid state if compressed; items that are caked with dried blood or OPIM and are capable of releasing the material during handling; contaminated sharps; and pathological and microbiological wastes containing blood or OPIM.

Resident flora: species of microorganisms that are always present on or in the body and are not easily removed by mechanical friction.

Retraction: the entry of oral fluids and microorganisms into water lines through negative water pressure.

Retrovirus: a type of virus that stores its genetic information in a single-stranded RNA molecule and then constructs a double-stranded DNA version of its genes using a special enzyme called reverse transcriptase. The DNA copy is then integrated into the host cell's own genetic material. HIV is an example of a retrovirus.

Reverse transcriptase (RT): an enzyme found in HIV and other retroviruses. RT converts single-stranded HIV RNA into double-stranded HIV DNA. Some anti-HIV drugs interfere with this stage of HIV's life cycle.

Ribonucleic acid (RNA): chemical structure that carries genetic instructions for protein synthesis. Although DNA is the primary genetic material of cells, RNA is the genetic material for some viruses.

Rinse-spray-rinse-spray: a disinfection method whereby an item that has been or potentially can be contaminated with oral secretions is rinsed under running water and then sprayed with disinfectant. This method is most appropriate for items that are not easily wiped as in the spray-wipe-spray method.

Semicritical: the category of medical devices or instruments (e.g., mouth mirror and amalgam condenser) that come into contact with mucous membranes and do not ordinarily penetrate body surfaces.

Seroconversion: the process by which a newly infected person develops antibodies to HIV. These antibodies are then detectable by an HIV test. Seroconversion may occur anywhere from days to weeks or months following HIV infection.

Single-use disposable item: a device intended to be used on one patient and then discarded appropriately; these items are not intended to be reprocessed (cleaned, disinfected, or sterilized) and used on another patient.

Spatter: visible drops of liquid or body fluid that are expelled forcibly into the air and settle out quickly, as distinguished from particles of an aerosol, which remain airborne indefinitely.

Spaulding classification: a strategy for sterilization or disinfection of inanimate objects and surfaces based on the degree of risk involved in their use. The three categories are: critical, semicritical, and noncritical. The system also established three levels of germicidal activity for disinfection: high, intermediate, and low.

Spore test: see "biological indicator."

Spray-wipe-spray: disinfection of environmental surfaces using a two-step procedure. In the first step ("spray-wipe"), contaminated surfaces are precleaned by vigorously wiping the surface with a cleaning agent. The second step involves applying a disinfectant (spray) over the entire precleaned surface and allowing it to remain moist for the contact time recommended by the manufacturer.

Standard precautions: Universal precautions were based on the concept that all blood and body fluids that might be contaminated with blood should be treated as infectious because patients with bloodborne infections can be asymptomatic or unaware they are infected. The relevance of universal precautions to other aspects of disease transmission was recognized, and in 1996 the CDC expanded the concept and changed the term to "standard precautions." Standard precautions integrate and expand the elements of universal precautions into a standard of care designed to protect healthcare personnel (HCP) and patients from pathogens that can be spread by blood or any other body fluid, excretion, or secretion. Standard precautions apply to contact with (a) blood; (b) all body fluids, secretions, and excretions (except sweat), regardless of whether they contain blood; (c) nonintact skin; and (d) mucous membranes. Saliva has always been considered a potentially infectious material in dental infection control; thus no operational difference exists in clinical dental practice between universal precautions and standard precautions.

Steam sterilization: a sterilization process that uses saturated steam under pressure, for a specified exposure time and at a specified temperature, as the sterilizing agent.

Sterilant: a liquid chemical germicide that destroys all forms of microbiological life, including high numbers of resistant bacterial spores.

Sterile/sterility: state of being free from all living microorganisms; in practice, usually described as a probability function (e.g., the probability of a surviving microorganism being 1 in 1,000,000).

Sterile water: water that is sterilized and contains no antimicrobial agents.

Sterilization: the destruction or removal of all forms of life, with particular reference to microbial organisms. The limiting factor and requirement for sterilization is the destruction of heat-resistant bacterial and mycotic spores.

Subclinical: a state in which an individual either does not experience all of the characteristic symptoms of a particular disease or the manifestations are less severe.

Substantivity: see persistent activity.

Subunit (component) vaccines: preparations used for immunization that use a portion of the bacteria or virus that is able to stimulate host protective immunity.

Surface barrier: material that prevents the penetration of microorganisms, particulates, and fluids. Barrier choices range from inexpensive plastic food wrap to commercially available custom-made covers.

Surfactants: surface-active agents that reduce surface tension. They help cleaning by loosening, emulsifying, and holding soil in suspension, which can then be more readily rinsed away.

Surgical hand scrub: an antiseptic-containing preparation that substantially reduces the number of microorganisms on intact skin; it is broad spectrum, fast acting, and persistent.

Tabletop steam sterilizer: a compact steam sterilizer that has a chamber volume of not more than 2 cubic feet and generates its own steam when distilled or deionized water is added by the user.

Transient flora: microorganisms that may be present in or on the body under certain conditions and for certain lengths of time; they are easier to remove by mechanical friction than resident flora.

Transmission-based precautions: a set of practices that apply to patients with documented or suspected infection or colonization with highly transmissible or epidemiologically important pathogens for which precautions beyond the standard precautions are needed to interrupt transmission in healthcare settings.

Tubercle: a small rounded nodule produced by infection with *Mycobacterium tuberculosis*, consisting of a mass of inflammatory cells and bacteria surrounded by connective tissue.

Ultrasonic cleaner: a device that uses waves of acoustic energy (a process known as "cavitation") to loosen and break up debris on instruments.

Unit dose: the amount of material that is sufficient to accomplish a particular procedure to prevent cross-contamination. The material is dispensed before patient contact, and any excess is discarded at completion.

Universal precautions: a set of practices and procedures based on the concept that all blood and all body fluids that might be contaminated with blood should be treated as infectious. (Also see "standard precautions.")

Unsaturated chemical vapor sterilization: a sterilization process that uses hot formaldehyde vapors under pressure.

Vaccination (or immunization): the act of artificially inducing immunity against a disease.

Vaccine: an administered immunologic preparation that stimulates the body's immune system to produce protective humoral immunity (antibodies) and/or cell-mediated immunity (sensitized T-lymphocytes) against a disease.

Viremia: the presence of viruses in the blood.

Volatile organic compounds (VOCs): compounds that have a high vapor pressure and low water solubility. Many VOCs are human-made chemicals that are used and produced in the manufacture of paints, pharmaceuticals, refrigerants, and building materials.

Washer-disinfector: an automatic unit designed to clean and thermally disinfect instruments. Such units use a high-temperature cycle rather than a chemical bath.

Wicking: absorption of a liquid by capillary action along a thread or through material (e.g., the enhanced penetration of liquids through undetected holes in a glove).

Wipe-discard-wipe: disinfection of environmental surfaces in a two-step procedure using disinfecting cloths or wipes. Two cloths must be used—one to clean and another to disinfect the surface.

Work practice controls: practices incorporated into the everyday work routine that reduce the likelihood of exposure by altering the manner in which a task is performed (e.g., prohibiting recapping of needles by a two-handed technique).

Index

AAMI. *See* Association for the Advancement of Medical Instrumentation

Abacavir, 39*t*

ACD. *See* Allergic contact dermatitis (ACD)

Acid-fast bacilli (AFB), 54

Acquired immune deficiency syndrome (AIDS), 32–44. *See also* Human immunodeficiency virus (HIV); People living with AIDS
  cause of, 34
  death attributed to, 36
  defining illnesses, 37*t*
  demographics in United States, 36–37
  emergence of, 34
  HCP concerns of, 14

Active immunity, 24

Active immunization, 91. *See also* Vaccination

Acute retroviral syndrome (ARS), 33, 35

Acute tracheobronchitis, 50–51
  clinical manifestations, 51
  diagnosis, 51
  treatment, 51

Acyclovir, 41*t*

ADA. *See* American Dental Association

Administrative strategies, for infection control, 55–57, 56*t*
  identification of patients with TB disease, 56
  isolation of patients with TB disease, 56
  referral of patients with TB disease, 67
  TB education and training for DHCP, 56, 56*t*
  TB infection control program, 56
  TB risk assessment, 56

Advisory Committee for Immunization Practices (CDC), 18, 94

Aerosols, 64, 70, 102, 109, 142, 213

AFB. *See* Acid-fast bacilli

AHA. *See* American Heart Association

AIDS. *See* Acquired immune deficiency syndrome

Air quality. *See* Dental air quality; Indoor air quality

Air removal test, 149, 154

Airborne microbial infections, 47*t*

Airborne transmission, 4, 5

Alcohol-based hand rubs, 124, 126, 133*t*, 136
  hand washing v., 132*t*
  pros and cons, 132*t*

Alcohols, 134–35, 178–79, 179*t*

Allergic contact dermatitis (ACD), 102, 108–9

Allergies. *See* Allergic contact dermatitis; Latex; Occupation-related allergies, in dentistry

American Dental Association (ADA), 6, 22
  Acceptance Program, 178
  on alcohol, 179
  Association Report, 71–72
  "Best Management Practices for Amalgam Waste," 266
  on cleaning, 187
  Council on Dental Therapeutics, 145, 178
  Council on Prosthetic Services and Dental Laboratory Relations, 145
  on dental waterline contamination, 67–68
  glove recommendations, 234
  sterilization, 150

American Heart Association (AHA), 145

American Society of Heating, Refrigerating and Air Conditioning Engineers (ASHRAE), 195, 199

Amikacin, 55*t*

Aminoglycosides, 55*t*

Aminosalicylic acid, 55*t*

Amphotericin, 40*t*

Anaphylaxis (immediate anaphylactic hypersensitivity), 102, 106

Ancillary equipment, 203

Andrews, Nancy, 123, 194

Andrews, Ross, 194

Anesthetic devices, safety, *217*

Anicteric, 14, 22

Anthrax, 47*t*

Antibody, 14, 19. *See also* HIV antibody
  HBV persistence, 26
  rapid-, testing for HIV, 216

Antigen, 14, 18

Antigenic drift, 46, 48

Antigenic shift, 46, 48

Anti-HIV. *See* HIV antibody

Antimicrobial chemical action, 177

Antimicrobial hand-hygiene agents
  alcohols, 134–35
  CHG, 133, 133*t*, 143, 144
  iodine compounds, 133*t*, 134
  iodophors, 133*t*, 134, 179–80, 179*t*
  PCMX, 134
  quaternary ammoniums, 134, 177–78, 178*t*
  spectrum and characteristics, 133*t*
  triclosan, 133*t*, 134–35

Antimicrobial mouth rinses
  characteristics of, 144*t*, 280
  ideal agent properties, 143, 143*t*
  preprocedural, 141–47, 280, 291
  rationale for, 142

Antimicrobial oral rinse. *See* Antimicrobial mouth rinses

Antimicrobial soap, 124, 127

Antimycobacterial agents, 55*t*

Antiretroviral therapy (ART), 33, 34, 36, 39, 39*t*, 42. *See also* Highly active antiretroviral therapy

Antisepsis. *See* Hand hygiene and antisepsis; Surgical antisepsis

Antiseptic, 124, 125

Antiseptic hand rub, 124, 128*t*, 132*t*

Antiseptic hand wash, 124, 128*t*, 133

AORN. *See* Association of Operating Room Nurses

ARS. *See* Acute retroviral syndrome

ART. *See* Antiretroviral therapy

Artificial fingernails, 124, 136

Asepsis, 4, 6, 179, 194–205, 278–79

Aseptic technique, 4, 6, 195, 196, 238. *See also* Environmental protection control
  in dental equipment selection, 201–4
  for parental medications, 280, 291

ASHRAE. *See* American Society of Heating, Refrigerating and Air Conditioning Engineers

Aspergillosis, 40*t*

Assistant secretary, 295

Association for the Advancement of Medical Instrumentation (AAMI), 163, 228

Association of Operating Room Nurses (AORN), 228

Association Report, of ADA, 71–72

Assumption-based guidelines evolution, 80, 82

Atazanavir, 39*t*

Attenuated (live) vaccines, 90, 92

Australia antigen, 18

Autoclave, 149, 151

Azithromycin, 41*t*

AZT, 39*t*

Bacille Calmette-Guerin (BCG) vaccine
strains, 54

Bacteria, 64, 68

Bacterial count, 64

Bacterial disease risks, 5*t*

Bacterial infection, 46*t*

Baker's yeast, 25

Barrier techniques. *See* Personal
protective equipment

Barrier-protected film, *240*

Barriers. *See* Physical barriers; Surface
barriers

BBP. *See* Bloodborne pathogens

BCG. *See* Bacille Calmette-Guerin vaccine
strains

Bead sterilizer (endodontic dry-heat
sterilizer), 149, 157

Bednarsh, Helene, 3, 79

"Best Management Practices for Amalgam
Waste" (ADA), 266

BI. *See* Biological indicator

Bioburden, 222, 223

Biofilm
dental infection control program,
279–80
dental waterline contamination,
65, 67
heterogeneity of, *66*
life cycle of, *66*

Biohazard bag, *249*

Biological indicator (BI), 149, 154, *163*.
See also Control biological
indicator
mailing envelopes, *164*
spore tests, 164*t*

Biological monitoring, 161–66

Biopsy specimen, handling, 281, 291

Bite registrations, 256–57

Blood, 265, 295
exposure prevention, 273
precautions, 81*t*
spills, 278, 289
transfusions, 38
waste, 265

Bloodborne disease transmission,
14–15

Bloodborne disease transmission
efficiency, 6, 10*t*

Bloodborne pathogen transmission
prevention, 273–74, 285–86

Bloodborne pathogens (BBPs), 80, 82,
210, 295. *See also* Hepatitis B
virus; Hepatitis C virus; Human
Immunodeficiency virus;
specific pathogen
aerosols and, 213
occupational-exposure risks of, 211,
212*t*, 213

Bloodborne Pathogens Standard (OSHA),
80, 83, 84, 112, 263, 263*t*, 265,
294–307

Board of Registration in Dentistry, 85

Body fluid waste, 265

Body substance isolation (BSI), 81*t*, 83,
278, 289

Boil water advisory, 64, 70, 280, 290

Bordetella pertussis, 50

Bordetella pertussis vaccine, 94

BSI. *See* Body Substance Isolation

Building code, 195, 196

Building systems, 195, 196
considerations, 199–200, *200, 201*
electrical/illumination, 195, 200
mechanical, 199
surface materials selection, 200

Built-in dispensers, *200*

Cancer, liver, 2

Candida oral, 40*t*

Capreomycin, 55*t*

Carrier, 14

Caseation necrosis, 46

CDC. *See* Centers for Disease Control

Cell-mediated immunity, 91. *See also*
Cellular immunity

Cellular immunity, 90

Centers for Disease Control and Prevention
(CDC), 6, 25, 34, 80, *175*
Advisory Committee for Immunization
Practices, 18, 94
AIDS date collection, 37
on alcohol, 179
cross-infection determination, 176
current guidelines and precautions,
84–85
on digital sensors barrier protection,
241
on flushing dental unit waterlines,
189–90
glove recommendations, 234
*Guidelines for Infection Control in
Dental Health-care Settings–2003,*
68, 84, 96, 145, 284–307
hand hygiene guidelines of, 125
HAV incidence, 15
hepatitis outbreaks, 234
housekeeping environmental surfaces
recommendations, 177
"Isolation Techniques for Use in
Hospitals," 82
management of occupational
exposures, 211, 213*t*, 215
positive spore test recommendation,
165*t*
"Recommended Infection Control
Practices for Dentistry," 83
saliva, 5, 210–11
on shelf life, 228
sterilization, 150, 163
TB recommendations, 54
transmission-based precautions of,
85
vaccinations cited by, 90

CFU. *See* Colony forming unit

Chemical disinfectants, 177–81
alcohols, 134–35, 178–79, 179*t*
chlorine-containing agents, 180, 180*t*
complex (synthetic) phenols,
180–81, 181*t*
detergents, 124, 127, 172, 177–78
hydrogen peroxide, 181, 181*t*
iodine, 179–80
iodophors, 133*t*, 134, 179–80, 179*t*
phenols and derivatives, 180

Chemical germicides, 157, 157*t*

Chemical indicators, 149, 159, *162*, 222, 226

Chemical monitoring, 159–60

Chemical sterilants, 149, 157, 157*t*, 172, 173

Chemical vapor sterilizer (chemiclave),
149, 155

Chemiclave. *See* Chemical vapor sterilizer

CHG. *See* Chlorhexidine gluconate

Chickenpox, 47*t*

Chlamydia pneumoniae, 50

Chlorhexidine gluconate (CHG), 133, 133*t*,
143, 144

Chlorine-containing agents, 180, 180*t*

Chloroxylenol parachlorometaxylenol
(PCMX), 134

Chronic, 14

Cidofovir, 41*t*

Ciprofloxacin, 55*t*

Cirrhosis, 14

CJD. *See* Creutzfeldt-Jakob disease

Clarithromycin, 41*t*

Cleaning, 6, 172, 173, 186, 222
ADA on, 187
in dental laboratory, 251
digital radiography, 238, 241–43,
242, 280
instruments, 223–25
in radiography and infection control,
239
surface, decision factors, 187*t*

Cleared barrier, of FDA, 238

Clinical contact surface, 172, 176, 176*t*,
278, 289

Clinical laboratory, 295

Clinical zones, 195, 197

Clothing, protective, 111–12, 275, 286–87
donning and removing, 112*t*

Clotrimazole, 40*t*

CMV. *See* Cytomegalovirus

Colony forming unit (CFU), 64, 65

Commercial dental laboratory, 250

Commissioning, 195, 200–201

Common cold, 47*t*
clinical manifestations, 47
diagnosis, 48
etiology and epidemiology, 47
treatment and prevention, 48

Complex (synthetic) phenols,
180–81, 181*t*

Compliance
of OSHA, 297–301
for single-use disposable items, 234–35

Component (subunit) vaccines, 95, 95*t*

Compound impressions, 255
Compressed air, microbial quality of dental, 71
Computer equipment, 242–43, *243*
Contact dermatitis, 275. *See also* Allergic contact dermatitis; Irritation contact dermatitis
Contamination, 222, 239*t*, 295. *See also* Decontamination; Dental waterline contamination; Internal contamination and equipment cleanability
    cross-, 4, 5, 113*t*
    dental equipment selection, 202–3
    laundry, 295
    patient-care items, 173–76, 222–23
    sharps, 264–65, 295
Contiguous located zones, 197
Contiguous zones, 195
Control biological indicator, 149, 162
Control panel, barrier-protected, *239*
Cottone, J. A., 5
Council on Dental Therapeutics (ADA), 145
Council on Prosthetic Services and Dental Laboratory Relations (ADA), 145
Countertop instrument washer, *225*
Covers, 189
    barrier, 172, 177, 177*t*, 189, 230–234, 239, 240
    head and shoe, 112, 275
Creutzfeldt-Jakob disease (CJD), 292–93
Critical, 149, 151, 151*t*. *See also* Noncritical; Semicritical
Cross-infection, 4, 5*t*, 176
Cryptococcal meningitis, 40*t*
Cryptosporidosis, 40*t*
Cuny, Eve, 123
Custom impression trays, 256–57
Cycloserine, 55*t*
Cytomegalovirus (CMV), 41*t*, 142
Dapsone, 40*t*
Darkrooms, infection control procedures in, 242*t*
Daylight loader, 238, 241, *241*, 242*t*
Decontamination, 172, 173, 295
    of instruments, 223–25
    methods of, 174*t*
Delavirdine, 39*t*
Delta Hepatitis. *See* Hepatitis D virus
Dental air quality, 63–75. *See also* Indoor air quality
    future research and development, 72
    microbial quality of compressed air, 71
    nitrous oxide exposure, 71–72
    respiratory hazards, 72
Dental appliances, 255–56
Dental casts, 257, *257*
Dental (rubber) dams, 112
Dental equipment selection, aseptic considerations, 201–4
    ancillary equipment, 203
    digital technology, 203
    equipment switches and controls, 202, *202*

external equipment design, 201–2, *202*
internal contamination and equipment cleanability, 202–3
manufacturer specifications and maintenance, 203
nonclinical area equipment, 203–4
removable components, 203
Dental handpieces, 157–58, *158*, 158*t*, 280, 290
Dental healthcare personnel (DHCP), 4, 34. *See also* Immunizations, for DHCP
    bare hands of, 83
    hepatitis concern of, 14–15
    immune compromised, 58
    OSHA guidelines for, 83–84
    personal protective equipment for, 101–19
    respiratory tract infections work restrictions of, 58, 58*t*
    TB disease postexposure, 57–58
    TB education and training for, 56, 56*t*
    TB infection control surveillance program for, 57–58
    vaccine-preventable disease risks, 91
Dental impressions, *251*, 251–55
    compound, 255
    disinfection method, 252*t*, *253*, 253–54, *254*
    elastomeric, 254–55
    hydrocolloid, 255
    ZOE, 255
Dental infection control program. *See also* Cleaning; Hand hygiene and antisepsis; Personal protective equipment
    administration/personnel health elements, 272–73
    aseptic technique for parental medications, 280, 291
    biofilm, 279–80
    biopsy specimen handling, 281, 291
    bloodborne pathogens transmission prevention, 273–74, 285–86
    contact dermatitis, 275
    dental radiography, 280
    dental unit waterlines, 189–90, 279–80
    environmental infection control, 57, 278–79
    extracted teeth handling, 265, 266, 266*t*, 281, 291
    handpieces and other devices, 157–58, *158*, 158*t*, 280, 290
    laboratory, 281
    latex hypersensitivity, 106, 275, 287
    oral surgical procedures, 281
    patient-care items sterilization and disinfection, 276–78
    preprocedural mouth rinses, 141–47, 280, 291
    radiography, 237–45
        digital radiography considerations, 238, 241–43, *242*, 280
        environmental, 238–39

        PPE and hand hygiene, 238
        processing procedures, 241
        supplies, 239
        treatment area to darkroom transition, 241
    single-use devices, *233*, 233–35, 280, 291
    TB, 281
    water quality, 279–80
Dental instruments, *159*
Dental laboratory, infection control, 246–60, 292
    cleaning, 251
    commercial lab, 250
    communication, 248–49
    consultation room, 251
    impressions, 251–55
    in-office lab, 249
    orthodontics, 257–58
    PPE, 248
    procedures for, 250–51
    production area, 250–51
    prostheses and appliances, 255–56
    prosthodontics, 257–58
    receiving area, 250
    shipping area, 251
    transported items, 252*t*
Dental practice regulations, state, 68–69
Dental prosthesis, 255–56
Dental radiography, 280. *See also* Infection control, in dental radiography
Dental radiology, 290–91
Dental treatment water, 64, 65, 69–70
Dental unit waterlines, 189–90, 279, 290. *See also* Waterlines, flushing
Dental waterline contamination, 64–70
    biofilm, 65, 67
    boil water advisories, 64, 70, 280, 290
    future research and development, 72
    guidelines and policy, 67–69
    influences on health, 67
    retraction, 70
    separate water reservoir, *68*
    source water concerns, 70
    sterile irrigating solutions, 69
    treatment water improvement, 64, 65, 69–70
DePaola, Louis G., 32
Derivatives, 180
    phenol, 133*t*
Dermatitis, 287. *See also* Allergic contact dermatitis
    gloves associated with, 106–9
    irritation contact, 106
    nonspecific irritation, 106
Dermatomycotic infection, *136*
Design and equipment selections, 194–205
Detergents, 124, 127, 172, 177–78
DHCP. *See* Dental healthcare personnel
Didanosine, 39*t*
Digital radiography, 238, 241–43, *242*, 280
Digital sensors, 238, 241
Digital technology, 203

Direct contact transmission, 4, 5
Disease risks, 5*t*, 91
Disinfectants, 149, 151, 172. *See also*
    Chemical disinfectants
    environmental surface, 185–93
    high-level, 149, 151, 172, 174
    hospital, 172, 175, 186, 187
    ideal, properties, 173*t*
    liquid, 188*t*
    low-level, 172, 175, 186, 187
    misuse potential, 188–90
Disinfection, 6, 149, 150, 172, 173, 186,
    276–78
    chemical class for process of, 174*t*
    decision factors, 187*t*
    of dental impressions, 252*t*, 253,
        253–54, *254*
    in dental laboratory, 248
    of incoming case, *250*
    of nonsterilizable surface, *190*
    of patient care items, 287
    procedures, 188
    strategies of environmental surfaces,
        176–77
    surface, suggestions, 189*t*
Dispensers, *200, 201*
Disposable item, 233, 280. *See also*
    Single-use disposable item
Division of Over-the-Counter Drug
    Products (FDA), 133
DNA viruses, 15*t*
Droplet microbial infections, 47*t*
Droplet nuclei, 46, 102, 110
Droplets, 102, 103
Dry heat, 149
Dry heat sterilization, 152*t*, 154–55.
        See also Forced air sterilization;
        static air sterilization
Dry-heat sterilizer, 149, 157
Durunavir, 39*t*
Efavirenz, 39*t*
EIA. *See* Enzyme linked immunoassay
Eklund, Kathy, 79
Elastomeric impressions, 254–55
Electrical/illumination systems, 195, 200
Electrosurgery plumes, 292
Emollients (humectants), 124, 127
Employee zone, 195, 198
Emtricitabine, 39*t*
Endodontic dry-heat sterilizer. *See* Bead
    sterilizer
Endotoxin, 64, 67
Enfuvirtide, 39*t*
Engerix-B, 25
Engineering controls, 210, 217, 273, 295
Entry inhibitor, 39*t*
Environmental infection control, 57, 278–79
Environmental Protection Agency (EPA),
    172, 173, 186, 187, 239, 262
Environmental protection control, 238–39
Environmental strategies, for infection
    control, 57
Environmental surface, 173–76
    categories of, 176*t*
    classification of, 176–77

as cross-infection sources, 176
    disinfectants, 185–93
Enzyme linked immunoassay (EIA), 38
EPA. *See* Environmental Protection
    Agency
Epstein-Barr virus, 142
Equipment. *See also* Dental equipment
    selection, aseptic
    considerations; Personal
    protective equipment (PPE)
    ancillary, 203
    computer, 242–43, *243*
    design and, 194–205
    external design of, 201–2, *202*
    nonclinical area, 203–4
    switches and controls, 202, *202*
Ethambutol, 55*t*
Ethionamine, 55*t*
Ethyl alcohol, 178–79
Ethylene oxide gas (ETO), 156
ETO. *See* Ethylene oxide gas
Event-related shelf life, 222, 228
Exposure control, 296–97
Exposure incident form, *214*, 295
Exposure time, 149, 155
External equipment design, 201–2, *202*
Extracted teeth, 265, 266, 266*t*, 281, 291
Extraoral radiographic procedures,
    239–40, 240*t*
Eyewear, protective, 111, 112*t*, 275, 286
Face shields, 275, 286
Famciclovir, 41*t*
Fast steam sterilization, 156
FDA. *See* Food and Drug Administration
Fingernails, 136. *See also* Artificial
    fingernails
First Obstetrics Clinic of the General
    Hospital of Vienna, 82, 125
Flammability, 136
Flash sterilization, 149, 156, 156*t*
Flavivirus, 26
Floor standing instrument washer, *225*
Flora, 124, 126, 142
Flow patterns, in office space, 199
Fluoroquinolones, 55*t*
Food and Drug Administration (FDA), 69,
    102, 124, 149, 172, 173, 222, 263
    -cleared barrier, 238, 241
    Division of Over-the-Counter Drug
        Products, 133
    glove manufacturing and labeling,
        104
    instrument-washing equipment
        regulations of, 224
    medical device clearance, 151
Forced air sterilization, 152*t*, 155
Fosamprenavir, 39*t*
Foscarnet, 41*t*
Fulminant, 14, 20
Fungal disease risks, 5*t*
Furnishings, 278, 289
Fusion, 35
Gallo, Robert, 34
Gamma globulin, 14
Ganciclovir, 41*t*

Gatifloxacin, 55*t*
Gay-related immune deficiency (GRID), 34
General Duty Clause, of OSHA, 83
Germ theory, Pasteur's, 82
German measles, 47*t*
German measles vaccine. *See* Rubella
    vaccine
Germicidal chemicals, *175*
Glass, B. J., 5
Gloves, 103–6, 174–75, 234, 275. *See also*
    Latex
    dermatitis conditions associated with,
        106–9
    donning and removing, 112*t*
    nonmedical, 105–6
    patient examination, 104, 105*t*
    surgeons, 105, 105*t*
    types of, 105*t*
Glycocalyx, 64, 65
Gravity displacement sterilizer, 149,
    152*t*, 154
GRID. *See* Gay-related immune deficiency
*Guidelines for Infection Control in Dental
    Health-care Settings–2003* (CDC),
    68, 84, 96, 145, 284–307
    bloodborne pathogen transmission
        prevention, 273–74, 285–86
    personnel health in infection control
        program, 284–85
*Guidelines for the Design and Construction
    of Health-care Facilities,* 195, 196
HAART. *See* Highly active antiretroviral
    therapy
Hand hygiene and antisepsis, 123–40, *198,*
    286. *See also* Antimicrobial
    hand-hygiene agents;
    Antimicrobial soap; Antiseptic
    hand rub; Antiseptic hand
    wash; Gloves
    active ingredients in antimicrobial
        agents, 133
    adherence to recommended
        procedures, 126–27
    artificial fingernails, 124, 136
    educational and motivational
        programs for, 137
    features of agents of, 132
    fingernails, 136
    flammability and alcohol-based hand
        rubs, 136
    flora found on skin, 126
    historical background, 125
    Infection control, in dental
        radiography, 238
    irritant dermatitis related to, 135
    jewelry, 136, *136*
    for nonsurgical dental procedures,
        127, *129, 130,* 131, *131*
    for oral surgical procedure, 131–32
    plain or non-antimicrobial soap,
        132–33
    preparations for, 132–35
    skin care, 136
    storage and dispensing of hand-care
        products, 136

transmission of diseases and, 125
types of, 128*t*
Hand washing, 82, 124, 125, 128*t*
alcohol-based hand rubs v., 132*t*
facilities, 295
general considerations, 126–27
for nonsurgical procedures, 127, *129, 130,* 131, *131*
for oral surgical procedure, 131–32
pros and cons, 132*t*
Hand-care products, 136
Hands
of DHCP, 83
diseases transmission through, 125
Harte, Jennifer A., 13, 101, 123, 148, 171, 185, 209, 221, 232, 237, 261
Harvey sterilizer, 155
HAV. *See* Hepatitis A virus
Havrix, 18
HBsAg. *See* Hepatitis B surface antigen
HBV. *See* Hepatitis B virus
HCP. *See* Healthcare personnel
HCV. *See* Hepatitis C virus
HDV. *See* Hepatitis D virus
Head and shoe covers, 112, 275
Healthcare Infection Control Practices Advisory Committee (HICPAC), 69
Healthcare personnel (HCP), 14
hand washing of, 125
HIV and, 38
occupational concerns of, 14
poor adherence to hand-hygiene procedures, 126
Healthcare professional, 210, 211, 295
Healthcare-associated infection, 4, 6, 11*t*
Heat sterilization methods, 152*t*
Heating, ventilation, and air conditioning (HVAC), 195, 196
Heat-sensitive items, processing, 156–57
Hemagglutinin (HI), 48
Hepatitis, 234. *See also* Viral hepatitis; *specific type*
associated antigen, 18
HCP concerns of, 14–15
terminology of, 19*t*
vaccines, 13–31
viral, 13–31, 15*t*, 16*t*
Hepatitis A vaccines, 17–18
Hepatitis A virus (HAV), 15, 16*t*, 17–18
characteristics, 17*t*
serology, 17*t*
transmission of, 17
Hepatitis B immune globulin (HBIG), 210
Hepatitis B surface antigen (HBsAg), 18
Hepatitis B three-injection vaccine series, 24*t*
Hepatitis B vaccine, 25–26, 97*t*, 98, 210, 273
antibody persistence, 26
booster dose, 26
declination, 307
injection site, 26
OSHA on, 303–4
plasma-derived, 24–25
recombinant DNA, 25

Hepatitis B virus (HBV), 6, 16*t*, 90, 234, 295, 301–3
antigens and, *18*
carrier state and dentistry, 23–24
among dental personnel, 23*t*
exposure risk, 23*t*
frequency of infection, 21–22
occupational exposure risk, 211, 215
onset of, 19
outcomes of, *21*
PEP recommendations for, 216*t*
prevalence of, in dental profession, 22–23
prevention via immunoprophylaxis, 24–26
properties and morphological components, 18–20
serologic pattern of acute, *20*
serologic profile of carrier state, *22*
serologic profiles interpretation, 20*t*
subclinical, 14, 22
transmission from carrier to dentist to patient, 23*t*
transmission modes, 20–21
undiagnosed cases of, 2
vaccine for, 21
Hepatitis C virus (HCV), 16*t*, 26–27, 234
acute, *27*
occupational exposure risk, 213, 215
vaccine not available for, 27
Hepatitis D virus (HDV), 16*t*, 28, *28*
Hepatitis E virus (HEV), 16*t*, 28–29
Hepatitis G virus (HGV), 16*t*
Herpes simplex virus disease, 41*t*, 142
Herpes zoster dermatomal, 41*t*
Heterotrophic bacteria, 64
Heterotrophic water bacteria, 68
HEV. *See* Hepatitis E virus
Hevea brasiliensis, 106
HGV. *See* Hepatitis G virus
HI. *See* Hemagglutinin
HICPAC. *See* Healthcare Infection Control Practices Advisory Committee
High-level disinfectant, 149, 151, 172, 174
Highly active antiretroviral therapy (HAART), 33, 36, 42
Histoplasmosis, 40*t*
HIV. *See* Human immunodeficiency virus
HIV antibody (anti-HIV), 35
Holmes, Oliver Wendell, 82, 125
Hospital disinfectant, 172, 175, 186, 187
Hospital steam sterilizer, *153, 161*
Housekeeping surface, 172, 176, 176*t*, 177, 278, 289
HTL-III. *See* Human T-cell leukemia virus-III
Human immunodeficiency virus (HIV), 25, 32–44, 295, 301–3. *See also* Acquired immune deficiency syndrome
cycle replication of, *35*
death attributed to, 36
demographics in United States, 36–37
diagnostic testing, 38–39
emergence of, 34
epidemiology of, 36–37

history of untreated, 35, *36*
medical management of, 39, 42
occupational exposure risk, 213, 215–16
occupational transmission risks, 38
opportunistic infections associated with, 40*t*–41*t*
oral manifestations of, 34
pathogenesis and history of, 34–36
PEP for percutaneous injuries, 217*t*
rapid, -antibody testing, 216
TB and, 53*t*, 54
transmission of, 37–38
Human T-cell leukemia virus-III (HTL- III), 34
Human vaccines, 93–94, 93*t*
Humectants. *See* Emollients (humectants)
Humoral immunity, 90, 91
HVAC. *See* Heating, ventilation, and air conditioning
Hydrocolloid impressions, 255
Hydrogen peroxide, 181, 181*t*
Hydrophilic viruses, 175*t*
Hygiene, general considerations, 126–27, 126*t*. *See also* Hand hygiene and antisepsis
Hypochlorites, 180, 180*t*
IAQ. *See* Indoor air quality
Iatrogenic, 4
Iatrogenic infections, 6
ICD. *See* Irritation contact dermatitis
Icteric, 14
IESNA. *See* Illumination Engineering Society of North America
Illumination Engineering Society of North America (IESNA), 195, 200
Illumination systems. *See* Electrical/ illumination systems
Immune serum globulin (ISG), 24
Immune-compromising diseases and conditions, 93*t*
Immunity
active, 24
cell-mediated, 91
cellular, 90
to HAV, 17
humoral, 90, 91
passive, 24
Immunizations, for DHCP, 89–100, 272, 284–85. *See also* Active immunization; Advisory Committee for Immunization Practices
history, 95–96
ideal vaccines, 92–93, 92*t*
mumps, 96, 98
principles of, 91–92
recommendations, 96, 97*t*–98*t*
recording, 96
rubella, 96
rubeola, 96
vaccine administration, 96
vaccine types, 93–94
Immunoprophylaxis, 24–26
Implantable device, 149, 163, 277
Impressions. *See specific type*

Inactivated polio vaccine (IPV), 94
Inactivated (killed) vaccines, 90, 94, 94*t*
Independent water reservoir, 64, 70
Indinivir, 39*t*
Indirect contact transmission, 4, 5
Indoor air quality (IAQ), 195, 199
Infection(s). *See also* Centers for Disease
    Control
  cross-, 4, 5*t*, 176
  droplet microbial, 47*t*
  healthcare-associated, 4, 6, 11*t*
  lower respiratory tract, 34, 40*t*,
    50–54, *90*
  mycotic, 46*t*
  nosocomial, 4, 6
  opportunistic, 4, 6, 33, 42
  respiratory, 45–62, 46*t*, 142
Infection control, 4, 5, 83, 242*t*. *See also*
    Centers for Disease Control;
    Dental infection control program
  administrative strategies for, 55–57,
    56*t*
    identification of patients with TB
      disease, 56
    isolation of patients with TB
      disease, 56
    referral of patients with TB
      disease, 67
    TB education and training for
      DHCP, 56, 56*t*
    TB infection control program, 56
    TB risk assessment, 56
  dental laboratory, 246–60
    biohazard bag, *249*
    flowchart of procedures, 247*t*
    labeled disinfected items, *249*
    sterilization v. disinfection, 248
  in dental radiography, 237–45
    cleaning, disinfecting and sterilizing
      instruments, 239
    digital radiography considerations,
      241–43
    environmental, 238–39
    intraoral and extraoral procedures,
      239–40
    patient preparation, 240*t*
    PPE and hand hygiene, 238
    processing procedures, 241
    supplies, 239
    treatment area to darkroom
      transition, 241
  of dental unit, 189–90
  environmental, 57, 289
  office zones, 195–99
  respiratory tract infections, 54–58
  respiratory-protection controls, 57
  TB, surveillance program for DHCP,
    57–58
  20th century accomplishments, 6, 10*t*
  zones, *197*, 197–99
Infectious aerosols. *See* Aerosols
Infectious disease, risks in dentistry, 5*t*
Infectious tuberculosis. *See* Tuberculosis
Infectious waste, 262
Inflammation, 14

Influenza, 47*t*, 90, 98–99
  aerosols spreading, 70
  clinical manifestations, 49
  diagnosis, 49
  etiology and epidemiology, 48
  prevention and treatment, 49
  types of, compared, 48*t*
  vaccine, 97*t*
In-office incubators, for BIs, *163*
In-office laboratories, 249
Institute of Medicine (IOM), 84
Instrument cassettes, *226*
Instrument processing and circulation
    area design, 222, 223*t*
    contaminated patient-care items
      handling, 222–23
    preparation and packaging, 225–27
    receiving, cleaning, and
      decontamination, 223–25
    sterilization, 164, 165*t*, 227–28
    storage of sterilized items, 228–29
Instrument washers, 222, 223, 224,
    224, 225
Instruments
  dental, *159*
  hinged, *227*
  sterilization of unwrapped,
    276–77, 288
  unwrapped, 156
Intermediate-level disinfectant, 172, 175,
    186, 187, 238, 239, 247, 248
Internal contamination and equipment
    cleanability, 202–3
Intradermal (Mantoux) test, 53
Intraoral radiographic procedures,
    239–40, 240*t*
Iodine, 133*t*, 134, 179–80
Iodophors, 133*t*, 134, 179–80, 179*t*
IOM. *See* Institute of Medicine
IPV. *See* Inactivated polio vaccine
Irrigating solutions, 69
Irritant dermatitis, 135
Irritation contact dermatitis (ICD), 102,
    106, 124, 135, *135*
ISG. *See* Immune serum globulin
Isolation or transmission-based guidelines
    evolution, 82–84
"Isolation Techniques for Use in Hospitals"
    (CDC), 82
Isoniazid, 55*t*
Itraconazole, 40*t*
Jaundice, 14, 15
Jenner, Edward, 90
Jewelry, 136, *136*
The Joint Commission, 228
Journal of Infectious Diseases, 23
Kanamycin, 55*t*
Kaposi's sarcoma (KS), 34
KS. *See* Kaposi's sarcoma
Lamivudine, 39*t*
Laryngitis
  clinical manifestations, 50
  diagnosis, 50
  etiology and epidemiology, 50
  treatment of, 50

Laser, 292
Latent tuberculosis infection (LTBI), 52
  preventative therapy, 57
  progressing to TB disease, 52–53, 53*t*
Latex, 102, 104. *See also* Type I natural
    latex hypersensitivity
  allergies, 102, 108
    safe treatment provisions for
      patients with, 109*t*
    summary and recommendations
      110*t*
  hypersensitivity, 106, 275, 287
LAV. *See* Lymphadenopathy-associated
    virus
Legionellosis, 47*t*
Legionnaires' disease, aerosols
    spreading, 70
Leuke, P., 5
Levofloxacin, 55*t*
Licensed healthcare professional, 295
Lipophilic viruses, 175*t*
Liquid disinfectants, 188*t*
Lister, Joseph, 90, 126
Live, attenuated vaccines, 94–95, 94*t*
Liver
  cancer, 2
  inflammation, 15
Lopinavir, 39*t*
Lower respiratory tract infections, 50–54
  acute tracheobronchitis, 50–51
  pneumonia, 34, 40*t*, 50, 51, 90
  TB, 51–54
Low-level disinfectant, 172, 175, 186, 187
LTBI. *See* Latent tuberculosis infection
Lymphadenopathy-associated virus
    (LAV), 34
Lymphocytes, 33, 34, 42
Maintenance protocols, 200–201
Masks, 109–11, 112*t*, 275, 286
Material Safety Data Sheet (MSDS), 266
Mavaviroc, 39*t*
MDRTB. *See* Multiple drug-resistant
    tuberculosis
Measles, 47*t*
Measles live-virus vaccine, 97*t*
Measles vaccine. *See* Rubeola vaccine
Mechanical indicator, 150, 159, *161*
Mechanical monitoring, 159
Medical waste, 262, *262*
  blood and body fluid, 265
  contaminated sharps management,
    264
  extracted teeth, 265, 266, 266*t*, 281,
    291
  managing, in dental healthcare setting,
    263, 263–64, 279
  needle disposal, 265*t*
  regulations and guidelines for, 262–63
  sharps container, 265*t*
  tissue, 265–66
  types of dental, 263
Medical waste management, 261–68, 264*t*
Meeks, Valli I., 32
Merchant, Virginia A., 246
Merck Sharp & Dohme, 24, 25

Microbial product vaccines, 95
Microbial respiratory infections.
    See Respiratory infections
Microbiological rationale
    historical perspectives and principles,
        3–12
    HIV/AIDS and related infections, 32–44
    tuberculosis and respiratory infections,
        45–62
    viral hepatitis and hepatitis vaccines,
        13–31
    water and air quality challenges in
        dental unit, 63–75
Molinari, Gail, 141
Molinari, John A., 3, 13, 45, 79, 89, 101,
        123, 148, 171, 185, 209, 221, 232,
        237, 261
Montagnier, Luc, 34
Mouth rinses. *See* Antimicrobial mouth
        rinses; Preprocedural mouth
        rinse
Moxifloxacin, 55*t*
MSDS. *See* Material Safety Data Sheet
Multiple drug-resistant tuberculosis
        (MDRTB), 46, 52
Multiresistant organisms, 124, 126
Mumps, 47*t*
Mumps live-virus vaccine, 97*t*
Mumps vaccine, 96, 98
Mycobacterium avium complex, 41*t*
Mycobacterium tuberculosis
        (M. tuberculosis).
        See Tuberculosis
Mycoplasm pneumoniae, 50
Mycotic infection, 46*t*
N-95 respirator, 71, 102, 111
NA. *See* Neuraminidase
NADL. *See* National Association of Dental
        Laboratories
National Association of Dental
        Laboratories (NADL), 248
National Center for Policy Analysis
        (NCPA), 234
National Childhood Vaccine Injury Act, of
        1986, 92
National Fire Protection Association
        (NFPA), 136
National Institute for Occupational
        Safety and Health (NIOSH),
        71, 102, 108
NCPA. *See* National Center for Policy
        Analysis
Needleless system, 295
Needles
    disposable safety, *234*
    disposal, 265*t*
    recapping, *218*
Needlestick Safety and Prevention Act, of
        2000, 84
Nelfinavir, 39*t*
Neuraminidase (NA), 48
Neveu, Kathy, 261
Nevirapine, 39*t*
NFPA. *See* National Fire Protection
        Association

NIOSH. *See* National Institute for
        Occupational Safety and Health
Nitazoxanide, 40*t*
Nitrous oxide exposure, 71–72
NNRTI. *See* Non-nucleoside reverse
        transcriptase inhibitor
Non-antimicrobial soap, 132–33
Nonclinical area equipment, 203–4
Noncritical, 150, 151, 151*t*
Nonmedical gloves, 105–6
Non-nucleoside reverse transcriptase
        inhibitor (NNRTI), 39*t*
Nonspecific irritation dermatitis, 106
Nonsurgical dental procedures, hand
        hygiene for, 127, *129, 130,*
        131, *131*
Nosocomial infection, 4, 6
NRTI. *See* Nucleoside reverse transcriptase
        inhibitor
Nucleoside reverse transcriptase
        inhibitor (NRTI), 39*t*
Nystatin pastilles, 40*t*
Occupational blood exposure management,
        211, 213–16, 213*t, 214*
Occupational exposure, 210–16, 295
Occupational risks, preventative
        measures, 216–18
Occupational Safety and Health
        Administration (OSHA), 6, 71,
        80, 102, 103, 248, 262
    Bloodborne Pathogens Standard, 80,
        83, 84, 112, 263, 263*t*, 265,
        294–307
    communication of hazards to
        employees, 304–6
    compliance methods, 297–301
    definitions, 295–96
    exposure control, 296–97
    Hepatitis B vaccination and
        post-exposure evaluation and
        follow-up, 303–4
    HIV and HBV research laborato-
        ries and production facilities,
        301–3
    recordkeeping, 306–7
    General Duty Clause, 83
    regulations, 83–84
Occupation-related allergies, in
        dentistry, 107*t*
Office space components, infection
        control zones and, 195–99
Ofloxacin, 55*t*
OI. *See* Opportunistic infection
One-handed safety scoop, *218*
OPIM. *See* Other potentially infectious
        materials
Opportunistic infection (OI), 4, 6, 33, 42
Oral manifestations, of HIV, 34
Oral microflora, 142
Oral surgical procedures, 64, 102, 105,
        124, 291
    dental infection control program, 281
    hand hygiene for, 131–32
Organization for Safety and Asepsis
        Procedures, 179

Orthodontics, 257–58
OSHA. *See* Occupational Health and
        Safety Administration
Other potentially infectious materials
        (OPIM), 102, 103, 186, 187, 210,
        262, 263, 273, 295
Packaging, of instruments, 151, 225–27,
        226, 226*t,* 227*t*
    label information, 227*t*
    sterilization method
        compatibility, 227*t*
Parachlorometaxylenol. *See* Chloroxylenol
        parachlorometaxylenol
Parasitic infection, 46*t*
Parenteral, 296
Parenteral antischistomal therapy
        (PAT), 83
Parenteral medications, 280
Paromomycin, 40*t*
Particulate respirator, 102
Particulate respirator mask (PRM), 111
Pass through cabinets, 197, *198*
Passive immunity, 24
Pasteur's germ theory, 82
PAT. *See* Parenteral antischistomal
        therapy
Patients
    care items, categories, 150, 151*t*
    examination gloves, 104, 105*t*
    flow, 199
PCMX. *See* Chloroxylenol
        parachlorometaxylenol
PCP. *See Pneumocystis carinii* pneumonia
PCR. *See* Polymerace chain reaction
Pentamidine, aerosolized, 40*t*
People living with AIDS (PLWA), 36
PEP. *See* Postexposure prophylaxis
Percutaneous injury, 210, 211
Perforated basket, *224*
Persistent activity, 124, 131
Personal protection
    immunizations for dental healthcare
        personnel, 89–100
    safe work practices, 113*t*
    standard precautions concept and
        application, 79–88
Personal protective equipment (PPE),
        101–19, 286–87, 296
    clothing, 111–12, 112*t,* 275, 286–87
    dental (rubber) dams, 112
    in dental laboratory, 248
    donning and removing, 112*t,* 113
    eyewear, 111, 112*t,* 275, 286
    gloves, 103–6
    head and shoe covers, 112, 275
    Infection control, in dental
        radiography, 238
    masks, 109–11, 112*t,* 275, 286
    surface barriers of, 172, 177, 177*t,* 189,
        233–34
Pestivirus, 26
Pharyngitis, 50
    clinical manifestations, 50
    diagnosis, 50
    treatment of, 50

Phenols, 180–81, 181*t*
  derivatives, 133*t*
Physical barriers, 197, *198*
PI. *See* Protease inhibitors
Plain soap, 124, 127, 132–33
Planktonic, 64, 65
Plasma-derived vaccine, 24–25
PLWA. *See* People living with AIDS
Pneumocystis carinii pneumonia (PCP), 34, 40*t*
Pneumonia, 50, 51, 90
  clinical manifestations, 51
  diagnosis, 51
  etiology and epidemiology, 51
  PCP, 34, 40*t*
  treatment, 51
Pneumonic plague, 47*t*, 70
Polio, 94
Polymerace chain reaction (PCR), 38
Postexposure management, 213–16, 272, 274, 285
Postexposure prophylaxis (PEP), 27, 210, 211, 216*t*, 217*t*
Potable (drinking) water, 64, 65
Pouches, self-sealing, *226*
Precautions, 4. *See also* Standard precautions; Universal precautions
  blood, 81*t*
  CDC current guidelines and, 84–85
  historical summary of isolation, 81*t*
  transmission-based, 80, 85
Pregnancy
  HEV during, 28–29
  HIV and, 38
Preprocedural mouth rinse, 141–47, 280, 291. *See also* Antimicrobial mouth rinses
Prevacuum steam sterilizer, 150
Prion diseases, 292–93
PRM. *See* Particulate respirator mask
Product vaccines, 90, 95
Production facility, 296
Prosthodontics, 257–58
Protease inhibitors (PI), 36, 39*t*
Protective equipment, 27, *250*. *See also* Personal protective equipment
Public zone, 195, 198
Pulmonary tuberculosis. *See* Tuberculosis
Pyrazinamide, 55*t*
Pyrimethamine, 40*t*
Qualified healthcare professional, 210, 211
Quarantine, 82
Quaternary, 133*t*
Quaternary ammoniums, 134, 177–78, 178*t*
Radiography and infection control, 237–45
  cleaning, disinfecting and sterilizing instruments, 239
  intraoral and extraoral procedures, 239–40
  patient preparation, 240*t*
  supplies, 239

Raltegravir, 39*t*
RCRA. *See* Resource Conservation and Recovery Act
Recombinant DNA vaccines, 25
"Recommended Infection Control Practices for Dentistry" (CDC), 83
Recording devices, for sterilizers, *161*
Regulated waste, 233, 262, 263, 289–90, 296
Removable components, 203
Research laboratory, 296
Resident flora, 124, 126
Resource Conservation and Recovery Act (RCRA), 263
Respirator
  N-95, 71, 102, 111
  particulate, 102
Respiratory infections, 45–62, 46*t*, 142. *See also* Tuberculosis; Upper respiratory tract infections; *specific type*
Respiratory tract infections, 54–58, 58*t*
Respiratory-protection strategies, for infection control, 57
Retraction, 64, 67, 70
Retrovirus, 33, 34
Reverse transcriptase (RT), 33, 34
Rhinosinusitis, 49–50
  clinical manifestations, 49
  diagnosis, 49–50
  etiology and epidemiology, 49
  treatment of, 50
Rhinoviruses, 47
Ribonucleic acid (RNA), 33
Rifabutin, 55*t*
Rifamate, 55*t*
Rifampin, 55*t*
Rifamycins, 55*t*
Rifapentin, 55*t*
Rifater, 55*t*
Rinse-spray-rinse-spray, 247, 257, *257*
Ritonavir, 39*t*
RNA. *See* Ribonucleic acid
RNA virus, 15*t*, 34
Room configuration, 196–97
RT. *See* Reverse transcriptase
Rubber dams. *See* Dental (rubber) dams
Rubella live-virus vaccine, 97*t*
Rubella vaccine, 96
Rubeola vaccine, 96
Saccharomyces cerevisiae (baker's yeast), 25
Safety anesthetic devices, *217*
Safety needles, disposable, *234*
Saliva, 5, 210–11
Salk, Jonas, 94
Saquinavir, 39*t*
SARS. *See* Severe acute respiratory syndrome
Scalpels, *217, 234*
Semicritical, 150, 151, 151*t*
Semmelweis, Ignaz, 82, 125, 126

Sensor faucets, *198*
Seroconversion, 33, 35
Severe acute respiratory syndrome (SARS), 33, 47*t*, 70
Sexual contact, HIV transmission and, 37–38
Sharps, 264–65, 265*t*, 295, 296
Shelf life. *See* Event-related shelf life
Shingles, 41*t*
Single-use disposable item, 233, 280, 291
  compliance of use, 234–35
  discarding properly, 234
  examples of, *233,* 233–34
Skin care, 136
Smallpox, 90
SmithKline Biologicals, Belgium, 25
Soap. *See* Antimicrobial soap; Non-antimicrobial soap; Plain soap
Source individual, 296
Spatter, 4, 5, 64, 70, 103, 142
Spaulding classification, 150, 151, 172, 173–74, 176
Special Project 91 Healthcare Facilities Design Guide (ASHRAE), 199
Spore test, 150, 161
  CDC recommendations for positive, 165*t*
  review after positive, 166*t*
  of small office sterilizers, 164*t*
Spray-wipe-spray, 186, 188
spread of, 52–53
Standard precautions, 4, 11, 103, 247
  assumption-based guidelines evolution, 80, 82
  CDC guidelines, 83
  concept and application, 79–88
  current recommendations, 81*t*
  isolation or transmission-based guidelines evolution, 82–84
  OSHA, 83–84
Staphylococcal pneumonia, 51
State dental practice regulations, 68–69
Static air sterilization, 152*t*, 155
Stavudine, 39*t*
Steam sterilization, 150, 151, 152*t*, *153*, 153–54
Sterilant, 156. *See also* Chemical sterilants
Sterile
  irrigating solutions, 69
  packaging, 151
  sterility, 150
  surgeons gloves, 105
  water, 64, 67
Sterilization, 6, 148–70. *See also* Dental infection control program; Heat sterilization methods; *specific method*
  of amalgam-free teeth for educational setting, 266*t*
  for circulation of instruments, 227–28
  dental handpieces, 157–58, *158*, 158*t*, 280, 290
  in dental laboratory, 248
  dry heat, 152*t*, 154–55

failure due to common errors, 165*t*
fast steam, 156
flash, 149, 156, 156*t*
forced air, 152*t*, 155
instrument processing, 164, 165*t*, 227–28
log, 166*t*
methods, 151, 153–56
monitoring, 158–59, 160*t*, 277, 288–89
overview, 150–51
packaging material compatibility with
    method of, 227*t*
of patient care items, 287
preventative maintenance, 165*t*
records, 166
static air, 152*t*, 155
steam, 150, 151, 152*t*, 153, 153–54
unsaturated chemical vapor, 150, 152*t*,
    155–56
of unwrapped instruments, 276–77, 288
Sterilize, 296
Sterilizers, 164*t*. *See also* Instrument
    washers; *specific type*
bead, 149, 157
chemical vapor, 149, 155
dry-heat, 149, 157
gravity displacement, 149, 152*t*, 154
Harvey, 155
hospital steam, *153, 161*
prevacuum steam, 150
tabletop steam, 150, 153, *153, 161, 228*
Storage
of hand-care products, 136
of sterilized items, 228–29, 278
Streptococcus pneumoniae infection, 90
Streptomycin, 55*t*
Subclinical, 14, 22
Substance isolation, blood, 81*t*. *See also*
    Body substance isolation
Substantivity, 133. *See also* Persistent
    activity
Subunit (component) vaccines, 90
Sulfamethoxazole, 40*t*
Surface active substances. *See* Detergents
Surface barriers, 172, 177, 177*t*, 189,
    233–34
Surface materials, selection, 200
Surfactants, 124, 133
Surgeons gloves, 105, 105*t*
Surgical antisepsis, 128*t*
Surgical hand scrubs, 124, 133
Surgical N-95 Respirators, 71, 102, 111
Surgical smoke, 292
Synthetic phenols, 180–81, 181*t*. *See also*
    Complex (synthetic) phenols
Tabletop steam sterilizer, 150, 153, *153,
    161, 228*
TB. *See* Tuberculosis
Tenofovir, 39*t*
Terézhalmy, Géza T., 45, 89
Tetanus-Diphtheria, 99
Timeline, of infectious disease and
    control, 6, 7*t*–10*t*
Tipranavir, 39*t*

Tissue waste, 265–66
Toxoplasmosis, 40*t*
Tracheobronchitis. *See* Acute
    tracheobronchitis
Transient flora, 124, 126
Transmissibility, 6, 11*t*
Transmission-based
    guidelines evolution, 82–84
    precautions, 80, 85
Triclosan, 133*t*, 134–35
Trimethoprim, 40*t*
TST. *See* Tuberculin skin test
Tube head, barrier-protected, *239*
Tubercle, 46
Tuberculin skin test (TST), 53, 53*t*
Tuberculosis (TB), 45–62, 47*t*, 102, 103,
    281, 292. *See also* Infection
    control; Multiple drug-resistant
    tuberculosis
    aerosols spreading, 70
    DHCP and, 56–58, 56*t*
    diagnosis of, 53–54
    drug-resistant disease, 54
    etiology and epidemiology, 51–52
    in HIV patients, 54
    latent infection of, 52, 53–54
    lower respiratory tract infections, 51–54
    MDRTB, 46
    persons at highest risk for
        exposure, 52*t*
    preventative measures, 111
Tuberculosis (TB) disease, 54, 56*t*
    DHCP post-exposure to, 57–58
    LTBI progressing to, 52–53, 53*t*
Twinrix, 18
Type I natural latex hypersensitivity, 106
Ultrasonic cleaner, 222, 223, *223*
    test protocol, 224*t*
Unit dose, 233
Unit dosing, 247, 249
United States FDA. *See* Food and Drug
    Administration
United States Public Health Service, 85
Universal precautions (UP), 4, 11, 80, 81*t*,
    83, 296
Unsaturated chemical vapor sterilization,
    150, 152*t*, 155–56
Unwrapped instruments, 156
UP. *See* Universal precautions
Upper respiratory tract infections, 47–50.
    See also Common cold;
    Influenza; Laryngitis;
    Pharyngitis; Rhinosinusitis
Vaccination, 90
Vaccine-preventable diseases, 91*t*
Vaccines, 90, 92. *See also* Immunizations,
    for DHCP; Vaccination; *specific
    vaccine*
    attenuated (live), 90, 92
    bordetalla pertussis, 94
    HAV, 17–18
    hepatitis, 13–31
    human, 93–94, 93*t*

ideal, 92–93, 92*t*
inactivated, 90, 94, 94*t*
IPV, 90, 94
live, attenuated, 94–95, 94*t*
measles live-virus, 97*t*
microbial product, 95
prevention and, 18, 91
product, 90, 95
rubella, 96
rubella live-virus, 97*t*
rubeola, 96
types of, 93–94
VAQTA, 18
Valacyclovir, 41*t*
Valganciclovir, 41*t*
VAQTA vaccine, 18
Varicella zoster immunoglobulin, 41*t*
Varicella-zoster live-virus vaccine, 97*t*, 99
Viral disease risks, 5*t*
Viral hepatitis, 13–31, 15*t*, 16*t*
Viral infection, 46*t*
Viremia, 14, 17
Viruses, 15*t*. *See also* Retrovirus; *specific
    types*
    major categories, 175*t*
    viral hepatitis caused by, 14, 15*t*
VOCs. *See* Volatile organic compounds
Volatile organic compounds (VOCs),
    195, 199
Voriconazole, 40*t*
Wall-mounted dispensers, *201*
Washer-disinfector, 222, 224. *See also*
    Instrument washers
Waste, 266. *See also* Medical waste
    blood, 265
    body fluid, 265
    container requirements, 263*t*
    extracted teeth, 265, 266, 266*t*, 281, 291
    infectious, 262
    regulated, 233, 262, 263, 289–90, 296
    tissue, 265–66
Waste management. *See* Medical waste
    management
Water contamination, 279, 290. *See also*
    Dental waterline contamination
Water quality, 63–75, 279–80
Waterlines, flushing, 189–90, *190*
Wax bites, *256,* 256–57
Wax rims, 256–57
WB. *See* Western blot
Western blot (WB), 38
Wicking, 103, 104
Wipe-discard-wipe, 186, 188
Work practice controls, 210, 217–18,
    273, 296
Work restrictions, respiratory tract
    infections, 58, 58*t*
Worker flow, 199
ZDV. *See* Zidovudine
Zidovudine (ZDV), 38, 39*t*
Ziehl-Neelson method, 54
Zinc Oxide Eugenol (ZOE) impressions, 255
ZOE. *See* Zinc Oxide Eugenol impressions

RRS0811